PRESENT KNOWLEDGE IN NUTRITION

Present Knowledge in Nutrition

Ninth Edition

Volume II

Edited by
Barbara A. Bowman
and Robert M. Russell

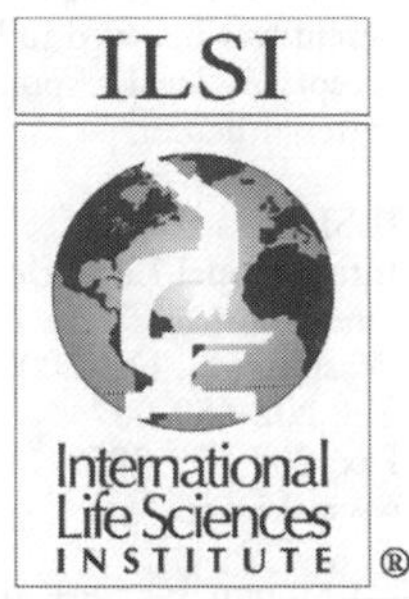

International Life Sciences Institute
Washington, DC 2006

ILSI Press
International Life Sciences Institute
One Thomas Circle, NW, Ninth Floor
Washington, DC 20005-5802, USA
Tel: 202-659-0074
Fax: 202-659-3859
www.ilsi.org

ISBN: 978-1-57881-199-1

Printed in the United States of America

Contents

Preface

Nutrition continues to be an evolving science, and *Present Knowledge in Nutrition* continues to be a favored ready reference—a constant companion on the professional bookshelf that is often turned to first when questions on nutrition arise, and known for its up-to-date, concise, authoritative chapters by distinguished experts. Each new edition represents tangible evidence of the growing scope and challenge of nutrition as a field, with an increasing number of chapters. Each chapter presents fresh perspectives from new disciplines as well as current research. In particular, this edition reflects the remarkable impact of genomics on the field of nutrition and growing realization of the potential for this new knowledge to transform the human condition.

The first edition of *Present Knowledge in Nutrition* was published in 1953, just a few years after the isolation of Vitamin B_{12}, which was the last of the vitamins to be identified. The fourth edition, edited by Dr. Mark Hegstead and published in 1976, contained 53 chapters, compared with 70 chapters in the current edition, reflecting the broad and interdisciplinary scope of nutrition science. For the first time, *Present Knowledge in Nutrition* is being published in two volumes—the first volume contains chapters on systems biology, energy physiology, and the nutrients (chapters 1-40), and the second volume contains chapters on nutrition and the life cycle, immunity, chronic diseases, diet and food, public health, and international nutrition. Volume II concludes with a section on emerging issues in nutrition, covering food-borne illness and food safety, food biotechnology, and bioactive components in food and supplements.

Collaborating as editors on this volume was a tremendous honor, but also a daunting task. Critical research questions have moved beyond the understanding of the role of inadequate nutrient intakes in deficiency to also include, often simultaneously, the role of nutrition in chronic disease prevention and the consequences of overnutrition. Most of the chapters in this edition conclude with a discussion of future directions, including research needs, to challenge and prepare the reader for developments in the years ahead.

Our task as editors was also challenged by *Present Knowledge in Nutrition*'s broad use in the field. Historically, the book has had an incredibly diverse readership including undergraduate, graduate, and post graduate students in nutrition, public heath, medicine, and related fields; dieticians, physicians, and other health professionals; and academic, industrial and government researchers. *Present Knowledge in Nutrition*'s readers range from food scientists and technologists to regulators, policy makers and members of the wider public. We expect the ninth edition to become a standard text and authoritative reference work in classrooms, libraries, laboratories, clinics, and offices around the world. We believe we have achieved a highly readable, well-organized, comprehensive, and timely summary of current nutrition science.

This edition of *Present Knowledge in Nutrition* reflects the dedication and hard work of many people. First, we want to thank our expert authors from seven countries around the world for their diligent efforts to present the essence of a topic, often condensing decades of specialized research into concise, accessible chapters with a manageable number of references. We wish to thank the members of our editorial board for their assistance in developing the framework for this book, our colleagues at the Jean Mayer USDA Human Nutrition Research Center on Aging at Tufts University and the Centers for Disease Control and Prevention, especially Sarah Peterson from Tufts. Fourth, we are indebted to Suzie Harris and the patient, professional, and dedicated staff at the International Life Sciences Institute (ILSI), especially Suzanne White and Eleanore Tapscott.

Finally, we dedicate this volume to our parents and families, mentors, colleagues and students from whom we have learned so much.

Barbara A Bowman, Atlanta, Georgia
Robert M. Russell, Boston, Massachusetts
Editors

These findings and conclusions are those of the authors and do not necessarily represent the views of the Centers for Disease Control and Prevention.

Contributors

Editors

Barbara Bowman, PhD
Centers for Disease Control and Prevention
Atlanta, Georgia, USA

Robert M. Russell, MD, PhD
Jean Mayer USDA Human Nutrition Research Center on Aging
Tufts University
Boston, Massachusetts, USA

Editorial Advisory Board

Benjamin Caballero, MD, PhD
Center for Human Nutrition
Johns Hopkins University
Baltimore, Maryland, USA

Paul Coates, PhD
Office of Dietary Supplements
National Institutes of Health
Bethesda, Maryland, USA

Fergus Clydesdale, PhD
Department of Food Sciences
University of Massachusetts
Amherst, Massachusetts, USA

Joseph G. Hautvast, MD
International Union of Nutritional Sciences
Wageningen, Netherlands

Janet King, PhD
Children's Hospital
Oakland Research Institute
Oakland, California, USA

Alfred H. Merrill, PhD
School of Biology
Georgia Institute of Technology
Atlanta, Georgia, USA

Penelope S. Nestel, PhD
International Food Policy Research Institute
Washington, DC, USA

Irwin H. Rosenberg, MD
Friedman School of Nutrition Science & Policy
Tufts University
Boston, Massachusetts, USA

Authors

Janice Albert, MS
Nutrition and Consumer Protection Division
Food and Agriculture Organization of the United Nations
Rome, Italy

Lindsay H. Allen, PhD
Department of Nutrition
University of California
Davis, California, USA

John J.B. Anderson, PhD
Department of Nutrition
School of Public Health and School of Medicine
University of North Carolina
Chapel Hill, North Carolina, USA

Jamy D. Ard, MD
Departments of Nutrition Sciences and Internal Medicine
University of Alabama
Birmingham, Alabama, USA

Lynn B. Bailey, PhD
Department of Food Science and Human Nutrition
University of Florida
Gainesville, Florida, USA

C.J. Bates, DPhil
Elsie Widdowson Laboratory
MRC Human Nutrition Research
Cambridge, United Kingdom

Charles Baum, MD
Department of Medicine
University of Illinois
Chicago, Illinois, USA

John Beard, PhD
Department of Nutrition
College of Health and Human Development
The Pennsylvania State University
University Park, Pennsylvania, USA

Gary R. Beecher, PhD
Food Composition Laboratory
Beltsville Human Nutrition Research Center
Agricultural Research Service
US Department of Agriculture
Beltsville, Maryland, USA

Jeffrey B. Blumberg, PhD
Antioxidants Research Laboratory
Jean Mayer USDA Human Nutrition
Research Center on Aging
Tufts University
Boston, Massachusetts, USA

Annalies Borrel, MSc
Friedman School of Nutrition Science & Policy
Tufts University
Boston, Massachusetts, USA

Ronette R. Briefel, DrPH, RD
Research Department
Mathematica Policy Research, Inc.
Washington, DC, USA

Mona S. Calvo, PhD
US Food and Drug Administration
Washington, DC, USA

Wayne W. Campbell, PhD
Department of Foods and Nutrition
Purdue University
West Lafayette, Indiana, USA

Gabriela Camporeale, PhD
Department of Nutrition and Health Sciences
University of Nebraska
Lincoln, Nebraska, USA

Robert Carter III, MD
Departments of Medicine and Microbiology
University of Alabama
Birmingham, Alabama, USA

Samuel N. Cheuvront, PhD
Thermal and Mountain Medicine Division
US Army Research Institute of Environmental Medicine
Natick, Massachusetts, USA

Paul M. Coates, PhD
Office of Dietary Supplements
National Institutes of Health
Bethesda, Maryland, USA

Robert J. Cousins, PhD
Department of Food Sciences and Human Nutrition
Center for Nutrition Sciences
University of Florida
Gainesville, Florida, USA

Sai Krupa Das, PhD
Jean Mayer USDA Human Nutrition
Research Center on Aging
Tufts University
Boston, Massachusetts, USA

Bess Dawson-Hughes, MD
Calcium and Bone Metabolism Laboratory
Jean Mayer USDA Human Nutrition
Research Center on Aging
Tufts University
Boston, Massachusetts, USA

Adam Drewnowski, PhD
Nutritional Sciences Prorgram
School of Public Health and Community Medicine
University of Washington
Seattle, Washington, USA

John W. Erdman, Jr., PhD
Department of Food Science
University of Illinois
Urbana, Illinois, USA

Guylaine Ferland, PhD
Centre de Recherche
Institut Universitaire de Géariatrie de Montréal
Montreal, Quebec, Canada

Edward A. Frongillo, Jr., PhD
Division of Nutritional Sciences
Cornell University
Ithaca, New York, USA

Daniel D. Gallaher, PhD
Department of Food Science and Nutrition
University of Minnesota
St. Paul, Minnesota, USA

Sanford C. Garner, PhD
Constella Group, Inc.
Durham, North Carolina, USA

Peter J. Gillies, PhD, FAHA
DuPont Central Research and Development and
Department of Nutrition Science
The Pennsylvania State University
University Park, Pennsylvania, USA

Amy Gorin, PhD
Department of Psychiatry and Human Behavior
Brown Medical School
Providence, Rhode Island, USA

Jesse F. Gregory III, PhD
Department of Food Science and Human Nutrition
University of Florida
Gainesville, Florida, USA

Olivier Guérin, MD
Service de Gériatrie
Hôpitaux de Nice
Nice, France

Sung Nim Han, PhD
Jean Mayer USDA Human Nutrition
Research Center on Aging
Tufts University
Boston, Massachusetts, USA

James M. Harnly, PhD
Food Composition Laboratory
Beltsville Human Nutrition Research Center
Agricultural Research Service
US Department of Agriculture
Beltsville, Maryland, USA

Susan L. Hefle, PhD
Department of Food Science and Technology
University of Nebraska
Lincoln, Nebraska, USA

William C. Heird, MD
Department of Pediatrics
Baylor College of Medicine
Houston, Texas, USA

Helen L. Henry, PhD
Department of Biochemistry
University of California, Riverside
Riverside, California, USA

Daniell B. Hill, MD
Department of Internal Medicine
University of Louisville
Louisville, Kentucky, USA

Joanne M. Holden, MS, RD
Nutrient Data Laboratory
Beltsville Human Nutrition Research Center
Agricultural Research Service
US Department of Agriculture
Beltsville, Maryland, USA

Robert A. Jacob, PhD, FACN
Grand Forks Human Nutrition Research Center
Agricultural Research Service
US Department of Agriculture
Grand Forks, North Dakota, USA

Carol S. Johnston, PhD
Department of Nutrition
Arizona State University East
Mesa, Arizona, USA

Peter J.H. Jones, PhD
School of Dietetics and Human Nutrition
Macdonald Campus of McGill University
Ste-Anne-de-Bellevue, Quebec, Canada

Heather I. Katcher,
Department of Nutrition Science
The Pennsylvania State University
University Park, Pennsylvania, USA

Young-In Kim, MD, FRCP(C)
Departments of Medicine and Nutritional Sciences
University of Toronto
Toronto, Ontario, Canada

Philip J. Klemmer, MD
School of Medicine
University of North Carolina
Durham, North Carolina, USA

Penny M. Kris-Etherton, PhD
Department of Nutrition
Pennsylvania State University
University Park, Pennsylvania, USA

Alice H. Lichtenstein, DSc
Cardiovascular Nutrition Research Program
Jean Mayer USDA Human Nutrition
Research Center on Aging
Tufts University
Boston, Massachusetts, USA

Brian L. Lindshield, BS
Division of Nutritional Sciences
University of Illinois
Urbana, Illinois, USA

Joanne R. Lupton, PhD
Department of Nutrition and Food Science
Texas A & M University
College Station, Texas, USA

Luis Marsano, MD
Department of Internal Medicine
University of Louisville
Louisville, Kentucky, USA

Reynaldo Martorell, PhD
Robert W. Woodruff Health Sciences Center
Emory University
Atlanta, Georgia, USA

Tahsin Masud, MD
Renal Division
Emory University School of Medicine
Atlanta, Georgia, USA

Craig J. McClain, MD
Department of Internal Medicine
University of Louisville
Louisville, Kentucky, USA

Donald B. McCormick, PhD
Department of Biochemistry
Emory University
Atlanta, Georgia, USA

Megan A. McCrory, PhD
School of Nutrition and Exercise Science
Bastyr University
Kenmore, Washington, USA

Heather McGuire, MD
Department of Nephrology
Billings Clinic
Billings, Montana, USA

Catherine McIsaac, MS, RD
Medical Center
University of Vermont
Burlington, Vermont, USA

Alfred H. Merrill, Jr., PhD
School of Biology
Georgia Institute of Technology
Atlanta, Georgia, USA

Simin Nikbin Meydani, DVM, PhD
Department of Pathology and Sackler
Graduate School of Biomedical Sciences
Jean Mayer USDA Human Nutrition
Research Center on Aging
Tufts University
Boston, Massachusetts, USA

Paul E. Milbury, MS, CFII
Antioxidants Research Laboratory
Jean Mayer USDA Human Nutrition
Research Center on Aging
Tufts University
Boston, Massachusetts, USA

Joshua W. Miller, PhD
Department of Medical Pathology
University of California
Davis, California, USA

John A. Milner, PhD
Nutrition Science Research Group
National Cancer Institute
National Institutes of Health
Rockville, Maryland, USA

William E. Mitch, MD
Renal Division
Emory University School of Medicine
Atlanta, Georgia, USA

Pablo Monsivais, PhD
Nutritional Sciences Program
School of Public Health and Community Medicine and
Dental Public Health Sciences
School of Dentistry
University of Washington
Seattle, Washington, USA

Scott J. Montain, PhD
Military Nutrition Division
US Army Research Institute of Environmental Medicine
Natick, Massachusetts, USA

Suzanne P. Murphy, PhD
Cancer Research Center
University of Hawaii
Honolulu, Hawaii, USA

Marguerite A. Neill, MD
Division of Infectious Diseases
Brown University Medical School
Memorial Hospital of Rhode Island
Pawtucket, Rhode Island, USA

Forrest H. Nielsen, PhD
Grand Forks Human Nutrition Research Center
Agricultural Research Service
US Department of Agriculture
Grand Forks, North Dakota, USA

Chizuru Nishida, PhD
Department of Nutrition for Health and Development
World Health Organization
Geneva, Switzerland

Anthony W. Norman, PhD
Department of Biochemistry
University of California, Riverside
Riverside, California, USA

Marga C. Ocké, PhD
Department of Chronic Diseases Epidemiology
National Institute for Public Health
and the Environment
Bilthoven, The Netherlands

Christine M. Olson, PhD
Division of Nutritional Sciences
Cornell University
Ithaca, New York, USA

Andrea A. Papamandjaris, PhD
Regulatory and Scientific Affairs
Nestlé, Inc.
North York, Ontario, Canada

David L. Pelletier, PhD
Division of Nutritional Sciences
Cornell University
Ithaca, New York, USA

Paul B. Pencharz, MD, PhD
Division of Gastroenterology/Nutrition
Hospital for Sick Children
Toronto, Ontario, Canada

Harry G. Preuss, MD
Division of Nephrology and Hypertension
Georgetown University Medical Center
Washington, DC, USA

Joseph R. Prohaska, PhD
Department of Biochemistry and Molecular Biology
University of Minnesota
Duluth, Minnesota, USA

Charles J. Rebouche, PhD
Department of Pediatrics
University of Iowa
Coralville, Iowa, USA

Patrick Ritz, MD
Service de Nutrition
Centre Hospitalier Universitaire
Angers, France

Richard S. Rivlin, MD
The American Health Foundation
New York, New York, USA

Susan B. Roberts, PhD
Jean Mayer USDA Human Nutrition Research Center on Aging
Tufts University
Boston, Massachusetts, USA

Lisa M. Rogers, PhD
Department of Nutrition
University of California
Davis, California, USA

Robert B. Rucker, PhD
Department of Nutrition
University of California
Davis, California, USA

Edward Saltzman, MD
Jean Mayer USDA Human Nutrition Research Center on Aging
Tufts University
Boston, Massachusetts, USA

Lisa M. Sanders, PhD
University of North Carolina
Chapel Hill, North Carolina, USA

Charles R. Santerre, PhD
Department of Foods and Nutrition
Purdue University
West Lafayette, Indiana, USA

Michael N. Sawka, PhD
Thermal and Mountain Medicine Division
US Army Research Institute of Environmental Medicine
Natick, Massachusetts, USA

Eva M. Schmelz, PhD
Department of Nutrition and Food Sciences and Karmanos Cancer Institute
Wayne State University
Detroit, Michigan, USA

Stéphane Schneider, MD
Archet University Hospital
Nice, France

Anuraj H. Shankar, MD
Helen Keller International/Indonesia
Jakarta, Indonesia

Noel W. Solomons, MD
Center for Studies of Sensory Impairment, Aging and Metabolism (CeSSIAM)
Guatemala City, Guatemala

Sally P. Stabler, MD
Department of Medicine
University of Colorado Health Sciences Center
Denver, Colorado, USA

Virginia A. Stallings, MD
Division of Gastroenterology and Nutrition
Children's Hospital of Philadelphia
Philadelphia, Pennsylvania, USA

Aryeh D. Stein, MPH, PhD
Rollins School of Public Health
Emory University
Atlanta, Georgia, USA

Barbara J. Stoecker, PhD
Department of Nutritional Sciences
Oklahoma State University
Stillwater, Oklahoma, USA

Roger A. Sunde, PhD
Department of Nutritional Sciences
University of Wisconsin
Madison, Wisconsin, USA

Paolo M. Suter, MD
Department of Internal Medicine
Medical Policlinic/University Hospital
Zurich, Switzerland

Deborah Tate, PhD
Department of Psychiatry and Human Behavior
Brown Medical School
Providence, Rhode Island, USA

Robert V. Tauxe, MD, MPH
Centers for Disease Control and Prevention
Atlanta, Georgia , USA

Christine L. Taylor, PhD
Science and Health Coordination
Food & Drug Administration
Rockville, Maryland, USA

Steve L. Taylor, PhD
Department of Food Science and Technology
University of Nebraska
Lincoln, Nebraska, USA

Howard C. Towle, PhD
Department of Biochemistry, Molecular Biology, and Biophysics
University of Minnesota
Minneapolis, Minnesota, USA

Maret G. Traber, PhD
Department of Nutrition and Food Management
Linus Pauling Institute
Oregon State University
Corvallis, Oregon, USA

Wija A. Van Staveren, PhD
Division of Human Nutrition and Epidemiology
Wageningen University
Wageningen, The Netherlands

Bruno J. Vellas, MD, PhD
Department of Internal Medicine and Gerontology
Centre Hospitalier Universitaire
Toulouse, France

Frank Vinicor, MD, MPH
Division of Diabetes Translation
Centers for Disease Control and Prevention
Atlanta, Georgia, USA

Stella Lucia Volpe, PhD
School of Nursing
University of Pennsylvania
Philadelphia, Pennsylvania, USA

May Dongmei Wang, PhD
The Wallace H. Coulter Department of Biomedical Engineering and The Petit Institute of Bioengineering and Bioscience
Georgia Institute of Technology
Atlanta, Georgia, USA

Mary Lee Sell Watts, MPH, RD
Legislative and Political Affairs
American Dietetic Association
Washington, DC, USA

Connie M. Weaver, PhD
Department of Foods and Nutrition
Purdue University
West Lafayette, Indiana, USA

Robert C. Weisell, PhD
Nutrition and Consumer Protection Division
Food and Agriculture Organization of the United Nations
Rome, Italy

Jonathan Wells, PhD
Lawrence Berkeley National Laboratory
Berkeley, Kitsap, California, USA

Rena R. Wing, PhD
Department of Psychiatry and Human Behavior
Brown Medical School
Providence, Rhode Island, USA

Judith Wylie-Rosett, EdD, RD
Department of Epidemiology and Social Medicine
Albert Einstein College of Medicine
Bronx, New York, USA

Helen Young, PhD
Famine Center
Friedman School of Nutrition Science & Policy
Tufts University
Medford/Somerville, Massachusetts, USA

Vernon R. Young, PhD, DSc
Laboratory of Human Nutrition
Massachusetts Institute of Technology
Cambridge, Massachusetts, USA

Steven H. Zeisel, MD, PhD
Department of Nutrition
University of North Carolina
Chapel Hill, North Carolina, USA

Janos Zempleni, PhD
Department of Nutritional Science and Dietetics
University of Nebraska
Lincoln, Nebraska, USA

Michael B. Zimmermann, MD, MSc
Laboratory for Human Nutrition
Swiss Federal Institute of Technology
Zurich, Switzerland

VII Nutrition and the Life Cycle

41 Pregnancy and Lactation

Lindsay H. Allen

Enabling pregnant women to meet their nutrient needs has long been a global public health priority, based on evidence that undernutrition during the period of reproduction can have serious, long-term adverse effects on the mother and child. Programs designed to improve maternal undernutrition can be cost-effective. In wealthier countries, an increasing amount of information is emerging about how variability in nutritional status and nutrient metabolism and requirements of individuals affects pregnancy weight gain, the risk of preterm delivery, and birth defects. Well-designed studies on undernourished women in developing countries have been particularly informative about the impact that improved maternal nutrition can have on maternal and infant health. However, rates of preterm delivery, low birth weight, birth defects, and other pregnancy complications are still unacceptably high even in wealthier countries, and there is much to be learned about optimal maternal nutrient requirements during pregnancy and lactation.

Changes in Maternal Physiology During Pregnancy

Hormonal Changes

In pregnancy, larger amounts of nutrients are required by the mother to support the growth and metabolism of maternal and fetal tissues, and for storage in the fetus. Some of this additional need for nutrients is met by increased maternal food intake, but, regardless of dietary intake, enormous metabolic adjustments in nutrient use support the development of the fetus. Some of the most important changes in serum hormone concentrations, and in tissue deposition and metabolism, are summarized in Table 1.

A few days after implantation, an increased secretion of hormones by the corpus luteum and placenta is present. These ensure the maintenance of pregnancy and prepare the mother for the development of the fetus. Human chorionic gonadotropin concentrations continue to rise to about 60 days after conception and serve to maintain the corpus luteum. After this time, they decline gradually but remain elevated throughout pregnancy. Human placental lactogen secretion starts as soon as the ovum is implanted to maintain the corpus luteum. Secretion of human placental lactogen continues to increase throughout pregnancy so that serum concentrations at term are 20 times higher than before conception. Human placental lactogen is a member of the growth hormone/prolactin gene family. It stimulates growth of the placenta and fetus, modulates fetal intrauterine growth factor production, and helps direct nutrients to the fetus by stimulating maternal fat breakdown and antagonizing the action of maternal insulin. It also stimulates mammary gland development in preparation for lactation.

The importance of corticotropin-releasing hormone (CRH) has been recognized recently. In the mid-1990s a report documented that, as early as 18 weeks of gestation, the risk of preterm delivery can be predicted from high maternal serum CRH concentrations, and that of post-term delivery can be predicted by low concentrations.[1] CRH is produced by the maternal and fetal components of the placenta by 8 weeks of conception, but, in most pregnancies, it is undetectable in maternal serum until about the third trimester when there is about a 50-fold increase in its release. Placental CRH stimulates the synthesis of corticotropin by the anterior pituitary of the fetus, and, subsequently, the production of cortisol by the fetal adrenals. Cortisol blocks the inhibitory effect of progesterone on placental synthesis of CRH and fetal cortisol. CRH and cortisol concentrations are increased in preeclampsia, and by maternal stress and infections, which may explain the higher risk of preterm delivery in these conditions.[2] Umbilical cord CRH and cortisol are elevated in growth-retarded fetuses.[3]

Table 1. Changes in Hormone Concentrations and in Tissue and Nutrient Deposition During Pregnancy

	Week of Gestation			
	10	**20**	**30**	**40**
Serum Placental Hormones				
Human chorionic gonadotropin (10^4 U/L)	1.3	4.0	3.0	2.5
Human placental lactogen (nmol/L)	23	139	255	394
Estradiol (pmol/L)	5	22	55	66
Products of Conception				
Fetus (g)	5	300	1,500	3400
Placenta (g)	20	170	430	650
Amniotic fluid (g)	30	250	750	800
Maternal Tissue Gain				
Uterus (g)	140	320	600	970
Mammary gland (g)	45	180	360	405
Plasma volume (mL)	50	800	1,200	1,500
Nutrient Metabolism and Accretion in Mother + Fetus				
Increase in basal metabolism	80*	170	260	400
	0.19†	0.41	0.62	0.95
Fat deposition (g)	328	2064	3594	3825
Protein deposition (g)	36	165	498	925
Iron accretion (mg)				565
Calcium accretion (g)				30
Zinc accretion (mg)				100
Hemoglobin (g/L)	125	117	119	130

From King 2000.[91] Used with permission from *The American Journal of Clinical Nutrition.* Copyright Am J Clin Nutr. American Society for Nutrition.
*Kcal
†MJ

Serum estrogen concentrations increase early in pregnancy. The higher concentrations of CRH and adrenocorticotropic hormone stimulate the fetal adrenal to produce dehydroepiandrosterone sulfate, which is converted to estrogen by the placenta. Estrogen then prepares the mother for delivery of the infant. It simulates synthesis of connexin molecules by: 1) the myometrial cells in the uterus so that they will work synchronously during labor; 2) oxytocin receptors in the uterus so that the uterine muscle cells can cause contractions during labor; and 3) prostaglandins, which digest collagen in the cervix and make it more flexible during delivery. Estrogens also alter carbohydrate and lipid metabolism, increase the rate of maternal bone turnover, and stimulate the conversion of somatotroph cells in the maternal pituitary to prolactin-secreting mammotrophs. Prolactin production by these cells is required for the initiation and maintenance of lactation. Progesterone comes initially from the corpus luteum and then from the placenta. Progesterone relaxes the smooth muscle cells of the gastrointestinal tract and uterus, stimulates maternal respiration, promotes the development of mammary gland lobules, and prevents milk secretion from occurring during pregnancy.

In general, pregnancy is a period of increasing resistance of pancreatic β cells to insulin. This occurs in parallel with the higher secretion of chorionic gonadotropin, progesterone, cortisol and prolactin, and serves to permit the flow of glucose, very-low-density lipoproteins, and amino acids to the fetus rather than being deposited in maternal tissues.

Although the weight of the fetus increases throughout pregnancy, about 90% of its growth occurs in the last 20 weeks (Table 1). Fetal growth is accompanied by expansion of the placenta, uterus, and mammary glands. The additional tissues cause maternal metabolic rate to be 60% higher during the last half of pregnancy, creating a need for additional dietary energy. The protein, fat, minerals, and vitamins deposited in the fetal and maternal tissues come from increased maternal food intake and/or more efficient intestinal absorption or renal reabsorption, depending on the specific nutrient.

Changes in Blood and Other Fluids

Plasma volume increases by about 50% (1.5 L) by the end of pregnancy. Red cell mass increases only by 15% to 20%. This "hemodilution of pregnancy" means that hemoglobin and hematocrit concentrations fall, especially during the second trimester when there is the largest rise in plasma volume (Table 1). To correct for this phenomenon, the recommended hemoglobin cutoff values that signify anemia fall to 110 g/L in the first and third trimesters and 105 g/L in the second trimester. The serum concentration of serum albumin and most nutrients is also lower in pregnancy because of hemodilution and alterations in turnover. In contrast, there is a higher maternal plasma concentration of most globulins, lipids (especially triacylglycerol), and vitamin E. Renal plasma flow increases by 75% and glomerular filtration rate by 50%, accompanied by a greater urinary excretion of glucose, amino acids, and water-soluble vitamins.

Weight Gain During Pregnancy

On average, the healthy, well-nourished woman gains about 12 to 15 kg (26 to 33 pounds) during pregnancy. Recognizing that earlier guidelines were low (9 to 11.5 kg) compared with current weight gains, in 1990, the Institute of Medicine revised the guidelines for pregnancy weight gain in the United States.[4] These recent guidelines recognize that the amount of weight gained is inversely related to the fatness, or body mass index (BMI = weight/height^2), of the woman at conception. Based on national surveillance data, the usual weight gain of healthy women who produced a full-term, healthy infant weighing between 3 and 4 kg was estimated for each BMI category. This produced the recommended weight gains shown in Table 2. Obese women tend to gain relatively low amounts of weight and yet produce a normal birth weight infant. For this reason, and to minimize excessive postpartum weight retention, such women are advised to gain less weight but at least 6 kg. Young adolescent and black women should gain amounts in the upper end of the recommended range, because this is more compatible with their producing a normal birth-weight infant. However, black women retain significantly more weight postpartum and tend to gain more weight in the postpartum period.[5] In contrast, shorter (<157 cm, or 62 inches) women should gain in the lower range of their BMI category. Because the risk of low birth weight is highest for thin women who gain low amounts of weight during pregnancy, this group should be a priority for targeting nutrition counseling and support. For women bearing twins, the recommended target weight gain is 16 to 20.5 kg (35 to 45 pounds), but there were insufficient data to recommend a gain based on prepregnancy BMI in a twin gestation.

Table 2. Pregnancy Weight Gain Recommendations

Body Mass Index Category	Recommended Weight Gain in Kilograms (Pounds)
Low (<19.8)	12.5–18 (28–40)
Normal (19.8–26.0)	11.5–16 (25–35)
High (>26.0–29.0)	7–11.5 (15–25)
Obese (>29.0)	≥6.0 (15)

Adapted with permission from Food and Nutrition Board, Institute of Medicine, 1990.[4]

The implementation guide published by the Institute of Medicine is one of the best sources of practical information about how to assess, monitor, and provide nutrition during pregnancy and lactation.[6] The guide includes grids for plotting actual weight gain and comparing actual weight gain to the expected rate, and a special chart for the rapid estimation of a woman's BMI category, based on her height and weight. The importance of monitoring weight change is emphasized, with advice on what to do if gain is less than 2 pounds (1 kg) in any month, more than 6.5 pounds (3 kg) in any month, or consistently above or below the recommended gain. Checklists are provided for evaluation of diets and nutritional status at each clinic visit in pregnancy and lactation, along with advice about appropriate counseling and interventions.

The Institute of Medicine guidelines have been adopted widely by the health profession, at least in part. A review found that the best pregnancy outcomes were indeed obtained when the Institute of Medicine weight gain guidelines were followed.[7] Weight gains below the recommendations were consistently associated with a greater risk of preterm delivery and low birth weight, whereas those above the suggested ranges had a higher risk of macrosomia, cesarean delivery, and excessive postpartum weight retention.

Metabolism and Recommended Intakes of Nutrients

The profound physiological changes that cause hemodilution, changes in the ratio of free to bound forms of nutrients, and alterations in nutrient turnover and homeostasis, affect our ability to assess nutritional status and requirements during pregnancy. For most nutrients, the recommended intake is calculated using a factorial approach. This involves adding estimates of the amount of the nutrient deposited in the mother and the fetus, and a factor to cover the inefficiency of use for tissue growth, to the requirements for nonpregnant women. For a few nutrients, including folate, there are some experimental data that permit the more satisfactory approach of basing recommendations on the amount needed to maintain tis-

Table 3. Recommended Intakes of Nutrients for Nonreproducing, Pregnant, and Lactating Women*

	Adult Woman	Pregnancy	Lactation (0–6 months)
Vitamin A (μg RE)	800	800	1300
Vitamin D (μg)	5	5	5
Vitamin E (mg α-tocopherol)	15	15	19
Vitamin C (mg)	75	85	120
Thiamin (mg)	1.1	1.2	1.4
Riboflavin (mg)	1.1	1.4	1.6
Vitamin B_6 (mg)	1.3	1.9	2.0
Niacin (mg NE)	14	18	17
Folate (μg dietary folate equivalents)	400	600	500
Vitamin B_{12} (μg)	2.4	2.6	2.8
Pantothenic acid (mg)	5	6	7
Biotin (μg)	30	30	35
Choline (mg)	425	450	550
Calcium (mg)	1000	1000	1000
Phosphorus (mg)	700	700	700
Magnesium (mg)	320	350	310
Iron (mg)	15	30	15
Zinc (mg)	12	11	12
Iodine (μg)	150	175	200
Selenium (μg)	55	60	70
Fluoride (mg)	3	3	3

Data from Food and Nutrition Board, Institute of Medicine, 1998,[25] 2000,[63] and 1997.[92]
*Values are recommended dietary intakes, except for vitamin D, pantothenic acid, biotin, cholin, and calcium, where value is an adequate intake.

sue levels and nutrient-dependent function. A summary of recommended nutrient intakes for pregnancy is provided in Table 3. The following discussion is limited to those nutrients that have been established as affecting human pregnancy outcome when they are consumed in inadequate or excessive amounts. However, in animal studies, many more nutrient deficiencies have adverse effects on fetal development and function, and these are likely to affect humans as well.

Energy

Changes in the body composition of well-nourished, normal weight women, include an average increase of 3.7 kg fat and 927 g protein. This amounts to nearly 40,000 kcal or 180 kcal/d across pregnancy. In addition, the total energy expenditure in metabolism and activity increases by 8 kcal/week. Because only small changes in total energy expenditure and weight gain occur in the first trimester, it is recommended that energy intakes increase only in the second and third trimesters.[8] For women ages 14 to 50, the recommended increases are 340 kcal/d in the second trimester and 452 kcal/d in the third.

The actual amount of energy required varies greatly among women. One study of 10 healthy North American women reported that the cumulative energy costs of tissue metabolism and deposition ranged from 60,000 to 170,000 kcal (252 to 714 MJ).[8] As described in the previous section, the amount of weight, especially of fat deposited, is strongly influenced by maternal fatness at conception. Thinner women gain more weight due, in part, to a relatively small increase in resting metabolic rate (RMR), whereas fatter women deposit less fat and have a much larger increase in their metabolic rate.[9]

The mechanism by which maternal fat mass is inversely associated with RMR during pregnancy appears to involve the hormone leptin, which is partially derived from the placenta. Serum leptin concentrations are strongly correlated with the BMI of mothers prior to pregnancy and in the second trimester.[10] Serum leptin concentrations are higher in fatter individuals, and leptin is normally associated with a greater metabolic rate.

It is unclear how this variability in energy deposition translates into recommended energy intakes. Higher energy intakes given during pregnancy to underweight, energy-restricted women can improve birth weight and length, and reduce stillbirths and perinatal mortality.[11,12] A higher energy intake causes more maternal fat deposition, as well as a higher metabolic rate, across well-nourished and poorly nourished populations.[13] In The Gambia, the mid-pregnancy RMR of undernourished women actually fell below pre-pregnancy values but was significantly increased by energy supplementation. Evidently, there are adaptations in energy expenditure and deposition, depending on energy availability.[13] However, these adaptations do not necessarily enable optimal fetal development. Substantial support exists for the concept that an individual who suffered nutritional restriction in utero has a "thrifty genotype." This may help survival in conditions of nutrient restriction, but may also increase the risk of obesity and type 2 diabetes when the food supply is plentiful.[14] Risk of coronary heart disease, hypercholesterolemia, and hypertension is higher for adults who were born small.[15] In utero, nutrition may also adversely affect later adult immunocompetence. Also in The Gambia, adults who had been born during the hungry season had an 11-fold higher risk of dying prematurely of infectious diseases than those born during the rest of the year.[12]

At present, the best strategy for managing energy intake in pregnancy may be to closely monitor weight gain and counsel women to either consume more or less dietary energy as needed. Because the requirement for most nutrients increases substantially more than that for energy, however, recommendations to lower intake must be made with caution. Advice to improve dietary quality and to obtain sufficient exercise is usually appropriate.

Essential Fatty Acids

Essential polyunsaturated fatty acids (PUFAs) must be consumed in the diet because they cannot be synthesized by humans. These include the parent essential fatty acids, linoleic acid (18:2n–6) and ∝-linolenic acid (18:3n–3), found mainly in seed oils, and their longer chain, more unsaturated derivatives called long-chain polyenes. Important long-chain polyenes, derived from linoleic acid, include arachidonic acid (AA) and dihomo-γ-linolenic acid. Those derived from linolenic acid include eicosapentaenoic acid and docosahexaenoic acid (DHA). The linoleic-acid-derived long-chain polyenes and eicosapentaenoic acid are precursors of prostanoids, AA is a structural fatty acid in the brain, and DHA and AA can be converted to biologically active hydroxy fatty acids. The fetal supply of PUFAs depends on maternal PUFA status, which declines as pregnancy progresses. Indeed, evidence shows that the PUFA status of some pregnant women is inadequate to support optimal neonatal status, especially if there are multiple births.[16] The DHA status of neonates is associated with their head circumference, birth length, and weight, and DHA supplementation of preterm infants caused more rapid visual information processing and attention, and affected retinal function. Research is ongoing to resolve the long-term consequences of neonatal essential fatty acid status for function. The major sources of AA are egg yolk and lean meat. DHA is found in meat and fatty fish. Higher intakes of trans fatty acids are associated with poorer maternal and neonatal PUFA status, so it may be beneficial to consume less of these during pregnancy.

Protein

From very early in pregnancy, there are adaptations in maternal nitrogen metabolism that increase nitrogen and protein deposition in the mother and the fetus. These include lower urea production and excretion, lower plasma α-amino nitrogen, and a lower rate of branched chain amino acid transamination.[17] The recommended dietary allowance for pregnancy is an increase of 25 g per day over the prepregnant requirement.[7] This allowance covers the deposition of protein in fetal and maternal tissues. Most pregnant women in industrialized countries, and probably the majority in developing countries, consume at least the recommended intake of protein.

Vitamins

Vitamin A

Vitamin A deficiency during pregnancy and lactation is not a public health problem in industrialized countries. More concern exists about the dangers of excessive supplementation with the vitamin, either as retinol or the analog isotretinoin, which is used to treat severe cystic acne. Ingestion of large amounts of retinol has been associated with birth defects, including abnormalities of the central nervous system, craniofacial and cardiovascular defects, and thymus malformations.[18] The first trimester is most critical because the malformations are derived from cranial neural crest cells. About 20 case reports of retinol toxicity occur during pregnancy, although their interpretation is confounded by the fact that the retinol was usually consumed as part of a multinutrient supplement.[19] Nevertheless, animal studies are clearly consistent with the teratogenic effects of even a single high dose of retinol. The upper safe limit has been set at 8000 or 10,000 IU/d (2400 retinol equivalents),[20] but, in well-nourished populations, the advice is to consume a total of only 3000 μg/d in pregnancy. Large intakes of β-carotene are not toxic.

Vitamin A deficiency is highly prevalent in developing countries. Weekly supplementation of pregnant women in Nepal, where vitamin A deficiency is endemic, reduced maternal mortality by about 44% due to less susceptibility to infections.[21] An equivalent amount of β-carotene had a similar effect. The supplements were started before conception, and it is unknown whether similar benefits would occur if the intervention were started later in pregnancy.

Vitamin D

In both pregnant and nonpregnant individuals, the serum concentration of 25-hydroxyvitamin D, the main circulating form of the vitamin, is the best indicator of vitamin D status. This form of the vitamin crosses the placenta and is converted to the active form, 1,25-dihydroxyvitamin D, by the neonate. The placenta synthesizes 1,25-dihydroxyvitamin D so that maternal serum levels are more than doubled by late pregnancy, and calcium absorption is increased several-fold. Maternal and fetal concentrations of free 1,25-dihydroxycholecalciferol are correlated at term. The main sources of vitamin D are synthesis in the skin through the action of ultraviolet light, and fortified milk and breakfast cereals in the United States. When milk is not fortified with the vitamin, or dairy product or fortified cereal intake is low, seasonal fluctuations in serum 25-hydroxyvitamin D are more evident. Little of the vitamin is synthesized in the skin during winter in more northern latitudes. In the National Health and Nutrition Examination Survey (1988–1994), low serum 25-hydroxyvitamin D concentrations were found in 42% of African-American women and 4% of Caucasian non-Hispanic women in seven states.[22] This results in mothers and their newborn infants having very low serum 25-hydroxyvitamin D concentrations. In France, about 24% of infants born to unsupplemented mothers in the winter or spring had signs of vitamin D deficiency, including poor mineralization of the fetal skeleton and teeth.[23] In China, the bones of infants born in the spring were less developed than those born after the summer.[24]

Vitamin B_6

Although plasma concentrations of pyridoxal and pyridoxal phosphate decline more than can be accounted for by hemodilution, the cause is probably hormonal changes rather than poor vitamin status.[25] Pyridoxal is transferred by active diffusion to the placenta, which converts it to pyridoxal phosphate.[26] In the United States, nonpregnant women's intakes of vitamin B_6 average about 1.5 mg/d. However, apart from older studies of women taking high-dose oral contraceptives that affected B_6 status, there is no evidence of significant problems being caused by vitamin B_6 deficiency during pregnancy in the United States. In Japan, 2 mg/d of the vitamin improved vitamin B_6 status and growth of the newborn.

Vitamin B_{12}

Low plasma vitamin B_{12} concentrations are very common in many countries and are reported to occur in about 40% of individuals of all ages in Latin America.[28] Urban pregnant women in Nepal had a 65% prevalence of low plasma B_{12}, which was associated with elevated plasma homocysteine (Hcy) and twice the risk of preeclampsia and preterm delivery.[29] Although it has long been recognized that strict vegetarian (vegan) diets will cause vitamin B_{12} deficiency because the vitamin is found only in animal products (or fortified foods), it is increasingly clear that lacto-ovo vegetarians are at higher risk of vitamin B_{12} depletion than omnivores.[30,31] Pregnant lacto-ovo vegetarian women had lower plasma vitamin B_{12} and higher Hcy concentrations than omnivores.[32] All vegan or lacto-ovo vegetarian women are advised to consume supplemental vitamin B_{12} during pregnancy, because poor maternal status has been associated with increased risk of early recurrent abortion, neural tube defects (NTDs),[33] and spina bifida.[34]

Folic Acid

There is a marked increase in folate use during pregnancy, due to the acceleration of reactions requiring single-carbon transfer, the rapid rate of cell division in maternal and fetal tissues, and deposition in the fetus. The recommended intakes for pregnancy are based on the amount that maintained erythrocyte concentrations in clinical trials.

Randomized, controlled trials have proven that taking folic acid supplements before conception and through about the first 4 weeks of pregnancy lowers the risk of genetically predisposed women having a baby with an NTD. Unfortunately, most women are unaware that they are pregnant at this stage. NTDs occur in about 0.1% of births in the United States and up to 0.9% in other countries, and tend to recur in subsequent pregnancies. A higher intake of folate from diet plus supplements,[35,36] or higher erythrocyte folate concentrations,[37] is inversely related to NTD risk. The metabolic defect that causes NTD, and the mechanisms by which folic acid lowers NTD risk, are not fully understood.[25] Women at risk of NTD presumably have a metabolic defect that affects folate metabolism, reducing the transport of folate or critical metabolites to the developing embryo. The folic acid may increase the amount of nucleotides, methionine, or S-adenosylmethionine available while the neural tube is closed. Also, women who had an NTD-affected pregnancy tend to absorb about 20% to 25% less folate from either supplements or food, compared to control women.[38] In China, the occurrence of NTDs was reduced up to 80% by a supplement providing only 400 μg/d of folic acid.[39] A daily supplement of 400 μg folic acid reduced the risk by 70% in New England[35] and by 35% in California.[36]

The recommendation is for pregnant women to consume 200 μg/d of synthetic folic acid, in addition to the recommended dietary allowance of 400 μg/d of dietary folate for nonpregnant women. The 200 μg of folic acid is equivalent to 400 μg of dietary folate, because food folates have only about half the bioavailability of the synthetic form. This recommendation is based on the amount of folate that will maintain normal folate status in pregnancy, including prevention of elevated plasma Hcy concentrations. To reduce the risk of NTDs, women capable of becoming pregnant should consume 400 μg of folate daily from supplements, fortified foods, or both, in addition to obtaining food folate from a varied diet.[25] Orange juice and dark-green leafy vegetables and legumes average about 75 to 100 μg of folate per serving, and many commercial fortified breakfast cereals provide 100 μg of folic acid (about 170 dietary folate equivalents).

B Vitamins and Homocysteinemia

Low serum or red blood cell folate and elevated plasma Hcy concentrations are often associated with other pregnancy complications.[40] For example, in a large, retrospective Norwegian study, women currently in the upper quartile of plasma Hcy compared with the lowest quartile had a 32% greater risk of preeclampsia, 38% higher risk of preterm delivery, and 101% higher risk of a very low birth weight infant.[41] Rates of club foot and placental abruption also tended to be higher in those with elevated plasma Hcy. In a smaller group of Spanish women and their infants, maternal plasma Hcy concentrations before conception and throughout pregnancy were correlated with fetal cord blood Hcy and negatively with birth weight.[42] Impressively, those women in the upper tertile of plasma Hcy at 2 months of gestation and at labor had a 3.3 and 4 times greater risk of their infant being born in the lowest tertile of birth weight, respectively. These results do not prove that folate deficiency was the underlying problem, because deficiencies of riboflavin, vitamin B_6, and vitamin B_{12} can also cause elevated plasma tHcy. However, a meta-analysis of intervention trials showed that of all of the vitamin and mineral supplements tested, only folic acid lowered the risk of preterm delivery.[43] Furthermore, folic acid supplementation of Spanish women during the second and third trimesters of pregnancy significantly lowered plasma Hcy; 500 to 600 μg per day produced a maximal response.[44] Further prospective studies of this question are needed, given that birth defects and preterm delivery are leading causes of infant mortality. Although the policy of fortifying grain products with folic acid in the United States and Canada and many other countries was based primarily on the potential of folic acid to lower NTD rates, the effect of this policy on other pregnancy complications may be significant.[45]

Minerals

Calcium

Mechanisms exist to ensure that an adequate amount of calcium is available to the fetus. Additional calcium is made available through a substantial increase in the efficiency of calcium absorption starting early in pregnancy. Calcium is carried across the placenta by an active transport mechanism that involves calcium binding protein and 1,25-dihydroxyvitamin D. Although bone resorption becomes increasingly elevated during pregnancy, there is no detectable change in bone mineral content between conception and parturition.[46] Very little additional dietary calcium is needed during pregnancy, so recommended intakes are not increased over those for nonpregnant women.

Pregnancy-induced hypertension affects about 10% of all pregnancies in the United States and increases the risk of maternal morbidity and mortality, and includes preeclampsia and eclampsia as well as hypertension. Based on epidemiological and experimental evidence of a link between calcium intake and pregnancy-induced hypertension, several clinical trials tested the benefit of calcium supplements for reducing this condition. A meta-analysis of 14 randomized, controlled trials showed that supplements providing 375 to 2000 mg of calcium significantly reduced maternal blood pressure and lowered the risk of gestational hypertension and preeclampsia to about 30% to 40% of that in controls.[47] A subsequent meta-analysis of many of the same trials revealed that the risk of preeclampsia was more reduced in the six populations with low calcium diets than in the four groups with higher calcium intakes.[48] In contrast, the more recent multicenter Calcium for Preeclampsia Prevention trial on 4589 pregnant women in the United States found no significant effect of a 2000 mg/d supplement on blood pressure, PIH, or preeclampsia.[49] This apparent inconsistency might be due to the fact that their usual dietary calcium intake averaged about 1100 mg/d, although even those whose median intake from foods was less than 422 mg/d did not benefit. Women at high risk of PIH, such as young teenagers and those consuming very low amounts of dietary calcium, may still benefit from calcium supplements during pregnancy, but this remains to be proven.

Iron

On average, an additional 6 mg/d of iron needs to be absorbed during pregnancy.[50] Iron is retained by the fetus (300 mg), deposited in the placenta (60 mg), and used for the synthesis of additional maternal red blood cells (450 mg). Blood loss during delivery accounts for another 200 mg. The mother retains about 200 mg in the increased red cell mass after parturition. Serum iron is carried by transferrin to transferrin receptors on the placenta, holotransferrin is endocytosed, iron is released, and apotransferrin is returned to the maternal circulation.[51] More is transferred to the fetus if the mother is iron deficient. Iron absorption increases several-fold during the second and third trimesters, and, unless the maternal diet is low in available iron, it has been calculated based on absorption data that the diet can supply sufficient iron to meet the needs of pregnancy.[52] However, the World Health Organization estimates that anemia affects about 18% of women in industrialized countries and from 35% to 75% of those in developing countries.[53] The Centers for Disease Control and Prevention estimate that about 10% of low-income women are anemic in the first trimester, 14% in the second, and 33% in the third.[54] This prevalence has been essentially unchanged for the past 20 years. In addition, a much higher percentage of women become iron depleted by the end of pregnancy. Because of the pattern of hemodilution, the hemoglobin cutoffs that signify anemia are 110 g/L in trimesters 1 and 3 and 105 g/L in trimester 2.[6] Serum ferritin concentrations fall, often to barely detectable levels, but transferrin concentrations are almost doubled.

In many countries, including the United States, iron supplementation is routinely recommended for all pregnant women. The current recommendation is for pregnant women to take an additional 30 mg of iron daily during pregnancy, starting around the 12th week. Because this amount of iron cannot be readily obtained in food, iron supplements should be taken between meals and without coffee or tea, which can impair iron absorption.[55] Anemic women with low plasma ferritin (<30 μg/L) should take 120 or 180 mg/d of supplemental iron until hemoglobin values become normal. Taking iron once a week can also improve hemoglobin concentrations and iron status. However, a meta-analysis that compared the efficacy of iron supplementation with 60 mg daily or 120 mg weekly concluded that the daily dose was more effective for pregnant women, probably because of the difficulty of consuming enough iron during the relatively short period of gestation.[56]

The advantages of maternal iron supplementation are somewhat controversial. Steer[57] argued that low hemoglobin concentrations at the end of the second trimester are normal and even beneficial because they signify appropriate plasma volume expansion, unless the mean corpuscular volume is elevated. On the other hand, benefits include improved maternal hemoglobin concentrations and a lower risk of anemia and iron depletion in late pregnancy, even in industrialized countries.[57] Increasing evidence shows that iron supplementation during pregnancy increases the iron stores of the infant through about 6 months of infancy, which could be an advantage, especially in developing countries, where complementary foods are low in available iron.[58,59] Severe anemia likely increases the risk of maternal mortality, but whether this is true for moderate anemia is uncertain.[60] Numerous studies report an association between preterm delivery and maternal anemia, but well-designed studies are still needed to confirm that this relationship is causal.[61]

Zinc

The estimated additional zinc required for pregnancy is about 100 mg, equivalent to 5% to 7% of the mother's body zinc.[62] About half of this zinc is deposited in the fetus, and one quarter in the uterus. The recommendation is to consume 11 mg/d during pregnancy.[63] Average intakes of pregnant women in the United States are close to 10 mg/d, with vegetarians consuming much less.[64]

Maternal zinc retention is increased primarily through greater intestinal absorption.[65] Zinc plays critical roles in cell division, hormone metabolism, protein and carbohydrate metabolism, and immunocompetence. Zinc deficiency during pregnancy in animals causes birth defects and intrauterine growth retardation. Because zinc status is thought to be marginal in the United States and many developing countries, especially where few animal products are consumed, several investigators have tested the benefits of zinc supplements for pregnancy outcome. The results of these trials have been mixed. Of 41 studies that described an association between maternal zinc status and birth weight, 17 found a positive association.[65,66] Ten of these were from industrialized countries and seven were from developing countries, and sometimes different studies from the same country found different results. The inconsistent results may be due to poor assessment of maternal zinc status and failure to control for confounding variables. Of 12 randomized, controlled intervention trials, two found an increase in birth weight, and six found no effect. The positive trials were in India and in the United States and included a reduction in preterm deliveries. The latter study enrolled only low-income African American women with below-average zinc concentrations, and only the nonobese women produced heavier infants as a result of the supplementation.[67] Surprisingly, there was no impact of 15 and 30 mg zinc daily on gestational age or size at birth in well-designed controls in Peru and Bangladesh.[68,69] Although the benefits of zinc supplementation for pregnancy need further resolution, it is prudent to ensure adequate zinc intake for women at higher risk of zinc deficiency. These are women with low intakes, high-fiber diets, high intakes of supplemental calcium or iron, and gastrointestinal diseases that lower zinc absorption.[65] Iron doses above 30 mg/d are likely to adversely affect zinc absorption. This may be an important consideration for women consuming the levels of dietary zinc often observed in developing countries, who are given high doses of iron to treat anemia. Maternal infection, smoking, and alcohol abuse may lower placental zinc transport.

Iodine

Iodine deficiency during pregnancy causes cretinism and has permanent adverse effects on the growth, development, and cognitive function of the infant. In areas of severe iodine deficiency, iodized oil injection prior to midpregnancy produced a marked reduction in cretinism and a 30% reduction in neonatal mortality.[70] Even mild maternal iodine deficiency, such as observed in Belgium, can have adverse effects on infant development.[71] In the United States and in many other countries, iodized salt provides sufficient iodine for pregnant women, although not all pregnant women consume this fortified salt.

Other Nutrition-Related Conditions

Pregnancy in the Obese Woman

A general agreement reveals that even a moderate degree of overweight increases the risk of pregnancy complications and rates of cesarean delivery.[72] Moderately overweight women (BMI 25–30) have about 2 to 6 times the risk of gestational diabetes of those with normal weight[73] and significantly more pregnancy hypertension. In obese women, these rates of diabetes and hypertension are even greater, and there is a higher risk of cesarean sections, postoperative complications, low Apgar scores, macrosomia, about 3 times more perinatal mortality, and inexplicably, a higher risk of NTD infants. Macrosomic infants are more likely to become obese in later years. Many of these problems are probably caused by the relatively higher plasma insulin concentrations in obese women. Preconceptional counseling about the risks of obesity during pregnancy, followed by dietary counseling and exercise for weight reduction, is clearly the best preventive strategy. Once obese women become pregnant, they need careful monitoring for diabetes and hypertension and should be advised to gain lower amounts of weight (Table 2) and to increase exercise. Activities at a low to moderate intensity level are usually safe, including walking, swimming, running, aerobic dancing, and exercising on a stationary bicycle. Games that increase risk of abdominal trauma or falling, weight lifting, anaerobic exercise are contraindicated, even in normal weight pregnant women.

Gestational Diabetes

Gestational diabetes is defined as an intolerance to carbohydrate that appears during pregnancy. It is characterized by higher fasting and postprandial plasma concentrations of glucose, amino acids (especially branched-chain), and lipids (fatty acids and especially triacylglycerol). Gestational diabetes may be an extreme manifestation of the normal insulin resistance of pregnancy, or it may reflect a predisposition to type 2 diabetes.[74] The Diabetes in Early Pregnancy Trial found that postprandial, but not fasting, concentrations of plasma glucose predicted birth weight.[75] To improve insulin sensitivity and reduce the risk of infant macrosomia, the American College of Obstetricians and Gynecologists recommends lower energy intakes for overweight and obese pregnant diabetic women, self-monitoring of glucose and urinary ketones, and exercise.[76] Insulin therapy is needed if fasting blood glucose is above 5 mmol/L or 1 hour postprandial glucose is greater than 7.2 mmol/L. Restricting the energy intake of obese women with gestational diabetes to 1200 to 1800 kcal (5020–7531 kJ) per day reduced the prevalence of macrosomia to 6% compared to 23% in unrestricted women.[77] However, excessive energy restriction will lead to ketonemia, which should be avoided because it is potentially harmful to infant mental development.[78]

Preeclampsia

Preeclampsia is a leading cause of maternal and perinatal mortality. The symptoms are the new development of hypertension with proteinuria, edema, or both, usually during the third trimester. It can end in eclampsia or severe and potentially fatal seizures. The syndrome involves reduced placental perfusion often secondary to abnormal implantation and maternal endothelial dysfunction. Increasing evidence shows that the endothelial dysfunction is caused by oxidative stress secondary to the poor placental perfusion.[79] Although the causes of preeclampsia are not yet understood, several risk factors are nutrition-related and include maternal obesity, diabetes, hypertension, and hyperhomocysteinemia. Moreover, maternal antioxidant nutrient status may be important: women with previous pregnancy complications or an abnormal ultrasound, and randomly assigned to supplementation with 1000 mg ascorbic acid and 400 IU of vitamin E from weeks 16 to 22 of gestation, experienced a 76% reduction in preeclampsia and a 21% decrease in indicators of endothelial activation and placental dysfunction.[80] Salt restriction is not advised for the prevention or treatment of preeclampsia.

Alcohol and Caffeine Abuse

Heavy alcohol consumption in pregnancy has teratogenic effects. Fetal alcohol syndrome affects about 1200 infants annually in the United States. Infants with this condition are typically growth retarded with facial defects and have abnormalities of the central nervous, cardiac, and genitourinary systems. This syndrome affects 10% of women consuming 1.5 to 8 alcoholic drinks per week (each containing 0.6 ounces of absolute alcohol) and 30% to 40% of those taking more than 8 drinks a week. The Surgeon General advises that no alcohol be consumed during pregnancy. Alcoholic drinks also displace other dietary items and can alter the absorption and metabolism of nutrients. Although little evidence supports that multivitamin-mineral supplements counteract the effects of alcohol, it is prudent to advise these supplements for women who continue to abuse alcohol when pregnant.

Caffeine crosses the placenta and affects fetal heart rate and respiration. Large amounts of caffeine are teratogenic in animals. Limited evidence shows that moderate coffee intake lowers birth weight in humans. It has not been proven without doubt that caffeine is safe for pregnant women, so the US Food and Drug Administration recommends avoiding or limiting coffee in pregnancy. Caffeine consumption should be limited to less than 300 mg/d, which is equivalent to two to three cups of coffee, four cups of tea, or six cola drinks.

Physiology of Lactation

At parturition, major hormonal changes lead to the onset of lactation. Estrogen and progesterone secretion fall markedly, while the elevated prolactin concentrations are maintained. Prolactin causes the breasts to begin milk secretion. During the first 2 to 7 days postpartum, colostrum is secreted, a thick yellow fluid containing large amounts of immune factors, protein, minerals, and carotenoids. Colostrum can provide the newborn infant with large amounts of maternal antibodies, which is particularly important because the immune system of the infant does not develop fully for some months. Between about 7 and 21 days postpartum the milk is transitional, and, after 21 days, mature milk is secreted.

Suckling is required for the continued synthesis of prolactin and the maintenance of milk production. The action of suckling inhibits the secretion of dopamine from the hypothalamus; dopamine usually inhibits prolactin production. Suckling also releases oxytocin from the posterior pituitary. Oxytocin causes the contraction of the smooth muscle cells that line the alveoli and ducts of the mammary gland, resulting in the contraction of the milk ducts so that the milk is moved down into sinuses near the nipple or even ejected from the breast (milk "let-down"). Emotions can affect oxytocin production, such that, when the mother hears her infant cry, milk let-down may occur. Once lactation is established, it appears that suckling once a day is sufficient to sustain the signals for milk production to continue, whereas milk synthesis stops within a few days once suckling stops. Continued suckling inhibits the release of luteinizing hormone and gonadotropin-releasing hormone so that the return of ovulation and menses is delayed; this provides very effective birth control.

The volume of breast milk secreted increases rapidly in the first postpartum days to about 500 mL on day 5, 650 mL at 1 month, and 700 mL at 3 months.[80-82] Afterward the volume is relatively stable but falls during the process of weaning. Although the infant is growing continuously larger, its rate of growth declines markedly during the period of lactation, causing a fall in nutrient requirements per unit body weight. Thus, breast milk production is usually adequate to meet the energy and protein requirements of the infant until at least age 6 months. In general, the mother can quite easily produce the amount of milk demanded by her infant and can feed two or more infants adequately. The recommendation is for exclusive breast-feeding of the infant until about 6 months of life, which means that no other fluids or foods should be given. Reasons for this recommendation include the fact that introducing other liquids or foods introduces sources of infection and contamination, can lower the quantity of nutrients consumed (especially if special infant foods are not used), and cause the premature disruption of milk production.

Milk Composition

For the purpose of estimating maternal and infant nutrient requirements, the Food and Nutrition Board estimates that the average volume of milk produced is 780 mL/d during the first 6 months and 600 mL for the second 6 months of lactation. Maternal malnutrition must be very severe, that is, BMI substantially below 18.5, before the volume of milk produced is adversely affected. However, some reports reveal that milk fat content is reduced by less severe malnutrition.[83]

The protein content of human milk is about 8 to 9 g/L and contains roughly equal amounts (about 25%) of lactalbumin and casein and substantial quantities of lactoferrin and immunoglobulin A. The content tends to decline slightly with duration of lactation but is not affected by maternal undernutrition. Cow's milk contains about 35 g of protein/L, which is mostly casein. Feeding undiluted cow's milk to young infants is inadvisable because of the large osmotic load produced by large amounts of protein and other solutes and the risk of occult fecal blood loss and subsequent iron deficiency.[84] About 25% of the total nitrogen in milk is nonprotein nitrogen, mainly urea. Lactose concentrations tend to increase throughout lactation, providing an osmotic balance as the content of protein and monovalent items falls slightly. Lactose provides energy, galactose for central nervous system development, and enhanced growth of lactobacilli in the infant intestine. Fat provides about half of the energy in breast milk. The average fat content is about 3.8% but varies greatly within a feed. Hind milk contains substantially more fat than fore milk and may serve as a signal to the infant to stop feeding. Fat content is also greater at the end of the day. The fatty acid content of the mother's diet affects the amount of fatty acids in her breast milk.

Vitamins and Minerals

The concentration of several vitamins and minerals in human milk is influenced by maternal diet and/or vitamin status. Table 4 summarizes the concentrations of these nutrients in normal milk, and the effect of maternal deficiency and supplementation on milk content and the infant.

For the purpose of predicting the risks caused by infant or maternal micronutrient deficiencies in lactation, and for planning interventions, it is useful to categorize nutrient deficiencies based on their effects on the nutrient in milk.[85] Priority nutrients include vitamin A, thiamin, riboflavin, vitamins B_6 and B_{12}, iodine, and selenium. These nutrients are of most concern because low maternal intake or stores reduce their content in milk, which affects the infant adversely.[86] The concentration in milk can be rapidly restored by maternal supplementation. Also, infant stores of these nutrients are more often low and readily depleted, increasing the infant's dependence on receiving an adequate supply from breast milk or complementary foods. Lower-priority nutrients include vitamin D, folic acid, calcium, iron, copper, and zinc. Maternal intake and stores of these nutrients have little effect on breast milk concentrations or infant status, or on the amount required from complementary foods. Consequently, the mother is less likely to become depleted. Maternal supplementation is more likely to benefit the mother than her infant.

The deficiencies described in Table 4 occur predominantly in developing countries, but several do occur in the United States. Examples include low milk vitamin B_{12} and subsequent infant deficiency as a result of strict maternal vegetarianism,[87] and low milk vitamin D and abnormal vitamin D status of infants receiving insufficient exposure to sunlight.[88] The American Academy of Pediatrics recommends that deeply pigmented African-American infants who are breast-fed and whose mothers did not take vitamin D supplements during pregnancy should receive 400 IU of vitamin D per day as a supplement. A high dose (200,000 to 300,000 IU) of vitamin A during the first 6 weeks postpartum, when there is a minimal chance of the woman being pregnant again, can increase breast milk retinol and improve infant vitamin A status in developing countries.[89] Human milk provides sufficient fluoride for the first 6 months of life, but the infant should be given 0.05 mg/kg/d starting at age 6 months.

Maternal Nutrient Requirements During Lactation

The daily nutrient requirements of the lactating woman are higher than her requirements during pregnancy. The recommended intakes are based on the amounts secreted in milk and, for energy and protein, the efficiency of milk synthesis. To estimate maternal energy requirements during lactation, it is assumed that breast milk contains 0.67 kcal/g, so that about 500 kcal/d are secreted in milk during the first 6 months and 400

Table 4. Effects of Maternal Micronutrient Deficiencies and Supplements During Lactation on Breast Milk and Infant Micronutrient Status

		Effects of			
Nutrient	**Normal Milk Concentration**	**Maternal Deficiency on Milk Content**	**Maternal Deficiency on Infant**	**Maternal Supplementation on Milk Content**	**Maternal Supplementation on Infant**
Vitamin A, μg RE/L	485	↓ to 290	Low serum retinol, depletion	↑	↑ Serum retinol and liver stores for 2–3 mo after massive dose
Vitamin D, μg/L	0.55	↓ to 0.25	↑ Risk of rickets, depending on UV light exposure	↑	↑ Serum 25(OH)D if dose >2,000 IU/d
Thiamin, mg/L	0.21	↓ to 0.16	Beriberi	↑ to normal	↓ Infant beriberi
Riboflavin, mg/L	0.35	↓ to 0.2	High EGRAC	↑	↓ EGRAC in mother and infant
Vitamin B_6, mg/L	0.13	↓ to 0.9	Neurological problems	↑	↓ Neurological problems
Folate, μg/L	85	No change	Unknown		None, but ↑ maternal status
Vitamin B_{12}, μg/L	0.42	↓ to 0.13–0.36	↑ Urine MMA, neurological problems, developmental delays	↑	↓ MMA
Ascorbic acid, mg/L	40	↓ to 25	Unknown	↑ (small)	—
Calcium, mg/L	280	↓ to 215	↓ Bone mineral but relative in utero vs. postpartum influence unclear		None
Iron, mg/L	0.3	No change	None	None	None
Zinc, mg/L	1.2	No change	None	None	None
Copper, mg/L	0.25	No change	None	None	None
Iodine, μg/L	146	↓ to 9–32	Uncertain; deficiency in pregnancy more important	↑	Unknown
Selenium, μg/L	18	↓ to ≤10	↓ Plasma and RBC content	↑	Unknown

EGRAC, erythrocyte glutathione reductase activity coefficient; MMA, methylmalonic acid; RBC, red blood cell.
Data from Brown et al., 1998[81]; Allen 1994[85]; and Allen and Graham, 2003.[86]

kcal/d during the second 6 months.[7] However, during the first 6 months of lactation, about 170 kcal daily are normally used from maternal fat stores accumulated during pregnancy, so that the additional energy intake for lactation should be about 330 kcal/d from 0 to 6 months and 400 kcal/d from 6 to 12 months. The recommended dietary allowance for protein is for an additional consumption of 25 g/d, to cover the protein secreted in breast milk and the efficiency of conversion from dietary to milk protein.

The recommended intake of most micronutrients is also increased to cover the amounts secreted in milk (Table 3). The only nutrient that is needed in lower amounts during lactation is iron, except for women who need to synthesize large amounts of blood to replace major blood losses during delivery. Bone mineral content and urinary calcium fall during lactation to meet the additional calcium requirements for milk production.[46] The loss in mineral is temporary, and it is gradually regained by about 3 months after weaning. Higher intakes of calcium than the recommended 1200 mg/d do not affect these lactation-associated changes in maternal bone turnover, bone mineral content, or the amount of calcium in breast milk.[90]

Conclusions and Future Directions

Research is still limited concerning the recommended energy intakes that will support optimal pregnancy outcome in women with different BMIs at conception; weight gain is clearly related to some inherent differences in metabolism between thinner and fatter women, but the extent to which this could or should be accompanied by differences in energy intake is unknown. Pregnant and lactating women are at risk of many micronutrient deficiencies because of poor nutrient status at conception, inadequate dietary quality and/or quantity, and the high nutrient requirements during this period. Much remains to be learned about how the genotype of the mother affects her risk of adverse outcomes, such as NTDs and the extent to which gene abnormalities can be overcome with nutritional supplementation. Clear evidence supports the benefits of maternal supplementation with folic acid (especially at conception), iron, and vitamin D, and iodine, in areas of endemic deficiency. Early prevention of vitamin B deficiencies may lower plasma homocysteine and reduce preterm deliveries and low birth weight, although intervention studies are needed to prove a causal role for homocysteinemia as a risk for poor pregnancy outcomes. More studies are needed to confirm whether improving maternal antioxidant status can reduce risk of preeclampsia. Finally, good maternal nutrition and, in some cases, supplementation, may be necessary to maintain the required concentrations of some micronutrients in breast milk. This is a neglected issue in both industrialized and developing countries.

References

1. McLean M, Bisits A, Davies J, et al. A placental clock controlling the length of human pregnancy. Nat Med. 1995;1:460–463.
2. Wolfe CD, Patel SP, Campbell EA, et al. Plasma corticotrophin-releasing factor (CRF) in normal pregnancy. Br J Obstet Gynaecol. 1988;95:997–1002.
3. Goland RS, Jozak S, Warren WB, et al. Elevated levels of umbilical cord plasma corticotropin-releasing hormone in growth-retarded fetuses. J Clin Endocrin Metab 1993;77:1174–1179.
4. Food and Nutrition Board. Institute of Medicine. *Nutrition During Pregnancy: Part I, Weight Gain. Part II, Nutrient Supplements.* Washington, DC: National Academy Press; 1990.
5. Scholl TO, Hediger ML, Schall JI, et al. Gestational weight gain, pregnancy outcome, and postpartum weight retention. Obstet Gynecol. 1995;86:423–427.
6. Institute of Medicine. *Nutrition During Pregnancy and Lactation: An Implementation Guide.* Washington, DC: National Academy Press; 1992.
7. Institute of Medicine. *Dietary Reference Intakes for Energy, Carbohydrate, Fiber, Fat, Fatty Acids, Cholesterol, Protein, and Amino Acids.* Washington, DC: National Academy Press; 2002/2005.
8. Kopp-Hoolihan LE, van Loan MD, Wong WW, et al. Fat mass deposition during pregnancy using a four-component model. J Appl Physiol. 1999;87: 196–202.
9. Bronstein MN, Mak RP, King JC. Unexpected relationship between fat mass and basal metabolic rate in pregnant women. Br J Nutr. 1996;75:659–668.
10. Williams MA, Havel PJ, Schwartz MW, et al. Preeclampsia disrupts the normal relationship between serum leptin concentrations and adiposity in pregnant women. Paediatr Perinat Epidemiol. 1999;13: 190–204.
11. Ceesay SM, Prentice AM, Cole TJ, et al. Effects on birth weight and perinatal mortality of maternal dietary supplements in rural Gambia: 5 year randomised controlled trial. Br Med J. 1997;315:786–790.
12. Moore SE. Nutrition, immunity and the fetal and infant origins of disease hypothesis in developing countries. Proc Nutr Soc. 1998;57:241–247.
13. Prentice AM, Goldberg GR. Energy adaptations in human pregnancy: limits and long-term consequences. Am J Clin Nutr. 2000;71:1226S–1232S.
14. Hales CN, Barker DJ. Type 2 (non-insulin-dependent) diabetes mellitus: the thrifty phenotype hypothesis. Diabetologia. 1992;35:595–601.
15. Godfrey KM, Barker DJ. Fetal nutrition and adult disease. Am J Clin Nutr. 2000;71:1344S–1352S.
16. Hornstra G. Essential fatty acids in mothers and their neonates. Am J Clin Nutr. 2000;71:1262S–1269S.
17. Kalhan SC. Protein metabolism in pregnancy. Am J Clin Nutr. 2000;71:1249S–1255S.
18. Rothman KJ, Moore LL, Singer MR, et al. Teratogenicity of high vitamin A intake. N Engl J Med. 1995; 333:1369–1373.
19. Azaïs-Braesco V, Pascal G. Vitamin A in pregnancy: requirements and safety limits. Am J Clin Nutr. 2000; 71:1325S–1333S.
20. World Health Organization. *Safe Vitamin A Dosage During Pregnancy and Lactation. Recommendations and Report from a Consultation.* Geneva; 1998.
21. West KP Jr, Katz J, Khatry SK, et al. Double blind, cluster randomised trial of low dose supplementation with vitamin A or beta carotene on mortality related to pregnancy in Nepal. The NNIPS-2 Study Group. Br Med J. 1999;318:570–575.
22. Nesby-O'Dell S, Scanlon KS, Cogswell ME, et al. Hypovitaminosis D prevalence and determinants

among African American and white women of reproductive age: third National Health and Nutrition Examination Survey, 1988–1994. Am J Clin Nutr. 2002;76:187–192.

23. Zeghoud F, Vervel C, Guillozo H, et al. Subclinical vitamin D deficiency in neonates: definition and response to vitamin D supplements. Am J Clin Nutr. 1997;65:771–778.
24. Specker BL, Ho ML, Oestreich A, et al. Prospective study of vitamin D supplementation and rickets in China. J Pediatr. 1992;120:733–739.
25. Food and Nutrtion Board. Institute of Medicine. *Dietary Reference Intakes for Thiamin, Riboflavin, Niacin, Vitamin B_6, Folate, Vitamin B_{12}, Pantothenic Acid, Biotin, and Choline.* Washington, DC: National Academies Press; 1998.
26. Schenker S, Johnson RF, Mahuren JD, et al. Human placental vitamin B_6 (pyridoxal) transport: normal characteristics and effects of ethanol. Am J Physiol. 1992;262:R966–R974.
27. Chang SJ. Adequacy of maternal pyridoxine supplementation during pregnancy in relation to the vitamin B_6 status and growth of neonates at birth. J Nutr Sci Vitaminol. 1999;45:449–458.
28. Allen LH. Folate and vitamin B_{12} status in the Americas. Nutr Rev. 2004;62:S29–S33; discussion S34.
29. Bondevik GT, Schneede J, Refsum H, et al. Homocysteine and methylmalonic acid levels in pregnant Nepali women. Should cobalamin supplementation be considered? Eur J Clin Nutr. 2001;55:856–864.
30. Helman AD, Darnton-Hill I. Vitamin and iron status in new vegetarians. Am J Clin Nutr. 1987;45: 785–789.
31. Herrmann W, Schorr H, Purschwitz K, et al. Total homocysteine, vitamin B_{12}, and total antioxidant status in vegetarians. Clin Chem. 2001;47:1094–1101.
32. Koebnick C, Hoffmann I, Dagnelie PC, et al. Long-term ovo-lacto vegetarian diet impairs vitamin B_{12} status in pregnant women. J Nutr. 2004;134: 3319–3326.
33. Ray JG, Blom HJ. Vitamin B_{12} insufficiency and the risk of fetal neural tube defects. Q J Med. 2003;96: 289–295.
34. Groenen PM, van Rooij IA, Peer PG, et al. Marginal maternal vitamin B_{12} status increases the risk of offspring with spina bifida. Am J Obstet Gynecol. 2004; 191:11–17.
35. Werler MM, Shapiro S, Mitchell AA. Periconceptional folic acid exposure and risk of occurrent neural tube defects. JAMA. 1993;269:1257–1261.
36. Shaw GM, Schaffer D, Velie EM, et al. Periconceptional vitamin use, dietary folate, and the occurrence of neural tube defects. Epidemiology. 1995;6:219–226.
37. Daly LE, Kirke PN, Molloy A, et al. Folate levels and neural tube defects. Implications for prevention. JAMA. 1995;274:1698–1702.
38. Boddie AM, Dedlow ER, Nackashi JA, et al. Folate absorption in women with a history of neural tube defect-affected pregnancy. Am J Clin Nutr. 2000;72: 154–158.
39. Berry RJ, Li Z, Erickson JD, et al. Prevention of neural-tube defects with folic acid in China. China-U.S. Collaborative Project for Neural Tube Defect Prevention. N Engl J Med. 1999;341:1485–1490.
40. Scholl TO, Hediger ML, Bendich A, et al. Use of multivitamin/mineral prenatal supplements: influence on the outcome of pregnancy. Am J Epidemiol. 1997;146:134–141.
41. Vollset SE, Refsum H, Irgens LM, et al. Plasma total homocysteine, pregnancy complications, and adverse pregnancy outcomes: the Hordaland Homocysteine Study. Am J Clin Nutr. 2000;71:962–968.
42. Murphy MM, Scott JM, Arija V, et al. Maternal homocysteine before conception and throughout pregnancy predicts fetal homocysteine and birth weight. Clin Chem. 2004;50:1406–1412.
43. Gülmezoglu M, de Onis M, Villar J. Effectiveness of interventions to prevent or treat impaired fetal growth. Obstet Gynecol Surv. 1997;52:139–149.
44. Murphy MM, Scott JM, McPartlin JM, et al. The pregnancy-related decrease in fasting plasma homocysteine is not explained by folic acid supplementation, hemodilution, or a decrease in albumin in a longitudinal study. Am J Clin Nutr. 2002;76:614–619.
45. Botto LD, Lisi A, Robert-Gnansia E, et al. International retrospective cohort study of neural tube defects in relation to folic acid recommendations: are the recommendations working? Obstet Gynecol Surv. 2005;60:563–565.
46. Ritchie LD, Fung EB, Halloran BP, et al. A longitudinal study of calcium homeostasis during human pregnancy and lactation and after resumption of menses. Am J Clin Nutr. 1998;67:693–701.
47. Bucher HC, Cook RJ, Guyatt GH, et al. Effects of dietary calcium supplementation on blood pressure. A meta-analysis of randomized controlled trials. JAMA. 1996;275:1016–1022.
48. Villar J, Belizán JM. Same nutrient, different hypotheses: disparities in trials of calcium supplementation during pregnancy. Am J Clin Nutr. 2000;71: 1375S–1379S.
49. Levine RJ, Hauth JC, Curet LB, et al. Trial of calcium to prevent preeclampsia. N Engl J Med. 1997; 337:69–76.
50. Hallberg L. Iron balance in pregnancy. In: Berger H, ed. *Vitamins and Minerals in Pregnancy and Lactation.* New York: Raven Press; 1988; 115–127.
51. Harris ED. New insights into placental iron transport. Nutr Rev. 1992;50:329–331.
52. Barrett JF, Whittaker PG, Williams JG, et al. Absorption of non-haem iron from food during normal pregnancy. Br Med J. 1994;309:79–82.
53. ACC/SCN. *Fourth Report on the World Nutrition Situation.* Geneva; 2000.
54. Kim I, Hungerford R, Yip R. Pregnancy nutrition

surveillance system—United States, 1979–1990. Morb Mortal Wkly Rep. 1992;41:26–42.

55. Food and Nutrition Board. Institute of Medicine. *Iron Deficiency Anemia: Recommended Guidelines for the Prevention, Detection, and Management Among US Children and Women of Child Bearing Age.* Washington, DC: National Academies Press; 1993.
56. Beard JL. Effectiveness and strategies of iron supplementation during pregnancy. Am J Clin Nutr. 2000; 71:1288S–1294S.
57. Steer PJ. Maternal hemoglobin concentration and birth weight. Am J Clin Nutr. 2000;71:1285S–1287S.
58. Allen LH. Anemia and iron deficiency: effects on pregnancy outcome. Am J Clin Nutr. 2000;71: 1280S–1284S.
59. Preziosi P, Prual A, Galan P, et al. Effect of iron supplementation on the iron status of pregnant women: consequences for newborns. Am J Clin Nutr. 1997;66:1178–1182.
60. Brabin BJ, Hakimi M, Pelletier D. An analysis of anemia and pregnancy-related maternal mortality. J Nutr. 2001;131:604S–614S.
61. Rasmussen K. Is there a causal relationship between iron deficiency or iron-deficiency anemia and weight at birth, length of gestation and perinatal mortality? J Nutr. 2001;131:590S–601S; discussion 601S–603S.
62. Swanson CA, King JC. Zinc and pregnancy outcome. Am J Clin Nutr. 1987;46:763–771.
63. Food and Nutrition Board. Institute of Medicine. *Dietary Reference Intakes for Vitamin A, Vitamin K, Arsenic, Boron, Chromium, Copper, Iodine, Iron, Manganese, Molybdenum, Nickel, Silicon, Vanadium, and Zinc.* Washington, DC: National Academies Press; 2000.
64. Apgar J. Zinc and reproduction: an update. J Nutr Biochem. 1992;3:266–278.
65. King JC. Determinants of maternal zinc status during pregnancy. Am J Clin Nutr. 2000;71: 1334S–1343S.
66. Tamura T, Goldenberg RL. Zinc nutriture and pregnancy outcome. Nutr Res. 1996;16:139–181.
67. Goldenberg RL, Tamura T, Neggers Y, et al. The effect of zinc supplementation on pregnancy outcome. JAMA. 1995;274:463–468.
68. Osendarp SJ, van Raaij JM, Arifeen SE, et al. A randomized, placebo-controlled trial of the effect of zinc supplementation during pregnancy on pregnancy outcome in Bangladeshi urban poor. Am J Clin Nutr. 2000;71:114–119.
69. Caulfield LE, Zavaleta N, Figueroa A, et al. Maternal zinc supplementation does not affect size at birth or pregnancy duration in Peru. J Nutr. 1999;129: 1563–1568.
70. Thilly CH, Delange F, Lagasse R, et al. Fetal hypothyroidism and maternal thyroid status in severe endemic goiter. J Clin Endocrin Metab. 1978;47: 354–360.
71. Delange F, Wolff P, Gnat D, et al. Iodine deficiency during infancy and early childhood in Belgium: does it pose a risk to brain development? Eur J Pediatr. 2001;160:251–254.
72. Galtier-Dereure F, Boegner C, Bringer J. Obesity and pregnancy: complications and cost. Am J Clin Nutr. 2000;71:1242S–1248S.
73. Abrams B, Parker J. Overweight and pregnancy complications. Int J Obes. 1988;12:293–303.
74. Butte NF. Carbohydrate and lipid metabolism in pregnancy: normal compared with gestational diabetes mellitus. Am J Clin Nutr. 2000;71:1256S–1261S.
75. Jovanavic-Peterson L, Peterson CM. New strategies for the treatment of gestational diabetes. Isr J Med Sci. 1991;27:510–515.
76. ACOG. ACOG Technical Bulletin. Diabetes and pregnancy. *Int J Gynaecol Obstet.* 1995;48:331–339.
77. Dornhorst A, Nicholls JS, Probst F, et al. Calorie restriction for treatment of gestational diabetes. Diabetes. 1991;40(Suppl 2):161–164.
78. Rizzo T, Metzger BE, Burns WJ, et al. Correlations between antepartum maternal metabolism and child intelligence. N Engl J Med. 1991;325:911–916.
79. Roberts JM, Hubel CA. Oxidative stress in preeclampsia. Am J Obstet Gynecol. 2004;190:1177–1178.
80. Chappell LC, Seed PT, Briley AL, et al. Effect of antioxidants on the occurrence of pre-eclampsia in women at increased risk: a randomised trial. Lancet. 1999;354:810–816.
81. Brown K, Dewey K, Allen L. Complementary feeding of young children in developing countries: a review of current scientific knowledge. Geneva; World Health Organization/UNICEF; 1998.
82. Neville MC, Allen JC, Archer PC, et al. Studies in human lactation: milk volume and nutrient composition during weaning and lactogenesis. Am J Clin Nutr. 1991;54:81–92.
83. Prentice AM, Goldberg GR, Prentice A. Body mass index and lactation performance. Eur J Clin Nutr. 1994;48(Suppl 3):S78–S86; discussion S86–S89.
84. Ziegler EE, Jiang T, Romero E, et al. Cow's milk and intestinal blood loss in late infancy. J Pediatr. 1999;135:720–726.
85. Allen LH. Maternal micronutrient malnutrition: effects on breast milk and infant nutrition, and priorities for intervention. SCN News. 1994;11:21–24.
86. Allen LH, Graham JM. Assuring micronutrient adequacy in the diets of young infants. In: Delange FM, West KP, eds. *Micronutrient Deficiencies in the First Six Months of Life.* Basel: Vevey/S. Karger AG; 2003; 55–88.
87. Specker BL, Black A, Allen L, et al. Vitamin B_{12}: low milk concentrations are related to low serum concentrations in vegetarian women and to methylmalonic aciduria in their infants. Am J Clin Nutr. 1990; 52:1073–1076.

88. Specker BL. Do North American women need supplemental vitamin D during pregnancy or lactation? Am J Clin Nutr. 1994;59:484S–490S; discussion 490.
89. Stoltzfus RJ, Hakimi M, Miller KW, et al. High dose vitamin A supplementation of breast-feeding Indonesian mothers: effects on the vitamin A status of mother and infant. J Nutr. 1993;123:666–675.
90. Prentice A. Maternal calcium metabolism and bone mineral status. Am J Clin Nutr. 2000;71: 1312S–1316S.
91. King JC. Physiology of pregnancy and nutrient metabolism. Am J Clin Nutr. 2000;71:1218S–1225S.
92. Food and Nutrition Board. Institute of Medicine. *Dietary Reference Intakes for Calcium, Phosphorus, Magnesium, Vitamin D, and Fluoride.* Washington, DC: National Academies Press; 1997.

42
Infant Nutrition

William C. Heird

The normal infant experiences a three-fold increase in weight and a two-fold increase in length during the first year of life, and these increases are accompanied by dramatic developmental changes in organ function and body composition. These rapid rates of growth and development impose unique nutritional needs over and above the relatively high maintenance needs incident to the higher metabolic and nutrient turnover rates of infants compared with adults. Despite these unique nutritional needs, reference intakes for the 0- to 6-month-old and the 7- to 12-month-old infant have been established for all nutrients. Some of these, as well as several specific issues relevant to infant nutrition—breast versus formula feeding, introduction of complementary foods, use of formula versus bovine milk, the need for preformed, long-chain polyunsaturated fatty acids (LC-PUFAs)—are discussed in the following sections. These discussions are preceded by a discussion of the differences among requirement, recommended intake, and reference intake.

Requirement versus Recommended or Reference Intakes

The "requirement" for a specific nutrient is the amount that results in some predetermined physiological end point. In infants, this end point is usually the maintenance of satisfactory rates of growth and development and/or the prevention of specific signs of deficiency. The requirement for a specific nutrient is usually defined experimentally, often in a relatively small study population. Thus, the mean requirement of a specific nutrient estimated in this way (the estimated average requirement or EAR) usually meets the needs of roughly half the population. Thus, for some it may be inadequate and for others it may be excessive.

In contrast, the recommended daily allowance (RDA) of a specific nutrient is the intake of that nutrient deemed by a scientifically knowledgeable group of individuals to meet the "requirement" of most healthy members of a population. If the EAR of a specific nutrient is normally distributed within the population in which it was established, the RDA usually is set at the EAR of the population plus two standard deviations. Since the EARs of many nutrients are not normally distributed, other considerations of population variability are often necessary. For example, if the EAR appears to be adequate for most of the study population, the RDA may be less than the requirement plus two standard deviations. RDAs are useful guides for nutrient intakes of individuals or groups, but they are not useful for ascertaining the adequacy or inadequacy of an individual's intake of a specific nutrient. Moreover, since the EAR of many nutrients is not known with certainty, it is often impossible to establish an RDA.

Because of the difficulties in establishing an EAR for many nutrients, and the uncertainty of an RDA based on limited information concerning requirement, the Food and Nutrition Board of the National Academies of Science has established Dietary Reference Intakes (DRIs). These include RDAs for those nutrients for which an EAR, and therefore an RDA, can reliably be established as well as other "reference intakes" such as Adequate Intake (AI) and Tolerable Upper Intake Level (UL). AI, which is used when a RDA cannot be determined, is the observed or approximated daily intake of a specific nutrient by a group of healthy individuals (e.g., the intake of the breast-fed infant, which is the basis for the majority of the most recent DRIs for infants under 6 months of age). The UL is the highest daily intake of a specific nutrient that is likely to pose no risk. It is not a recommended level of intake, but rather an aid in avoiding adverse effects secondary to excessive intake.

The DRIs established by the Food and Nutrition Board[1-6] for 0- to 6-month-old and 7- to 12-month-old infants are summarized in Table 1, and some are discussed in the following paragraphs.

Table 1. Reference Intakes of Nutrients for Normal Infants[1-6]

	Intake per Day	
Nutrient*	Age 0–6 Months	Age 7–12 Months
Energy (kcal or kJ)†		
Males	570 (2385)	743 (3109)
Females	520 (2176)	676 (2829)
Fat (g)	31	30
Carbohydrate	60	95
Protein (g)	9.1	13.5
Electrolytes and Minerals:		
Calcium (mg)	210	270
Phosphorus (mg)	100	275
Magnesium (mg)	30	75
Sodium (mg)	115	368
Chloride (mg)	178	568
Potassium (mg)	390	702
Iron (mg)	0.27	11‡ (5)
Zinc (mg)	2	3‡ (5)
Copper (μg)	200	220
Iodine (μg)	110	130
Selenium (μg)	15	20
Manganese (mg)	0.003	0.6
Fluoride (mg)	0.01	0.5
Chromium (μg)	0.2	5.5
Molybdenum (μg)	2	3
Vitamins:		
Vitamin A (μg)	400	500
Vitamin D (μg)	5	5
Vitamin E (mg α-TE)	4	6
Vitamin K (μg)	2.0	2.5
Vitamin C (mg)	40	50
Thiamine (mg)	0.2	0.3
Riboflavin (mg)	0.3	0.4
Niacin (mg NE)	2	4
Vitamin B_6 (μg)	0.1	0.3
Folate (μg)	65	80
Vitamin B_{12} (μg)	0.4	0.5
Biotin (μg)	5	6
Pantothenic Acid (mg)	1.7	1.8
Choline (mg)	125	150

* Unless indicated otherwise, values are Adequate Intake (AI): mean intake of normal breast-fed infants 0–6 months of age or mean intake of 7–12 month old infants from human milk plus complementary foods.

† Estimated Energy Requirement (EER)

‡ Recommended Daily Allowance (RDA)

DRIs of Specific Nutrients

Energy

Since an energy intake that is adequate for all or almost all individuals will result in excessive weight gain by individuals with a low or an average requirement, the reference energy intakes reflect the estimated energy requirement (EER) for each population, or the dietary energy intake predicted to maintain energy balance in a healthy individual of a defined age, gender, weight, height, and level of physical activity. The EERs are based on predictive equations for normal-weight individuals that include daily energy expenditure measured by the doubly labeled water method plus an allowance for energy deposition. Since an RDA by definition will exceed the EER of many individuals and result in excessive weight gain, setting an RDA for energy would only contribute to the growing prevalence of overweight and obesity. Similarly, the UL is not appropriate for energy because any intake above the EER will result in excessive weight gain.

Expressed per unit of body weight, the EER of the normal newborn infant is about twice that of the normal adult. The greater energy requirement of the infant reflects primarily the higher metabolic rate and the special needs for growth and development. The inefficient intestinal absorption of the infant compared with the adult contributes only minimally to the higher energy requirement of infants fed human milk or modern infant formula.

There is no evidence that either carbohydrate or fat is a superior source of energy. Sufficient carbohydrate to prevent ketosis and/or hypoglycemia is necessary (approx. 5.0 g/kg body wt/d), as is enough fat to provide essential fatty acid requirements (0.5–1.0 g/kg body wt/d of linoleic acid plus a smaller amount of α-linolenic acid). Currently, there is concern that infants may also require LC-PUFA ω3 and perhaps ω6 fatty acids. This issue is discussed in a separate section and in the chapter on fat metabolism (Chapter 10).

The minimum needs for carbohydrate and fat amount to no more than about 30 kcal (125.5 kJ)/kg body wt/d, or only approximately one-third of the infant's total energy need. Whether the remainder should be comprised predominantly of fat or of equicaloric amounts of each is not known. The acceptable macronutrient distribution range (AMDR) for carbohydrate and fat specified by the Food and Nutrition Board is 20% to 25% of total energy as fat and 45% to 65% of total energy as carbohydrate. While appropriate for older children and adults, the "acceptable" range for fat is lower than most would endorse for infants. Human milk and most currently available formulas contain equicaloric amounts of fat and carbohydrate. This distribution, about 45% of total energy as carbohydrate and about 45% as fat, seems appropriate.

The AI for ω6 fatty acids (linoleic acid) is 4.4 g/d for the 0- to 6-month-old and 4.6 g/d for the 7- to 12-month-old infant. The AI for ω3 fatty acids (α-linolenic acid) is 0.5 g/d for both the 0- to 6-month-old and the 7- to 12-month-old infant. These reference intakes are based on the average intake of these fatty acids in the average volume of human milk ingested from 4 to 6 months of age and the average intake from human milk plus complementary foods from 7 to 12 months of age.

Protein

The protein requirement of the normal infant is also higher per unit of body weight than that of the adult. In addition, it is thought that the infant requires a higher proportion of essential amino acids than the adult. These include the amino acids recognized as essential (or indispensable) for the adult (leucine, isoleucine, valine, threonine, methionine, phenylalanine, tryptophan, lysine, and histidine) as well as cysteine and tyrosine. The need for cysteine is thought to reflect the fact that the hepatic activity of cystathionase, a key enzyme in conversion of methionine to cysteine, does not reach adult levels until at least 4 months of age.[7,8] The reason for the infant's apparent need for tyrosine is not clear; the hepatic activity of phenylalanine hydroxylase, the rate-limiting enzyme for conversion of phenylalanine to tyrosine, is at or near adult levels early in gestation.[9] Furthermore, recent studies show that even preterm infants can convert phenylalanine to tyrosine.[10,11]

Human milk protein and all proteins currently used in infant formulas contain adequate amounts of all essential amino acids (including cysteine and tyrosine), which are the amounts of each in the volume of human milk necessary to provide the AI for protein intake of the 0- to 6-month-old infant and the RDA for protein intake of the 7- to 12-month-old infant, which is set at the amount deposited in body protein by infants of this age corrected for efficiency plus the same maintenance needs as the adult.

The required intake of a specific protein depends upon its quality, or how closely its amino acid pattern resembles that of human milk. Further, the overall quality of a specific protein can be improved by supplementing it with the essential amino acid(s) that results in its quality being low (the limiting amino acid). Native soy protein, for example, has insufficient methionine, but when fortified with methionine, the quality of soy protein approaches or equals that of bovine milk protein.[12]

The protein sources of most infant formulas, usually bovine milk protein or modern preparations of soy protein such as human milk protein, are very high-quality proteins. Furthermore, if properly processed, these proteins are utilized nearly as well as human milk protein. Thus, as reflected by recent DRIs for protein, the amounts of these proteins needed are not much, if at all, higher than the amount of human milk protein needed.[13] The recent DRIs for protein are considerably lower than previous RDAs (approx. 1.5 g/kg body wt/d versus 2.2 g/kg body wt/d) throughout the first year of life.

Electrolytes, Minerals, and Vitamins

The normal infant's needs for electrolytes, minerals, and vitamins are not as well defined as those for energy and protein. Nonetheless, reference intakes, usually the mean intake of each by normally growing 0- to 6-month-old infants or the mean intake of each from human milk and complementary food by the 7- to 12-month-old infant, have been established (Table 1).

Although the normal newborn infant is thought to have sufficient stores of iron to meet the requirements for 4 to 6 months, iron deficiency remains the most common nutrient deficiency syndrome in infancy. This reflects the fact that iron stores at birth and the absorption of iron are quite variable. Interestingly, although human milk contains less iron than most formulas, iron deficiency is less common in breast-fed infants. However, to prevent iron deficiency, routine iron supplementation of breast-fed infants and the use of iron-fortified formulas for formula-fed infants are recommended.[14] The increasing use of iron-fortified formulas over the past decade has dramatically reduced the incidence of iron deficiency.

If protein intake is adequate, vitamin deficiencies are rare; if it is inadequate, deficiencies of nicotinic acid and choline, which are synthesized from tryptophan and methionine, respectively, may develop. In contrast, if bovine milk and bovine milk formulas were not supplemented with vitamin D, hypovitaminosis D would be endemic among formula-fed infants, particularly those with limited exposure to sunlight. Since breast-fed infants may be even more susceptible to the development of vitamin D deficiency, routine vitamin D supplementation of breast-fed infants is recommended, particularly if exposure to sunlight is limited.[14]

Routine perinatal administration of vitamin K is recommended as prophylaxis against hemorrhagic disease of the newborn. Thereafter, deficiency of this vitamin is uncommon except in infants with conditions associated with fat malabsorption.

Water

The normal infant's absolute requirement for water probably is considerably less than the DRIs. The requirement is 700 mL/d for the 0- to 6-month-old and 800 mL/d for the 7- to 12-month-old infant. These are the amounts provided by the mean human milk intake of the 0- to 6-month-old and the mean intake of the 7- to 12-month-old from human milk plus complementary food. Because of higher obligate renal, pulmonary, and dermal water losses and a higher overall metabolic rate, the infant is more susceptible to dehydration, particularly with vomiting and/or diarrhea, and especially if solute intake is high, as it is in bovine milk. Thus, the intake of high-solute foods, (e.g., bovine milk) before 1 year of age is discouraged. The typical breast-fed or formula-fed infant usually consumes at least 150 mL/kg body wt/d for the first several weeks of life. Although somewhat higher than the AI, there is no reason to believe that a fluid intake of this amount is excessive.

The Second Six Months of Life

By 4 to 6 months of age, the infant's capacity to digest and absorb a variety of dietary components and to metabolize, utilize, and excrete the absorbed products of digestion is near the capacity of the adult.[15] Moreover, at this time, teeth are beginning to erupt and the infant is more active and beginning to explore his/her surroundings. With the eruption of teeth, the role of dietary carbohydrate in the development of dental caries must be considered.[16] Consideration of the long-term effects of inadequate or excessive intake during infancy also assumes greater importance, as does consideration of the psychosocial role of foods during development.

These considerations, rather than concerns about delivery of adequate amounts of nutrients, are the basis for many feeding practices advocated for the formula-fed infant during the second 6 months of life. While it is clear that all nutrient needs during this period can be met with reasonable amounts of currently available infant formulas, the addition of other foods after 4 to 6 months of age is recommended. In contrast, the volume of milk produced by many women is not adequate to meet all nutrient needs of the breast-fed infant beyond 4 to 6 months of age. Thus, for these infants complementary foods are an important source of nutrients.

By approximately 12 months of age, most infants have graduated successfully to table food and are content with three meals plus two to three snacks daily. Once a few teeth have erupted and tolerance of solid foods has been demonstrated, weaning can be completed. Weaning or "follow-on" formulas have been popular in Europe for some time and have recently become available in the United States. These formulas contain somewhat more protein than standard infant formulas. They also may have a somewhat lower fat content and a somewhat higher carbohydrate content. The types of fat and carbohydrate present are similar to those of standard infant formulas (vegetable oils and lactose plus corn syrup solids). There is no convincing evidence that these formulas, which have not been particularly popular in the United States, are superior to standard infant formulas or bovine milk (after 12 months of age).

Aside from the association of bottle feeding with dental caries,[16] little is known about either the potential hazards or the non-nutritional role of diet during the latter half of the first year of life. Thus, feeding practices during this period vary widely. Nonetheless, most recent surveys indicate that infants fed according to current practices receive the reference intakes for most nutrients.[17]

Human Milk versus Artificial Formula

The ready availability and safety of human milk, coupled with the possibility that it may enhance intestinal development, resistance to infection, and bonding between the mother and infant, make human milk the perfect food for the normal infant. Most authorities recommend exclusive breast-feeding for the first 6 months of life, with continued breast-feeding throughout the first year or longer.[18,19] This recommendation is supported by evidence that breast-fed infants in both affluent and developing societies have fewer common and serious infections during early life than formula-fed infants.[20,21] However, as publicized a few years ago in the lay press,[22] it cannot automatically be assumed that maternal milk supply will be adequate and/or constant. Thus, it is essential that breast-fed infants, particularly first-born infants, be followed closely over the first few days to weeks of life to ensure that growth and development are proceeding normally. With proper counseling, most problems can be corrected and/or avoided.

In large part, the historical problems associated with artificial feeding have been solved. In fact, the safety and easy digestibility of modern infant formulas approach the safety and digestibility of breast milk. Furthermore, the clear economic advantages and microbiological safety of breast-feeding are of lesser importance for affluent, developed societies with ready access to a clean water supply and refrigeration than for less developed, less affluent societies. Thus, a reasonable and conservative approach is to allow the mother to make an informed choice of how she wishes to feed her infant and support her in that decision. As stated by Fomon[23]:

> "...in industrialized countries, any woman with the least inclination toward breast feeding should be encouraged to do so, and all assistance possible should be provided by nurses, physicians, nutritionists and other health workers. At the same time, there is little justification for attempts to coerce women to breast feed. No woman in an industrialized country should be made to feel guilty because she elects not to breast feed her infant."

A number of formulas are available for feeding the normal infant. The composition of those used most commonly in the United States is shown in Table 2. The composition of those commonly used in other countries is similar. Most are available in both a "ready-to-use" and a concentrated liquid form. Powdered products, which are lower in cost, also are available and are being used with increasing frequency. These products usually are the only ones available in many parts of the world.

The most commonly used formulas contain mixtures of bovine whey proteins and caseins at a total protein concentration of about 1.5 g/dL. Thus, the infant who receives 150 to 180 mL/kg body wt/d receives a protein intake of 2.25 to 2.7 g/kg body wt/d. This is as much as 50% more than the intake of the breast-fed infant and, hence, the recent DRI for protein.

At one time, unmodified bovine milk protein, which has a whey-to-casein ratio of 18:82, was the protein source for all bovine milk formulas. Today, however, the majority of bovine milk formulas contain mixtures of bovine milk protein and bovine whey proteins, or mixtures of bovine whey proteins and caseins with whey-to-casein ratios of 60:40 and 48:52, respectively. These proteins appear to be equally efficacious for the normal-term infant. Formulas containing soy protein are available for feeding infants who are intolerant of bovine milk proteins, and formulas containing partially hydrolyzed bovine milk proteins are available for feeding infants who are intolerant of both bovine milk and soy protein (Table 3).

Although lactose-free bovine milk formulas are available, the major carbohydrate of most formulas is lactose. Soy protein formulas usually contain either sucrose or a glucose polymer. Thus, these formulas or lactose-free bovine milk protein formulas are useful for the infant with either transient or congenital lactase deficiency.

The fat content of both bovine milk and soy protein formulas accounts for about 50% of the non-protein energy, and the blend of vegetable oils present in most formulas results in absorption of at least 90% of the ingested fat. The formulas currently available in the United States provide adequate intakes of the essential fatty acids linoleic and α-linolenic acid. Most also contain the longer-chain, more unsaturated derivatives of these fatty acids (LC-PUFAs) that are thought to contribute to the better neurodevelopmental outcome of breast-fed compared with formula-fed infants (see below).

The electrolyte, mineral, and vitamin contents of most formulas are similar and, when fed in adequate amounts (150–180 mL/kg body wt/d), all provide the DRIs of these nutrients. Both iron-supplemented (approx. 12 mg/L) and non-supplemented (approx. 1 mg/L) formulas are available, but as mentioned above, iron-supplemented formulas are recommended. Many favor making non-supplemented formulas unavailable.

The goal of both breast-feeding and formula-feeding is to deliver enough nutrients to support normal growth and development. As a rule of thumb, the normal-term infant's weight should double by 4 to 5 months of age and triple by 12 months of age. In general, unless an infant has other problems, normal growth is accompanied by normal development. Demand feeding is considered preferable, particularly during the early weeks of life. However, most infants easily adjust to being fed every 3 or 4 hours and, after 2 months of age, rarely demand night feedings.

Complementary Feeding

Although it is clear that all nutrient needs for the first year of life can be met with reasonable amounts of currently available infant formulas, the addition of other foods after 4 to 6 months of age is recommended. In contrast, the volume of milk produced by many women may not be adequate to meet all of the nutrient needs of the breast-fed infant beyond about 6 months of age. This is particularly true for iron. Thus, for breast-fed infants,

Table 2. Composition (Amount/100 kcal) of Standard Formulas for Normal Infants

Component	Similac*	Enfamil†	Good Start‡
Protein (g)	2.07 (bovine milk) casein, 48% whey)	2.1 (bovine milk, whey)	2.4 (bovine whey)
Fat (g)	5.4 (high-oleic safflower, coconut, and soy oils)	5.3 (palmolein, soy, coconut, and high-oleic sunflower oils)	5.1 (palmolein, soy, coconut, and high-oleic safflower oils)
Carbohydrate (g)	10.8 (lactose)	10.9 (lactose)	11.0 (lactose, maltodextrin)
Electrolytes and minerals:			
Calcium (mg)	78	78	64
Phosphorus (mg)	42	53	36
Magnesium (mg)	6	8	6.7
Iron (mg)	1.8	1.8	1.5
Zinc (mg)	0.75	1	0.75
Manganese (μg)	5	15	7
Copper (μg)	90	75	80
Iodine (μg)	6	10	8
Selenium (μg)	–	2.8	–
Sodium (mg)	24	27	24
Potassium (mg)	105	108	98
Chloride (mg)	65	63	59
Vitamins:			
Vitamin A (IU)	300	300	300
Vitamin D (IU)	60	60	60
Vitamin E (IU)	3.0	2	2
Vitamin K (μg)	8	8	8.2
Thiamine (μg)	100	80	60
Riboflavin (μg)	120	140	135
Vitamin B_6 (μg)	60	60	75
Vitamin B_{12} (μg)	0.25	0.3	0.22
Niacin (μg)	1050	1000	750
Folic acid (μg)	15	16	9
Pantothenic acid (μg)	450	500	450
Vitamin C (mg)	9	12	8
Biotin (μg)	4.4	3	2.2
Choline (mg)	16.0	12	12
Inositol (mg)	4.7	6	18

* Ross Laboratories, Columbus, Ohio
† Mead-Johnson Nutritionals, Evansville, Indiana
‡ Carnation Nutritional Products, Glendale, California

complementary foods are an important source of nutrients.

Complementary foods (i.e., the additional foods, including formulas, given to the breast-fed infant) or replacement foods (i.e., food other than formula given to formula-fed infants) should be introduced in a stepwise fashion beginning about the time the infant is able to sit unassisted, usually between 4 and 6 months of age. Rice cereal is usually the first such food given. It and other grain cereals are good sources of iron, but the other cereals are more allergenic and could cause problems, particularly if there is a family history of food and other allergies. Vegetables and fruits are introduced next, followed shortly by meats and, finally, eggs. The order in which

Table 3. Composition (Amount/100 kcal) of Soy and Hydrolyzed Protein Formulas

Component	Isomil*	Prosobee†	Nutramigen†	Pregestimil†	Alimentum*
Protein (g)	2.45 (soy protein isolate)	2.5 (soy protein isolate; methionine)	2.8 (casein hydrolysate; cystine, tyrosine and tryptophan)	2.8 (casein hydrolysate; cystine, tyrosine and tryptophan)	2.75 (casein hydrolysate; cystine; tyrosine and tryptophan)
Fat (g)	5.46 (soy and coconut oils)	5.3 (palmolein; soy; coconut and high-oleic sunflower oils)	5.0 (palmolein, soy, coconut and high oleic sunflower oils)	5.6 medium-chain triglycerides; corn, soy and high oleic safflower oils)	5.54 (medium-chain triglycerides; safflower and soy oils)
Carbohydrate (g)	10.3 (corn syrup; sucrose)‡	10.6 (corn syrup solids)	11 (corn syrup solids)	10.2 (corn syrup solids; dextrose)	10.2 (sucrose, modified tapioca starch)
Electrolytes and Minerals					
Calcium (mg)	106	105	94	115	105
Phosphorus (mg)	75	83	63	75	75
Magnesium (mg)	7.5	11	11	11	7.5
Iron (mg)	1.8	1.8	1.8	1.8	1.8
Zinc (mg)	0.75	1.2	1	1	0.75
Manganese (μg)	25	25	25	25	8
Copper (μg)	75	75	75	75	75
Iodine (μg)	15	15	15	15	15
Selenium (μg)	–	2.8	2.8	2.8	2.8
Sodium (mg)	44	36	47	47	44
Potassium (mg)	108	120	110	110	118
Chloride (mg)	62	80	86	86	80

Vitamins					
Vitamin A (IU)	300	300	300	380	300
Vitamin D (IU)	60	60	6	50	45
Vitamin E (IU)	3	2	2	4	3.0
Vitamin K (IU)	11	8	8	12	15
Thiamine (μg)	60	80	80	80	60
Riboflavin (μg)	90	90	90	90	90
Vitamin B_6 (μg)	60	60	60	60	60
Vitamin B_{12} (μg)	0.45	0.3	0.3	0.3	0.45
Niacin (μg)	1350	1000	1000	1000	1350
Folic acid (μg)	15	16	16	16	15
Pantothenic acid (μg)	750	500	500	500	750
Biotin (μg)	4.5	3	3	3	4.5
Vitamin C (mg)	9	12	12	12	9.0
Choline (mg)	8	12	12	12	8
Inositol (mg)	5	6	17	17	5

* Ross Laboratories, Columbus, Ohio
† Mead Johnson Nutritionals, Evansville, Indiana
‡ Isomil-SF (sucrose free) has similar composition with the exception that glucose polymers are substituted for corn syrup and sucrose.

these foods are introduced probably is not crucial unless there is a family history of food or other allergies. However, it is recommended that only one new food be introduced at a time and that additional new foods should be spaced apart by at least 3 to 4 days to allow detection of any adverse reaction.

Either home-prepared or manufactured complementary or replacement foods can be used. The latter are convenient and also likely to contain less salt. Many such products also have supplemental nutrients (e.g., iron) and are available in different consistencies to match the infant's ability to tolerate larger-size particles as he or she matures.

Prepared dinners and soups containing a meat and one or more vegetables are quite popular. However, the protein content of these products is not as high as that of strained meat. Puddings and desserts also are popular items, but, aside from their milk and egg content, are poor sources of nutrients other than energy, so intakes of these should be limited. Moreover, the intake of egg-containing products generally should be delayed, especially if there is a family history of food or other allergies, until after the infant has demonstrated tolerance to eggs (either a mashed, hard-boiled egg yolk or a commercial egg yolk preparation).

Infant Formula versus Bovine Milk

Although current recommendations are to limit the intake of bovine milk and to avoid low-fat or skim milk before at least a year of age,[24] surveys suggest that many (albeit fewer than two decades ago[25,26]) 6- to 12-month-old infants are fed bovine milk rather than infant formula.[27] More important, many of these infants are fed low-fat or skim milk—often, interestingly, on the advice of their physician. The consequences of this practice are not known with certainty. However, on average, infants fed bovine milk ingest three to four times the DRI of protein and considerably more than the DRI for sodium, but less than the DRIs for iron and linoleic acid. The ingestion of bovine milk also increases intestinal blood loss and therefore contributes to the development of iron-deficiency anemia.[28]

Infants fed skim rather than whole bovine milk have protein and sodium intakes that are even higher; furthermore, the iron intake is equally low and the intake of linoleic acid is very low. Ironically, while the most common reason for substituting low-fat or skim milk for whole milk or formula is to reduce fat and energy intakes, the total energy intake of infants fed skim milk is not necessarily lower than that of infants fed whole milk or formula.[26] It appears that the infants compensate for the lower energy density of low-fat or skim milk by taking more of it or by increasing their intake of other foods.

Whether the protein and sodium intakes of infants fed whole or skim bovine milk warrant concern is not known with certainty. The low iron intake clearly is undesirable, but medicinal iron supplementation should prevent the development of iron deficiency. The low intake of linoleic acid may be more problematic. While signs or symptoms of essential fatty acid deficiency appear to be uncommon in infants fed whole or skim milk, an exhaustive search for such symptoms has not been made. Moreover, since essential fatty acid deficiency develops in both younger and older infants fed formulas with a low content of linoleic acid,[29] it is likely that such a search would reveal a reasonably high incidence of biochemical essential fatty acid deficiency. On the other hand, infants who were breast-fed or fed formulas with a high linoleic acid content early in life may have sufficient body stores to limit the consequences of a low intake later. However, since essential fatty acid deficiency in animals is associated with long-term deleterious effects on development,[30] it is not wise to assume that biochemical essential fatty acid deficiency without clinically detectable symptoms is without consequences.

Resolving the issues concerning the use of bovine milk in feeding the 6- to 12-month-old infant is important for economic as well as health reasons. Since the cost of bovine milk is less than half that of infant formula, replacing formula with homogenized bovine milk obviously would have important economic advantages for most families, particularly those with limited income. In addition, if the Federal Food Assistance programs could provide homogenized bovine milk rather than formula to infants over 6 months of age, the program's current funds would permit expansion of benefits to many more of the country's most needy infants. Clearly, this cannot be considered without further data concerning the consequences of feeding bovine milk.

The apparently common practice of substituting skim or low-fat milk for whole milk or formula raises a number of more complex questions. For example, the suggestion that infants fed skim milk increase their intake of milk or other foods to maintain the same energy intake raises the important question of whether the amount of food intake during infancy may in some way imprint intake patterns throughout life. If so, this apparent attempt to improve longevity, or at least cardiovascular health, is paradoxically likely to be more detrimental to both than a less prudent diet during infancy.

LC-PUFAs

LC-PUFAs by definition are fatty acids that are more than 18 carbons in length and have more than two double bonds. There are several such fatty acids, but those that are most relevant to infant nutrition are arachidonic acid (20:4n-6) and docosahexaenoic acid (22:6n-3) acid. These two fatty acids are the most prevalent n-6 and n-3 fatty acids, respectively, in the central nervous system, and the latter comprise up to 40% of the fatty acid content of retinal photoreceptor membranes.[31] Both arachidonic acid and docosahexaenoic acid are synthesized, respectively, from the essential fatty acids linoleic (18:2n-6) and α-linolenic acid (18:3n-3). The two essential fatty acids undergo a series of desaturation and elongation reactions catalyzed by the same enzymes. Thus, the two families of fatty acids compete with each other for the desaturases and elongases involved. These enzymes prefer the n-3 fatty acids, but the ratio of the two essential fatty acids in the diet can be an important determinant of the amount of each LC-PUFA synthesized.

Both term and preterm infants are capable of converting linoleic acid and α-linolenic acid, respectively, to arachidonic acid and docosahexaenoic acid.[32-37] However, the content of arachidonic acid and docosahexaenoic acid in plasma and erythrocyte lipids of infants fed unsupplemented formulas is lower than that in plasma and erythrocyte lipids of breast-fed infants,[38] and autopsy studies show that the low erythrocyte lipid content of docosahexaenoic acid, but not arachidonic acid, is accompanied by a lower concentration in brain.[39] These differences are assumed to reflect the presence of both fatty acids in human milk but not formula, suggesting that the synthetic pathway, while intact, does not synthesize enough docosahexaenoic acid. The generally better cognitive development of breast-fed compared with formula-fed infants also has been attributed to the presence of arachidonic acid and docosahexaenoic acid in human milk but not formula.[40,41] In addition, since studies in both rodents and primates have shown that deficiency of n-3 fatty acids compromises visual function,[42,43] a number of studies have addressed differences in visual function of breast-fed compared with formula-fed infants.

Since human milk contains a number of factors other than LC-PUFAs that might be important for development, the specific role of LC-PUFAs in visual and cognitive development cannot be determined by studies of breast-fed compared with formula-fed infants. Moreover, there are major psychosocial and socioeconomic differences between mothers who choose to breast-feed rather than formula-feed their infants. Thus, over the past decade, many studies have addressed differences in visual function and/or neurodevelopmental status of infants fed LC-PUFA-supplemented compared with unsupplemented formulas. Some of these have shown distinct advantages of LC-PUFA supplementation, but others have not, and the reasons for the different findings are not clear.[44] The magnitude of the advantage of LC-PUFA supplementation of formulas on visual function of term infants, if any, equates to no more than approximately one line on the Snellen chart, and this advantage is not apparent at all ages. Data concerning the effects of LC-PUFAs on neurodevelopmental outcome are equally unclear. One small study showed an advantage of about 0.5 standard deviation in the Bailey Mental Development Index at 18 months of age in infants fed supplemented formula for the first 4 months of life over those not supplemented.[45] Others have shown no advantages of supplementation,[46,47] but none has shown disadvantages.

Because of this uncertainty concerning the functional effects of LC-PUFAs, along with criticisms of methods used in most studies to assess visual function and neurodevelopmental status and concern about the safety of many of the sources available for supplementation of formulas, a panel of experts chosen by the Life Sciences Research Organization to make recommendations for the nutrient content of term infant formulas did not recommend the addition of LC-PUFAs to formulas manufactured and marketed in the United States.[48] On the other hand, panels appointed by other national and international agencies evaluating the same data recommended that formulas for term infants, and particularly for preterm infants, be supplemented with LC-PUFAs,[49,50] and such formulas have been available in many parts of the world for approximately a decade. Supplemented formulas also are now available in the United States and appear to be safe. Whether they are efficacious remains to be determined.

Future Directions

Although most infants in modern industrialized countries, whether breast-fed or formula-fed, grow and develop normally, a number of important issues relative to infant nutrition remain unresolved. Some of these have been discussed briefly in this chapter. However, since it is impossible to discuss all of the relevant issues, only those which the author feels should receive the highest priority have been discussed.

One such issue is the impact of size at birth and at 1 year of age on subsequent cardiovascular health. Epidemiological studies have shown a reasonably strong association between low birth weight and low weight at 1 year of age and the incidence of obesity, hypertension, diabetes, and/or cardiovascular disease in adulthood.[51,52] Subsequent studies suggested that the risk of adult disease may be even greater in those who are small at birth or at 1 year of age but grow rapidly thereafter.[53] Even more recent studies show that preterm infants fed formulas that promote more rapid growth for a period of only 4 weeks prior to hospital discharge have higher neurodevelopmental scores at 18 months[54] and 7 years[55] than those fed a less nutrient-dense formula during initial hospitalization; however, they have a higher incidence of risk factors for cardiovascular health at 14 to 16 years of age.[56] Unraveling these issues obviously will yield important insights concerning optimal nutrition during early life.

A somewhat related issue concerns the effect of intake during early life and intake thereafter. For example, do infants who are overfed tend to eat excessively once they begin feeding themselves? If so, could this contribute to the current epidemic of obesity in children and adults?

A final issue of particular relevance is the reasonably

low prevalence of exclusive breast-feeding for the first 4 to 6 months of life and the even lower prevalence of breast-feeding for a year or longer, as is currently recommended.[18,19] While as many as 75% of mothers in the United States begin by breast-feeding, fewer than half of these are still doing so 3 months later. This is not surprising. The majority of modern mothers work outside the home, many of economic necessity, and today's maternity leave policies make it necessary for many to return to work long before the infant is 4 months old. The lack of facilities for collecting breast milk at work and the scarcity of on-site child care facilities are additional factors making it difficult for women to continue breast-feeding after returning to work.

While the need to return to work and the difficulty of continuing to breast-feed after doing so is a logical explanation for the low prevalence of breast-feeding as currently recommended, definitive proof for this explanation is lacking. This is unfortunate because business executives and government officials are unlikely to be enthusiastic about supporting expensive changes in maternity leave and child care policies that may not increase the prevalence of breast-feeding. These officials also are likely to want data substantiating the advantages of exclusive breast-feeding for the first 4 to 6 months of life and continued breast-feeding for the next 6 months or longer. Such advantages are easy to substantiate for infants in developing countries, where alternatives to breast-feeding are either prohibitively expensive or actually hazardous; however, they are much more difficult to substantiate for infants in more affluent countries. Nonetheless, until we can do so, it is unlikely that the expensive social changes that might increase the duration of breast-feeding will be instituted or that the prevalence of breast-feeding as currently recommended will increase.

Acknowledgments

This work is a publication of the USDA/ARS Children's Nutrition Research Center, Department of Pediatrics, Baylor College of Medicine, Houston, Texas, and has been funded in part with federal funds from the US Department of Agriculture, Agricultural Research Service under Cooperative Agreement No. 38-6250-1-003. The contents of this publication do not necessarily reflect the views or policies of the US Department of Agriculture, nor does the mention of trade names, commercial products, or organizations imply endorsement by the United States Government.

References

1. Food and Nutrition Board, Institute of Medicine. *Dietary Reference Intakes for Calcium, Phosphorus, Magnesium, Vitamin D, and Fluoride.* Washington, DC: National Academies Press; 1997.
2. Food and Nutrition Board, Institute of Medicine. *Dietary Reference Intakes for Thiamin, Riboflavin, Niacin, Vitamin B6, Folate, Vitamin B12, Pantothenic Acid, Biotin, and Choline.* Washington, DC: National Academies Press; 1998.
3. Food and Nutrition Board, Institute of Medicine. *Dietary Reference Intakes for Vitamin C, Vitamin E, Selenium, and Carotenoids.* Washington, DC: National Academies Press; 2000.
4. Food and Nutrition Board, Institute of Medicine. *Dietary Reference Intakes for Vitamin A, Vitamin K, Arsenic, Boron, Chromium, Copper, Iodine, Iron, Manganese, Molybdenum, Nickel, Silicon, Vanadium, and Zinc.* Washington, DC: National Academies Press; 2001.
5. Food and Nutrition Board, Institute of Medicine. *Dietary Reference Intakes for Energy, Carbohydrate, Fiber, Fat, Fatty Acids, Cholesterol, Protein, and Amino Acids (Macronutrients).* Washington, DC: National Academies Press; 2002.
6. Food and Nutrition Board, Institute of Medicine. *Dietary Reference Intakes for Water, Potassium, Sodium, Chloride, and Sulfate.* Washington, DC: National Academies Press; 2004.
7. Sturman JA, Gaull GA, Räihä NC. Absence of cystathionase in human liver: is cystine essential? *Science.* 1970;169:74–76.
8. Gaull G, Sturman JA, Räihä NC. Development of mammalian sulfur metabolism: absence of cystathionase in human fetal tissues. Pediatr Res. 1972;6: 538–547.
9. Räihä NC. Phenylalanine hydroxylase in human liver during development. Pediatr Res. 1973;7:1–4.
10. Kilani RA, Cole FS, Bier DM. Phenylalanine hydroxylase activity in preterm infants: is tyrosine a conditionally essential amino acid? Am J Clin Nutr. 1995;61:1218–1223.
11. Denne SC, Karn CA, Ahlrichs JA, Dorotheo AR, Wang J, Liechty EA. Proteolysis and phenylalanine hydroxylation in response to parenteral nutrition in extremely premature and normal newborns. J Clin Invest. 1996;97:746–754.
12. Fomon SJ, Thomas LN, Filer LJ Jr, Anderson TA, Bergmann KE. Requirements for protein and essential amino acids in early infancy. Studies with a soy-isolate formula. Acta Pediatr Scand. 1973;62:33–45.
13. Räihä NC. Nutritional proteins in milk and the protein requirement of normal infants. Pediatrics. 1985; 75(1 part 2):136–141.
14. Committee on Nutrition, American Academy of Pediatrics. Iron deficiency. In: Kleinman RE, ed. *Pediatric Nutrition Handbook.* 5th ed. Elk Grove, IL: American Academy of Pediatrics; 2004; 299–312.
15. Montgomery RK. Functional development of the gastrointestinal tract: the small intestine. In: Heird WC, ed. *Nutritional Needs of the Six to Twelve Month*

Old Infant. New York: Raven Press; 1991; 1–17.
16. Mandel ID. The nutritional impact on dental caries. In: Heird WC, ed. *Nutritional Needs of the Six to Twelve Month Old Infant.* New York: Raven Press; 1991; 89–107.
17. Devaney B, Ziegler P, Pac S, Karwe V, Barr SI. Nutrient intakes of infants and toddlers. J Am Diet Assoc. 2004;104(suppl 1):S14–S21.
18. Work Group on Breastfeeding, American Academy of Pediatrics. Breastfeeding and the use of human milk. Pediatrics. 1997;100:1035–1039.
19. World Health Organization. The World Health Organization's infant-feeding recommendations. *WHO Weekly Epidemiological Record.* 1995;70: 119–120.
20. Kovar MG, Serdula MK, Marks JS, Fraser DW. Review of the epidemiologic evidence for an association between infant feeding and infant health. Pediatrics. 1984;74(4 part 2):S615–S638.
21. Brown KH, Black RE, Lopez de Romana G, Creed de Kanashiro H. Infant-feeding practices and their relationship with diarrheal and other diseases in Hauscar (Lima), Peru. Pediatrics. 1989;83:31–40.
22. *The Wall Street Journal,* July 22, 1994; page 1.
23. Fomon SJ. Recommendation for feeding normal infants. In: Fomon SJ, ed. *Nutrition of Normal Infants.* St. Louis: Mosby; 1993; 455–458.
24. Committee on Nutrition, American Academy of Pediatrics. The use of whole cow's milk in infancy [policy statement]. AAP News. 1992;8:8–22.
25. Ryan AS, Martinez GA, Krieger FW. Feeding lowfat milk during infancy. Am J Phys Anthropol. 1987; 73:539–548.
26. Martinez GA, Ryan AS, Malec DJ. Nutrient intakes of American infants and children fed cow's milk or infant formula. Am J Dis Child. 1985;139: 1010–1018.
27. Fox MK, Pac S, Devaney B, Jankowski L. Feeding infants and toddlers study: What foods are infants and toddlers eating? J Am Diet Assoc. 2004;104(1 suppl 1):S22–S30.
28. Ziegler EE, Fomon SJ, Nelson SE, et al. Cow milk feeding in infancy: further observations on blood loss from the gastrointestinal tract. J Pediatr. 1990;116: 11–18.
29. Pettei MJ, Daftary S, Levine JJ. Essential fatty acid deficiency associated with the use of a medium-chain-triglyceride infant formula in pediatric hepatobiliary disease. Am J Clin Nutr. 1991;53: 1217–1221.
30. Crawford MA, Hassam AG, Stevens PA. Essential fatty acid requirements in pregnancy and lactation with special reference to brain development. Prog Lipid Res. 1981;20:31–40.
31. Martinez M. Tissue levels of polyunsaturated fatty acids during early human development. J Pediatr. 1992;120:S129–S138.
32. Carnielli VP, Wattimena DJ, Luijendijk IH, Boerlage A, Degenhart HJ, Sauer PJ. The very low birth weight premature infant is capable of synthesizing arachidonic and docosahexaenoic acids from linoleic and linolenic acids. Pediatr Res. 1996;40:169–174.
33. Demmelmair H, von Schenck U, Behrendt E, Sauerwald T, Koletzko B. Estimation of arachidonic acid synthesis in full term neonates using natural variation of ^{13}C content. J Pediatr Gastroenterol Nutr. 1995; 21:31–36.
34. Salem N Jr, Wegher B, Mena P, Uauy R. Arachidonic and docosahexaenoic acids are biosynthesized from their 18-carbon precursors in human infants. Proc Natl Acad Sci U S A. 1996;93:49–54.
35. Sauerwald TU, Hachey DL, Jensen CL, Chen H, Anderson RE, Heird WC. Intermediates in endogenous synthesis of C22:6ω3 and C20:4ω6 by term and preterm infants.Pediatr Res. 1997;41:183–187.
36. Sauerwald TU, Hachey DL, Jensen CL, Chen H, Anderson RE, Heird WC. Effect of dietary α-linolenic acid intake on incorporation of docosahexaenoic and arachidonic acids into plasma phospholipids of term infants. Lipids. 1996;31(suppl):S131–S135.
37. Uauy R, Mena P, Wegher B, Nieto S, Salem N Jr. Long chain polyunsaturated fatty acid formation in neonates: effect of gestational age and intrauterine growth. Pediatr Res. 2000;47:127–135.
38. Putnam JC, Carlson SE, DeVoe PW, Barness LA. The effect of variations in dietary fatty acids on the fatty acid composition of erythrocyte phosphatidylcholine and phosphatidylethanolamine in human infants. Am J Clin Nutr. 1982;36:106–114.
39. Makrides M, Neumann MA, Byard RW, Simmer K, Gibson RA. Fatty acid composition of brain, retina, and erythrocytes in breast- and formula-fed infants. Am J Clin Nutr. 1994;60:189–194.
40. Pollock JI. Long-term associations with infant feeding in a clinically advantaged population of babies. Dev Med Child Neurol. 1994;36:429–440.
41. Rogan WJ, Gladen BC. Breast-feeding and cognitive development. Early Hum Dev. 1993;31:181–193.
42. Benolken RM, Anderson RE, Wheeler TG. Membrane fatty acids associated with the electrical response in visual excitation. Science. 1973;182: 1253–1254.
43. Neuringer M, Connor WE, Lin DS, Barstard L, Luck S. Biochemical and functional effects of prenatal and postnatal ω3 fatty acid deficiency on retina and brain in rhesus monkeys. Proc Natl Acad Sci U S A. 1986;83:4021–4025.
44. Heird C, Lapillonne A. The role of essential fatty acids in development. Ann Rev Nutr. 2005;25: 549–571.
45. Birch EE, Garfield S, Hoffman DR, Uauy R, Birch DG. A randomized controlled trial of early dietary supply of long-chain polyunsaturated fatty acids and

mental development in term infants. Dev Med Child Neurol. 2000;42:174–181.
46. Auestad N, Halter R, Hall RT, et al. Growth and development in term infants fed long-chain polyunsaturated fatty acids: a double-masked, randomized, parallel, prospective, multivariate study. Pediatrics. 2001;108:372–381.
47. Makrides M, Neumann MA, Simmer K, Gibson RA. A critical appraisal of the role of dietary long-chain polyunsaturated fatty acids on neural indices of term infants: a randomized, controlled trial. Pediatrics. 2000;105:32–38.
48. [No authors listed.] Assessment of nutrient requirements for infant formulas. J Nutr. 1998;128(suppl 11):2059S–2293S.
49. British Nutrition Foundation. Recommendation for intakes of unsaturated fatty acids. In: *Unsaturated Fatty Acids: Nutritional and Physiological Significance.* London: Chapman and Hull; 1992; 152–163.
50. Food and Agriculture Organization/World Health Organization Expert Committee. *Fats and Oils in Human Nutrition. Food and Nutrition Paper.* Rome: Food and Agriculture Organization; 1994; 57.
51. Barker DJ, ed. *Fetal and Infant Origins of Adult Disease.* London: BJM Publishing; 1992.
52. Eriksson JG, Forsén T, Tuomilehto J, Winter PD, Osmond C, Barker J. Catch-up growth in childhood and death from coronary heart disease: longitudinal study. BMJ. 1993;318:427–431.
53. Hales CN, Ozanne SE. The dangerous road of catch-up growth. J Physiol. 2003;547(part 1):5–10.
54. Lucas A, Morley R, Cole TJ, et al. Early diet in preterm babies and developmental status at 18 months. Lancet. 1990;335:1477–1481.
55. Lucas A, Morley R, Cole TJ. Randomised trial of early diet in preterm babies and later intelligence quotient. BMJ. 1998;317:1481–1487.
56. Singhal A, Cole TJ, Fewtrell M, Deanfield J, Lucas A. Is slower early growth beneficial for long-term cardiovascular health? Circulation. 2004;109:1108–1113.

43 Adolescence

Virginia A. Stallings

Adolescence

Adolescence is an important period during which major biologic, social, physiologic, and cognitive changes take place. Adolescents have special nutritional needs because of rapid growth (lean body mass, fat mass, bone mineralization) and maturational changes associated with the onset of puberty. Dietary surveys show that many adolescents do not meet nutrient recommendations for their age group and have inadequate dietary intake of calcium, iron, thiamin, riboflavin, and vitamins A and C.[1] Clinically, however, despite their poor dietary intakes, the only biochemical nutrient deficiency commonly seen among adolescents is iron-deficiency anemia. An increasing number of adolescents have problems with dietary excesses and obesity. For adolescent girls and young adult women who become pregnant, their preconceptional nutritional status is critical to their health and the health of their babies. In this chapter, we will discuss growth changes that occur during adolescence, nutritional needs, nutritional assessment, and nutrition-related issues applicable to adolescence.

Growth During Adolescence

Children vary considerably as to age at onset of puberty and rate of progression through puberty.[2] The hormonal changes of puberty result in characteristic alterations in body size, body composition (muscle, fat, bone), and skeletal and sexual maturation. Such alterations are the basis for the increased dietary requirements associated with adolescence for energy, protein, and most micronutrients. The adolescent growth spurt occurs approximately 2 years later in boys than in girls, and so boys and girls of similar age often differ in nutritional requirements. Undernutrition and many chronic diseases can delay the onset of puberty.[3-5] Furthermore, growth is not a continuous process, but proceeds as a series of small growth spurts that vary in amplitude and frequency.[6] All of these factors influence an individual adolescent's nutritional needs, which will vary between and within individuals over time. Above all, it is important to recognize that adequate nutritional intake is necessary to ensure normal growth and maturation.

The onset of puberty occurs at an earlier age than previously thought, with variability among ethnic groups. Among a national sample of US boys and girls (Third National Health and Nutrition Examination Survey [NHANES III]) evaluated at 8 to 19 years of age,[7] the median ages of onset of pubic hair development were 11.2, 12.0, and 12.3 years for non-Hispanic black, non-Hispanic white, and Mexican-American boys, respectively, and 9.4, 10.6, and 10.4 years for non-Hispanic black, non-Hispanic white, and Mexican-American girls, respectively. In another large sample of US girls evaluated at ages 3 to 12 years, the average age at menarche was 12.2 years for African Americans and 12.9 years for whites.[8] Menarche usually occurs just after the adolescent growth spurt.[2] At the peak of the adolescent linear growth spurt, the rate of increase in height is approximately 10.3 cm/year for boys (range 7.2–13.4) and 9.0 cm/year for girls (range 7.0–11.0).[2] From the onset of the adolescent growth spurt to the attainment of adult stature, both boys and girls gain approximately 17% of their final height.[9]

The adolescent growth spurt in height is followed by rapid accrual of bone mass. Peak bone mass, the maximum amount of bone gained during the life cycle, is achieved by the end of adolescence or in early adulthood.[10,11] Epidemiologic evidence suggests that a higher peak bone mass is associated with both greater dietary calcium intake and lower rates of hip fracture later in life.[11] Thus, adequate calcium intake to ensure optimal accrual of bone mass during childhood and adolescence may have important lifelong health implications.[12]

Bone mineral density increases through puberty.[10] A longitudinal growth study by Bailey et al.[13] showed that the peak accrual in whole body bone mineral content occurred after the adolescent growth spurt in height. Ac-

Table 1. Recommended Calcium Intake (mg/d) Levels from Three Sources

Age Range (y)	RDA (1989)[14]	AI (1997)[15]	NIH (1994)[16]
4–8	800	800	800–1200
9–13	800–1200†	1300	1200–1500†
14–18	1200	1300	1200–1500

† Changes at age 11 y.

cordingly, to accommodate these rapid adolescent gains, calcium requirements are considerably higher for adolescents than for children or adults (Table 1). Compared with the 1989 Recommended Dietary Allowances (RDA),[14] the 1997 Dietary Reference Intakes[15] recommendations increased the recommended amount and decreased the age at which the calcium requirements increased.

Similarly, the National Institutes of Health consensus report[16] recommends a range (1200–1500 mg calcium) rather than a single recommended amount for adolescents to accommodate the interindividual and intraindividual variability in calcium requirements associated with the timing of puberty and the adolescent growth spurt. Although recommended calcium intake is 63% higher for adolescents than children, results from the NHANES III show that actual dietary calcium intake in the United States declines as children become adolescents (Table 2), and that calcium intake is lower in non-Hispanic black compared with non-Hispanic white and Mexican-American children and adolescents.[17] In a more recently published survey of a mixed ethnic sample from the NHANES (1999–2000),[18] girls still showed a decline in dietary calcium intake from childhood to adolescence; however, calcium intake in boys remained stable, and well below the 1300 mg/d recommended during adolescence.[15] Net calcium absorption is highest in infancy and adolescence.[19] However, it is unlikely that increased calcium absorption efficiency in the context of inadequate dietary calcium intake is sufficient to optimize peak bone mass. Calcium supplementation can increase bone mineral density in children,[20] a finding that underscores the importance of adequate calcium intake. Increased calcium intake must be sustained to maintain the effect on bone mineral density.

Other factors that influence bone mass accrual during growth include vitamin D status and physical activity. Adequate vitamin D levels are necessary to facilitate calcium absorption in the gut. Although casual daily sunlight exposure to the hands and face is sufficient to achieve adequate vitamin D levels in healthy adolescents,[21] seasonal fluctuations in sunlight exposure and health status may affect vitamin D status.[22] Also, weight-bearing physical activity is important to strengthen bone and increase muscle mass.[23] Exercise before and during adolescence is also of great importance to bone formation.[24]

Nutritional Needs of Adolescents

Nutritional needs of adolescents are higher than those of children because of the growth spurt, sexual maturation, changes in body composition, skeletal mineralization, and changes in physical activity. Physical activity is not necessarily increased, but total energy needs are increased because of larger body size. Unlike children, adolescent males and females differ in their nutritional needs, and these sex-based differences continue into adulthood. Reasons include the earlier maturation of females and the considerable variability of puberty and nutrient requirements.[25] Nutrient needs are increased for protein, energy, calcium, iron, and zinc. In addition, increased nutritional requirements occur with pregnancy, many chronic diseases, and rigorous physical conditioning. Some common adolescent illnesses, such as the eating disorders anorexia nervosa and bulimia, may have profound effects on nutritional status and maturation. Rec-

Table 2. Calcium Intake (mg/d) for Males and Females, from the National Health and Nutrition Examination Surveys 1988 to 1991[17] and 1999 to 2000[18]

	Males		Females	
1988–1992*	**6–11 y**	**12–15 y**	**6–11 y**	**12–15 y**
Non-Hispanic white	994	822	822	744
Non-Hispanic black	761	688	688	613
Mexican American	986	890	890	790
1999–2000†	**6–11 y**	**12–19 y**	**6–11 y**	**12–19 y**
All race/ethnic groups	843	956	812	661

ommended dietary intakes for adolescents[26] often represent interpolations based on known requirements for children and adults rather than evidence based on adolescent research subjects. Nutrient requirements are usually greater for males than females and for pregnant and lactating females than nonpregnant females.

Often, adolescents' dietary habits differ from those of children and adults. Adolescents tend to skip meals, eat more meals outside their home, and eat snacks, especially soda, candy, and diet or fast foods. Some develop strong food beliefs, adopt food fads, or become vegetarians. These diet preferences may reflect an expression of independence, a busy lifestyle, problems with body image, or a search for self-identity, or they may be secondary to peer and social pressures.

Typically, dietary intake data show insufficient intake of calcium, iron, and vitamins A and C in the diets of US adolescents. The average intake for boys was closer to the RDA than that for girls. Adolescents often have high intakes of soda, coffee, tea, and alcohol, and low intakes of milk and juice, a pattern seen more often in white adolescents.[25] In a large survey of 12,500 children aged 11 to 18 years, Gavadini et al.[27] showed that total energy intake, as well as the proportion of energy from total fat and saturated fat, decreased from 1965 to 1996. Total milk consumption decreased, accompanied by an increase in soft drinks and noncitrus juices. Among US high school students surveyed between 1999 and 2003, only 16% to 18% reported drinking more than three glasses of milk daily.[28] Vegetable intake was lower than the recommended five servings per day, and folate, iron, and calcium intakes were lower than recommendations for girls.[15,26,27,29] In adolescent females and low-income youth, vitamins B_6, A, E, iron, calcium, and zinc intakes were low.[30] In the typical American adolescent's diet, french-fried potatoes make up 25% of all the vegetables consumed, intake of simple sugars exceeds the intake of complex carbohydrates, and more than one-third of the dietary fat (which accounts for >33% of calories consumed) is saturated fat. Junk food and high-fat fast food account for more than 33% of the daily caloric intake.[31,32] Although the food guide pyramid suggests that an appropriate intake of fruit and vegetables is five or more servings per day, adolescents have lower intakes. Only 22% to 24% of high school students surveyed between 1999 and 2003 in the National Youth Risk Behavior Survey[28] ate five or more servings of fruits and vegetables per day. In an earlier survey, fruit and vegetable intake was found to be higher in whites than in adolescents from other ethnic groups.[25]

Recommendations for adolescent nutrient intake from various sources stress the following: increased intake of calcium-rich and iron-containing foods in adolescent girls; limitation of foods high in simple sugars; decrease in the intake of complex carbohydrate foods that could be retained in the mouth and contribute to dental caries; use of fluoridated water, dentifrices, topical treatments, and rinses to prevent dental caries; limitation of fat intake to less than 30% of energy intake, with saturated fat intake less than 10% and dietary cholesterol less than 300 mg/d; and limitation of salt intake to less than 6 g/d and daily protein intake less than two times the RDA. The American Academy of Pediatrics recommends a fat intake of approximately 20% to 30% of energy because of the rapid growth that occurs.[33]

Energy

Exact energy requirements of the individual growing adolescent are difficult to determine.[34] The new Dietary Reference Intake recommendations provide a method to estimate the requirement for energy as Estimated Energy Requirements (kcal/d) prediction equations (Table 3).[35] In addition, an activity factor should be used to account for the potentially very different levels of physical activity for individual categories. Peak energy requirements occur in girls at approximately 15 to 16 years of age and in boys at approximately 18 years, and correspond to the increased needs of later pubertal growth and development. Active adolescent females require approximately 2300 kcal/d, whereas males require 2600 to 3300 kcal/d. Energy needs increase and vary during the second and third trimester of pregnancy and during the first and second 6 months of lactation.[35] Mathematic formulas are available to calculate the Estimated Energy Requirements-based energy needs for obese adolescent females and males.[35]

Data from the NHANES III show that energy intakes were higher for males than for females, and that intakes peaked in late adolescence.[36] Although dietary intakes in some adolescents were less than the RDAs, there has been an increase in the number of overweight adolescents. Despite a trend toward decreasing dietary fat intake, that intake is still higher than recommended.[25]

Protein. Recently revised protein recommendations are shown in Table 4. Most adolescents easily achieve these levels in the United States, as seen in the NHANES III.[36] Exact data on adolescent protein requirements are not available, and the recommendations come from data interpolated from results of studies in infants and adults. Peak protein intake coincides with peak energy intake. Protein should account for 12% to 14% of energy intake. Adolescents at risk for low protein intake are those with eating disorders, malabsorption, chronic disease, and socioeconomic limitations resulting in food insecurity. In the event of inadequate energy intake, protein is used for energy needs, and may result in protein calorie malnutrition.

Minerals. Some adolescents have inadequate intakes of minerals, including calcium, iron, zinc, and magnesium. Calcium and phosphorus are essential for good bone health. Although dietary phosphorus intake is usu-

Table 3. Estimated Energy Requirement for Boys and Girls Aged 13 to 18 Years

Boys Age	Reference Weight	Reference Height	Sedentary PAL	Low Active PAL	Active PAL	Very Active PAL
(y)	*kg(lb)*	*m(in)*				
13	45.6 (100.4)	1.56 (61.4)	1935	2276	2618	3038
14	51.0 (112.3)	1.64 (64.6)	2090	2459	2829	3283
15	56.3 (124.0)	1.70 (66.9)	2223	2618	3013	3499
16	60.9 (134.1)	1.74 (68.5)	2320	2736	3152	3663
17	64.6 (142.3)	1.75 (68.9)	2366	2796	3226	3754
18	67.2 (148.0)	1.76 (69.3)	2383	2823	3263	3804
Girls Age	**Reference Weight**	**Reference Height**	**Sedentary PAL**	**Low Active PAL**	**Active PAL**	**Very Active PAL**
13	45.8 (100.4)	1.57 (61.8)	1684	1992	2281	2762
14	49.4 (112.3)	1.60 (63.0)	1718	2036	2334	2831
15	52.0 (124.0)	1.62 (63.8)	1731	2057	2362	2870
16	53.9 (134.1)	1.63 (64.2)	1729	2059	2368	2883
17	55.1 (142.3)	1.63 (64.2)	1710	2042	2353	2871
18	56.2 (148.0)	1.63 (64.2)	1690	2024	2336	2858

Adapted with permission from Food and Nutrition Board, Institute of Medicine, 2002.[35]
PAL, physical activity level.

ally adequate, calcium intake is often inadequate in adolescents. National surveys show that calcium intake is less than recommended and has either declined or not increased over the last 20 years. Among girls aged 15 to 18 years, the average calcium intake decreased from 680 mg/d in 1980 to 600 mg/d in 1990.[37] Among girls ages 12 to 19 years in the NHANES (1999–2000),[18] median calcium intake was 611 mg/d, which is only 51% of the currently recommended amount of 1300 mg/d.[15] The best way to meet nutritional requirements for calcium is through foods rather than through calcium supplements, and calcium is more efficiently absorbed in combination with lactose. Dairy products provide approximately 55% of the calcium intake in the US diet. Calcium absorption from other dietary sources is important, however, especially in communities where dairy products are not easily available and for adolescents who have lactose intolerance.

Table 4. Dietary Reference Intakes for Protein

	Males		Females	
	g/kg/d	*g/d*	*g/kg/d*	*g/d*
9–13 y	0.95	34	0.95	34
14–18 y	0.85	52	0.85	46
Pregnancy*	—	—	1.10	+25

Adapted with permission from Food and Nutrition Board, Institute of Medicine, 2002.[35]
* For pregnant adolescents, an additional 25 g of protein daily is recommended. For a 14- to 18-year-old pregnant adolescent girl, 71 g of protein daily (46 + 25 g/d) is recommended.

Despite the iron fortification of many cereal grains, iron deficiency remains common. Iron needs are higher during adolescence because of increases in blood volume and muscle mass. Girls' needs are further increased by menstrual losses. The adolescent girls who are at increased risk for iron deficiency include the older adolescent female, the pregnant adolescent, and female athletes. Median iron intake for 12- to 19-year-old girls in the NHANES (1999–2000) was 11.7 mg/d, 78% of the 15 mg/d recommended for girls ages 14 to 18 years.[18,29] Iron deficiency during pregnancy results in an increased risk of preterm birth and low birth weight infants. Because of their rapid growth, young pubertal boys are also at risk for iron-deficiency anemia. Iron needs decrease with slower growth after puberty. Iron deficiency is more common among low-income youth and is seen more often in adolescent females than in adolescent males.[25] The prevalence of iron-deficiency anemia among adolescents varies from 2% to 10% and is more frequent in boys aged 11 to 14 years and in girls aged 15 to 19 years.[30]

Increased zinc is needed for growth and puberty, and zinc intake is often low in adolescents. Zinc deficiency is associated with growth retardation and hypogonadism, and zinc supplementation results in reversal of these clinical manifestations. Data from the NHANES (1999–2000)[18] show that magnesium intake among US adolescents ages 12 to 19 years did not meet recommendations.[15]

Vitamins. The vitamins that are usually consumed in insufficient amounts in the diets of adolescents include vitamins A, B_6, E, D, C, and folic acid. Because girls have lower food intakes than boys, dietary deficiencies are more common among them. Data from the NHANES (1999–2000)[38] show that median intake of vitamins A, E, C, and folic acid for adolescents ages 12 to 19 years, in general, do not meet recommendations.[26,29]

Fiber. Adolescents ingest less than recommended amounts of fiber. Average fiber intake is approximately 12 g/d in comparison with the 25 g/d recommended by the American Heart Association for blood cholesterol reduction and the 35 to 45 g/d recommended for reduction of colon cancer risk.[39] Recent Dietary Reference Intake[35] recommendations are for males ages 9 to 13 years to consume 31 g/d of total fiber, and ages 14 to 18 years to consume 38 g/d. Female intake is recommended as 26 g/d for ages 9 to 18 years. Data from the NHANES III (1988–1994) show that adolescent fiber intake was 11 to 16 g/d for adolescents ages 12 to 19 years, much less than the recommended 26 to 38 g/d.[36,40]

Nutritional Assessment

During the adolescent years, anthropometric assessment of nutritional status is complicated by the influence of puberty on weight, height, and body composition. Still, it is an important period for careful monitoring of nutritional status because of the heightened risk of nutritional disorder such as obesity and anorexia nervosa. In addition to standard growth charts,[41] height and height velocity growth charts,[42] which include a classification for early and late onset of puberty, are useful to assess height growth relative to maturity status. For early or late-maturing children whose growth deviates significantly from their previous growth status or from the standard growth curve, these charts are important for the interpretation of growth measurements. Assessment of sexual maturity status is classified according to the stages described by Tanner[2] for pubic hair growth and genital development in boys and for breast development in girls. A self-assessment pictorial questionnaire can be used to establish puberty stage.[43] For assessment of weight-for-height status, the body mass index (BMI; expressed in kilograms per square meter) may be used. Growth charts for children include a BMI chart. By using these charts, a sex- and age-specific BMI percentile can be plotted in the same manner as for weight and height. There are no clear guidelines on how to assess BMI relative to early or late sexual maturity.[44] For assessment of overweight and obesity, BMI should be combined with triceps skin-fold measurements.[45]

Special Nutrition-related Issues

Obesity. The prevalence of obesity in children and adolescents has increased dramatically over the last several decades. According to national surveys, the prevalence of overweight (defined as having a BMI ≥ 95th percentile)[46] in adolescents ages 12 to 19 years, remained fairly stable at 5% to 6% from 1963 to 1980, and then increased to 10.5% from 1988 to 1994, and further increased to 15.5% from 1999 to 2000.[47] This is a tripling of the rate of overweight adolescents over a 20-year period. Data from the NHANES completed from 1976 to 2002 (Table 5) show that this significant increase in the prevalence of overweight has occurred among 12- to 19-year-old adolescents from all race and ethnic groups surveyed, with the greatest increases occurring among non-Hispanic black and Mexican adolescents.[48] Furthermore, in the NHANES (1999–2000), 31% of male adolescents and 30% of female adolescents were overweight or at risk for overweight (BMI ≥ 85th percentile).[46] A greater proportion of non-Hispanic black boys (36%) and girls (46%), and Mexican boys (43%) and girls (44%) were at risk for overweight as adolescents than non-Hispanic white boys (27%) and girls (25%).[47] The risk of becoming obese as a child, and remaining obese as an adult, is influenced by family history and the child's age. Forty percent of children with one overweight parent are overweight, and 80% of children with two overweight parents are overweight. Only 10% of children with no overweight parents become overweight. Older children, more obese children, and children with an obese mother or father are much more likely to be obese as young adults (21–29 years old).[49] For example, an obese or very obese 3- to 5-year-old child

Table 5. Prevalence of Overweight in Adolescents (Ages 12–19 Years) Prevalence ≥ 95th Percentile Body Mass Index

	Non-Hispanic White	Non-Hispanic Black	Mexican
Boys			
1976–1980	3.8	6.1	7.7
1988–1994	11.6	10.7	14.1
1999–2002	14.6	18.7	24.7
Girls			
1976–1980	4.6	10.7	8.8
1988–1994	8.9	16.3	13.4
1999–2002	12.7	23.6	19.6

Data from Ogden et al., 2002[47] and Hedley et al., 2004.[48]

is four times as likely to become an obese adult (compared with a nonobese child), whereas an obese or a very obese 10- to 14-year-old child is 28 times as likely to become an obese adult. This age relationship defines the need to prevent and treat obesity in adolescence.

Obesity is caused by an energy imbalance in which individuals expend less energy than they consume. A chronic, small positive energy imbalance can have a large effect on weight gain. Finding such a small energy surplus makes the prevention and treatment of obesity very challenging. In general, the search for the causes for obesity has focused on four areas: genetics, environment, energy expenditure, and dietary factors.

Genetics. Although some genetic syndromes (e.g., Prader-Willi syndrome, Down syndrome) and clinical syndromes of other cause (e.g., Cushing's syndrome) are associated with obesity, these represent less than 1% of the cases of obesity in children. Most adolescents with a medical cause of obesity may be identified earlier in life, but acquired clinical syndromes (e.g., hypothyroidism) may present in adolescence. Genetic influence on obesity is supported by the clustering of obesity within families and by studies of adopted and twin children. The relative weight of adults who were adopted as children is positively associated with the relative weight of their biologic parents, but no such relationship exists between them and their adoptive parents.[50] Similarly, the relative weights of adoptive twins reared apart in different family environments are similar to that of twins reared together. The discovery of leptin and the leptin gene raised the hope that obesity genes would be identified; however, the search has not yet been fruitful in humans.

Socioeconomic factors, parental education, family size, season, region of the country, and urban versus rural factors are all associated with obesity. An important environmental influence is the amount of time spent watching television. A relationship between television watching and obesity has been clearly described in older children, including a dose response.[51] Preadolescents and young adolescents were 5.5 times as likely to be overweight if they watched more than 5 hours of television a day compared with those who watched less than 2 hours a day.

Altered resting energy expenditure, energy of physical activity, and total energy expenditure are potential causes for excessive weight gain. Many obese adolescents and their families believe they must have a low metabolic rate, but data do not consistently support this. Although these studies specifically evaluated children and adults, similar findings would be expected in adolescents. A recent finding has been a lower resting energy expenditure among African-American children and adults. Decreased energy expenditure through a pattern of decreased physical activity could induce a positive energy balance, resulting in excessive weight gain. Obese children may be less physically active than nonobese children, but it seems that obese individuals expend extra energy to carry their excess body mass. Therefore, they expend as much or more total energy completing these activities as do nonobese children. Despite these mixed findings, the improved clinical outcome with weight management that includes exercise[52,53] supports the influence of the pattern of sedentary and physical activity on the development and treatment of obesity.

Dietary Intake. Data on dietary intake and obesity suggest that obese children tend to eat higher-fat diets and thus higher-energy diets. Humans also have a taste preference for energy-dense foods. In our current environment, in which most people have easy access to an abundance of high fat, energy-dense foods, this preference may underlie the increasing prevalence of obesity. Assessing dietary intake and energy needs is difficult. Obese adolescents may underreport energy intake by 40% to 60%.[54] New standardized prediction equations to calculate energy requirements of obese children are available.[35] The measurement of resting energy expenditure is possible in some clinical settings and provides an accurate estimates of energy needs.

Health Consequences of Obesity. Medical problems that require immediate intervention (e.g., sleep apnea, type 2 diabetes, significant hypertension) are increasingly common in obese adolescents (Table 6). Abdominal and visceral fat patterning have been shown to be associated with cardiovascular disease risk in children and adults.[55,56] Most commonly, obesity is associated with elevations in triglyceride levels and decreases in high-density lipoprotein cholesterol levels. However, even a small reduction (10%) in weight has been associated with improvement in cardiovascular disease risk in adults.[57] Although the data are more limited in children and adolescents, it seems that relatively small reductions in weight have similar effects on cardiovascular disease risk in children.

Table 6. Medical Conditions Associated with Obesity in Adolescents

Hypertension
Lipid disorders (especially hypertriglyceridemia and low levels of high-density lipoprotein)
Insulin resistance and type 2 diabetes
Acanthosis nigricans
Orthopedic problems
Slipped capital femoral epiphysis
Blount's disease
Cholelithiasis
Nonalcoholic steatohepatitis
Sleep apnea
Polycystic ovary syndrome
Pseudotumor cerebri
Psychosocial dysfunction

Type 2 diabetes was once a rare problem in children, but it is now becoming more common. For example, the incidence of type 2 diabetes in adolescents was estimated to increase 10-fold from 1982 to 1994 in the greater Cincinnati area.[58] The mean age of the newly diagnosed adolescents was 13.8 years, and the mean BMI was 37.7. The high relative weight of these adolescents, along with the known association between obesity and type 2 diabetes, suggests that this rapid increase in type 2 diabetes among adolescents is related to the well-documented rapid increase in obesity in the United States. Adolescents from certain ethnic groups—African Americans, Mexican Americans, and Native Americans—are especially at risk for developing type 2 diabetes. The reasons for the increased risk in these groups are not known.

Ten percent of obese adolescents have been shown to have elevated liver function test results, which may be a sign of nonalcoholic steatohepatitis. The liver function test result abnormalities have been associated with lower serum antioxidant levels. Normalization of these abnormalities has been reported with vitamin E therapy in an open-label trial. Obesity-related nonalcoholic steatohepatitis has been reported to progress to cirrhosis and liver failure requiring liver transplantation.

Obesity is often associated with psychosocial complications for children and adolescents, including low self-esteem, poor body image, depression, and learning problems. Obese individuals are frequently the targets of social discrimination and stigmatization.[59] Obese adolescents more frequently have low self-esteem than do overweight preadolescents, perhaps because of the greater influence of peers on self-esteem for adolescents.

Evaluation and Treatment. True assessment of adiposity is difficult. One of the most commonly used measures to assess relative weight is BMI. In adults, a BMI greater than 25 defines overweight and greater than 30 defines obesity. However, BMI normally increases as children grow in height and weight, so a particular BMI cutoff point cannot be set to define obesity in adolescents. For adolescents, a BMI greater than the 95th percentile (for age and sex) identifies obesity, and a BMI greater than the 85th percentile identifies overweight. The 2000 Centers for Disease Control growth charts include age- and sex-specific BMI percentile curves and will allow the clinical use of BMI to assess relative weight.[41] On these curves, the area between the 85th and 95th percentiles is defined as at risk for overweight, whereas points above the 95th percentile are defined as overweight.[46] Skin-fold thickness measurements specifically provide a more direct indication of adiposity.

The assessment of an obese child should include a routine history and physical examination, which includes a review for signs of obesity-related syndromes or conditions. Screening for associated important clinical conditions (e.g., hyperlipidemia, insulin resistance) or contributing processes (e.g., low metabolic rate) should be considered, as indicated from the history and physical examination. Significant family dysfunction or adolescent psychologic problems need to be evaluated as part of the weight-management program.

Several treatment methods, including behavioral modification, diet, exercise, and school-based programs, have been devised in an effort to help obese adolescents. Most pediatric weight-management programs have targeted younger age groups. Treatment is more successful when a comprehensive behavioral program, in conjunction with specific diet and exercise prescriptions, is used.[60,61] An important component of adolescent treatment is parental participation. In addition to attending group sessions, the parent must work with the adolescent to restructure the home and play environments and to monitor progress.

In the treatment of adolescents, the potential risk of an eating disorder should be considered. It has been suggested that energy restriction may trigger binge eating and eating disorders in adults. Although following a low-energy diet does not seem to exacerbate binge eating in those obese adults already identified as binge eaters, evidence suggests the behavior could develop in adults on a low-energy diet who have not binged before. Interventions for weight management must encourage healthy eating habits that promote gradual weight loss in the growing adolescent.

Hyperlipidemia

Adult cardiovascular disease has its roots in children and young adults. American casualties in the Korean and Vietnam wars were found to have a significant prevalence of atherosclerosis on autopsy, despite their young age.[62] The Bogalusa Heart Study and the Pathobiological Determinants of Atherosclerosis in Youth Research Group have found significant correlations between early atherosclerotic changes seen at autopsy and both total and low-density lipoprotein (LDL) cholesterol levels.[63] These and other studies suggest that adolescents at risk for developing premature atherosclerosis should be identified to try to reduce the risk of premature heart disease. There is now a consensus that adolescents with cholesterol levels greater than the 75th percentile should be considered clinically hypercholesterolemic and potentially at risk for adult heart disease.[64,65]

Blood cholesterol levels track over time. Thus, adolescents with high cholesterol levels tend to have higher levels as young adults, and those with low levels tend to have lower levels as adults. However, tracking is not perfect for any one individual.[65,66] A significant degree of biologic and laboratory variation in cholesterol measurements contributes to this deviation from pattern. Lifestyle changes of participants (e.g., weight loss, changes in diet) in longitudinal surveys of cholesterol levels may also contribute to the lower observed degree of tracking.[67] Adolescents may have elevated cholesterol levels for a variety of reasons. Primary genetic defects or familial hyperlipidemia, along with secondary medical causes of hyperlipoproteinemia, should be considered. Inappropriate dietary habits, by themselves or by interaction with any of the above factors, can contribute to moderately increased cholesterol levels. Although a few children do have well-defined familial hyperlipidemia, most individuals with hyperlipidemia do not have such specific syndromes.

Screening for Hypercholesterolemia. Children with unavailable family histories, or those with other risk factors for coronary heart disease, should be screened for hypercholesterolemia at approximately 2 years of age (Table 7).[64,65] The currently recommended approach to screening is based on LDL cholesterol and is outlined in Figure 1. Adolescents with a family history of premature coronary heart disease, defined as disease before the age of 55 years in a parent, grandparent, or aunt or uncle, should have a fasting lipid profile completed. Use of the average values from two lipid profile measurements is recommended to make a clinical diagnosis because of the biologic and laboratory variability in lipid values. Adolescents with average LDL cholesterol levels greater than 3.36 mmol/L (>130 mg/dL) are considered to have elevated levels; LDL cholesterol levels less than 2.84 mmol/L (<110 mg/dL) are considered acceptable. Levels of 2.84 to 3.36 mmol/L (110–130 mg/dL) are borderline elevated. Two of the more common familial conditions, familial hypercholesterolemia and familial combined hyperlipidemia, are autosomal dominantly inherited. Therefore, every generation in the family should have at least one affected individual who can be identified by a thorough review of the family history.

Treatment of Hyperlipidemia. Dietary modification is the best initial intervention for hypercholesterolemic adolescents. Dietary goals include 30% or less (and ≥20%) of total energy as fat (distributed approximately equally among saturated, monounsaturated, and polyunsaturated fat), and 100 mg or less of cholesterol per 1000 kcal (2.4 mg/MJ) consumed (maximum 300 mg/d).[64,65] The initial goal is to achieve an LDL cholesterol level less than 3.36 mmol/L (<130 mg/dL), but the ideal goal is to decrease it to less than 2.84 mmol/L (<110 mg/dL). If these goals are not reached by dietary modification, greater dietary modification should be attempted (<7% calories as saturated fat and cholesterol at <66 mg per 1000 kcal [2.4 mg/MJ] to a maximum of 200 mg/d). Other considerations include increasing dietary fiber and decreasing dietary transfatty acid intake. In general, LDL cholesterol levels decrease 10% to 15% as a result of dietary modification, although the response varies. To ensure a complete and balanced diet that promotes normal growth and development, any diet modification in adolescents should be completed under appropriate supervision by a pediatric registered dietitian with appropriate experience and knowledge. In addition to dietary modification, other cardiovascular disease risk factors such as sedentary lifestyle, obesity, diabetes, hypertension, and smoking should be evaluated and minimized.

Some adolescents require drug therapy. They include those whose LDL cholesterol remains greater than 4.5 mmol/L (190 mg/dL); those whose LDL cholesterol remains greater than 4.1 mmol/L (160 mg/dL) and who have a positive family history of premature coronary heart disease; and those who have two or more other cardiovascular disease risk factors. Approved medication for the treatment of hyperlipidemia in children and young adolescents include cholestyramine and statins with some age and health restrictions. Cholestyramine is considered safe, although gastrointestinal-related side effects commonly make long-term compliance unsuccessful. The safety and efficacy of the statin mediators 3-hydroxy-3-methylglutaryl-coenzyme A reductase inhibitors have been suggested by limited trials in adolescents.[68]

Table 7. Screening Guidelines for Hypercholesterolemia

Indication for Screening	Screening Test
Total cholesterol > 6.2 mmol/L (240 mg/dL) in parents	Nonfasting total cholesterol
Family history of premature heart disease or total cholesterol > 5.2 mmol/L (200 mg/dL)	Two fasting lipid profiles (total cholesterol, triglycerides, HDL, calculated LDL); average the results
Total cholesterol > 4.4–5.2 mmol/L (170–199 mg/dL)	Repeat total cholesterol; if average > 4.4 mmol/L (170 mg/dL), proceed with lipid profile screening

HDL, high-density lipoprotein; LDL, low-density lipoprotein.

Unhealthy Eating Practices and Eating Disorders

One of the changes that occurs during puberty is an increased awareness and preoccupation with body image and size. In the Western world, the epitome of beauty is for girls to be tall and thin and for boys to be tall and muscular. With these expectations, many adolescents often are dissatisfied with their body image. Body dissatisfaction is more commonly found among girls than boys. In a study of US high school students, approximately 40% wanted to lose weight; by sex, the percentages were 61% of the girls and 22% of the boys. Attempts to lose weight were more common among white and Hispanic

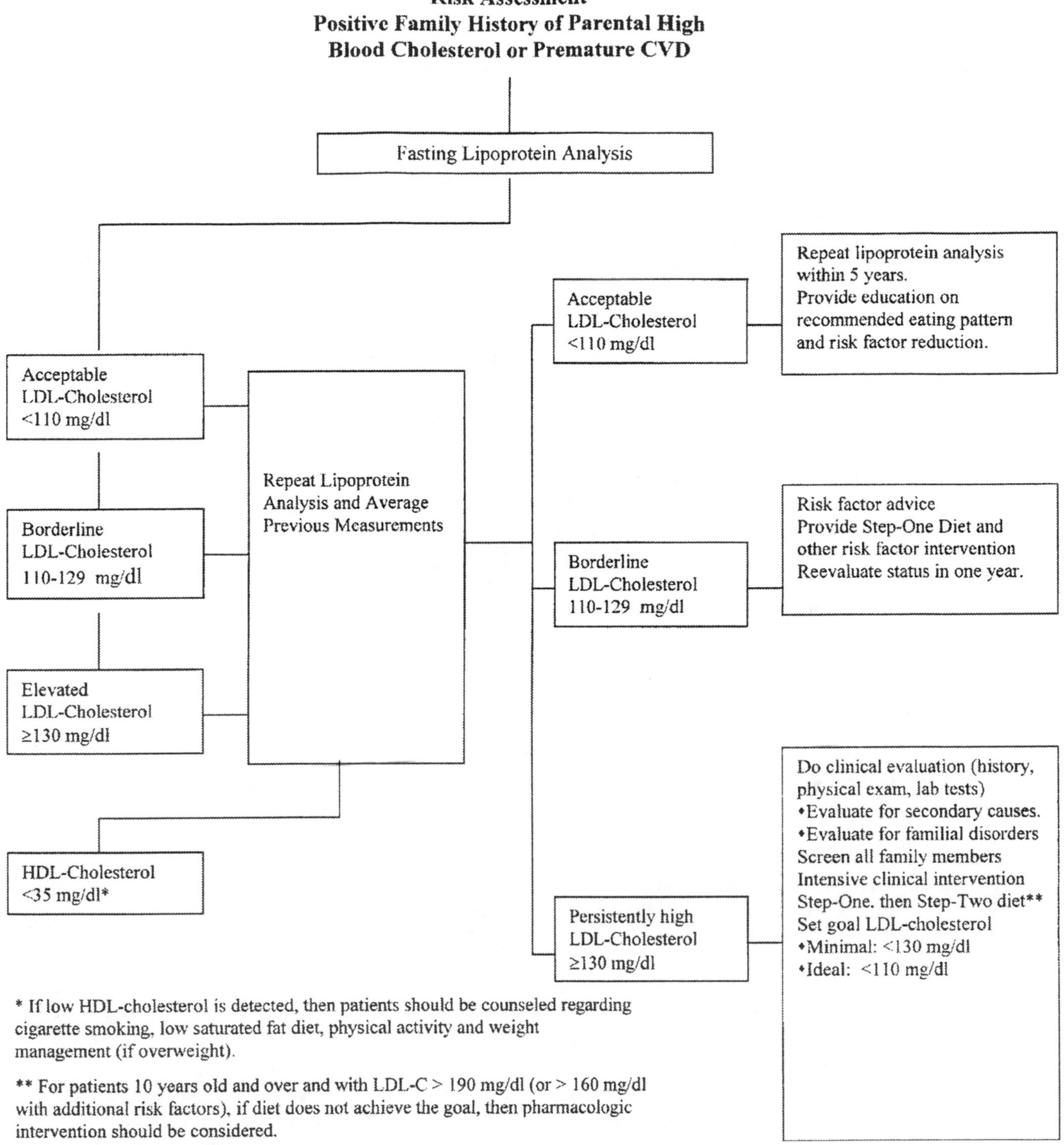

Figure 1. Flowchart of classification, education, and follow-up of children based on LDL cholesterol levels. (Adapted with permission from *AHA Scientific Statement: Cardiovascular Health in Childhood.*[65] Copyright 2002 American Heart Association.)

girls than among black girls.[69] More recent data from the National Youth Risk Behavior Survey (1999–2003) show that 29% to 30% of high school students described themselves as overweight and that 43% to 46% were actively trying to lose weight.[70] Although most students used healthy measures to achieve weight loss, such as eating less food overall, consuming less calories or fat in their meals (40%–44%), or exercising more frequently (57%–60%), a surprising proportion of students reported using more drastic and unhealthy methods to achieve weight loss such as not eating for more than 24 hours at least once within the 30 days before the survey (13%–14%), or vomiting and using laxatives at least once within the past month (5%–6%).[28] Worldwide, eating disorders increase as countries shift to a more affluent economy. Problems associated with dieting and decreased energy intake include weight loss, delayed sexual maturation, menstrual irregularities, constipation, weakness, irritability, sleep problems, poor concentration, and impulses to binge eat.[30]

Eating disorders (anorexia nervosa and bulimia) are relatively common in older adolescents. Psychosocial issues such as environmental problems, low self-esteem, abnormal family dynamics, and depression are often associated with eating disorders.[71] Anorexia nervosa is characterized by a persistent, progressive, and severe restriction of energy intake, often combined with excessive physical activity. Bulimia is characterized by binge eating that is followed by purging, induced vomiting, diuretic use, exercise, or fasting. Although patients with eating disorders usually belong to the middle- or upper-income group, recent trends suggest that eating disorders also occur in other economic groups. Biologic factors include a familial increased incidence of eating disorders and neurotransmitter imbalance of serotonin and other neurotransmitters. Groups at risk for developing eating disorders include gymnasts, runners, ballet dancers, and some other athletes. Societal factors include stereotypical and unrealistic body images, women's role in society, and media pressure. The nutritional changes seen with eating disorders are those of malnutrition and starvation. Although most patients with binge-eating disorders are thin, some may be obese. Amenorrhea is usually seen in anorexia nervosa. In the malnourished patient, bradycardia, orthostatic hypotension, hypothermia, wasting, thin and pale-colored hair, dry skin, alopecia, acrocyanosis, and poor capillary refill may be evident. Parotid gland enlargement, erosion of dental enamel, and abrasions over the metacarpophalangeal joints (Russell's sign) may also be seen, partly related to induced vomiting. Laboratory evaluation reveals electrolyte abnormalities (hypokalemic alkalosis), anemia, and mildly elevated liver enzymes (consistent with fatty infiltration of the liver seen with malnutrition).

The management of the patient with eating disorders is multidisciplinary and involves a dietitian, a psychologist, a physician specializing in adolescence, and the family. A weight goal has to be determined and the patient educated about healthy diet choices and stepwise energy increase to a diet goal. In addition, cognitive-behavioral therapy has been shown to be very effective in the treatment of eating disorders. Selective serotonin reuptake inhibitors have been used for their antidepressive effects and have decreased binge eating and purging in patients with bulimia. When used for patients with anorexia, selectiveserotonin reuptake inhibitors help with weight maintenance and relapse prevention, but are not helpful for patients who are very malnourished. Hospitalization is required for those patients with severe malnutrition, electrolyte abnormalities, or moderate-to-severe dehydration, or those at risk for refeeding syndrome. The prognosis for patients with anorexia nervosa is better than that for those with bulimia.[71]

Pregnancy

Sexual activity among American adolescents has increased over the past decades. Predictive factors for sexual activity in early adolescent years include early puberty, poverty, history of sexual abuse, cultural and family patterns of early sexual experience, poor school performance, lack of school goals, and lack of attentive and nurturing parents.[72] Most of the one million teenagers in the United States who become pregnant are 18 to 19 years old. The general trend for birth rates over the last several years has been a gradual decrease, mainly for black and white teenagers over 15 years of age. The birth rate has remained steady for adolescents less than 15 years of age. Twenty-five percent of female teenagers who have babies have more than one pregnancy as a teen. The United States has the highest adolescent birth rate of all developed countries. Although the reasons for this rate are unknown, poverty is a significant factor in adolescent pregnancy.[72] Recent studies have described an association between low birth weight and adult cardiovascular risk factors such as hyperlipidemia, hyperinsulinemia, and hypertension. It has been suggested that the nutritionally stressed intrauterine environment induces adaptations that, in a non-nutritionally stressed extrauterine environment, are associated with a higher level of cardiovascular disease risk factors.[73] Because many adolescent females who become pregnant are psychosocially at risk, efforts to optimize the nutritional support of pregnant teens may have long-term positive health effects on their children.

There is an increased incidence of medical complications in adolescent pregnancy, especially among adolescents less than 17 years of age. The maternal mortality rate is twice that of adult pregnant women. Other medical problems include poor maternal weight gain, prematurity, hypertension, anemia, sexually transmitted diseases, low-birth-weight infants, and increased neonatal death. These latter two complications are more common in adolescent mothers less than 14 years of age and in the black population. Factors responsible for all of the above complications include low prepregnancy weight and height, parity, poor pregnancy weight gain, poverty, unmarried status, low educational levels, drug use, and inadequate prenatal care. Evidence indicates that adolescent mothers continue to grow in stature and fat-free mass during pregnancy. This growth may occur at the expense of the fetus and result in decreased birth weight despite increased maternal weight gain, or in suboptimal maternal nutritional status and growth. Reduced maternal ferritin, cord ferritin, and folate blood levels have been noted in adolescents who grew during pregnancy.[74,75] The fact that pregnant adolescent girls still grow implies that nutrient needs for pregnant adolescents are even greater than those for nonadolescent pregnant women. To accommodate the potential growth of the pregnant adolescent, it is recommended that pregnant teens gain weight at the upper end of the recommended range for their prepregnancy weight.[76] Weight gain in the first and second trimesters is related to improved birth weight.[77] Pregnant and lactating teens also need additional calories[35] and protein (Table 4), calcium, iron, vitamins B_6, C, A, D, and folate. A prenatal supplement that contains vitamins A, D, zinc, calcium, folate, and iron is recommended. Nutritional education and counseling are an important part of pregnant adolescents' prenatal care.

Vegetarianism

Adolescents may become vegetarians for different reasons including peer pressure, religious expression, humanitarian feelings, and self-expression, and these decisions should be respected. However, if their diets are not balanced and adjusted for the increased requirements of their age group, adolescent vegetarians are at increased risk for the development of malnutrition in addition to deficiencies of vitamins D and B_{12}, riboflavin, protein, calcium, iron, zinc, iodine, and essential fatty acids. The high fiber and low fat content of vegetarian foods can result in decreased energy intake. As a result, dietary protein may be used for energy, thus negatively affecting protein status. Because a purely vegetarian diet is deficient in vitamin B_{12}, a supplement is needed. High intakes of grains can decrease intestinal absorption of iron, calcium, and zinc. Thus, the adolescent who wants to be vegetarian should learn about the dietary principles, and care must to be taken to plan a diet that is sufficient in energy, protein, and micronutrients. A daily multivitamin supplement may be beneficial.

Data on adolescent vegetarians indicate that they have a low intake of energy, with cereals being their main source. When the diets of omnivorous adolescents were compared with those of lacto-ovo vegetarians and semivegetarians, a lower intake of energy, protein, calcium, iron, and zinc was found in the two vegetarian groups. In fact, 33% of the semivegetarians were at risk for inadequate intakes of iron and zinc.[78] In a group of 107 adolescent vegetarians compared with 214 nonvegetarian control subjects, the vegetarians were twice as likely to consume fruits and vegetables and less likely to consume sweets and salty snack foods. Vegetarians were more likely to have potential disordered eating behaviors such as dieting, intentional vomiting, and laxative use.[79] When growth, development, and physical fitness were evaluated in a group of 82 Flemish vegetarian children, the adolescent vegetarians had lower relative body weights and skinfold thickness and lower physical strength, but higher cardiorespiratory endurance, than did the nonvegetarians. The latter finding could have been related to the type of sports the vegetarians played. Normal height was achieved in female adolescent vegetarians but not in their male counterparts. Generally, the vegetarians were leaner than nonvegetarians. Puberty and sexual maturation were normal. Energy intake was lower in the vegetarian group.[80] With appropriate knowledge and guidance, a vegetarian diet for growing adolescents can be designed to meet their nutritional needs and to fit into the complex set of changes in their social, economic, and biologic environments.

Physical Activity and Sports Medicine

Many American adolescents are not physically active. In 2003, only 28% of students in grades 9 to 12 participated in daily physical education classes, and only 56% were enrolled in a physical education class that met 1 or more days in an average week.[81] Of these students, approximately 25% participated in moderate physical activity, and approximately 65% participated in vigorous physical activity.[81,82] Current physical activity recommendations include a minimum of 60 minutes of moderate physical activity on most (preferably all) days of the week.[83] The goal of Healthy People 2010 is to increase the proportion of adolescents who participate in daily school physical education to 50% and to increase the proportion of adolescents who engage in moderate physical activity ($\geq$30 minutes on $\geq$5 of the previous 7 days) and vigorous physical activity that promotes cardiorespiratory fitness on 3 or more days per week for 10 or more minutes per occasion.[82]

The incidence of eating disorders or inappropriate weight control measures among athletes is greater than that among non-athletes. Female athletes are at increased risk for abnormal eating patterns, amenorrhea, and loss of bone mineralization, predisposing them to osteoporosis later in life. The incidence of menstrual disorders (delayed puberty, oligomenorrhea, and secondary amenorrhea) is increased in girls participating in competitive sports and is caused by excessive training and athletic activity. Delays in puberty, scoliosis, and stress fractures are seen most often in athletes who start their training before menarche and are in competitive sports. There is also pressure in certain sports to stay small (gymnastics) and lean (ballet).[25] Diets of these athletes are usually low in calories, fat, and zinc. It is recommended that the amenorrheic athlete who is within 3 years of menarche decrease her level of physical activity and improve her nutritional status, especially for calcium and protein. Older athletes who are more than 16 years of age or more than 3 years after menarche may benefit from estrogen replacement therapy. For thin female athletes, it may be beneficial to check bone health status by dual-energy x-ray absorptiometry scans.

For adolescent athletes, who have increased energy needs, carbohydrates are the main fuel source; however, after glycogen stores are depleted, fat is used as an energy source. In general, for the adolescent athlete's diet, excessive protein intakes may be harmful and may actually decrease physical performance.[84] Competitive athletes' diets commonly are deficient in calcium, which is important for bone health, and iron. Iron needs are higher because of the decreased absorption during strenuous activity and increased losses in sweat and stool. Iron deficiency can lead to anemia with decreased endurance.[84] The recommended distribution of energy intake for an athlete is 60% to 75% energy from carbohydrates (500–600 g/d), 15% to 20% energy from protein (≤1.5 g/kg/d), and 20% to 30% energy from fat.[85] Hydration is very important during physical activity.[86] A variety of nutritional products (drinks, bars, and gels) are marketed for athletes, but no advantages in performance have been noted with excessive vitamin, mineral, or protein intake. Use of anabolic steroids and other drugs to enhance an athlete's performance is increasing. Side effects include accelerated sexual maturation, premature closure of the epiphysis, hypertension, clotting abnormalities, hypercholesterolemia, feminization in males and masculinization in females, and cardiac damage. Adolescent athletes should be strongly discouraged from using any unknown or untested supplements.

Chronic Illness and Disability

Chronic illness can have a significant impact on growth, development, and nutritional status during adolescence, potentially resulting in anorexia, malnutrition, delayed puberty, and nutrient deficiencies. Poor nutritional status can negatively affect disease severity and response to therapy. Decreased appetite is a relatively common symptom of chronic illness and occurs with some medications. Increased energy requirements resulting from increased resting energy expenditure, increased nutrient losses, and malabsorption can also occur. Delayed puberty is common among many chronic diseases of childhood.[5] Consequently, growth measures as indicators of nutritional status are difficult to interpret during adolescence.[44] Delayed puberty may result from chronic undernutrition or other independent disease-related factors. For example, delayed puberty is common in children with cystic fibrosis, and resting energy requirements are increased, even among those with mild pulmonary manifestations of the disorder.[87] To accommodate the increased energy needs of children with cystic fibrosis, their recommended energy intake is 120% of the RDA.[88] However, energy intake in affected children and adolescents rarely reaches this goal.[89] Osteoporosis has also been reported in patients with cystic fibrosis,[90] and so it is important to achieve the recommended intake of calcium and to be sure that vitamin D status is normal. Adolescents with sickle cell disease also experience delayed puberty[91] that may be related to malnutrition. In addition, greater resting energy expenditure occurs in children with sickle cell disease[92] compared with healthy children, without a concomitant increase in energy intake. Increased protein turn-over has also been reported in patients with sickle cell disease,[93] and adequate protein intake to sustain the adolescent growth spurt and puberty-related changes in body composition are important. Vitamins A, D, and E, and selenium, zinc, and calcium requirements may be increased in children with sickle cell disease,[94] but recommended levels have not been established.

Children with developmental disabilities frequently have nutritional problems, including obesity (24%), underweight (22%), feeding problems (23%), and nutrient deficiency states (13%).[30] Swallowing disorders, feeding disorders resulting in decreased energy intake, increased energy needs from abnormal movements and spasticity, and increased energy losses because of vomiting and feeding losses are all potential contributing factors.

Alcohol and Substance Abuse

Alcohol, tobacco, and marijuana are the substances most often abused by adolescents. Alcoholism is a documented problem in adolescence. A national survey of adolescents more than 10 years ago found a 19% incidence of alcohol use and a 10% incidence of marijuana use.[95] Among high school students participating in the National Youth Risk Behavior Survey in 2003, 45% reported current alcohol use, 22% reported current marijuana use, and 4% reported current cocaine use ("current" defined as one or more times in the 30 days before the survey).[96,97] In terms of potential alcohol abuse, 28% reported episodic heavy drinking of five drinks or more in a row on 1 or more days within the past 30 days before the survey.[96] The negative effects of alcoholism on nutritional status depend on the amount of alcohol ingested, duration of alcohol use, and effect on food habits. Teenage males who are alcohol and marijuana abusers have decreased intakes of milk, fruits, and vegetables, and increased snack food intake. Females who become pregnant and consume alcohol run the risk of fetal alcohol syndrome. The incidence of cigarette smoking among high school students is high; however, unlike alcohol and marijuana use, which have both increased among adolescents, cigarette smoking has decreased from 35% in 1999 to 22% in 2003.[82,98] There is no direct nutritional effect of cigarette smoking other than to affect vitamin C status. Indirect effects include contributions to chronic lung disease and, in pregnant adolescent females, increased risk of miscarriages and premature delivery.

Summary

Because adolescence is such an extremely important period in development, the increasing rates of obesity, hypercholesterolemia, low physical activity, adolescent pregnancy, eating disorders, and unhealthy diets (high dietary intake of total and saturated fat, low fruit and vegetable intake, low intake of calcium-rich foods) are alarming. Food habits get established early in life and have a major effect on the risk of chronic disease later in life. Poor dietary practices during adolescence can affect final adult height, puberty, bone health, hyperlipidemia, heart disease, cancer, and obesity. Adolescents need to be assessed nutritionally and screened for unhealthy eating behaviors and nutrition-related pathology. Health care providers should be vigilant to identify unhealthy eating habits and nutrition-associated health and behavioral issues, and provide age-appropriate and timely counseling.

Acknowledgment

Maria R. Mascarenhas, Babette Zemel, and Andrew M. Tershakovec contributed to the chapter on adolescence in the 8th edition, which was updated for the 9th edition, and Joan I. Schall contributed to the most recent update for this edition.

References

1. Skiba A, Logmani E, Orr DP. Nutritional screening and guidance for adolescents. Adolesc Health Update, Clin Guide Ped. 1997;9:1–8.
2. Tanner JM. *Growth at Adolescence.* Oxford: Blackwell Publications; 1962.
3. Zemel BS, Jenkins C. Dietary change and adolescent growth among the Bundi (Gende-speaking) people of Papua New Guinea. Am J Human Biol. 1989;1: 709–718.
4. Ramakrishnan U, Barnhart H, Schroeder DG, et al. Early childhood nutrition, education and fertility milestones in Guatemala. J Nutr. 1999;129:2196–2202.
5. Zeitler PS, Travers S, Kappy MS. Advances in the recognition and treatment of endocrine complications in children with chronic illness. Adv Pediatr. 1999;46:101–149.
6. Lampl M, Johnson ML. A case study of daily growth during adolescence: a single spurt or changes in the dynamics of saltatory growth? Ann Hum Biol. 1993; 20:595–603.
7. Sun SS, Schubert CM, Chumlea WC, et al. National estimates of the timing of sexual maturation and racial differences among US children. Pediatrics. 2002; 110:911–919.
8. Herman-Giddens ME, Slora EJ, Wasserman RC, et al. Secondary sexual characteristics and menses in young girls seen in office practice: a study from the Pediatric Research in Office Settings Network. Pediatrics. 1997;99:505–512.
9. Abbassi V. Growth and normal puberty. Pediatrics. 1998;102:507–511.
10. Theintz G, Buchs B, Rizzoli R, et al. Longitudinal monitoring of bone mass accumulation in healthy adolescents: evidence for a marked reduction after 16 years of age at the levels of lumbar spine and femoral neck in female subjects. J Clin Endocrinol Metab. 1992;75:1060–1065.
11. Matkovic V. Calcium and peak bone mass. J Intern Med. 1992;231:151–160.
12. Weaver CM, Peacock M, Johnston CC Jr. Adolescent nutrition in the prevention of postmenopausal osteoporosis. J Clin Endocrinol Metab. 1999;84: 1839–1843.
13. Bailey DA, McKay HA, Mirwald RL, et al. A six-year longitudinal study of the relationship of physical activity to bone mineral accrual in growing children: the University of Saskatchewan bone mineral accrual study. J Bone Miner Res. 1999;14:1672–1679.
14. Food and Nutrition Board. Institute of Medicine. *Recommended Dietary Allowances, 10th ed.* Washington, DC: National Academies Press; 1989.
15. Food and Nutrition Board. Institute of Medicine. *Dietary Reference Intakes for Calcium, Phosphorus, Magnesium, Vitamin D, and Fluoride.* Washington, DC: National Academies Press; 1997.
16. NIH Consensus Development Panel on Optimal Calcium Intake. Optimal calcium intake. JAMA. 1994;272:1942–1948.
17. Alaimo K, McDowell MA, Breifel RR, et al. *Dietary Intake of Vitamins, Minerals, and Fiber of Persons Ages 2 Months and Over in the United States: Third National Health and Nutrition Examination Survey, Phase 1, 1988–1991. Advance Data from Vital and Health Statistics, no. 258. U.S. Department of Health and Human Services.* Hyattsville, MD: National Center for Health Statistics; 1994.
18. Ervin RB, Wang CY, Wright JD, Kennedy-Stephenson J. *Dietary Intake of Selected Minerals for the United States Population: 1999–2000. Advance Data from Vital and Health Statistics, no 341.* Hyattsville, MD: National Center for Health Statistics; 2004.
19. Matkovic V. Calcium metabolism and calcium requirements during skeletal modeling and consolidation of bone mass. Am J Clin Nutr. 1991;54(suppl): 245S–260S.
20. Johnston CC, Miller JZ, Slemenda CW, et al. Calcium supplementation and increases in bone mineral density in children. N Engl J Med. 1992;327:82–87.
21. Holick MF. Photobiology of vitamin D. In: Feldman D, Glorieux FH, Pike JW, eds. *Vitamin D.* San Diego: Academic Press; 1997:33–39.
22. Docio S, Riancho JA, Perez A, et al. Seasonal deficiency of vitamin D in children: a potential target for osteoporosis-preventing strategies? J Bone Miner Res. 1998;13:544–548.
23. Specker BL. Evidence for an interaction between calcium intake and physical activity on changes in bone mineral density. J Bone Miner Res. 1996;11:1539–1544.
24. Marcus R. Exercise: moving in the right direction. J Bone Miner Res. 1998;13:1793–1796.

25. Dwyer JT. Adolescence. In: Zeigler EE, Filer LJ, eds. *Present Knowledge in Nutrition, 7th ed.* Washington, DC: ILSI Press; 1996:404–413.
26. Food and Nutrition Board. Institute of Medicine. *Dietary Reference Intakes for Thiamin, Riboflavin, Niacin, Vitamin B6, Folate, Vitamin B12, Pantothenic Acid, Biotin and Choline.* Washington, DC: National Academies Press; 1998.
27. Gavadini C, Siega-Riz AM, Popkin BM. U.S. adolescent food intake trends from 1965 to 1996. Arch Dis Child. 2000;83:18–24.
28. Department of Health and Human Services. Trends in the prevalence of dietary behaviors and weight control practices. National Youth Risk Behavior Survey: 1991–2003. DHHS, Centers for Disease Control and Prevention. Available at: http://www.cdc.gov/yrbss. 2005.
29. Food and Nutrition Board. Institute of Medicine. *Dietary Reference Intakes for Vitamin A, Vitamin K, Boron, Chromium, Copper, Iodine, Iron, Manganese, Molybdenum, Nickel, Vanadium, and Zinc.* Washington, DC: National Academies Press; 2001.
30. Story M, Alton I. Adolescent nutrition: current trends and critical issues. Top Clin Nutr. 1996;11: 56–69.
31. Krebs-Smith SM, Cook A, Subar AF, et al. Fruit and vegetable intakes of children and adolescents in the United States. Arch Pediatr Adolesc Med. 1996; 150:81–86.
32. Munoz KA, Krebs-Smith SM, Ballard-Barbash R, Cleveland LE. Food intakes of US children and adolescents compared to recommendations. Pediatrics. 1997;100:323–329.
33. Committee on Nutrition. Adolescent nutrition. In: Kleinman R, ed. *Pediatric Nutrition Handbook, 5th ed.* Elk Grove Village, IL: American Academy of Pediatrics; 2004:149–154.
34. Gong EJ, Heald FP. Diet, nutrition and adolescence. In: Shils ME, Olson JA, Shike M, eds. *Modern Nutrition in Health and Disease, 9th ed.* Malvern, PA: Lea & Febiger; 1999:857–869.
35. Food and Nutrition Board. Institute of Medicine. *Dietary Reference Intakes for Energy, Carbohydrate, Fiber, Fat, Fatty Acids, Cholesterol, Protein and Amino Acids.* Washington DC: National Academies Press; 2002.
36. Bialostosky K, Wright JD, Kennedy-Stephenson J, et al. Dietary intake of macronutrients and other dietary constituents: United States 1988–94. National Center for Health Statistics. Vital Health Stat 11. 2002; (245):1–158.
37. Albertson AM, Tobelman RC, Marquart L. Estimated dietary calcium intake and food sources for adolescent females: 1980–1992. J Adolesc Health. 1997;20:20–26.
38. Ervin RB, Wright JD, Wang CY, Kennedy-Stephenson J. *Dietary Intake of Selected Vitamins for the United States Population: 1999–2000. Advance Data from Vital and Health Statistics; no. 339.* Hyattsville, MD: National Center for Health Statistics; 2004.
39. Nicklas TA, Myers L, Berenson GS. Dietary fiber intake of children: the Bogalusa Heart Study. Pediatrics. 1995;96:988–994.
40. Williams CL, Bollella M, Wynder EL. A new recommendation for dietary fiber in childhood. Pediatrics. 1995;96:985–988.
41. Kuczmarski RJ, Ogden CL, Grummer-Strawn LM, et al. CDC growth charts: United States. Advance Data from Vital and Health Statistics. Hyattsville, MD: National Center for Health Statistics; 2000: no. 314. Available at: http://www.cdc.gov/growthcharts.
42. Tanner JM, Davies PSW. Clinical longitudinal standards for height and weight velocity for North American children. J Pediatr. 1985;107:317–329.
43 Morris NM, Udry JR. Validation of a self-administered instrument to assess stage of adolescent development. J Youth Adolesc. 1980;9:271–280.
44. Himes JH. Growth reference data for adolescents: maturation-related misclassification and its accommodation. In: Johnston FE, Zemel BS, Eveleth PB, eds. *Human Growth in Context. Auxology Advances in the Study of Human Growth and Development, no. 2.* London: Smith-Gordon; 1999:95–100.
45. Must A, Dallal GE, Dietz WH. Reference data for obesity: 85th and 95th percentiles of body mass index (wt/ht2) and triceps skinfold thickness. Am J Clin Nutr. 1991;53:839–846.
46. Kuczmarski RJ, Ogden CL, Guo SS, et al. 2000 CDC growth charts for the United States: methods and development. Vital Health Stat 11. 2002;246: 1–190.
47. Ogden CL, Flegal KM, Carroll MD, Johnson CL. Prevalence and trends in overweight among US children and adolescents, 1999–2000. JAMA. 2002;288: 1728–1732.
48. Hedley AA, Ogden CL, Johnson CL, Carroll MD, Curtin LR, Flegal KM. Prevalence of overweight and obesity among US children, adolescents and adults, 1999–2002. JAMA. 2004;291:2847–2850.
49. Whitaker RC, Wright JA, Pepe MS, et al. Predicting obesity in young adulthood from childhood and parental obesity. N Engl J Med. 1997;337:869–873.
50. Stunkard AJ, Sorensen TIA, Hanis C, et al. An adoption study of human obesity. N Engl J Med. 1986;314:193–198.
51. Andersen RE, Crespo CJ, Bartlett SJ, et al. Relationship of physical activity and television watching with body weight and level of fatness among children. JAMA. 1998;279:938–942.
52. Epstein LH, Wing RR, Penner BC, Kress MJ. Effect of diet and controlled exercise on weight loss in obese children. J Pediatr.1985; 107:358–361.
53. Shick SM, Wing RR, Klem ML, et al. Persons successful at long-term weight loss and maintenance

continue to consume a low-energy, low-fat diet. J Am Diet Assoc. 1998;98:408–413.
54. Bandini LG, Schoeller DA, Cyr HN, Dietz WM. Validity of reported energy intake in obese and non-obese adolescents. Am J Clin Nutr. 1990;52: 421–425.
55. Freedman DS, Srinivasan SR, Harsha DW, et al. Relation of body fat patterning to lipid and lipoprotein concentrations in children and adolescents: the Bogalusa Heart Study. Am J Clin Nutr. 1989;50: 930–939.
56. Freedman DS, Srinivasan SR, Burke GL, et al. Relation of body fat distribution to hyperinsulinemia in children and adolescents: the Bogalusa Heart Study. Am J Clin Nutr. 1987;46:403–410.
57. Van Gaal LF, Wauters MA, De Leeuw IH. The beneficial effects of modest weight loss on cardiovascular risk factors. Int J Obes. 1997;21(Suppl):S5-S9.
58. Pinhas-Hamiel O, Dolan LM, Daniels SR, et al. Increased incidence of non-insulin-dependent diabetes mellitus among adolescents. J Pediatr. 1996;128: 608–615.
59. Gortmaker SL, Must A, Perrin JM, et al. Social and economic consequences of overweight in adolescence and young adulthood. N Engl J Med. 1993;329: 1008–12.
60. Epstein LH, Myers MD, Raynor HA, Saelens BE. Treatment of pediatric obesity. Pediatrics. 1998;101: 554–570.
61. Wilson GT. Behavioral treatment of obesity: thirty years and counting. Adv Behav Res Ther. 1993;16: 31–75.
62. Strong JP. Coronary atherosclerosis in soldiers: a clue to the natural history of atherosclerosis in the young. JAMA. 1986;256:2863–2866.
63. Strong JP, Malcom GT, McMahan CA, et al. Prevalence and extent of atherosclerosis in adolescents and young adults: implications for prevention from the Pathobiological Determinants of Atherosclerosis in Youth Study. JAMA. 1999; 281:727–735.
64. Committee on Nutrition. Cholesterol in childhood. Pediatrics. 1998;101:141–147.
65. Williams CL, Hayman LL, Daniels SR, et al. Cardiovascular health in childhood: a statement for health professionals from the Committee on Atherosclerosis, Hypertension, and Obesity in the Young (AHOY) of the Council on Cardiovascular Disease in the Young, American Heart Association. Circulation. 2002;106:143–160.
66. Lauer RM, Clarke WR. Use of cholesterol measurements in childhood for the prediction of adult hypercholesterolemia: the Muscatine Study. JAMA. 1990; 264:3034–3038.
67. Stuhldreher WL, Richard TJ, Donahue RP, et al. Cholesterol screening in childhood: sixteen-year Beaver County Lipid Study experience. J Pediatr. 1991;119:551–556.
68. Stein EA, Illingworth DR, Kwiterovich PO, et al. Efficacy and safety of lovastatin in adolescent males with heterozygous familial hypercholesterolemia: a randomized controlled trial. JAMA. 1999;281: 137–144.
69. Kann L, Warren CW, Harris WA. Youth risk behavior surveillance-United States, 1993. MMWR Morb Mortal Wkly Rep. 1995;273:1429–1435.
70. Department of Health and Human Services. Trends in the prevalence of overweight. National Youth Risk Behavior Survey: 1991–2003. DHHS, Centers for Disease Control and Prevention. Available at: http://www.cdc.gov/yrbss. 2005.
71. Kreipe RE, Dukarm CP. Eating disorders in adolescents and older children. Pediatr Rev. 1999;20: 410–420.
72. American Academy of Pediatrics, Committee on Adolescence. Adolescent pregnancy-current trends and issues 1998. Pediatrics. 1999;103:516–520.
73. Barker DJP. The fetal and infant origins of disease. Eur J Clin Invest. 1995;25:457–463.
74. Scholl TO, Hediger ML, Schall JI. Maternal growth and fetal growth: pregnancy course and outcome in the Camden Study. Ann NY Acad Sci. 1997;817: 292–301.
75. Scholl TO, Hediger ML. A review of the epidemiology of nutrition and adolescent pregnancy: maternal growth during pregnancy and its effect on the fetus. J Am Coll Nutr. 1993;12:101–107.
76. Food and Nutrition Board. Institute of Medicine. *Nutrition During Pregnancy.* Washington, DC: National Academies Press; 1990.
77. Hediger ML, Scholl TO, Schall JI. Implications of the Camden study of adolescent pregnancy: interactions among maternal growth, nutritional status, and body composition. Ann NY Acad Sci. 1997;817: 281–291.
78. Donovan UM, Gibson RS. Dietary intakes of adolescent females consuming vegetarian, semi-vegetarian, and omnivorous diets. J Adolesc Health. 1996;18: 292–300.
79. Neumark-Sztainer D, Story M, Resnick MD, Blum RW. Adolescent vegetarians: a behavioral profile of a school-based population in Minnesota. Arch Pediatr Adolesc Med. 1997;151:833–838.
80. Hebbelinck, Calrys P, Malsche AD. Growth, development, and physical fitness of Flemish vegetarian children, adolescents and young adults. Am J Clin Nutr. 1999;70(suppl):579S–585S.
81. Department of Health and Human Services. *Trends in the Prevalence of Physical Activity. National Youth Risk Behavior Survey: 1991–2003.* DHHS, Centers for Disease Control and Prevention. Available at: http://www.cdc.gov/yrbss. 2005.
82. Healthy People 2010. *National Health Promotion and Disease Prevention Objectives.* Available at: http://www.health.gov/healthypeople. Accessed February 28, 2005.

83. U.S. Department of Agriculture, U.S. Department of Health and Human Services. *Nutrition and Your Health: Dietary Guidelines for Americans,* 2005. Washington, DC: USDA; 2005.
84. Committee on Nutrition. Sports nutrition. In: Kleinman R, ed. *Pediatric Nutrition Handbook, 5th ed.* Elk Grove Village, IL: American Academy of Pediatrics; 2004:155–166.
85. Probart CK, Bird PJ, Parker KA. Diet and athletic performance. Med Clin North Am. 1993;77: 757–772.
86. Kleiner SM. Nutrition advisor; eating for peak performance. Phys Sports Med. 1997;25:123–124.
87. Zemel BS, Kawchak DA, Cnaan A, et al. Prospective evaluation of resting energy expenditure, nutrition status, pulmonary function, and genotype in children with cystic fibrosis. Pediatr Res. 1996;40:578–586.
88. Ramsey BW, Farrell PM, Pencharz PB. Nutritional assessment and management in cystic fibrosis: a consensus report. Am J Clin Nutr. 1992;55:108–116.
89. Kawchak DA, Zhao H, Scanlin TF, et al. Longitudinal, prospective analysis of dietary intake in children with cystic fibrosis. J Pediatr. 1996;129:119–129.
90. Henderson RC, Specter BB. Kyphosis and fractures in children and young adults with cystic fibrosis. J Pediatr. 1994;125:208–212.
91. Platt OS, Rosenstock W, Espeland MA. Influence of sickle hemoglobinopathies on growth and development. N Engl J Med. 1984;311:7–12.
92. Barden EM, Zemel BS, Kawchak SA, et al. Total and resting energy expenditure in children and adolescents with sickle cell disease. J Pediatr. 2000;136: 73–79.
93. Borel MJ, Buchowski MS, Turner EA, et al. Alterations in basal nutrient metabolism increase resting energy expenditure in sickle cell disease. Am J Physiol. 1998;274(2 Pt 1):E357–E364.
94. Reed JD, Redding-Lallinger R, Orringer EP. Nutrition and sickle cell disease. Am J Hematol. 1987;24: 441–455.
95. Johnston LD, O'Malley PM, Bachman JG. *National Survey Results on Drug Use from the Monitoring the Future Study, 1975–1995.* Rockville, MD: U.S. Department of Health and Human Services; 1996.
96. Department of Health and Human Services. Trends in the prevalence of alcohol use. National Youth Risk Behavior Survey: 1991–2003. DHHS, Centers for Disease Control and Prevention. Available at: http://www.cdc.gov/yrbss. 2005.
97. Department of Health and Human Services. Trends in the prevalence of marijuana, cocaine, and other illegal drug use. National Youth Risk Behavior Survey: 1991–2003. Washington, DC: DHHS, Centers for Disease Control and Prevention, 2005.
98. Department of Health and Human Services. *Trends in the Prevalence of Cigarette Use. National Youth Risk Behavior Survey: 1991–2003.* Washington, DC: DHHS, Centers for Disease Control and Prevention; 2005.

44 Aging and Nutrition

Olivier Guérin, Patrick Ritz, Stéphane Schneider, and Bruno Vellas

Life expectancy at birth is 77.6 years in the United States.[1] The average age and the proportion of the older population increase each year. Individuals more than 65 years of age now comprise 12.5% of the population, compared with 4% in 1900. This percentage is expected to increase to 20% by the year 2030. According to projections from the US Census Bureau, the population more than 65 years of age will be approximately 60 million by the middle of the 21st century.[2]

Aging is a complex phenomenon that includes molecular, physiologic, and psychologic changes. Health problems and physiologic decline develop gradually and partly result from a lifetime of poor health habits. Direct effects from the aging process seem to be less important than previously reported, and some very old individuals can stay healthy and have good nutritional status. However, year after year, an increasing proportion of elderly persons become frail, with some diminution of sensorial functions, increase of cognitive impairments, and deterioration of functional status. Thus, 42% of the population more than 65 years of age have a disability[2] in the United States.

Much research has been conducted in recent years to determine how to keep elderly individuals fully functional physically, mentally, and socially, but much more information will be required before consensus can be reached on recommendations that will enhance people's lives throughout their late years. This chapter examines some of the areas of aging research currently being conducted and addresses promising areas of research for the future.

Effects of Aging on Nutritional Status

Evaluation of the Nutritional Status in the Older Population

Many geriatric assessment instruments have been developed to diagnose and treat high-risk situations in elderly patients. At the present time, the major components of a good geriatric assessment comprise four major domains (physical health, functional ability, psychologic health, and socioenvironmental factors), each composed of several subdomains.[3] As noted by Rubenstein,[3] use of the following well-validated instruments that encompass the major assessment domains makes the geriatric assessment more reliable and considerably easier: Activities of Daily Living,[4] Instrumental Activities of Daily Living,[5] Mini-Mental State Examination,[6] Geriatric Depression Scale,[7] Tinetti Balance and Gait Evaluation,[8] and nutritional examination.

Assessing the nutritional status of the older population requires clinical parameters to evaluate physical signs of nutritional health or disease, dietary parameters to evaluate nutrient intakes compared with the accepted standards, and laboratory investigations to provide data about quantities of particular nutrients in the body or to evaluate certain biochemical functions that depend on an adequate supply of a particular nutrient. Because use of a single measure is rarely sufficient to establish the level of malnutrition in a population, nutritional assessment is best accomplished with a combination of these methods. The greater the number of measurements outside the standard range, the more likely a population is to have poor nutritional status.

Body weight is a useful parameter to collect. A very low body weight can be considered a sign of malnutrition. Skin-fold thicknesses and waist and thigh girths are easy to measure. However, skin-fold thicknesses cannot be used to assess changes in body fat mass because of age-related fat redistribution. Waist and thigh girths, rather than skin-fold thicknesses, should be considered for use in longitudinal studies in the elderly because the changes in these girths capture increased abdominal adiposity and sarcopenia, respectively.[9]

To assess nutritional status as part of a geriatric evaluation in elderly patients in clinics, nursing homes, and hospitals, or in those who are frail, a single and rapid nutritional assessment, the Mini-Nutritional Assessment (MNA), was defined and validated.[10] The aim of the MNA is to evaluate the risk of malnutrition to permit early nutritional intervention when needed, without the need for specialized investigators. The following requirements were considered in developing the test: a reliable scale, definition of thresholds, compatible with the skills of a generalist assessor, minimal bias introduced by the data collector, acceptable to patients, and inexpensive. The MNA instrument is composed of simple measurements and questions to be completed in less than 15 minutes. The MNA has been validated by several studies performed on elderly subjects in a variety of settings. This tool has 18 items, including anthropometric elements (calf circumference and mid-arm circumference), body mass index (BMI), polymedication research, recent acute infections, presence of pressure ulcers, motion ability, appetite, food habits, and subjective health, which is a straightforward picture of an elderly patient's health status. The MNA is performed in two steps. The first step is case finding and comprises six items, with a maximum score of 14. A score of 12 or more indicates a sufficient nutritional status that does not require the next step. A score of 11 or less is an indication to continue with the whole MNA, and both scores of these two first steps are added together to form the total score. A total score between 17.5 and 23.5 indicates a nutritional risk, and a total score less than 17.5 indicates an existing malnutrition. A score more than 23.5 indicates a stable and satisfying nutritional status.

Weight Loss and Malnutrition

Malnutrition is a dynamic phenomenon that starts when nutritional intake is insufficient to match requirements. It can only occur if intake does not match needs. Most of the time, malnutrition refers to energy and protein, but the same reasoning can be applied to other nutrients (e.g., specific lipids, vitamins, and micronutrients). The negative balance between intake and requirements exists regardless of the requirement level. This is the case in patients with increased energy expenditure (e.g., patients with fever or burns), but also when energy expenditure is not increased (e.g., most disease situations).

Because malnutrition is a dynamic process, diagnosis can be made on either dynamic symptoms or when a status is considered at its lower threshold. Primarily, this concerns body weight and composition, together with various functions. Dynamic criteria to diagnose malnutrition are weight loss and reduction in energy intake (probably <20 kcal/kg of body weight/d). Weight status is considered in the malnutrition range when BMI is less than 20 kg/m^2, although there can be no ongoing weight change. This means that the change in weight is the dynamic indicator, but weight does not decrease any more after a period of time, and the subject remains wasted. There is a demonstrated increased mortality for BMI levels less than 22 kg/m^2, although functional status can be impaired between 22 and 27 kg/m^2.[11] Recent recommendations[11] suggest that malnutrition can be diagnosed with a 10% weight loss (either within 6 months or in comparison with weight recorded at a previous visit), a 5% weight loss in 1 month, a BMI less than 22 kg/m^2, or an MNA score less than 17.5. There is no consensus on the albumin concentration as a diagnostic tool and whether a concentration of transthyretin less than 110 mg/L (without arguments of inflammation) can be considered a good indicator of malnutrition. Malnutrition is considered severe when weight loss is greater than 15% in absolute terms (or >10% during 1 month), albumin concentration is less than 25 g/L, or transthyretin is less than 50 mg/L.

Functional consequences of malnutrition include impaired immunity, muscle mass, and cognitive function. Impaired immunity is particularly worrisome because of the natural consequences of aging on the immune system,[12] and because it is further impaired by the fasting and calorie restriction that often accompany disease.[13] This leads to an increased mortality that is well demonstrated, especially in neurodegenerative disease and various cancers.[11] Even in populations who appear to be healthy, a weight loss of 4% or more multiplies the risk of death by 2.7.[14] In patients with cancer, although malnutrition is present in two-thirds of the cases, cancer cachexia is considered responsible for death in more than 30% of the cases. Malnutrition is also associated with impaired healing after surgical procedures and is a risk factor for pressure sores.[15]

Muscle mass decrease is directly responsible for functional impairment with loss of strength, increased likelihood of falls, and loss of autonomy. Respiratory function can also be impaired with a reduced vital capacity that increases the risk of infection further. Malnutrition is often associated with heart failure, and is difficult to diagnosis because edema and fluid retention may mask weight loss. There is a close relationship between cognitive performance and weight changes accompanying Alzheimer's disease.

Malnutrition is also costly for the healthcare system, because the average length of stay increases by approximately 5 days, and it is estimated that the 50% of hospitalized patients who are malnourished are responsible for 75% of the expenditures.[16]

The prevalence of malnutrition depends on where the elderly person lives. Probably 5% or fewer of healthy elderly people living at home are malnourished. This level increases from 10% to 38% when at home and with disease from 28% to 65% when hospitalized. This prevalence varies with the criteria used for the diagnosis of malnutrition.

Weight loss affects more lean mass (mainly muscle) and water than fat.[17] This is particularly alarming because natural aging already affects those compartments (see "Sarcopenia" in this chapter), and body water mass is less well regulated in the elderly.

Causes of Malnutrition

Anorexia is frequent during disease and reduces food intake. Anorexia is associated with aging because of impaired taste and smell capacities. Poor dental health, digestive disorders, and dementia are also reasons for anorexia. Roberts has clearly demonstrated that after a period of over- or undernutrition, elderly people do not recover usual intake as well as young persons do.[18] A vicious circle begins in patients with aging-induced anorexia in whom disease adds another bout of anorexia, decreasing energy intake further. With the difficulties to recover usual intake, a downward step-by-step decay procedure is then initiated. Other nonphysiologic causes can be considered, such as isolation (e.g., dementia), poverty, various handicaps, and drug side effects (dryness of the mouth, changes in smell and taste). Between the ages of 20 and 80 years, the decrease in food intake is approximately 1200 kcal/d for men and approximately 800 kcal/d for women.[19] Reduced intake associated with natural aging does not seem to change weight, which is stable until it starts to decrease in persons more than 70 years of age. It is only in the very old and those with disease that weight changes are associated with functional impairments.[19] Appetite regulation by macronutrients is poorly studied in the elderly. The hypothesis that a hierarchy exists whereby fat suppresses appetite very little and glucose and most proteins do so much better is poorly studied. This hypothesis has been proven in healthy elderly persons.[20] However, the hierarchy disappears in malnourished elderly persons and those with disease.[20] In those cases, a change in subjective sensations of appetite are demonstrated, but changes in intake are not parallel to those indicators. Further studies are necessary to understand changes in appetite in elderly persons with disease. Indeed, this could lead to the development of useful strategies to improve appetite and energy intake. The digestive functions are maintained with aging, but oral problems (e.g., tooth loss and lack of saliva) play a role in reduced food intake.

Energy requirements decrease with age because of loss in muscle and lean mass and reduced physical activity.[21] It is often said that energy requirements increase in various situations; this remains to be demonstrated in most cases for total energy expenditure. Measurements of resting energy expenditure are useful but not sufficient to prove that requirements are increased.

Obesity

The prevalence of obesity decreases in extreme old age, but remains a common problem in the elderly. As Kennedy et al.[22] noted, decreased physical activity and decreased energy expenditure with aging predispose one to fat accumulation and fat redistribution. Reduction in muscle mass (sarcopenic obesity) is a major determinant of physical function and metabolic rate, and an important determinant of health status in the elderly. Chronic inflammation and endocrine changes contribute to the changes in metabolism and body composition that accompany aging, and are potential therapeutic targets. Body weight and BMI are imperfect indicators of the risk of obesity. The focus of treatment should be on the reduction of intra-abdominal fat and the preservation of muscle mass and strength. Recent studies have confirmed the effectiveness of exercise interventions in the elderly.[23,24] Reduced function and decreased quality of life accompany development of the complications of obesity such as diabetes and vascular disorders. There is considerable scope to impede the development of these complications in the elderly with lifestyle interventions. A strong association exists between obesity and type 2 or noninsulin-dependent diabetes mellitus (NIDDM). Indeed, 80% of middle-aged persons with NIDDM are obese. NIDDM is common, occurring in up to 18% of individuals more than 65 years of age. In approximately 50% of these subjects, however, the diagnosis of NIDDM is not made. The prevalence of diagnosed diabetes in elderly people is expected to increase by 44% in the next 20 years.[25] In addition, obesity is now a well-known risk factor for vascular dementia and Alzheimer's disease.[26]

Sarcopenia

Sarcopenia is defined as the loss of muscle mass and function associated with aging. In numerical terms, it is considered as a value below a mean of −2 standard deviations of the distribution in healthy young persons of similar weight.[27] Sarcopenia is present in twice as many patients more than 80 years of age than in those under 80; 29% of men and 16% of women more than 80 years of age have sarcopenia. Sarcopenia is responsible for most of the age-associated loss in lean mass. Sarcopenia is accompanied and aggravated by a cachectic component when stress occurs (surgery, sepsis, inflammation, or cancer). Proteolysis is dramatically increased, and muscle wasting is responsible for most of the weight loss.

Functional impairment is greater than expected for a given muscle mass change. It is estimated that a 30% mass decrease in muscle corresponds to a 50% function loss. This is a key factor for loss of autonomy. Sarcopenia multiplies the odds of walking with a stick by 2.3, of falling by 2.6, of having equilibrium disorders by 3.2, and of loss of autonomy by 3.7. The strength decline is estimated to be 1% per year, and is influenced by gender and the maintenance of physical activity.

A recent study by Janssen et al.[28] showed that the estimated direct health care cost attributable to sarcopenia in the United States was $18.5 billion in 2000, which represented approximately 1.5% of the total health care expenditures for that year. The excess health care expenditures were $860 for each man with sarcopenia and $933 for each woman with sarcopenia. A 10% reduction in sarcopenia prevalence could result in a savings of $1.1 billion ($2000) per year in US health care costs.

Muscle mass can be estimated with simple tools: anthropometric (muscle circumference) and instrumental (bioelectrical impedance analysis). Measurements with the latter technique have been validated against state-of-the-art methods.[29] Thresholds are defined that show an increased risk of loss of autonomy or functional impairment. In the National Health and Nutrition Examination Survey cohort, an index of muscle mass (mass divided by height squared) less than 5.75 kg/m^2 in women and 8.5 kg/m^2 in men multiplies the risk of loss of autonomy by approximately 3.[29] Similar results with a similar threshold were obtained in the European population (P. Ritz, personal communication, 2004).

Sarcopenia results from intrinsic muscle impairment, lesions in the central nervous system, and the consequences of behavioral changes (usual physical activity) and environmental changes (disease is associated with being bed-, room-, or house-bound).[19] Both the absolute and relative amounts of type II fibers in muscle are reduced (glycolytic and mostly used during intense and acute exercise), together with the myosin heavy chain content. Healthy aging is associated with a decrease in muscle protein synthesis[30] and the impaired postprandial fate of amino acids.

Some suggest that there is an hypercatabolic status during aging.[31] Interleukin-6 production by white blood cells and plasma interleukin-6 concentrations increase, and are correlated with the odds of sarcopenia in the Framingham cohort.[31] The cause-and-effect relationship remains to be established. Activation of proinflammatory cytokines after an episode of stress in the elderly is frequent (interleukin-1 and interleukin-6, tumor necrosis factor), and may indicate a chronic state of mild inflammation. Those parameters are known as proteolytic, especially in muscle. Caspase 3 activity, together with other proapoptotic markers, increase with age and are also known to be candidates for muscle hypercatabolism.[32]

The effect of sex steroids was reviewed by Bhasin.[33] The decreased concentrations in sex steroids accelerate muscle wasting during disease. Testosterone treatment increases muscle mass in patients (or volunteers) with hypogonadia. This is observed with more than 50 mg of testosterone enanthate per week. Increase in mass is dose-dependent in young subjects, is correlated with plasma concentrations, and is accompanied by an increase in strength. This effect is increased by exercise. In elderly persons free of disease, things are less clear. It seems that hormonal treatment only mildly increases plasma concentrations and muscle mass, and has a weak effect on muscle strength.[33] Sex steroid treatment in the very elderly is limited by the risk of prostate cancer and cardiovascular disease, although this has not been thoroughly evaluated. The contribution of a growth hormone deficiency has not been clearly established.

Resistance exercise (when muscle works against an external force) increases muscle strength at all ages, but in a heterogeneous manner.[34] A systematic review of 27 trials[34] showed that functional improvement is modest (number of falls, capacity to stand from a chair), as is the favorable effect on autonomy. Some programs can be implemented at home and seem to improve functional capacity and autonomy without affecting muscle strength and fitness. Side effects of exercise (cardiovascular) require that further evaluations be performed before any systematic promotion of exercise is implemented in the very old person.

Hydration Disorders

Water is the most abundant component of the body and represents 45% to 70% of body weight. This proportion varies with age, hydration, weight, and disease, and is the most difficult component to measure. Because of the dramatic consequences of dehydration (both personal and for the health care system), estimated to be responsible for 5% of hospital expenditure, diagnosis and treatment of hydration disorders should be a priority. The dramatic heat wave in the summer of 2003 in France showed the vulnerability of elderly people to extreme heat. Elderly people are exposed to an increased risk of dehydration for many reasons.

Water reserve in elderly persons is lower than in younger adults. Most water is contained in fat-free mass weight and represents approximately 70% to 75% of lean mass. A small amount is contained in the fat mass (5%–10%). Because the lean mass decreases with age (see above), total body water reserve decreases. This is even more the case when malnutrition occurs because of the changes in muscle mass.

The ratio of intracellular to extracellular water remains constant during healthy aging, although absolute quantities decrease. During disease, there is an expansion of the extracellular space at the expanse of the intracellular space. This means that in addition to a natural reduction in water reserve with aging, there is an added impairment in the repartition of water between its reserves during disease.

Elderly people have an impaired sensation of thirst, which is the main drive to drink fluids. In young adults the threshold for thirst is approximately 294 mOsm/L. It increases to 297 to 300 mOsm/L in the healthy elderly, whereas the amount to drink to quench thirst is lower in the elderly.[35] In the case of mild dehydration, elderly people are therefore less able to compensate with adequate fluid intake.

These modifications in thirst are minimal in healthy elderly persons but are always present in patients with neurologic disorders (Alzheimer's disease and other dementias; stroke). Furthermore, handicapped persons may not have easy access to water and may have impaired vision and communication skills. Sedative drugs impair the desire to drink. The fear of incontinence is another reason elderly persons may avoid drinking water.

Reduction in food intake is a disregarded cause of water shortage. It is estimated that 1000 kcal provides 400 mL of water (100 mL for an apple or a yogurt), whereas oxidation of macronutrients produces a significant amount of water (1.4 g/g fat and 0.6 g/g of glucose). It is therefore obvious that a reduction in appetite (naturally occurring with age or promoted by disease) is a risk factor for dehydration.

The kidneys play a key role in water retention. With aging, the maximal capacity to concentrate urine is reduced. After a 12-hour water deprivation, urine osmolarity is approximately 1200 mOsm/L in a young adult, whereas it is only 800 mOsm/L in a healthy elderly person. This is because the number of active nephrons decreases, which reduces the glomerular filtration rate by half between 20 and 70 years of age. There is also a decrease in the gradient between maximal and minimal values of osmolarity along the nephrons. In the elderly, despite an increased capacity to secrete antidiuretic hormone in response to hypovolemia (or hyperosmolarity), there seems to be a resistance to vasopressin.

During disease, water losses may be increased (diarrhea, vomiting, diuretic treatment, fever). It is estimated that water losses are increased by 300 mL per degree of central temperature greater than 38°C.

Because water spaces are difficult to measure, it is difficult to accurately diagnose hydration disorders. Diagnosis still relies on clinical symptoms that are neither specific nor precise. The state-of-the-art technique for the measurement of water space is tracer dilution, but this requires multiple sampling and time (minimum 4–5 hours for total body water), which is not compatible with the necessity to treat patients in a timely manner. Bioelectrical impedance analysis is an easy means of measuring body water spaces, but has attracted debate. We can say that valid equations have been proposed in the elderly (healthy or with disease).[36,37] However precise the measurements are, there is no database of theoretic values with which to compare observations. Until this database is produced and distributions of water spaces are known, there is no way for a measurement to be compared with theoretic values, therefore impeding any therapeutic evaluation. Until then we are left with clinical symptoms and treatment based on experience.

Conclusion

Sarcopenia predisposes to functional impairment and loss of autonomy. Anorexia and metabolic consequences of disease further impair muscle mass and function. A vicious circle appears with a step-by-step decline. Most strategies to improve food intake lead to an increase in fat mass; very few improve lean mass. Physical training may be an alternative because it is possible until a very old age[34] and has a positive interaction with improved nutrition,[38] but it should be used with caution. Hormonal treatment may be considered. A preventive attitude to promote lifelong physical activity and to correct any change in weight is recommended. Many factors contribute to hydration disorders. Today, the main barrier preventing an improvement in the quality of professional practices is the inability to define the ideal water composition of an individual. Until then, there is no way to improve care for hydration disorders with a scientifically based evaluation.

Effects of Nutritional Deficiencies on the Older Population

Nutrition and Longevity

As Heilbronn and Ravussin noted,[39] caloric restriction is the most robust and reproducible means of slowing aging, extending lifespan, and retarding age-related chronic diseases in a variety of species, including rats, mice, fish, flies, and yeast. The mechanisms by which this occurs are unclear. Caloric restriction reduces metabolic rate in oxidative stress, improves insulin sensitivity, and alters neuroendocrine and sympathic nervous system function in animals. Whether prolonged caloric restriction increases lifespan (or improves biomarkers of aging) in humans is unknown. In experiments of nature, humans have been subjected to periods of nonvolitional partial starvation. However, in almost all of these cases the diets were of poor quality. The absence of adequate information on the effects of good-quality, calorie-restricted diets in non-obese humans reflects the difficulties involved in conducting long-term studies in an environment that promotes overfeeding. Such studies in free-living persons also raise ethical and methodologic issues. Future studies in non-obese humans should focus on the effects of prolonged caloric restriction on metabolic rate, neuroendocrine adaptations, diverse biomarkers of aging, and predictors of chronic age-related diseases.

Nutrition and Frailty

It is thought that between 10% and 25% of people aged 65 years and more are frail, with the proportions increasing dramatically with increasing age; after age 85, 46% of those living in the community are frail.[40] The most widely agreed-on definition of frailty is the age-related physiologic vulnerability resulting from impaired homeostatic reserve and the reduced capacity of the organism to withstand stress.[40] Frail individuals are older persons with a higher risk of falls, injuries, acute illness, hospitalization, slow recovery, dependency, institutionalization, and mortality. Signs of frailty include weight loss, weakness, fatigue, inactivity, decreased food intake, sarcopenia, balance and gait abnormalities, and decreased bone mass. There is evidence that aging is associated with a decreased ability to appropriately modulate food intake to match total energy expenditure, and thus an increased likelihood of inadequate dietary intakes.[40] Energy intake lower than energy requirement in frail elderly persons can lead to a state of chronic protein-energy malnutrition. This chronic state increases the loss of lean body mass (or sarcopenia), contributes to the loss of muscle strength, and increases the risk of falls and fractures.

Nutrition and Cognitive Decline

Alzheimer's disease has major consequences on nutritional status. Among the complications of the disease, weight loss is frequent and occurs in approximately 40% of patients at all stages, including even the early stages before diagnosis is possible.[14] Malnutrition contributes to the alteration of general status, the frequency and gravity of complications (especially infectious), and a faster loss of independence. These states of malnutrition can be prevented or at least improved if an early intervention strategy is instituted, but management must be rapid and appropriate.[41] Weight loss is a phenomenon for which kinetics may vary, as observed in clinical practice. It can be a dramatic loss of several kilograms in a few months or a more moderate but continuous loss as the disease progresses. In a recent study,[42] two distinct modes of weight loss in Alzheimer's disease were identified in a large population with different risk factors: a progressive loss related to the evolution and worsening of Alzheimer's disease, and a rapid loss often related to concurrent medical or social events. Because the prognosis of these two modes of weight loss may be different, with nutritional support probably useless if too late in the former and necessary in the latter, a rigorous, early, and regular follow-up of nutritional variables is mandatory in patients with Alzheimer's disease.

On the other hand, correlations have been found between nutritional intakes and cognitive function for 10 years.[43] The theory underlying research on nutrition and Alzheimer's disease relates to free radicals. Peroxidation of membrane polyunsaturated fatty acids after damage by free radicals could be involved in brain deterioration and cause alteration of enzyme activity, transport functions, and receptor-ligand interaction, as well as loss of membrane lipid bilayer asymmetry and thus of membrane fluidity. Such changes may alter ion channels and neurotransmitter transport and thus be an underlying cause of brain dysfunction. Vitamins A, C, and E, and minerals such as zinc or selenium could thus play a protective role in Alzheimer's disease through their antioxidant properties. Morris et al.[44] performed a longitudinal study of 2889 elderly subjects (mean age 74 years) who completed a food-frequency questionnaire between 1993 and 2000 (mean follow-up 3.2 years). A cognitive study was carried out at 3 years with neuropsychologic tests. In subjects with the greatest intake of vitamin E, whether from foods or supplements (highest quintile), there was a 36% reduction in the rate of cognitive decline compared with subjects in the lowest quintile ($P = .05$). Vitamins A and C did not have a protective effect. A recent interventional study[45] concluded that vitamin E had no benefit in patients with mild cognitive impairment. The rate of progression to Alzheimer's disease after 3 years was not lower among patients treated with vitamin E than among those given placebo. These results have to be confirmed.

Another element that may enable prevention through nutrition is the vascular determinant. Alzheimer's disease and vascular lesions are found in association more frequently than would be the case by chance. The brains of patients without dementia who died of coronary disease were found to contain more senile plaque than the brains of patients who died of other causes.[46] The most recent works implicate homocysteine as a probable risk factor for Alzheimer's disease through microvascular lesions. Interesting results were obtained in the largest and longest study carried out on the subject, the Framingham study.[47] A total of 1092 subjects without dementia (667 women and 425 men with a mean age of 76 years) were followed for a mean of 8 years with a Mini-Mental State examination every 6 months and a battery of neuropsychologic tests yearly. Measurements of plasma homocysteine, vitamins B_6 and B_{12}, and folate were taken and apolipoprotein E typing was performed. At the end of the follow-up, dementia had developed in 111 patients, 83 of whom had Alzheimer's disease. The results showed that plasma homocysteine levels greater than 14 μmol/L were an independent risk factor for Alzheimer's disease (relative risk [RR] 1.9; confidence interval [CI] 1.3–2.8). This relation was strong and proportional. Seshadri et al.[47] found that a 5 μmol/L increase in plasma homocysteine increased the risk of Alzheimer's disease by 40% ($P < .001$), with no effect of sex or age. On the other hand, serum levels of vitamins B_6 and B_{12} and folate did not seem to be independent risk factors. Elevated plasma homocysteine thus seems to be significantly involved in the development and progression of Alzheimer's disease. In addition, arterial hypertension, diabetes, and hypercholesterolemia are factors not only of vascular dementia but also of Alzheimer's disease. In the Rotterdam study,[48] increased total fatty acid intake was a risk factor for dementia (RR 2.4; CI 1.1–5.2), as was increased saturated fatty acid intake (RR 1.9; CI 0.9–3.2). High consumption of fish, an important source of n-3 unsaturated fatty acids, decreased the risk of dementia (RR 0.4; CI 0.2–0.9). In a prospective study in Finland of 1449 volunteers ages 65 to 79 years with a mean follow-up of 21 years Kivipelto et al.[49] studied among other parameters the initial total cholesterol level, systolic blood pressure, apolipoprotein E genetic typing, and development of Alzheimer's disease. Fifty-seven participants (4%) were diagnosed with dementia at the follow-up visit at 11, 16, 21, or 26 years. Forty-eight participants fulfilled the criteria for possible Alzheimer's disease. It should be noted that 82 participants (6.1%) were classified with mild cognitive impairment, but were not taken into account in the rest of the study. Results showed that elevated total cholesterol (>6.5 mmol/L) was a risk factor for Alzheimer's disease (odds ratio 2.8; CI 1.2–6.7), as was elevated systolic blood pressure (odds ratio 2.6; CI 1.1–6.6). It is now time to institute large interventional studies to validate these hypotheses. Some studies are already under way, and some conclusions are available. Others are in preparation. Such studies are cumbersome and costly to set up, but are indispensable as long as we are confronted with a public health scourge as devastating as Alzheimer's disease. If nutritional intervention is found to have the impact we hope for, it will then be put into general use, fulfilling the aim of prevention that is so sought after in modern health systems. A policy of nutritional advice similar to that proposed to patients at risk of cardiovascular disease could then be envisaged.

Nutrient Requirements for Older Adults

Nutritional status is very different in elderly people in good health compared with elderly people with severe diseases or who are frail. Several factors contribute to an increased risk for nutrient deficiencies in people more than 60 years of age.[50] Mineral and vitamin deficiencies are also more frequent. Inadequate vitamin D and calcium intakes are well documented in elderly persons.[50] Other vitamin deficiencies are frequently related to overall poor nutritional intake. Chronic medication use can significantly affect the nutritional status of older adults and increase the potential for drug-nutrient interactions. Poor nutritional status, in turn, can alter drug use, absorption, and metabolism. Thus, nutritional recommendations for the elderly must not only prevent nutrient deficiencies, but also prevent or delay the development of chronic disease.

An excellent review by Russell and Rasmussen[50] provides reliable information about macronutrient and micronutrient requirements for elderly individuals and is recommended for readers who want to pursue this topic further.

The Dietary Reference Intake recommendations for vitamin D, calcium, and vitamin B_6 are higher for older people than for younger adults.[50] Studies examining vitamin D nutriture and metabolism suggest that current intakes are low in the majority of elderly people. Increased sun exposure during the summer months and the consumption of vitamin D-fortified food may help to improve overall vitamin D nutriture. The prevalence of poor vitamin B_6 status in elderly people is high, consistently found in different populations, and caused mainly by low dietary intakes. Calcium differs from most other minerals in that the plasma calcium concentration is not a guide to an individual's calcium nutriture. The quantification of bone density itself might provide a criterion of nutritional calcium status. However, the wide individual variation in bone density, along with hormonal and other factors, affects bone density. Recommendations for calcium intake in postmenopausal women are now higher than in the past, approaching 1200 to 1500 mg/d.

In regard to protein intakes in the elderly, the Dietary Reference Intake of 0.8 g of protein/kg body wt/d seems adequate even though it is still a much-debated issue; some elderly individuals continue to lose muscle mass even when receiving 0.8 g of protein/kg body wt/d. That is why the Toulouse group suggested that an ideal protein intake for the elderly should be 1 to 1.2 g of protein/kg body wt/d.[51] The requirements of elderly persons who are sick are higher (1.2–1.5 g/kg body wt/d.

One of the great challenges in the future will be to define nutritional recommendations during all stages of life for better health in the elderly by preventing chronic disease and preserving functional status.

References

1. Hoyert DL, Kung HC, Smith BC. Deaths: preliminary data for 2003. Natl Vital Stat Rep. 2005;53: 1–48.
2. United States Bureau of the Census. *Statistical Abstract of the United States: ed 2000.* US Government Printing Office; Washington DC: 2000.
3. Rubenstein LZ. Assessment instruments. In: Abrams WB, Berkow R (eds). *The Merck Manual of Geriatrics.* Rahway NJ: Merck Sharp & Dohme Research Laboratories, Division of Merck & Co; 1990:1189–2000.
4. Katz S. Assessing self maintenance: activities of daily living, mobility and instrumental activities of daily living. J Am Geriatr Soc. 1983;31:721–727.
5. Lawton MP, Brody EM. Assessment of older people: self-maintaining and instrumental activities of daily living. Gerontologist. 1969;9:179–186.
6. Folstein MF, Folstein SE, McHugh PR, et al. 'Mini-mental test'. A practical method for grading the cognitive state of patients for the clinician. J Psychiatry Res. 1975;12:189–198.
7. Yesavage J, Brink T, Rose T, et al. Development and validation of a geriatric depression screening scale: a preliminary report. J Psychiatr Res. 1983;17:37–49.
8. Tinetti ME. Performance-oriented assessment of mobility problems in the elderly. J Am Geriatr Soc. 1986;36:613–616.
9. Hugues VA, Roubenoff R, Wood M, et al. Anthropometric assessment of 10-years changes in body composition in the elderly. Am J Clin Nutr. 2004; 80:475–482.
10. Vellas B, Guigoz Y, Baumgartner M, et al. Relationships between nutritional markers and the Mini-Nutritional Assessment in 155 older persons. J Am Geriatr Soc. 2000;48:1300–1309.
11. Evaluation diagnostique de la dénutrition protéino-énergétique chez les adultes hospitalises. Agence Nationale pour l'Evaluation en Santé (ANAES): data for 2003, September.
12. Lesourd B, Mazari L. Nutrition and immunity in the elderly. Proc Nutr Soc. 1999;58:685–695.
13. Walrand S, Moreau K, Caldefie F, et al. Specific and nonspecific immune responses to fasting and refeeding differ in healthy young adult and elderly persons. Am J Clin Nutr. 2001;74:670–678.
14. Wallace JI, Schwartz RS, LaCroix AZ, Uhlmann RF, Pearlman RA. Involuntary weight loss in older outpatients: incidence and clinical significance. J Am Geriatr Soc. 1995;43:329–337.

15. Dambach B, Salle A, Marteau C, et al. Energy requirements are not greater in elderly patients suffering from pressure ulcers. J Am Geriatr Soc. 2004;53: 478–482.
16. Tucker HN, Miguel SG. Cost containment through nutrition intervention. Nutr Rev. 1996;54:111–121.
17. Schneider SM, Al-Jaouni R, Pivot X, et al. Lack of adaptation to severe malnutrition in elderly patients. Clin Nutr. 2002;21:499–504.
18. Roberts SB. Regulation of energy intake in relation to metabolic state and nutritional status. Eur J Clin Nutr. 2000;54(Suppl 3):S64–S69.
19. Bales CW, Ritchie CS. Sarcopenia, weight loss, and nutritional frailty in the elderly. Annu Rev Nutr. 2002; 22:309–323.
20. Irvine P, Mouzet JB, Marteau C, et al. Short-term effect of a protein load on appetite and food intake in diseased mildly undernourished elderly people. Clin Nutr. 2004;23:1146–1152.
21. Blanc S, Schoeller DA, Bauer D, et al. Energy requirements in the eighth decade of life. Am J Clin Nutr. 2004;79:303–310.
22. Kennedy RL, Chokkalingham K, Srinivasan R. Obesity in the elderly: who should be treating, and why, and how? Curr Opin Clin Nutr Metab Care. 2004; 7:3–9.
23. Jensen GL, Roy MA, Buchanan AE, et al. Weight loss intervention for obese older women: improvements in performance and function. Obes Res. 2004; 12:1814–1820.
24. Rolland Y, Lauwers-Cances V, Pahor M, et al. Muscle strength in obese elderly women: effect of recreational physical activity in a cross-sectional study. Am J Clin Nutr. 2004;79:552–557.
25. Stanga Z, Allison S, Vandewoude M. Nutrition in the elderly. In: Sobotka L, ed. *Basic in Clinical Nutrition, 3rd ed.* Galen. 2005:363–383.
26. Gustafson D, Rothenberg E, Blennow K, et al. An 18-year follow-up of overweight and risk of Alzheimer disease. Arch Intern Med. 2003;163: 1524–1528.
27. Baumgartner RN, Koehler KM, Gallagher D, et al. Epidemiology of sarcopenia among the elderly in New Mexico. Am J Epidemiol. 1998;147:755–763.
28. Janssen I, Heymsfield SB, Ross R. Low relative skeletal muscle mass (sarcopenia) in older persons is associated with functional impairment and physical disability. J Am Geriatr Soc. 2002;50:889–896.
29. Janssen I, Baumgartner RN, Ross R, et al. Skeletal muscle cutpoints associated with elevated physical disability risk in older men and women. Am J Epidemiol. 2004;159:413–421.
30. Proctor DN, Balagopal P, Nair KS. Age-related sarcopenia in humans is associated with reduced synthetic rates of specific muscle protein. J Nutr. 1998; 128(2 Suppl):351S–355S.
31. Roubenoff R. Catabolism of aging: is it an inflammatory process? Curr Opin Clin Nutr Metab Care. 2003;6:295–299.
32. Leeuwenburgh C. Role of apoptosis in sarcopenia. J Gerontol A Biol Sci Med Sci. 2003;58:999–1001.
33. Bhasin S. Testosterone supplementation for aging-associated sarcopenia. J Gerontol A Biol Sci Med Sci. 2003;58:1002–1008.
34. Latham NK, Bennett DA, Stretton CM, et al. Systematic review of progressive resistance strength training in older adults. J Gerontol A Biol Sci Med Sci. 2004;59:48–61.
35. Phillips PA, Rolls BJ, Ledingham JG, et al. Reduced thirst after water deprivation in healthy elderly men. N Engl J Med. 1984;311:753–759.
36. Ritz P: Investigators of the Source Study and of the Human Nutrition Research Centre-Auverne. Chronic cellular dehydration in the aged patient. J Gerontol A Biol Sci Med Sci. 2001;56: M349–M352.
37. Ritz P. Bioelectrical impedance analysis estimation of water compartments in elderly diseased patients: the source study. J Gerontol A Biol Sci Med Sci. 2001;56:M344–M348.
38. Ritz P. Factors affecting energy and macronutrient requirements in elderly people. Public Health Nutr. 2001;4:561–568.
39. Heilbronn LK, Ravussin E. Calorie restriction and aging: review of the literature and implications for studies in humans. Am J Clin Nutr. 2003;78: 361–369.
40. Fried LP, Watson J. Frailty and failure to thrive. In: Hazzard WR, Blass JP, Ettinger WH, et al, eds. *Principles of Geriatric Medicine and Gerontology, 4th ed.* New-York: McGraw Hill; 1998:1387–1402.
41. Rivière S, Gillette-Guyonnet S, Voisin T, et al. A nutritional education program could prevent weight loss and slow cognitive decline in Alzheimer's disease. J Nutr Health Aging. 2001;5:295–299.
42. Guerin O, Andrieu S, Schneider SM, et al. Different modes of weight loss in Alzheimer disease: a prospective study of 395 patients. Am J Clin Nutr. 2005;82: 435–441.
43. La Rue A, Koehler KM, Wayne S, et al. Nutritional status and cognitive functioning in a normally aging sample: a 6-y reassessment. Am J Clin Nutr. 1996; 65:20–29.
44. Morris MC, Evans D, Bienias J, et al. Vitamin E and cognitive decline in older persons. Arch Neurol. 2002;59:1125–1132.
45. Petersen RC, Thomas RG, Grundman M, et al. Vitamin E and donepezil for the treatment of mild cognitive impairment. N Engl J Med. 2005;352: 2439–2441.
46. Sparks DL, Hunsaker JC, Scheff SW, et al. Cortical senile plaques in coronary artery disease, aging and Alzheimer's disease. Neurobiol Aging. 1990;11:601–607.

47. Seshadri S, Beiser A, Selhub J, et al. Plasma homocysteine as a risk factor for dementia and Alzheimer's disease. N Engl J Med. 2002;346:476–483.
48. Engelhart MJ, Geerlings MI, Ruitenberg A, et al. Diet and risk of dementia: does fat matter? The Rotterdam Study. Neurology. 2002;59:1915–1921.
49. Kivipelto M, Helkala EL, Laakso M, et al. ApoE4, elevated midlife total cholesterol level, and high midlife systolic blood pressure are independent risk factors for late-life Alzheimer disease. Ann Intern Med. 2002;137:149–155.
50. Russell RM, Rasmussen H. The impact of nutritional needs of older adults on recommended food intakes. Nutr Clin Care. 1999;2:164–176.
51. Nicolas AS, Faisant C, Nourhashemi F, et al. The nutritional intake of a free-living healthy French population: a four-year follow-up. J Nutr Health Aging. 2000;4:77–80.

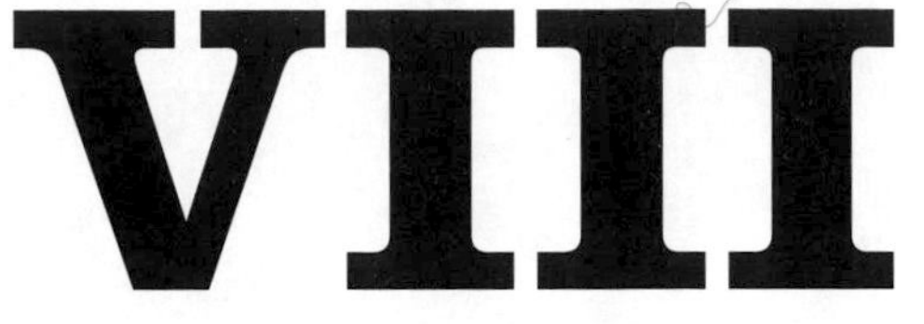

VIII Nutritional Immunity

45

Nutrient Regulation of the Immune Response: The Case of Vitamin E

Simin Nikbin Meydani and Sung Nim Han

The influence of nutrition on immune function was recognized in the early 1800s by Menkel when he described the thymic atrophy associated with severe malnutrition. Discovery of vitamins in the early 1900s was followed by reports on their contribution to host defenses, including immune responses.[1] These early observations were continued in several laboratories by the use of more advanced immunologic techniques. Vitamin E is perhaps the most studied nutrient related to the immune response. Evidence accumulated over the years and in many species indicates that vitamin E is an essential nutrient for the normal function of the immune system. Furthermore, results from several studies suggest that beneficial effects of certain nutrients, such as vitamin E on reducing disease risk, might be through their effects on the immune response. In this chapter, the regulatory roles of nutrients on immune function and their clinical significance will be discussed using vitamin E as an example.

Overview of the Immune System and Immunologic Methods

The immune system is a complex system involving various cells and lymphoid organs. Lymphoid organs can be classified as central (or primary) lymphoid organs—where lymphocytes arise and mature—and peripheral (or secondary) lymphoid organs—where mature lymphocytes respond to foreign antigens. Central lymphoid organs include bone marrow (where B and T lymphocytes originate and B lymphocytes mature) and the thymus (where T lymphocytes mature). Peripheral lymphoid organs include lymph nodes, the spleen, gut-associated lymphoid tissues such as tonsils, Peyer patches, adenoids, and the appendix. The immune system comprises different types of cells, including lymphocytes, granulocytes, and monocytes.

Lymphocytes (B and T lymphocytes and natural killer [NK] cells) are the major players of the immune response. B lymphocytes, when activated, differentiate into plasma cells that secrete antibodies. T lymphocytes can be subdivided into cytotoxic T lymphocytes (CTLs), which are recognized by surface protein marker CD8, and T helper cells, which are recognized by protein marker CD4. CTLs kill cells infected with viruses and tumor cells. T helper cells can be further divided into T helper 1 (Th1) and T helper 2 (Th2) cells according to their cytokine production. Interferon (IFN)-γ is the signature cytokine of Th1 cells, and Th1 cells mainly promote cellular immunity and activate macrophages. Th2 cells produce interleukin-4 (IL-4), IL-5, and IL–10 and promote humoral immune responses by stimulating B-cell growth and differentiation. NK cells (also called large granular lymphocytes) can lyse tumor cells and virus-infected cells without overt antigenic stimulation. Granulocytes containing abundant cytoplasmic granules are classified into three types according to the staining characteristics of the predominant granules: neutrophils, basophils, and eosinophils. Monocytes circulate in the blood and differentiate into macrophages once they have migrated to tissues. Macrophages play an important role in the innate immune response as phagocytes and in the inflammatory response by producing soluble molecules such as cytokine, prostaglandins, and nitric oxide.

Immune responses are classified as innate and specific (or acquired) immune responses. The innate immune response provided by phagocytes—macrophages and neutrophils—and NK cells is a first line of defense against many common microorganisms. Phagocytes engulf and digest many microorganisms to combat a wide range of bacteria. In innate immune responses, there is no discrimination among foreign substances (lack of specificity) and prior exposure does not enhance subsequent exposure (lack of memory). Specific immune response is mediated by lymphocytes and provides long-term protection against specific antigens. Specific immune responses are classified into two types based on the components of the immune system that mediate the responses: humoral immunity is mediated by antibodies produced by plasma cells (effector cells of B lymphocytes) and cell-mediated immunity is mediated by T lymphocytes. In humoral immune responses, antibodies eliminate extracellular microbes; in cell-mediated immune responses, T lymphocytes activate macrophages to kill intracellular microbes or CTLs are activated to destroy viral-infected or tumor cells.

Various techniques are used to measure immune responses and to understand their underlying mechanisms. Immune response can be determined in vitro using specific immune cells by evaluating the different cytokines produced, the ability of immune cells to proliferate in response to antigens or mitogens, their ability to kill target cells, and their ability to help other immune cells. Immune status is evaluated in vivo by determining protection or resistance against challenge with infections, antibody response after vaccination, delayed type hypersensitivity (DTH) reactions, and phenotypic enumeration of lymphocyte subpopulations.

The lymphocyte proliferation assay is the most commonly used technique for evaluating cell-mediated immunity. Although this assay can provide information related to overall immunologic competence, it provides little information about the functional capabilities of the responding cells. In this assay, polyclonal mitogens (e.g., phytohemagglutinin [PHA], concanavalin A [ConA], pokeweed mitogen, lipopolysaccharide [LPS]), anti-CD3, or direct triggering of intracellular activation pathways with phorbol ester and calcium ionophore are used to initiate the growth response; proliferating lymphocytes are then quantitated by measuring incorporation of [^{3}H]thymidine. These stimuli induce many or all lymphocytes of a given type to proliferate, and therefore the response of a heterogeneous population of cells is measured.

Determination of types and amounts of cytokines produced can provide information about the potential effector mechanisms of T cells (functional capabilities) and inflammatory responses of the host over the course of a disease. For example, the quantity of IL-2 synthesized is an important determinant of the magnitude of the T-cell-dependent immune response. Cytokines are hormone-like soluble proteins produced by different cell types that are involved in growth and differentiation of lymphocytes, communication between cells, and regulation of immune and inflammatory responses. Many cytokines have been discovered; those often used in studying the effects of nutrition on immune responses are briefly described in Table 1. Levels of cytokines can be determined by bioassay, radioimmunoassay, or enzyme-linked immunosorbent assay.

The effector function of CTLs can be determined by the ^{51}Cr release assay, which measures the ability of CTLs to kill target cells radioactively labeled with sodium chromate. CTLs kill target cells on the basis of cell-surface antigen recognition. The development and activity of

Table 1. Functions of Selected Cytokines Commonly Measured in Nutritional Immunology

Cytokine	Cell Source	Functions
IL-2	T cells	T-cell growth
IFN-γ	Th1 cells, CTLs, NK cells	Activation of macrophages and NK cells
		Antiviral activity
		B-cell differentiation
IL-4	Th2 cells	Production of IgE by B cells
		Inhibition of macrophage activation
		Growth and differentiation of Th2 cells
IL-1α or IL-1β	Macrophages, epithelial and endothelial cells	Mediation of local inflammation
		Induction of acute phase response
TNF-α	Macrophages, T cells, NK cells	Activation of macrophages and induction of nitric oxide production
		Induction of acute phase response
IL-6	Macrophages, T cells, vascular endothelial cells, fibroblasts, etc.	T- and B-cell growth and differentiation
		Induction of acute phase response

IL, interleukin; Th1, T helper 1; IFN, interferon; CTL, cytotoxic T lymphocyte; NK, natural killer; IgE, immunoglobulin E; Th2, T helper 2; TNF, tumor necrosis factor.

CTLs against specific pathogens can be detected by the use of appropriate target cells.

The fluorescence-activated cell sorter is a powerful tool for defining and enumerating the lymphocyte population. Each lymphocyte can be identified with the use of fluorescent dyes. Size and granularity of lymphocytes, changes in lymphocyte population, developmental stages of lymphocytes, cellular production of cytokines, and cell cycle status can be determined by fluorescence-activated cell sorter analysis.

The DTH response has been widely used to assess cell-mediated immunity in vivo. When small amounts of antigens are injected into subcutaneous tissue, a T-cell-mediated local inflammatory reaction occurs over 24 to 72 hours after the challenge, resulting in local skin swelling, erythema, and induration. The intensity of the DTH reaction is determined by measuring the diameter of the induration area and the number of positive responses to different antigens. In animal models, antigens are injected subcutaneously into the footpad of a previously challenged animal and the extent of footpad swelling is measured with a caliper.

B lymphocytes contribute to acquired immunity by secreting antibodies, and the in vivo response of B cells is often determined by analyzing specific antibody production after immunization. Antibody response to most antigens requires help from antigen-specific T cells. However, some antigens, such as bacterial polysaccharides, can directly induce B cells to produce antibody in the absence of help from T cells. Therefore, depending on the type of antigen used—T-cell dependent or independent—analysis of antibody production can also provide information on the functional capabilities of T cells.

Nutrient Regulation of the Immune Response

Nutritional deficiency leads to increased susceptibility to infection because of the effect on immune function. In humans, malnutrition usually includes deficiencies of several nutrients and rarely deficiency of a single nutrient. However, the effect of individual nutrient deficiencies on immune function has been reported with the use of animal models and clinical studies. Nutrients reported to affect immune function include zinc, iron, selenium, copper, magnesium, folic acid, β-carotene, and vitamins A, B_6, B_{12}, C, D, and E. The effects of zinc, iron, selenium, copper, and vitamins A, B_6, C, D, and E on immune function have been extensively studied. Detailed review articles are available on the effects of zinc,[2] iron,[3] selenium,[4] copper,[5] β-carotene,[6] vitamin B_6,[7,8] vitamin C,[9,10] and vitamin D,[11] and several books include in-depth information on individual nutrients and immune function.[12,13] Effects of deficiencies of some individual nutrients on immune functions are summarized in Table 2.

Vitamin E Deficiency Impairs Immune Response

Studies with different species of experimental animals indicate that vitamin E deficiency impairs both humoral and cell-mediated immune functions. Immunologic changes observed in animals with vitamin E deficiency include lower antibody response to sheep red blood cells (SRBCs),[14,15] depressed lymphocyte response to mitogens,[16] and impaired chemotaxis in response to bacterial culture filtrate.[17]

Tengerdy et al.[14] showed that vitamin-E-deficient mice had fewer plaque-forming cells and a lower hemagglutination titer in response to SRBC injection than did mice fed a diet containing vitamin E at 50 to 60 mg/kg diet. The addition of vitamin E (2035 mg/kg diet) to the diet significantly increased the response to SRBCs. A lower response to SRBCs in vitamin-E-deficient mice was reportedly due to impaired accessory cell function.[15] Macrophages from vitamin-E-deficient mice expressed less Ia antigen and acted as suppressor cells. The effect of vitamin E deficiency on cell-mediated immune response was demonstrated in experiments in which lymphocyte proliferation in response to T-cell mitogens (ConA and PHA) was shown to be depressed in vitamin-E-deficient rats.[16] F344 rats fed a vitamin-E-deficient diet for 7 weeks had significantly fewer thymocytes, lower mitogenic response to PHA and ConA, and lower IL-2 production.[18] Vitamin E deficiency also affected phagocyte function and bactericidal activity. Polymorphonuclear cells from peritoneal exudates of vitamin-E-deficient rats showed lower chemotactic and ingestive activities.[17] Furthermore, vitamin E deficiency augmented the adverse effect of prolonged low-level exposure to ozone on pulmonary bactericidal capacity.[19] Recently, vitamin E deficiency was shown to increase the virulence of the otherwise amyocarditic strain of coxsackievirus.[20] This increase in virulence was shown to be due to specific nucleotide changes in the viral genome in the vitamin-E-deficient host.

In contrast to the well-documented need for vitamin E in the maintenance of immune function in animals, limited studies have evaluated the effect of vitamin E deficiency in humans. The immune response is seldom mentioned when manifestations of vitamin E in humans are described, mainly because in humans, except for premature low-birth-weight infants, a primary severe deficiency of vitamin E rarely occurs. However, a secondary deficiency of vitamin E does occur in subjects with certain diseases such as primary biliary cirrhosis,[21] chronic cholestasis,[22] cystic fibrosis,[23] and intestinal fat malabsorption.[24] Unfortunately, when Horwitt's group[25,26] conducted the most extensive study of the effect of vitamin E deficiency in humans, a comprehensive evaluation of immune response was not performed. Furthermore, most studies of vitamin E deficiency secondary to other causes have focused on red blood cell hemolysis and neurologic

Table 2. Nutrient Deficiency and Immune Function

Nutrient Deficiency	Effects of Deficiency on Immune Function	Possible Mechanism	References
Protein-energy malnutrition	Thymic atrophy ↓ DTH ↓ No. of rosette-forming T lymphocytes ↓ NK activity	Unavailability of essential nutrients; altered metabolism	Cunningham-Rundles, 1982[93]
Vitamin B_6 deficiency	↓ Antibody response ↓ DTH ↓ IL-1β, IL-2, IL-2 receptor ↓ NK activity ↓ Lymphocyte proliferation	Effects on rate of production of 1-carbon units and capabilities to synthesize nucleic acids and proteins; serine-hydroxymethyl transferase is B_6-dependent enzyme	Chandra and Sudhakaran, 1990[7]; Trakatellis et al.,1997[8]
Copper deficiency	↓ DTH ↓ Lymphocyte proliferation ↓ T-cell–dependent production of antibody ↓ IL-2 production ↓ IL-2 mRNA Neutropenia	Effects on copper-dependent cellular antioxidant enzymes that affect transcriptional factors sensitive to redox status	Failla and Hopkins, 1998[5]
Iron deficiency	↓ Lymphoid cell development ↓ NK activity ↓ IL-1 production ↓ DTH ↓ Bactericidal capacity	Effects on enzymes such as mitochondrial aconitase and ribonucleotide reductase of which iron is a cofactor; effects on production of reactive oxygen species	Dallman, 1987[3]
Selenium deficiency	↓ IgG, IgM titers ↓ Antibody production ↓ Neutrophil chemotaxis ↑ Virulence of coxsackievirus	Antioxidant	McKenzie et al., 1998[4]; Turner and Finch, 1991[94]; Spallhoz et al., 1990[95]
Zinc deficiency	Thymic activity (↓ Thymulin activity) Depletion of developing B cells in marrow ↓ T- and B-cell proliferation ↓ DTH ↓ NK activity ↓ IL-2, IFNγ production Impaired chemotactic response	Effects on activity of enzymes involved in replication and transcription, binding of NF-κB to DNA	Fraker et al., 2000; Shankar and Prasad, 1998[96]; Fraker and King, 2004[97]

DTH, delayed-type hypersensitivity; IFN, interferon; Ig, immunoglobulin; IL, interleukin; NF, nuclear factor; NK, natural killer.

symptoms of vitamin E deficiency with no attention to immunologic changes. As a result, erythrocyte hemolysis and neurologic function are the most often used markers of vitamin E deficiency.[22,26]

A negative response to DTH skin response, low mitogenic response to PHA and ConA, low IL-2 production, and polyneuropathy were observed in a patient with severe vitamin E deficiency secondary to an intestinal malabsorptive disorder.[24] After vitamin E supplementation by intramuscular injection of vitamin E, mitogenic response and IL-2 production increased significantly and DTH response to three of the antigens became positive (Table 3). In a case report by Adachi et al.,[27] decreased NK activity was observed in a 16-month-old boy with Shwachman syndrome associated with severe vitamin E deficiency. Oral supplementation of 100 mg/d vitamin E for 8 weeks normalized the NK activity, which decreased again when vitamin E supplementation was discontinued for 16 weeks. A lower mitogenic response to pokeweed mitogen and ConA was observed in children with low serum vitamin E levels (<10th percentile) compared with those with higher vitamin E levels (>90th percentile).[28] Although the results obtained from human studies are limited, when put together with extensive and reproduci-

Table 3. Vitamin E Deficiency and the Immune Response in Humans

	Date		
Parameter	**July 7**	**July 14**	**November 14**
Plasma α-tocopherol (μmol/L)	9.3	21	27
Mitogenic response (cpm)			
PHA	846	35,520	54,215
ConA	338	13,125	29,828
IL-2 (U/mL)			
PHA	2.6	114.9	ND
ConA	<1	11.2	ND
DTH (No. of positive responses/total mm induration)	ND	0/0	3/11.5

ConA, concanavalin A; DTH; delayed-type hypersensitivity; IL, interleukin; ND, not determined; PHA, phytohemagglutinin.
Adapted from Kowdley et al., 1992[24]; copyright 1992, with permission from the American Gastroenterological Association.

ble data from different animal species, they strongly indicate that impairment of immune function should be included among the biologic effects of vitamin E deficiency.

Vitamin E Supplementation Enhances Immune Function

Dietary supplementation of vitamin E above the recommended levels has been shown to enhance both cell-mediated and humoral immune responses in various species of animals (Table 4). One of the most commonly used in vitro indices of cell-mediated immune response is the proliferative response of lymphocytes to mitogens such as ConA and PHA. Higher lymphocyte proliferation in response to ConA, PHA, or LPS stimulation was observed in rodents fed diets supplemented with vitamin E ranging from 50 to 2500 mg/kg diet.[29-32] Meydani et al.[30] also showed that old mice fed a vitamin-E-supplemented diet (500 mg/kg diet vs. a control diet with 30 mg/kg) for 6 weeks had significantly higher DTH response and IL-2 production and lower immunosuppressive prostaglandin E_2 (PGE_2) production. In a short-term study, young F344 rats were fed diets containing vitamin E at 50 (control group), 100, 250, 500, or 2500 mg/kg diet for 10 days.[31] Lymphocyte responses to PHA, ConA, and LPS, phagocytic activity of alveolar macrophages, and splenic NK activity were measured. Significantly higher lymphocyte responses to ConA were observed in rats fed diets containing >100 mg vitamin E/kg diet compared with the control group. The maximal proliferative response to ConA was observed in rats fed the diet with 500 mg vitamin E/kg diet. The response to PHA was not significantly different among groups. Splenic NK activity and phagocytosis of opsonized SRBCs by alveolar macrophages were higher in animals fed >250 and >100 mg vitamin E/kg diet, respectively. Bendich et al.[29] investigated the requirement of vitamin E for several different parameters in spontaneously hypertensive rats (SHR/NcrlBR). The dietary requirement for optimal lymphocyte response to mitogens was >50 mg/kg diet, which was higher than the requirement for prevention of erythrocyte hemolysis (50 mg/kg), prevention of myopathy (15 mg/kg), or normal growth and spleen-body weight ratio (7.5 mg/kg). In vitro supplementation of vitamin E also influences the mitogenic response of lymphocytes. Beharka et al.[33] showed that in vitro addition of vitamin E increased ConA-stimulated cell proliferation when macrophages from old mice were co-cultured with purified T cells from either old or young mice or when macrophages from young mice were co-cultured with purified T cells from old mice. IL-2 production was also increased with vitamin E supplementation in cocultures of macrophages from old mice and purified T cells from either old or young mice.

Vitamin E supplementation enhances the humoral response. Tanaka et al.[34] showed that vitamin E enhances antibody response to immunization with a hapten-carrier conjugate when mice have been primed with the same carrier. A shift from immunoglobulin M (IgM) to IgG was also reported. Vitamin E can also act as an adjuvant. When added to inactivated and emulsified vaccines, replacing 20% or 30% of mineral oil, vitamin E can induce more rapid and higher antibody response than control vaccines in chicks.[35]

The immunostimulatory effect of vitamin E supplementation was shown to be transferred to the offspring. Chicks fed diets supplemented with vitamin E had significantly higher tetrahydrofuran-stimulated bursal lymphocyte proliferation and higher ConA- and phorbol 12-myristate 13 acetate-stimulated splenic lymphocyte proliferation than did control chicks.[36]

Table 4. Vitamin E Supplementation and Immune Responses in Animals

Species	Dosage and Duration	Results	Reference
Young rats (N = 6/group)	50 or 200 mg/kg diet for 8–10 weeks	↑ Lymphocyte proliferation (ConA, LPS)	Bendich et al., 1986[29]
Old mice (N = 10/group)	500 mg/kg diet for 6 weeks	↑ Lymphocyte proliferation (ConA, LPS) ↑ DTH response ↑ IL-2 production ↓ PGE_2 production	Meydani et al., 1986[30]
Young and old mice (N = 5/group)	500 IU for 9 weeks	↑ Lymphocyte proliferation (ConA) in young ↔ Lymphocyte proliferation (ConA) in old ↑ IFN-γ in young under restraint stress ↔ IFN-γ in old under restraint stress	Wakikawa et al., 1999[98]
Young rats (N = 10/group)	50, 100, 250, 500, or 2500 mg/kg diet for 7 days	↑ Lymphocyte proliferation (>100 mg/kg diet, ConA) (>250 mg/kg diet, LPS) ↑ NK activity (>250 mg/kg diet)	Moriguchi et al., 1990[31]
Old rats (N = 5/group)	585 mg/kg diet for 12 months	↑ Lymphocyte proliferation (ConA, PHA) ↑ IL-2 production	Sakai and Moriguchi, 1997[32]
Young calves (N = 8/group)	125, 250, or 500 IU/d for 24 weeks	↑ Lymphocyte proliferation (PHA, ConA, pokeweed mitogen) ↑ Antibovine herpesvirus antibody titer to booster in 125–IU/d group	Reddy et al., 1987[99]
Young mice (N = 8/group)	200 mg/kg diet for 6–12 weeks	↑ Antibody response ↑ Helper T-cell activity	Tanaka et al., 1979[34]
Young pigs (N = 10/group)	100,000 IU/ton for 10 weeks	↑ Antibody response to *Escherichia coli*	Ellis and Vorhies, 1976[100]
Mice (N = 10/group)	500 mg/kg diet for 6 months	↓ IL-6 and PGE_2 (unstimulated) production by macrophages ↓ nitric oxide production (LPS) by macrophages	Beharka et al., [44]

ConA, concanavalin A; DTH, delayed-type hypersensitivity; IFN, interferon; IL, interleukin; LPS, lipopolysaccharide; PGE_2, prostaglandin E_2; PHA, phytohemagglutinin.

Over the past 15 years, several double-blind, placebo-controlled trials investigated the effects of vitamin E supplementation on immune functions (Table 5). These studies suggest that vitamin E supplementation is more effective in improving the immune response in elderly subjects, who have a dysregulated immune response, compared with that in young subjects.

Does Vitamin E Enhance Immune Response in the Aged?

Age-associated dysregulation of immune function has been clearly demonstrated in both animals and humans. Immunologic changes observed with aging include a decrease in lymphocyte proliferation, DTH response, and IL-2 production; a shift toward Th2 response; an increase in T cells expressing memory phenotype; a decrease in antibody response to vaccination; and an increase in the production of suppressive factors such as PGE_2.[37,38] T cells are considered to be the immune cells most vulnerable to the deleterious effects of aging. The impairment of T-cell functions—including a decline in T-cell proliferation and IL-2 production—is related to an increase in memory cells and to changes in signal transduction pathways such as defects in immediate calcium mobilization and protein phosphorylation after contact with an activating stimulus. Increased production of immunosuppressive PGE_2 by macrophages has also been shown to contribute to the age-associated decline of T-cell function.[37,39]

Vitamin E supplementation has an immunostimulatory effect in aged mice,[30] rats,[32] and humans.[40-42] In an early study by Meydani et al.,[40] 32 healthy elderly men and women >60 years were supplemented daily with either placebo or 800 mg *dl*-α-tocopheryl acetate for 30

Table 5. Vitamin E Supplementation and Immune Responses in Humans

Subjects	Age	Amount and Duration of Supplementation*	Effects	Reference
Adults and teenagers (N = 18)	25–30; 13–18	300 mg/d for 3 weeks	↓ Lymphocyte proliferation ↔ DTH ↓ Bactericidal activity	Prasad, 1980[47]
Adults (N = 31) and premature infants (N = 10)	24–31	600 mg/d for 3 months† 40 mg/kg body weight for 8–14 days	↓ Chemiluminescence	Okano et al., 1991[53]
Cigarette smokers (N = 60)	33 + 4	900 IU/d for 6 weeks	↓ Chemiluminescence	Richards et al., 1990[52]
Sedentary young and elderly (N = 21)	22–29; 55–74	800 IU/d for 48 days	↓ IL-6 secretion ↓ Exercise-enhanced IL-1β secretion	Cannon et al., 1991[45]
Adults (N = 26)	25–35	233 mg/d for 28 days‡	↑ Lymphocyte proliferation ↑ Total T cells, CD4 T cells ↓ Plasma malondialdehyde ↓ Urinary 8-OHDG	Lee and Wan, 2000[43]
Institutionalized elderly	63–93	200 mg/d for 4 months	↑ Total serum protein; α-2 and β-2 globulin fractions	Ziemlanski et al., 1986[48]
Institutionalized adults and elderly (N = 103)	24–104	200 or 400 mg /d for 6 months	↔ Antibody development to influenza virus	Harman and Miller, 1986[62]
Elderly (N = 32)	≥60	800 mg/d for 30 days	↑ Lymphocyte proliferation ↑ DTH ↑ IL-2 production ↓ PGE_2 production	Meydani et al., 1990[40]
Elderly (N = 88)	≥65	60, 200, or 800 mg/d for 235 days‡	↑ DTH and antibody titer to hepatitis B with 200 and 800 mg	Meydani et al., 1997[41]
Elderly (N = 74)	≥65	100 mg/d for 3 months	↔ Lymphocyte proliferation ↔ IgG, IgA levels	De Waart et al., 1997[46]
Elderly (N = 161)	65–80	50 or 100 mg/d for 6 months	↑ No. of positive DTH responses with 100 mg ↑ Diameter of induration of DTH response in a subgroup with 100 mg ↔ IL-2 production	Pallast et al., 1999[42]
Hypertriglyceridemic (N = 12) and normolipidemic (N = 8) adults	49.5 + 9.6 55.8 + 12.1	600 IU/d for 6 weeks†	↓ Superoxide production ↓ TNF-α, IL-1β, IL-8 production	van Tits et al., 2000[101]

*Supplemented with *dl*-α-tocopheryl acetate unless indicated.
†Supplemented with RRR-α-tocopherol.
‡Supplemented with *dl*-α-tocopherol.
DTH, delayed-type hypersensitivity; 8-OHDG, 8-hydroxydeoxyguanosine; Ig, immunoglobulin; IL, interleukin; PGE_2, prostaglandin E_2; TNF, tumor necrosis factor.

days. Vitamin E supplementation was associated with increased DTH response, proliferative response to ConA, and IL-2 production. Decreased PHA-stimulated PGE_2 production by peripheral blood mononuclear cells and decreased plasma lipid peroxide concentration were observed with vitamin E supplementation (Figure 1). In a more recent study, the effect of 4.5 months of vitamin E supplementation on in vivo indices of immune function was investigated in healthy elderly men and women >65 years; 88 subjects were supplemented daily with placebo or 60, 200, or 800 mg *dl*-α-tocopherol.[41] All three vitamin-E-supplemented groups showed a significant increase in DTH response compared with baseline. When DTH was expressed as median percentage change, subjects in the 200 mg/d group had a 65% increase, significantly greater ($P = 0.04$) than that of the placebo group (17%). Although the median percentage changes in the 60 and 800 mg/d groups (41% and 49%, respectively) were similar to the change in the 200 mg/d group (65%), these changes were not statistically different from that of the placebo group. A significant increase in antibody titer to hepatitis B was observed in the 200 and 800 mg/d groups. The 200 mg/d group also had a significant increase in antibody titer to tetanus vaccine. Lee and Wan[43] reported a significant increase in proliferative response to PHA or LPS and a significant decrease in plasma malondialdehyde and urinary DNA adduct 8-hydroxy-2′-deoxyguanosine after short-term supplementation with vitamin E (233 mg *dl*-α-tocopherol/d for 28 days) in Chinese adults. In addition to its effect on cell-mediated immunity, vitamin E may have anti-inflammatory effects; it has been shown to reduce production of proinflammatory mediators such as IL-1, IL-6, PGE_2, and nitric oxide in animals[44] and humans.[45] Long-term supplementation of vitamin E (55 mg/kg diet for 6 months) decreased the production of unstimulated IL-6 and LPS-stimulated

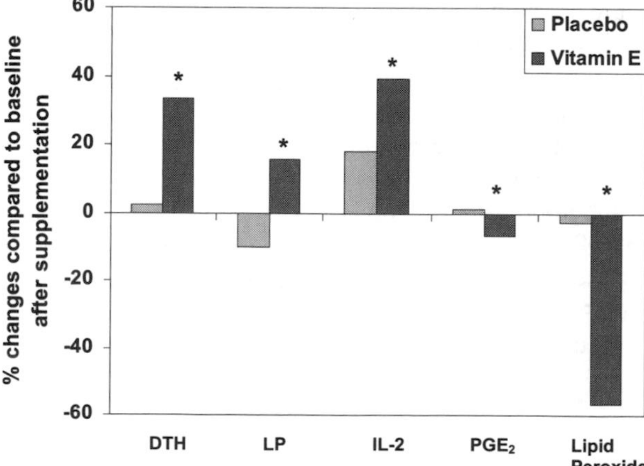

Figure 1. Effect of vitamin E supplementation (800 mg/d for 30 days) on immune responses of healthy older adults. *Significant changes from baseline at $P < 0.05$. Abbreviations: DTH, delayed-type hypersensitivity response; LP, lymphocyte proliferation; IL-2, interleukin-2; PGE_2, prostaglandin E_2. (Data adapted from Meydani et al., 1990.[40])

nitric oxide by peritoneal macrophages in mice.[44] In humans, supplementation with 800 mg vitamin E for 60 days prevented exercise-induced elevation of IL-1 and significantly decreased the production of IL-6.[45]

De Waart et al.[46] observed no significant changes in mitogenic response to ConA and PHA; IgG and IgA levels against *Penicillium*; and IgG4 levels against egg, milk, and wheat proteins after 3 months of supplementation with vitamin E at 100 mg/d. The lower dose of vitamin E and the use of previously frozen lymphocytes for determination of mitogenic response and elevation of antibody levels without previous specific vaccination may have contributed to the discrepancy observed between the results from De Waart et al.[46] and Meydani et al.[41] Prasad[47] measured mitogenic response to PHA, DTH response to PHA, and bactericidal activity against *Escherichia coli* of leukocytes in 13 young adults (25–30 years) and 5 young boys (13–18 years) after 3 weeks of supplementation with vitamin E at 300 mg/d. Bactericidal activity and mitogenic response were measured in the young adults, and DTH was measured in the young boys. DTH was tested by measuring induration after intradermal injection of PHA. Bactericidal activity and mitogenic response decreased after 3 weeks of supplementation, and there was no significant difference in DTH response after supplementation. However, only a few subjects were used and no placebo group was included. Pallast et al.[42] supplemented healthy elderly subjects 65 to 80 years of age with 50 or 100 mg vitamin E for 6 months. Subjects in the vitamin-E-supplemented group showed a significant increase in DTH (induration diameter and number of positive reactions) compared with their own baseline values. Only the change in the number of positive DTH reactions tended to be larger in the 100-mg-supplemented group than the placebo group ($P = 0.06$). A significantly greater improvement in cumulative DTH score and number of positive DTH reactions was observed in a subgroup of subjects who received 100 mg vitamin E and had low baseline DTH reactivity (≤positive DTH reactions). There was no significant difference in PHA-stimulated IL-2 production in the vitamin-E-treated groups compared with the placebo group, and IFN-γ production tended to be lower in groups receiving vitamin E. Significant increases in total serum protein and α-2 and β-globulin fractions were observed in older subjects supplemented with vitamin E at 2000 mg/d for 4 months.[48]

Differences in results among these human studies may reflect the difference in age of subjects, doses of supplementation (resulting in varied levels of changes in plasma vitamin E levels) (Table 6, Figure 2), and methodology, as well as subjects' vitamin E status at baseline. Mean plasma vitamin E level changes after supplementation with 19.3 μmol/L, an increase from baseline level of 17.9 μmol/L by 300 mg/d supplementation of young subjects in the study by Prasad[47]; 16.7 μmol/L, an increase from the baseline level of 33.0 μmol/L by 100-mg/d supplementation in the study by De Waart et al.[46]; and 10.1 and 15.8 μmol/L, an increase from baseline level of 28.8 and 31.1 μmol/L by 50

Table 6. Changes in Plasma Vitamin E Levels and DTH Responses

Vitamin E Dose (mg/d)	Change in Blood Vitamin E Levels (μmol/L)	Vitamin E Levels After Supplementation (μmol/L)	Change in Diameter of Induration (mm)	Reference
0	−1.2	23.3	2.0	Meydani et al., 1997[41]
50	10.1	38.9	4.6	Pallast et al., 1999[42]
60	11.2	38.4	5.0	Meydani et al., 1997[41]
100	15.8	46.9	6.0	Pallast et al., 1999[42]
200	25.4	51.0	10.0	Meydani et al., 1997[41]
800	45.7	71.5	11.0	Meydani et al., 1997[41]

and 100 mg/d supplementation, respectively, in the study by Pallast et al.[42] On the other hand, in the studies by Meydani et al.,[40,41] plasma vitamin E levels increased from 25.6 to 70.9 μmol/L with 800 mg/d supplementation for 30 days, and serum vitamin E levels increased from 25.6 and 25.8 μmol/L to 51.0 and 71.5 μmol/L with 200 and 800 mg/d supplementation, respectively, for 4.5 months. Considering the results from the study by Meydani et al.,[41] in which subjects in the upper tertile of serum vitamin E concentration (>48.4 μmol/L) after supplementation had higher antibody response to hepatitis B and higher DTH responses than those in the lower tertile of serum vitamin E, the amount of increase in vitamin E level achieved in the studies by others[42,46,47] might not have been adequate to observe a highly significant effect. It is also noteworthy that Lee and Wan[43] observed a significant increase in cell-mediated immune response with a 13.4-μmol/L increase in plasma vitamin E level, a level of increase comparable to those observed by others,[42,46] with 100 mg supplementation. However, De Waart et al.[46] observed no significant change, and Pallast et al.[42] observed significant improvement only in a subgroup of subjects with low baseline vitamin E status. This discrepancy in findings might be due to differences in vitamin E status of subjects at baseline among the various studies. Subjects in the study by Lee and Wan[43] had significantly lower plasma vitamin E levels of 14.25 μmol/L at baseline compared with vitamin E levels of 33.0 μmol/L and 31.3 μmol/L in the studies by De Waart et al.[46] and Pallast et al.,[42] respectively.

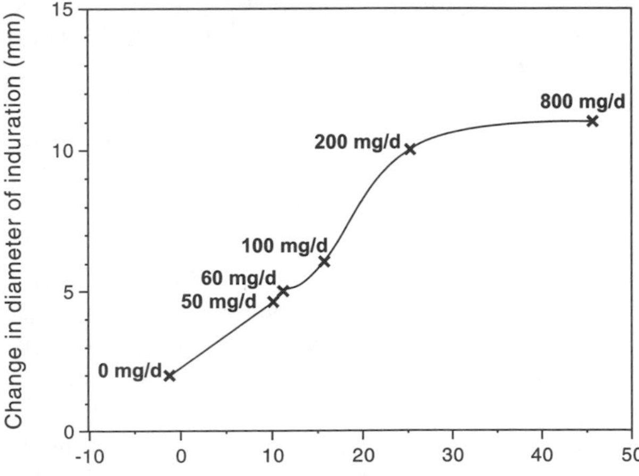

Figure 2. Relationship between changes in DTH and changes in blood vitamin E levels after different amounts of vitamin E supplementation. (Data adapted from Meydani et al., 1997[41] and Pallast et al., 1999.[42])

Concern has been raised that consuming high amounts of vitamin E may negatively affect phagocytosis and bactericidal activity of polymorphonuclear cells or increase autoantibody formation. Administration of 1600 IU vitamin E for 7 days resulted in less effective killing of *Staphylococcus aureus* 502A.[49] The results of this study need to be interpreted with caution because there were only three subjects supplemented with vitamin E and no control group. In a recent study[50] on the effect of vitamin E supplementation on secondary bacterial infection following influenza infection, vitamin E supplementation did not have a significant effect on *S. aureus* infection alone. However, vitamin E supplementation prevented the priming effect of influenza infection on *S. aureus* infection. The cytotoxic ability of neutrophils against *Candida albicans* was not compromised after 4.5 months of supplementation with 60, 200, and 800 IU vitamin E in a double-blind, placebo-controlled study with 88 subjects.[51] In addition, vitamin E supplementation did not increase the serum levels of two autoantibodies—anti-DNA and anti-thyroglobulin—in healthy elderly subjects.[51] Richards et al.[52] reported inhibition of oxidant generation by phagocytes after supplementation of cigarette smokers with 900 IU/d for 6 weeks. Oxidant generation was measured by the luminol-enhanced chemiluminescence response of phagocytes activated with PMA or *N*-formyl-L-methionyl-L-leucyl-L-phenylalanine with cytochalasin B. Suppressed production of superoxide by polymorphonuclear cells was observed with both very low and high levels (by in vitro addition or intramuscular injection) of vitamin E.[53] Opsonized zymosan-stimulated superoxide generation in polymorphonuclear cells was detected by chemiluminescence using a *Cypridina* luciferin analog. However, supplementation of young adult subjects (24–31 years) with 600 mg/d for 3 months or premature infants with 40 mg/kg/d for 8 to 14 days did not affect chemiluminescence, indicating that oral administration of vitamin E does not impair polymorphonuclear cell function.

Is the Immunostimulatory Effect of Vitamin E Associated with Increased Resistance to Infectious Diseases?

The immunostimulatory effect of vitamin E has been shown to be associated with increased resistance against several pathogens in different species of animals.[54] A lower incidence of mortality from *E. coli* infection was observed in chicks supplemented with vitamin E at 300 mg/kg diet for 6 weeks.[55] Furthermore, a 37% reduction in incidence of clinical mastitis and a 44% reduction in the duration of clinical symptoms were observed in cows receiving 740 mg/d of vitamin E.[56] Vitamin E supplementation at 180 mg/kg diet for 4 weeks increased the survival of nonimmunized mice from 20% to 80% when they were challenged with 20 organisms of *Diplococcus pneumoniae* type I, and of immunized mice from 15% to 70% when they were challenged with 20,000 organisms. The increased protection against *D. pneumoniae* type I seemed to result principally from increased macrophage activity and antibody production.[57]

Hayek et al.[58] showed that supplementation with vitamin E at 500 mg/kg diet for 6 weeks can lower the pulmonary viral titer in old mice infected with influenza virus. Old mice fed a diet high in vitamin E had a significantly lower lung viral titer than did those fed a diet containing an adequate level of vitamin E (30 mg/kg diet) on 2, 5, and 7 days after influenza virus infection (Figure 3). The mechanism for the antiviral effect of vitamin E was not fully described in this study; however, higher NK activity and preserved antioxidant nutrient status were found to contribute in part to the vitamin-E-induced reduction of viral titer. A subsequent study showed that IL-2 and IFN-γ production (Th1 response) by splenocytes increased significantly after influenza infection in vitamin-E-supplemented (500 mg/kg diet for 8 weeks) old mice, whereas old mice fed the control diet were unable to induce efficient Th1 response.[59] Old mice fed the vitamin E diet produced 100% more IFN-γ than did those fed the control diet. In addition, there was a significant inverse correlation between viral titer and IFN-γ production (Figure 4). Dysregulation of Th1 and Th2 functions are observed with aging; these changes in Th1/Th2 balance can contribute to the delayed clearance and recovery from influenza infection as Th1 clones are cytolytic in vitro and protective against lethal challenges in vivo, whereas Th2 clones are noncytolytic and not protective.[60] These studies indicate that the protective effect of vitamin E against

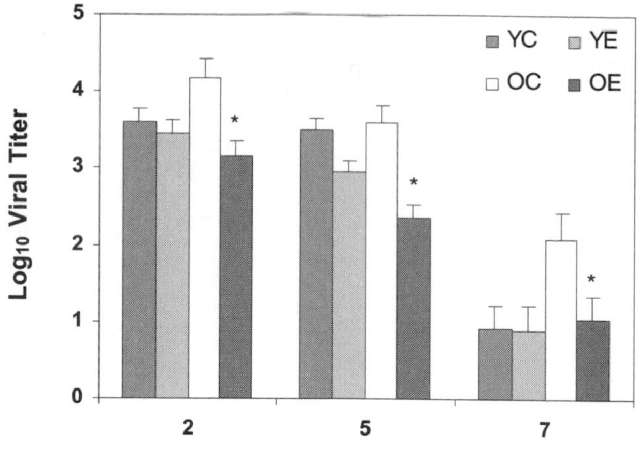

Figure 3. Pulmonary virus titers of young (4 months) and old (22 months) C57BL/6NIA mice fed 30 ppm (control) or 500 ppm (supplemented) vitamin E and given a total respiratory tract infection with H3N2 influenza virus. Mice were fed a diet for 6 weeks, infected intranasally, and killed 0, 2, 5, and 7 days after infection. Lungs were excised and homogenized, and virus titer was measured from the supernatants. Means ± SE are shown. N = 4–8. Abbreviations: OC, old mice fed the control diet; OE, old mice fed the vitamin-E–supplemented diet; YC, young mice fed the control diet; YE, young mice fed the vitamin-E–supplemented diet. *Significantly lower virus titer compared with OC ($P<0.05$). (Adapted from Hayek et al., 1997[58]; used with permission from The University of Chicago Press.)

influenza infection is mediated through reducing the viral load partly by enhancing NK activity and partly by enhancing Th1 response. Vitamin E supplementation was also shown to prevent retrovirus-induced suppression of splenocyte proliferation and NK activity and to partially restore production of IL-2 and IFN-γ by splenocytes.[61]

The clinical significance of vitamin E supplementation in regard to protection against infectious diseases in humans has been investigated in several studies published recently (Table 7). Harman and Miller[62] investigated the effect of vitamin E supplementation at 200 or 400 mg/d for 6 months on the incidence of infectious diseases in 103 patients in a chronic care facility. There was no effect of vitamin E on antibody titer to influenza vaccine or the incidence of pulmonary, urinary tract, and other infections. Because data on the subjects' health status, medication use, and other relevant variables were not reported, it is difficult to draw conclusions from this study. Furthermore, the number of subjects may not have been adequate to determine a significant difference.

In two separate articles published from the α-Tocopherol β-Carotene Cancer Prevention study,[63,64] the long-term effects of vitamin E (50 mg/d) and gb-carotene (20 mg/d) supplementation on the incidence of the common cold and hospital-treated pneumonia were evaluated. Vitamin E did not have an overall effect on the incidence of common cold episodes during a 4-year follow-up period in a cohort of 21,796 male smokers. Vitamin E did, however, show a beneficial effect in reducing the incidence of colds among older (>65 years) city dwellers who

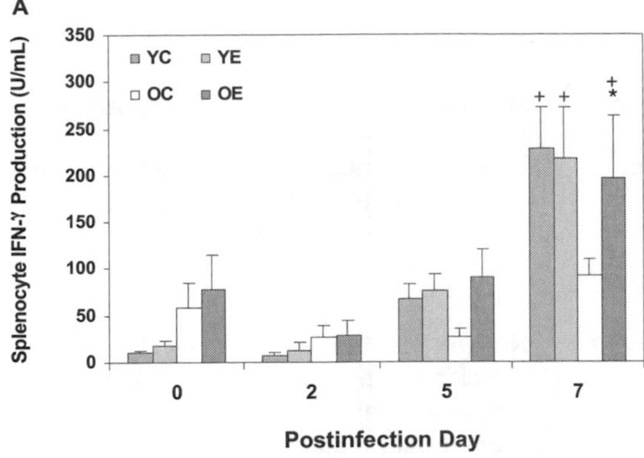

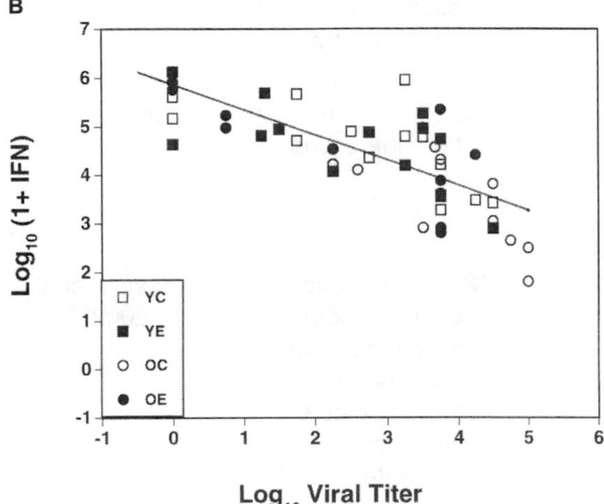

Figure 4. Interferon-γ (IFN-γ) production after influenza infection by splenocytes from young and old mice fed diets containing 30 ppm (control) or 500 ppm (supplemented) vitamin E for 8 weeks (A) and correlation between IFN-γ levels and pulmonary viral titers on days 5 and 7 (B). A: Splenocytes (5×10^6 cells/well) were stimulated with concanavalin A (ConA; 5 mg/L) for 24 hours. Values are means ±SEM. N = 4–9. *Significantly different from mice of the same age fed the control diet by the Fisher least significant test at $P < 0.05$. Abbreviations: OC, old mice fed the control diet; OE, old mice fed the vitamin-E–supplemented diet; YC, young mice fed the control diet; YE, young mice fed the vitamin-E–supplemented diet. B: A significant inverse correlation was observed between IFN-γ levels and viral titers ($r = -0.721$; $P < 0.001$; N = 49) by Pearson correlation. (From Han et al., 2000[59]; used with permission from Blackwell Publishing.)

smoked fewer than 15 cigarettes per day. The results from this study need to be interpreted with caution, as the dose of vitamin E used (50 mg/d) is not optimal for improving the immune response in the elderly. Furthermore, the data was based on self-reported incidence collected 3 times per year.[63] In another study,[64] vitamin E had no overall effect on the incidence of hospital-treated pneumonia during 6.1-year (median) follow-up in a cohort of 29,133 male smokers. Again, vitamin E did show a beneficial effect in a subpopulation of subjects, in this case, those who had initiated smoking at a later age (>21 years) with a relative risk of 0.65. These findings indicate that supplementation with 50 mg/d of vitamin E might not be adequate to observe a beneficial effect in elderly smokers, as any beneficial effect of vitamin E was observed in subgroups who smoked less or had initiated smoking at a later age (fewer smoking years).

Graat et al.[65] reported the effect of vitamin E and multivitamin–mineral supplementation on the incidence and severity of acute respiratory tract infections in elderly, noninstitutionalized individuals. A total of 652 individuals more than 60 years (mean age 73 years) were supplemented with placebo; 200 mg of vitamin E alone; multivitamin-mineral capsule containing retinol (600 μg), β-carotene (1.2 mg), ascorbic acid (60 mg), vitamin E (10 mg), cholecalciferol (5 μg), vitamin K (30 μg), thiamin mononitrate (1.4 mg), riboflavin (1.6 mg), niacin (18 mg), pantothenic acid (6 mg), pyridoxine (2.0 mg), biotin (150 μg), folic acid (200 μg), cyanocobalamin (1 μg), zinc (10 mg), selenium (25 μg), iron (4.0 mg), magnesium (30 mg), copper (1.0 mg), iodine (100 μg), calcium (74 mg), phosphorous (49 mg), manganese (1.0 mg), chromium (25 μg), molybdenum (25 μg), and silicon (2 μg); or vitamin E in combination with the multivitamin-mineral supplement for 15 months. Mean incidence of infections per year was 1.53, 1.73, 1.48, and 1.63 for placebo, vitamin E alone, multivitamin-mineral, and vitamin E plus multivitamin-mineral groups, respectively. When effects of multivitamin-mineral or vitamin E supplements were analyzed according to the 2 × 2 factorial design, there was no significant effect of multivitamin-mineral supplementation on the incidence rate ratio (0.95) and severity of infections. There was no significant difference in incidence rate ratio between vitamin-E-supplemented groups (1.12) and no vitamin E groups (1.00). However, this study also has limitations because the incidence and severity of acute respiratory tract infections were self-reported (1024 reports by 443 subjects), and only a small portion of reported infections were confirmed by microbiologic tests. There was also a difference in risk factors pertinent to respiratory infections such as chronic obstructive pulmonary disease, asthma, allergy, and smoking status among placebo and intervention groups. Furthermore, no differentiation was made between upper and lower respiratory infections, which have different microbial causes (mainly viral for upper and bacterial for lower respiratory infections).

In a randomized, double-blind study, 617 people >65 years residing at 33 nursing homes in the Boston, Massachusetts area received either a placebo or 200 IU of vitamin E (*dl*-α-tocopherol) daily for 1 year.[66] All participants received a capsule containing half the recommended daily allowance of essential vitamins and minerals. The results of this clinical trial showed that significantly fewer vitamin-E-supplemented subjects acquired ≥1 respiratory infections ($r^2 = 0.88$; $P = 0.04$) or upper respiratory infections ($r^2 = 0.81$; $P = 0.01$). However, supplementation with vitamin E had no significant effect on incidence or number of subjects acquiring lower respiratory infections. Further analysis on the foremost upper respiratory infection, the common cold, indicated that the vitamin E group had a lower incidence of common colds (0.66 vs. 0.83 per sub-

Table 7. Vitamin E Supplementation and Infectious Diseases in Humans

Subjects	Age (years)	Supplementation Dose	Duration	Results	Reference
Elderly nursing home residents (N = 617)	>65 (mean age 84–85)	200 IU (plus 0.5 dose of RDA of essential vitamins and minerals)	1 year	Lower incidence of common cold; no significant effect on lower respiratory infections	Meydani et al., 2004[66]
Male smokers (N = 29,133)	50–69	50 mg/d vitamin E (2 × 2 factorial design: 20 mg/d β-carotene)	6.1 years	No overall effect on incidence of pneumonia; decreased risk of pneumonia in subjects who started smoking at a later age	Hemila et al., 2004[64]
Noninstitutionalized elderly (N = 652)	>60 (mean age 73–74)	200 mg vitamin E (2 × 2 factorial design: multi-vitamin–mineral supplement)	15 months	No effect on respiratory tract infections	Graat et al., 2002[65]
Male smokers (N = 21,796)	>50–69	50 mg/d vitamin E (2 × 2 factorial design: 20 mg/d β-carotene)	4 years	No overall effect on common cold incidence; lower incidence of colds in older subjects who smoked <15 cigarettes per day	Hemila et al., 2002[63]
Adults in chronic care facility	24–104	200 or 400 mg/d	6 months	No effects on serum Ab titer to influenza vaccine; no effects on incidence of infectious diseases	Harman and Miller, 1986[62]

Ab, antibody; RDA, recommended daily allowance.

ject-year, $r^2 = 0.80$; $P = 0.04$) and fewer subjects in the vitamin E group acquired ≥1 common colds (46% vs. 57%, $r^2 = 0.80$; $P = 0.02$). There was also a nonsignificant trend for shorter duration of the common cold in vitamin-E-supplemented subjects. In conclusion, the results of this clinical trial show that vitamin E supplementation significantly reduces the risk for acquiring respiratory infections in the elderly. In particular, vitamin E supplementation reduced the incidence rate of common colds and the number of subjects who acquire a cold among elderly nursing home residents. A nonsignificant reduction in the duration of colds was also observed. Because of the high rate and more severe morbidity associated with common colds in this age group, these findings have important implications for the well-being of the elderly and for the economic burden associated with their care.

Colds are common afflictions, accounting for 30% of absenteeism in the United States across all age groups.[67] Rhinoviruses and coronaviruses represent the majority of the documented causes of colds.[68] They exacerbate chronic obstructive pulmonary disease[69] and are known to be associated with lower respiratory infections in the elderly.[68,70,71] For example, a prospective cohort study of community-based elderly found that rhinoviruses were associated with lower respiratory symptoms in nearly two-thirds of episodes: about one-fifth of patients were confined to bed, and 26% were unable to perform routine household activities.[71] Constitutional and lower respiratory tract symptoms and signs have been reported to be more common in the elderly compared with younger adults infected with cold viruses.[70] Nursing home populations may also be at risk for epidemic outbreaks of rhinovirus infections.[72] The common cold is generally less severe than influenza. However, its much higher incidence and its recognized morbidity in the elderly[68,70-72] make it an important public health problem in this age group.[73] This is particularly relevant because at present no clinically useful vaccine or antiviral therapy is available to combat colds. The economic impact of non-influenza-related viral upper respiratory infections in general, and in the elderly in particular, has been overlooked. Because of their high attack rate, these diseases are responsible for an economic burden that approaches $40 billion annually.[73] Thus, our finding that E supplementation reduces the common cold by 22% has significant implications for the elderly in reducing the burden of diseases and associated health care costs. Currently, there are 34 million elderly in the United States. The observation that vitamin E reduced the risk for acquiring any respiratory infections by 20% will translate into approximately 7 million fewer elderly acquiring respiratory infections. Thus, the findings from this study could have significant impact for improving the health status of the elderly and need to be considered in relation to their vitamin E requirement.

Mechanisms for the Immunostimulatory Effect of Vitamin E

Several mechanisms are possible for the immunostimulatory effect of vitamin E: it can enhance the immune response by influencing membrane integrity, influencing signal transduction, reducing the production of suppressive factors such as PGE_2, or directly influencing T-cell functions.

Vitamin E is a potent peroxyl radical scavenger that can prevent the propagation of free radical damage in biologic membranes. This antioxidant function of vitamin E can affect signal transduction pathways that are regulated by redox status.[74] Transcriptional factors such as nuclear factor κB (NF-κB) and activator protein-1 (AP-1) are important regulators of nuclear gene expression in immune cells and are sensitive to the antioxidant-oxidant balance. Reduction and oxidation can either up- or down-regulate DNA binding and transactivation activities in a transcriptional-activator-dependent and cell-type-dependent manner. In general, oxidants increase and reductants decrease NF-κB activity, but AP-1 activity is dramatically increased by reductants.[75] NF-κB is activated by various agents, including IL-1 and TNF-α, viruses, double-stranded RNA, endotoxins, phorbol esters, ultraviolet light, and hydrogen peroxide. Antioxidants may affect NF-κB function through suppression of NF-κB activation by various inducers.[76] The vitamin E derivatives α-tocopherol acetate and succinate inhibited NF-κB activation induced by TNF-α in human Jurkat T cells.[77] In contrast, both oxidative and reducing signals can activate AP-1. Prooxidants (e.g., hydrogen peroxide, ultraviolet irradiation) can induce AP-1 activation. On the other hand, AP-1-dependent transactivation was strongly enhanced by thioredoxin, cellular protein oxidoreductase with antioxidant activity, and other structurally unrelated antioxidants such as pyrrolidine dithiocarbamate and butylated hydroxyanisole.[78] Vitamin E might also regulate cellular reaction through its nonantioxidant functions by inhibiting protein kinase C activity.[79]

Many cytokines, including IL-1, IL-2, IL-6, and TNF-α, contain NF-κB and AP-1 binding sites in the promoter and enhancer regions of the genes encoding them. AP-1, nuclear factor of activated T cells, octamer proteins, and NF-κB were shown to play integral roles in the regulation of the *IL-2* gene. The production of IL-2 by activated T cells is critical for T-cell proliferation and differentiation and the development of T-cell-dependent immune response.[80] Both animal[30,32] and human[40] studies reported increased IL-2 production with vitamin E supplementation, but the effect of vitamin E on *IL-2* gene regulation was not tested.

PGE_2, the cyclooxygenase (COX) product of arachidonic acid metabolism, plays an important regulatory role in controlling immune function. PGE_2 has a direct inhibitory effect on the early stages of T-cell activation, resulting in decreased IL-2 production and decreased IL-2 receptor expression.[81] In addition, PGE_2 can modulate Th1 and Th2 responses through its effect on IL-12, which plays a central role in increasing Th1 responses by promoting the differentiation of Th0 cells into a population of Th1 cells.[82] In a co-culture study, the addition of PGE_2 at concentrations produced by macrophages from old mice decreased proliferation and IL-2 production by T cells from young mice; the addition of vitamin E decreased PGE_2 production and improved T-cell proliferation and IL-2 production.[33] Wu and collaborators[83] showed that in vivo vitamin E supplementation decreased PGE_2 production by LPS-stimulated macrophages from old mice (Figure 5). This effect of vitamin E was me-

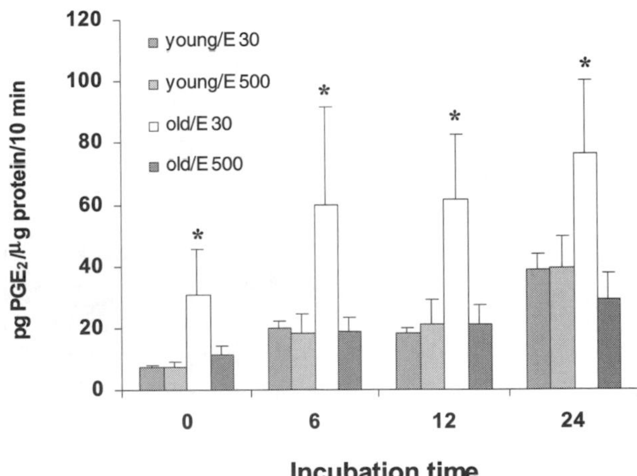

Figure 5. Cyclooxygenase (COX) activity in peritoneal macrophages isolated from young and old mice fed diets containing either 30 or 500 ppm vitamin E for 30 days. Peritoneal macrophages were isolated and cultured (5×10^5 cells/well) in the presence of lipopolysaccharide at 5 mg/L for 0, 6, 12, or 24 hours at 37°C. After removal of supernatants for assay of accumulated prostaglandin E_2 (PGE_2) production at each time point, cells were layered with 1 mL of endotoxin-free RPMI 1640 containing arachidonic acid at 30 μmol/L. After 10 minutes of incubation at 37°C, aspirin (2.1 mmol/L) was added to stop reaction. Supernatants were then collected for PGE_2 analysis, cells were lysed with NaOH (1 mol/L), and total cell protein was measured with a protein assay kit. COX activity (means ± SE for N = 10 in each age and diet group) is expressed as conversion of arachidonic acid to PGE_2 (pg/μg protein/10 min). *Significantly higher COX activity compared with young mice fed 30 or 500 ppm vitamin E containing diets and old mice fed 500 ppm vitamin E containing diet ($P < 0.05$). (Adapted with permission from Wu et al., 1998.[83])

A

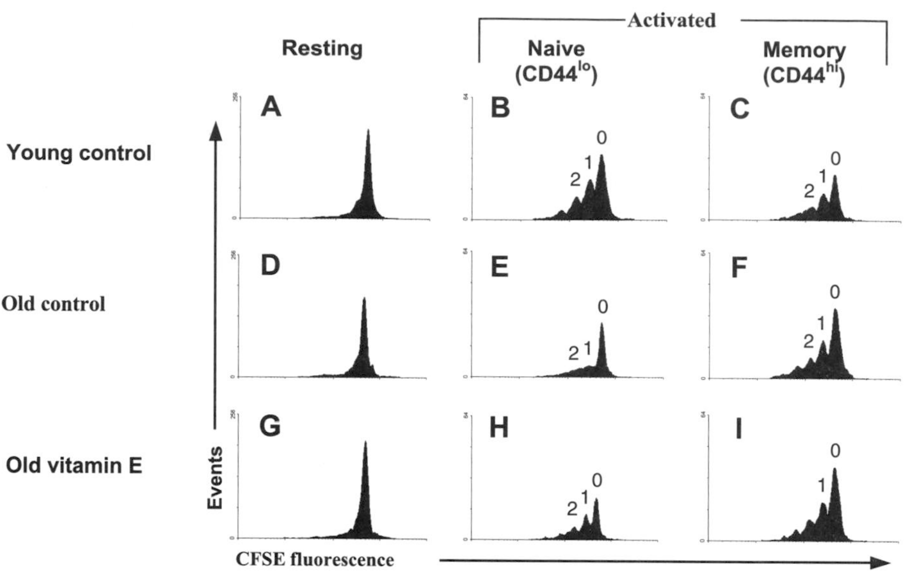

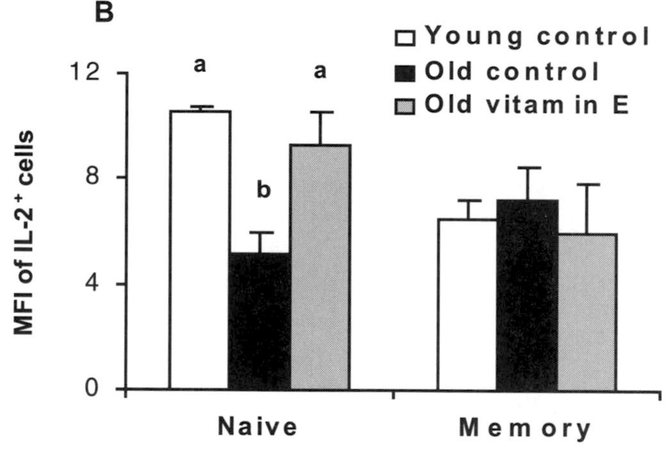

Figure 6. A. Effects of age and vitamin E on the progression of T cells through cell cycle division. Purified T cells were preincubated with 46 μM vitamin E for 4 hours, labeled with carboxyfluoroscein succinimidyl ester, and activated with immobilized anti-CD3 and soluble anti-CD28 mAbs for 48 hours. Cells were harvested, stained for CD44 expression, and analyzed on a flow cytometer. One representative histogram for each of young control (A, B, and C), old control (D, E, and F), and old preincubated with vitamin E (G, H, and I) are shown. Cell cycle division patterns are shown for unactivated T cells (A, D, and G), activated naive ($CD44^{lo}$) T cells (B, E, and H), and activated memory ($CD44^{hi}$) T cells (C, F, and I). Peaks representing cell division cycles 0, 1, and 2 are also indicated. B: Effects of age and vitamin E on intracellular IL-2 production by naive and memory T cell subsets. Purified T cells (N = 5) were preincubated with 46 μM vitamin E for 4 hours and activated with immobilized anti-CD3 and soluble anti-CD28 mAbs for 48 hours. Cells were treated with monensin, an inhibitor of IL-2 secretion, for the last 10 hours of activation. Harvested cells were stained with fluorochrome-conjugated anti-CD44 mAb, permeabilized, and stained with fluorochrome-conjugated anti-IL-2. T cells were divided into naive and memory phenotypes based on low or high expression of the CD44 antigen, respectively. Cell fluorescence was measured on a flow cytometer. Bars represent the linearized mean fluorescence intensity of IL-2+ T cells. Bars with different letters within each phenotype are significantly different ($P < 0.05$) by an ANOVA followed by the Tukey HSD post-hoc procedure. Abbreviations: ANOVA, analysis of variance; HSD; highly significant difference; IL, interleukin; mAb, monoclonal antibody. (From Adolfsson et al., 2001[81]; copyright 2001 The American Association of Immunologists, Inc.)

diated mainly through inhibition of COX activity, the rate-limiting enzymes in PGE_2 production—a 60% decrease in Cox activity was observed with vitamin E supplementation. Vitamin E appears to affect COX activity post-translationally; there was no effect of vitamin E on protein or mRNA levels of COX. COX activity requires the presence of oxidant hydroperoxides for its activation.[84] It has been suggested that free radical nitric oxide is involved in the regulation of COX activity.[85] Nitric oxide can be further metabolized to peroxynitrite in the presence of superoxide, and peroxynitrite has been shown to increase the activity of COX without affecting its expression.[86] Vitamin E is an effective biologic antioxidant and a chain-breaking free radical scavenger and therefore may attenuate COX activity by scavenging the oxidant hydroperoxide necessary for COX activation. Dietary supplementation of vitamin E resulted in reduced production of nitric oxide in macrophages from old mice.[87] When a nitric oxide donor was added in the presence of superoxide to elevate peroxynitrite levels in the culture, vitamin-E-induced inhibition of COX activity in the macrophages from old mice was diminished. These results suggest that vitamin E reduces COX activity in old macrophages by decreasing nitric oxide production, which results in lower production of peroxynitrite in macrophages from old mice.

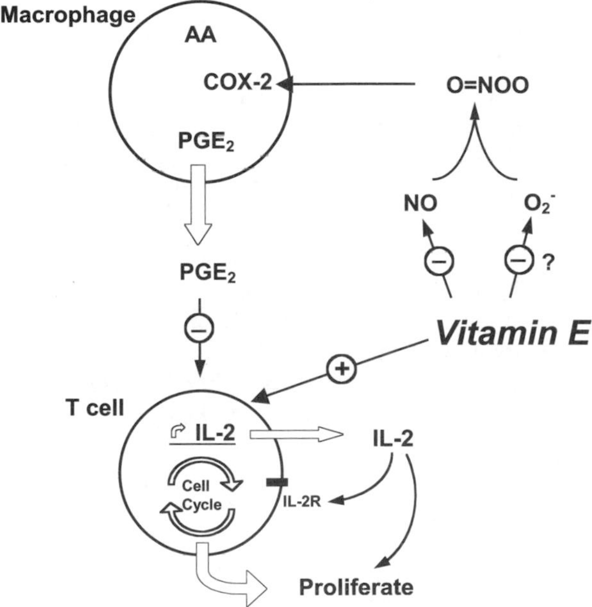

Figure 7. Mechanisms of vitamin E's influence on immune responses. Vitamin E reduces cyclooxygenase (COX) activity in old macrophages by decreasing nitric oxide production, which results in lower production of peroxynitrite in macrophages from old mice. Peroxynitrite has been shown to increase the activity of COX. Decreased COX activity by vitamin E results in decreased production of T-cell-suppressive prostaglandin E_2 (PGE_2) by macrophages, leading to enhancement of T-cell functions. Vitamin E can also directly (independent of its effect of PGE_2) enhance T-cell proliferation and IL-2 production by increasing cell-dividing capability, the number of IL-2+ T cells, and the amount of IL-2 produced per T cell. Vitamin E may also affect cell proliferation by affecting expression of cell-cycle-related molecules. AA, arachidonic acid; COX, cyclooxygenase; PGE_2, prostaglandin E_2; O=NOO, peroxynitrite; NO, nitric oxide; O_2^-, superoxide; IL-2, interleukin-2; IL-2R, interleukin-2 receptor.

Vitamin E was also shown to have a direct effect on T-cell functions independent of its effect on macrophage PGE_2 production.[33,88] When purified T cells from old mice were incubated in vitro with vitamin E at 46 μM prior to activation, a significant improvement was observed in cell-dividing capability, total IL-2 production and the number of IL-2+ T cells, and the amount of IL-2 produced per naive T cell[88] (Figure 6). Preliminary results indicate that vitamin E may improve effective immune synapse formation in naive T cells from old mice.[89] In addition, it may also increase the expression of cell-cycle-related proteins.[90] Schematic mechanisms of vitamin E's influence on T-cell function are presented in Figure 7.

Conclusion

The recommended daily intake for vitamin E was recently increased from 10 mg/d[91] to 15 mg/d of α-tocopherol for adults (ages >19 years).[92] The current recommendation is based largely on induced vitamin E deficiency in humans and the correlation between hydrogen-peroxide-induced erythrocyte lysis and plasma α-tocopherol concentrations. The Food and Nutrition Board had acknowledged the growing body of evidence for beneficial effects of a high intake of vitamin E on some chronic diseases; however, they stated that clinical evidence is limited and not conclusive to warrant a recommendation for higher vitamin E intake.[92]

Several studies in different species of animals have demonstrated an improvement in immune response when animals are supplemented with more than the recommended level of vitamin E. In addition, clinical trials in humans have shown significant improvement in the immune response of the elderly with vitamin E supplementation. The dose-response relationship shown in this age group suggests that 200 IU/d of α-tocopherol is the optimal level for improving the immune response in the elderly. This enhancement of immune response is associated with increased resistance to infectious diseases in animal models. Results from a recent clinical trial indicate that vitamin E supplementation reduces the risk of acquiring upper respiratory infections in elderly subjects. These findings should be taken into consideration when determining the vitamin E requirement of the elderly. Further studies are needed to determine if vitamin E supplementation is effective in improving the immune response and resistance to infectious diseases in young subjects as well.

Results from cellular and molecular mechanistic studies have shown that immunoregulatory effects of vitamin E are mediated indirectly by reducing the production of suppressive factors such as PGE_2 by macrophages and directly by increasing cell division capacity and IL-2 production by naive T cells.

References

1. Beisel WR. History of nutritional immunology: introduction and overview. J Nutr. 1992;122:591–596.
2. Fraker PJ, King LE, Laakko T, Vollmer TL. The dynamic link between the integrity of the immune system and zinc status. J Nutr. 2000;130: 1399S–1406S.
3. Dallman PR. Iron deficiency and the immune response. Am J Clin Nutr. 1987;46:329–334.
4. McKenzie RC, Rafferty TS, Beckett GJ. Selenium: an essential element for immune function. Immunol Today. 1998;19:342–345.
5. Failla ML, Hopkins RG. Is low copper status immunosuppressive? Nutr Rev. 1998;56:S59–S64.
6. Meydani SN, Wu D, Santos MS, Hayek MG. Antioxidants and immune response in aged persons: overview of present evidence. Am J Clin Nutr. 1995; 62:1462s–1476s.
7. Chandra RK, Sudhakaran L. Regulation of immune responses by vitamin B6. Ann N Y Acad Sci. 1990; 585:404–423.
8. Trakatellis A, Dimitriadou A, Trakatelli M. Pyridoxine deficiency: new approaches in immunosuppression and chemotherapy. Postgrad Med J. 1997; 73:617–622.
9. Jariwalla RJ, Harakeh S. Mechanisms underlying the action of vitamin C in viral and immunodeficiency disease. In: Packer L, Fuchs J, eds. *Vitamin C in Health and Disease.* New York: Marcel Dekker; 1997; 309–322.
10. Hemilä H. Vitamin C and infectious diseases. In: Packer L, Fuchs J, eds. *Vitamin C in Health and Disease.* New York: Marcel Dekker; 1997; 471–504.
11. Cantorna MT, Zhu Y, Froicu M, Wittke A. Vitamin D status, 1,25-dihydroxyvitamin D3, and the immune system. Am J Clin Nutr. 2004;80: 1717S–1720S.
12. Hughes DA, Darlington LG, Bendich A. *Diet and Human Immune Function.* Totowa, NJ: Humana Press; 2004; 400 pp.
13. Gershwin ME, Nestel P, Keen CL. *Handbook of Nutrition and Immunity.* Totowa, NJ: Humana Press; 2004; 365 pp.
14. Tengerdy RP, Heinzerling RH, Brown GL, Mathias M. Enhancement of the humoral immune response by vitamin E. Intern Arch Allergy. 1973;44: 221–232.
15. Gebremichael A, Levy EM, Corwin LM. Adherent cell requirement for the effect of vitamin E on in vitro antibody synthesis. J Nutr. 1984;114: 1297–1305.
16. Eskew ML, Scheuchenzuber WJ, Scholz RW, Reddy CC, Zarkower A. The effects of ozone inhalation on the immunological response of selenium- and vitamin E-deprived rats. Environ Res. 1986; 40:274–284.
17. Harris R, Boxer L, Baehner R. Consequences of vitamin E deficiency on the phagocytic and oxidative functions of the rat polymorphonuclear leukocyte. Blood. 1980;55:338–343.
18. Moriguchi S, Miwa H, Okamura M, Maekawa K, Kishino Y, Maeda K. Vitamin E is an important factor in T cell differentiation in thymus of F344 rats. J Nutr Sci Vitaminol. 1993;39:451–463.
19. Warshauer D, Goldstein E, Hoeprich PD, Lippert W. Effect of vitamin E and ozone on the pulmonary antibacterial defense mechanisms. J Lab Clin Med. 1974;83:228–240.
20. Beck MA, Kolbeck PC, Rohr LH, Shi Q, Morris VC, Levander OA. Vitamin E deficiency intensifies the myocardial injury of coxsackievirus B3 infection of mice. J Nutr. 1994;124:345–358.
21. Munoz SJ, Heubi JE, Balistreri WF, Maddrey WC. Vitamin E deficiency in primary biliary cirrhosis: gastrointestinal malabsorption, frequency and relationship to other lipid-soluble vitamins. Hepatology. 1989;9:525–531.
22. Sokol RJ, Guggenheim MA, Iannaccone ST, et al. Improved neurologic function after long-term correction of vitamin E deficiency in children with chronic cholestasis. N Engl J Med. 1985;313: 1580–1586.
23. Sitrin MD, Lieberman F, Jensen WE, Noronha A, Milburn C, Addington W. Vitamin E deficiency and neurologic disease in adults with cystic fibrosis. Ann Intern Med. 1987;107:51–54.
24. Kowdley KV, Mason JB, Meydani SN, Cornwall S, Grand RJ. Vitamin E deficiency and impaired cellular immunity related to intestinal fat malabsorption. Gastroenterology. 1992;102:2139–2142.
25. Horwitt MK, Harvey CC, Duncan GD, Wilson WC. Effects of limited tocopherol intake in man with relationship to erythrocyte hemolysis and lipid oxidation. Am J Clin Nutr. 1956;4:408–419.
26. Horwitt MK. Vitamin E and lipid metabolism in man. Am J Clin Nutr. 1960;8:451–461.
27. Adachi N, Migita M, Ohta T, Higashi A, Matsuda I. Depressed natural killer cell activity due to decreased natural killer cell population in a vitamin E-deficient patient with Shwachman syndrome: reversible natural killer cell abnormality by α-tocopherol supplementation. Eur J Pediatr. 1997;156: 444–448.
28. Vobecky JS, Vobecky J, Shapcott D, Rola-Pleszczynski M. Nutritional influences on humoral and cell-mediated immunity in healthy infants. J Am Coll Nutr. 1984;3:265.
29. Bendich A, Gabriel E, Machlin LJ. Dietary vitamin E requirement for optimum immune response in the rat. J Nutr. 1986;116:675–681.
30. Meydani SN, Meydani M, Verdon CP, Shapiro

AA, Blumberg JB, Hayes KC. Vitamin E supplementation suppresses prostaglandin E_2 synthesis and enhances the immune response of aged mice. Mech Ageing Dev. 1986;34:191–201.

31. Moriguchi S, Kobayashi N, Kishino Y. High dietary intakes of vitamin E and cellular immune functions in rats. J Nutr. 1990;120:1096–1102.
32. Sakai S, Moriguchi S. Long-term feeding of high vitamin E diet improves the decreased mitogen response of rat splenic lymphocytes with aging. J Nutr Sci Vitaminol. 1997;43:113–122.
33. Beharka AA, Wu D, Han SN, Meydani SN. Macrophage prostaglandin production contributes to the age-associated decrease in T cell function which is reversed by the dietary antioxidant vitamin E. Mech Ageing Dev. 1997;93:59–77.
34. Tanaka J, Fujiwara H, Torisu M. Vitamin E and immune response. I. Enhancement of helper T cell activity by dietary supplementation of vitamin E in mice. Immunology. 1979;38:727–734.
35. Franchini A, Bertuzzi S, Tosarelli C, Manfreda G. Vitamin E in viral inactivated vaccines. Poultry Sci. 1995;74:666–671.
36. Haq A-U, Bailey CA, Chinnah A. Effect of β-carotene, canthaxanthin, lutein, and vitamin E on neonatal immunity of chicks when supplemented in the broiler breeder diets. Poultry Sci. 1996;75: 1092–1097.
37. Miller RA. The aging immune system: primer and prospectus. Science. 1996;273:70–74.
38. Lesourd B, Mazari L. Nutrition and immunity in the elderly. Proc Nutr Soc. 1999;58:685–695.
39. Hayek MG, Meydani SN, Meydani M, Blumberg JB. Age differences in eicosanoid production of mouse splenocytes: effects on mitogen-induced T-cell proliferation. J Gerontol. 1994;49:B197–B207.
40. Meydani SN, Barklund MP, Liu S, et al. Vitamin E supplementation enhances cell-mediated immunity in healthy elderly subjects. Am J Clin Nutr. 1990;52:557–563.
41. Meydani SN, Meydani M, Blumberg JB, et al. Vitamin E supplementation and in vivo immune response in healthy elderly subjects. A randomized controlled trial. JAMA. 1997;277:1380–1386.
42. Pallast EG, Schouten EG, deWaart FG, et al. Effect of 50- and 100-mg vitamin E supplements on cellular immune function in noninstitutionalized elderly persons. Am J Clin Nutr. 1999;69:1273–1281.
43. Lee C-YJ, Wan JM-F. Vitamin E supplementation improves cell-mediated immunity and oxidative stress of Asian men and women. J Nutr. 2000;130: 2932–2937.
44. Beharka AA, Han SN, Adolfsson O, et al. Long-term dietary antioxidant supplementation reduces production of selected inflammatory mediators by murine macrophages. Nutr Res. 2000;20:281–296.
45. Cannon JG, Meydani SN, Fielding RA, et al. Acute phase response in exercise. II. Associations between vitamin E, cytokines, and muscle proteolysis. Am J Physiol. 1991;260:R1235–R1240.
46. De Waart F, Portengen L, Doekes G, Verwaal CJ, Kok FJ. Effect of 3 months vitamin E supplementation on indices of the cellular and humoral immune response in elderly subjects. Br J Nutr. 1997;78: 761–774.
47. Prasad JS. Effect of vitamin E supplementation on leukocyte function. Am J Clin Nutr. 1980;33: 606–608.
48. Ziemlanski S, Wartanowicz M, Klos A, Raczka A, Klos M. The effects of ascorbic acid and alpha-tocopherol supplementation on serum proteins and immunoglobulin concentration in the elderly. Nutr Int. 1986;2:1–5.
49. Baehner RL, Boxer LA, Allen JM, Davis J. Autooxidation as a basis for altered function by polymorphonuclear leukocytes. Blood. 1977;50:327–335.
50. Gay R, Han SN, Marko M, Belisle S, Bronson R, Meydani SN. The effect of vitamin E on secondary bacterial infection after influenza infection in young and old mice. Ann N Y Acad Sci. 2004;1031: 418–421.
51. Meydani SN, Meydani M, Blumberg JB, et al. Assessment of the safety of supplementation with different amounts of vitamin E in healthy older adults. Am J Clin Nutr. 1998;68:311–318.
52. Richards GA, Theron AJ, van Rensburg CEJ, et al. Investigation of the effects of oral administration of vitamin E and beta-carotene on the chemiluminescence responses and the frequency of sister chromatid exchanges in circulating leukocytes from cigarette smokers. Am Rev Respir Dis. 1990;142: 648–654.
53. Okano T, Tamai H, Mino M. Superoxide generation in leukocytes and vitamin E. Int J Vitam Nutr Res. 1991;61:20–26.
54. Han SN, Meydani SN. Vitamin E and infectious diseases in the aged. Proc Nutr Soc. 1999;58: 697–705.
55. Tengerdy RP, Nockels CF. Vitamin E or vitamin A protects chickens against E. coli infection. Poultry Sci. 1975;54:1292–1296.
56. Smith K, Harrison J, Hancock D, Todhunter D, Conrad H. Effect of vitamin E and selenium supplementation on incidence of clinical mastitis and duration of clinical symptoms. J Dairy Sci. 1984; 67:1293–1300.
57. Heinzerling RH, Tengerdy RP, Wick LL, Lueker DC. Vitamin E protects mice against Diplococcus pneumonia type I infection. Infect Immunity. 1974; 10:1292–1295.
58. Hayek MG, Taylor SF, Bender BS, et al. Vitamin E

supplementation decreases lung virus titers in mice infected with influenza. J Infect Dis. 1997;176: 273–276.
59. Han SN, Wu D, Ha WK, et al. Vitamin E supplementation increases T helper 1 cytokine production in old mice infected with influenza virus. Immunology. 2000;100:487–493.
60. Graham MB, Braciale VL, Braciale TJ. Influenza virus-specific CD4$^+$ T helper type 2 T lymphocytes do not promote recovery from experimental virus infection. J Exp Med. 1994;180:1273–1282.
61. Wang Y, Huang DS, Liang B, Watson RR. Nutritional status and immune responses in mice with murine AIDS are normalized by vitamin E supplementation. J Nutr. 1994;124:2024–2032.
62. Harman D, Miller RW. Effect of vitamin E on the immune response to influenza virus vaccine and the incidence of infectious disease in man. Age. 1986; 9:21–23.
63. Hemila H, Kaprio J, Albanes D, Heinonen OP, Virtamo J. Vitamin C, vitamin E, and beta-carotene in relation to common cold incidence in male smokers. Epidemiology. 2002;13:32–37.
64. Hemila H, Virtamo J, Albanes D, Kaprio J. Vitamin E and beta-carotene supplementation and hospital-treated pneumonia incidence in male smokers. Chest. 2004;125:557–565.
65. Graat JM, Schouten EG, Kok FJ. Effect of daily vitamin E and multivitamin-mineral supplementation on acute respiratory tract infections in elderly persons: a randomized controlled trial. JAMA. 2002;288:715–721.
66. Meydani SN, Leka LS, Fine BC, et al. Vitamin E and respiratory tract infections in elderly nursing home residents: a randomized controlled trial. JAMA. 2004;292:828–836.
67. Monto AS, Ullman BM. Acute respiratory illness in an American community. The Tecumseh study. JAMA. 1974;227:164–169.
68. Nicholson KG, Kent J, Hammersley V, Cancio E. Acute viral infections of upper respiratory tract in elderly people living in the community: comparative, prospective, population based study of disease burden. BMJ. 1997;315:1060–1064.
69. Seemungal T, Harper-Owen R, Bhowmik A, et al. Respiratory viruses, symptoms, and inflammatory markers in acute exacerbations and stable chronic obstructive pulmonary disease. Am J Respir Crit Care Med. 2001;164:1618–1623.
70. Falsey AR, McCann RM, Hall WJ, et al. The "common cold" in frail older persons: impact of rhinovirus and coronavirus in a senior daycare center. J Am Geriatr Soc. 1997;45:706–711.
71. Nicholson KG, Kent J, Hammersley V, Cancio E. Risk factors for lower respiratory complications of rhinovirus infections in elderly people living in the community: prospective cohort study. BMJ. 1996; 313:1119–1123.
72. Wald TG, Shult P, Krause P, Miller BA, Drinka P, Gravenstein S. A rhinovirus outbreak among residents of a long-term care facility. Ann Intern Med. 1995;123:588–593.
73. Fendrick AM, Monto AS, Nightengale B, Sarnes M. The economic burden of non-influenza-related viral respiratory tract infection in the United States. Arch Intern Med. 2003;163:487–494.
74. Traber MG, Packer L. Vitamin E: beyond antioxidant function. Am J Clin Nutr. 1995;62: 1501S–1509S.
75. Sun Y, Oberley LW. Redox regulation of transcriptional activators. Free Radic Biol Med. 1996;21: 335–348.
76. Sen CK, Packer L. Antioxidant and redox regulation of gene transcription. FASEB J. 1996;10: 709–720.
77. Suzuki YJ, Packer L. Inhibition of NF-κB activation by vitamin E derivatives. Biochem Biophys Res Comm. 1993;193:277–283.
78. Schenk H, Klein M, Erdbrugger W, Droge W, Schulze-Osthoff K. Distinct effects of thioredoxin and antioxidants on the activation of transcription factors NF-κB and AP-1. Proc Natl Acad Sci U S A. 1994;91:1672–1676.
79. Azzi A, Ricciarelli R, Zingg J-M. Non-antioxidant molecular functions of α-tocopherol (vitamin E). FEBS Lett. 2002;519:8–10.
80. Foletta VC, Segal DH, Cohen DR. Transcriptional regulation in the immune system; all roads lead to AP-1. J Leukoc Biol. 1998;63:139–152.
81. Vercammen C, Ceuppens J. Prostaglandin E2 inhibits T-cell proliferation after crosslinking of the CD3-Ti complex by directly affecting T cells at an early step of the activation process. Cell Immunol. 1987;104:24–36.
82. van der Pouw Kraan TCTM, Boeije LCM, Smeenk RJT, Wijdenes J, Aarden LA. Prostaglandin-E2 is a potent inhibitor of human interleukin 12 production. J Exp Med. 1995;181:775–779.
83. Wu D, Mura C, Beharka AA, et al. Age-associated increase in PGE2 synthesis and COX activity in murine macrophages is reversed by vitamin E. Am J Physiol. 1998;275:C661–C668.
84. Smith WL, Eling TE, Kulmacz RJ, Marnett LJ, Tsai A-L. Tyrosyl radicals and their role in hydroperoxide-dependent activation and inactivation of prostaglandin endoperoxide synthase. Biochemistry. 1992;31:3–7.
85. Salvemini D, Settle SL, Masferrer JL, Seibert K, Currie MG, Needleman P. Regulation of prostaglandin production by nitric oxide; an in vivo analysis. Br J Pharmacol. 1995;114:1171–1178.
86. Landino LM, Crews BC, Timmons MD, Morrow JD, Marnett LJ. Peroxynitrite, the coupling product

of nitric oxide and superoxide, activates prostaglandin biosynthesis. Proc Natl Acad Sci U S A. 1996; 93:15069–15074.

87. Beharka A, Wu D, Serafini M, Meydani SN. Mechanism of vitamin E inhibition of cyclooxygenase activity in macrophages from old mice: role of peroxynitrite. Free Radic Biol Med. 2002;32: 503–511.
88. Adolfsson O, Huber BT, Meydani SN. Vitamin E-enhanced IL-2 production in old mice: naive but not memory T cells show increased cell division cycling and IL-2-producing capacity. J Immunol. 2001;167:3809–3817.
89. Ahmed T, Marko M, Wu D, Chung H, Huber B, Meydani SN. Vitamin E supplementation reverses the age-associated decrease in effective immune synapse formation in $CD4^+$ T cells. Ann N Y Acad Sci. 2004;1031:412–414.
90. Han SN, Adolfsson O, Lee C-K, Prolla TA, Ordovas J, Meydani SN. Vitamin E and gene expression in immune cells. Ann N Y Acad Sci. 2004;1031: 96–101.
91. National Research Council. *Fat-Soluble Vitamins. Recommended Dietary Allowances.* Washington, DC: National Academies Press; 1989; 78–114.
92. Institute of Medicine. *Dietary Reference Intakes for Vitamin C, Vitamin E, Selenium, Carotenoids.* Washington, DC: National Academies Press; 2000; 529 pp.
93. Cunningham-Rundles S. Effects of nutritional status on immunological function. Am J Clin Nutr. 1982;35:1202–1210.
94. Turner RJ, Finch JM. Selenium and the immune response. Proc Nutr Soc. 1991;50:275–285.
95. Spallholz JE, Boylan LM, Larsen HS. Advances in understanding selenium's role in the immune system. Ann N Y Acad Sci. 1990;587:123–139.
96. Shankar AH, Prasad A. Zinc and immune function: the biological basis of altered resistance to infection. Am J Clin Nutr. 1998;68:447s–463s.
97. Fraker PJ, King LE. Reprogramming of the immune system during zinc deficiency. Annu Rev Nutr. 2004;24:277–298.
98. Wakikawa A, Utsuyama M, Wakabayashi A, Kitagawa M, Hirokawa K. Vitamin E enhances the immune functions of young but not old mice under restraint stress. Exp Gerontol. 1999;34:853–862.
99. Reddy PG, Morrill JL, Minocha HC, Stevenson JS. Vitamin E is immunostimulatory in calves. J Dairy Sci. 1987;70:993–999.
100. Ellis RP, Vorhies MW. Effect of supplemental dietary vitamin E on the serologic response of swine to an *Escherichia coli* bacterin. J Am Vet Med Assoc. 1976;168:231–232.
101. van Tits LJ, Demacker PN, de Graaf J, Hak-Lemmers HL, Stalenhoef A. α-tocopherol supplementation decreases production of superoxide and cytokines by leukocytes ex vivo in both normolipidemic and hypertriglyceridemic individuals. Am J Clin Nutr. 2000;71:458–464.

46

Nutritional Modulation of Immune Function and Infectious Disease

Anuraj Shankar

It has long been suspected that poorly nourished people are more susceptible to infectious diseases than well-nourished people. Ancient Greek writings indicated the importance of good nutrition in resistance to infection, and associations between famine and disease epidemics have been noted throughout history. In the late 1800s, experimental animal models were developed that documented effects of specific vitamins and minerals on disease resistance.[1] Subsequent human studies, particularly from the 1930s onward, prompted review by the World Health Organization Expert Committee on Nutrition and Infection and led to publication of the comprehensive monograph, *Interactions of Nutrition and Infection,* in 1968.[2] The authors concluded that:

> Infections are likely to have more serious consequences among persons with clinical or subclinical malnutrition, and infectious diseases have the capacity to turn borderline nutritional deficiencies into severe malnutrition. In this way, malnutrition and infection can be mutually aggravating and produce more serious consequences for the patient than would be expected from a summation of the independent effects of the two.

The clarity and breadth of that review established nutrition as a primary determinant of resistance to infection. In addition, it formalized the vicious cycle paradigm of nutrition and infection in which poor nutrition leads to suppressed immunity that predisposes to infections that further exacerbates malnutrition. Subsequent work by many nutritional immunologists began to establish a mechanistic basis for the debilitating effects of malnutrition on immunity and the effects of infection on malnutrition.[3-6] Moreover, the observation that specific nutrients selectively influence certain parts of the immune system became more clear.[7]

Continuing advances in nutritional immunology have revealed an increasingly complex relationship among nutrition, immunity, and infection. Poor nutrition, or selective nutrient deficiencies, does not simply suppress immune function but causes dysregulation of a normally coordinated host response to infection. This leads to the development of an ineffective response and, in some cases, exacerbation of immunopathologic sequelae. In addition, some evidence indicates that undernutrition may enhance the virulence of pathogens.

The consequences of these effects of nutrition on immune function are well documented in an informative series of recent articles related to the role of both micro- and macronutrient status in the global burden of disease morbidity and mortality.[8-11] Overall, the emerging data indicate more than ever that nutritional status is a predominant factor determining immune competence and plays a central role in infectious disease outcome.

The purpose of this chapter is to give the reader an understanding of the general principles of nutrition and immunity and to provide supporting evidence from studies in humans of the profound interaction among nutrition, infection, and health. These concepts will be illustrated primarily through examination of the effects of vitamin A and zinc as central modulators of the immune response. Some supportive data for other nutrients will also be discussed. As case studies to illustrate the strong interactions with infectious diseases, details will be presented on the relationship between nutrition and malaria, diarrheal disease, and respiratory disease. These sections are by no means exhaustive, and the reader is encouraged to consult additional summaries and discussions of the immune system,[12] nutrition and immune function,[12-14] and nutrition and health in developing countries.[16] Moreover, the reader is directed within each section to additional materials of interest. First, however, it is important to understand basic immune function and the pathways through which nutrients influence resistance to infection.

Overview of Immune Function

Immunity encompasses all measures taken by the body to defend itself against toxins, foreign organisms, or malignant cells. From a conceptual standpoint, the remarkable reliability of host immunity lies in the ability to quickly activate and coordinate redundant and synergistic strategies that are qualitatively diverse. These are generally classified as innate immunity, which provides barriers to infection and a rapid first line of defense with broad specificity, and adaptive immunity, which provides a very high degree of targeted specificity and "memorization" to enhance the speed of the response during any future reinfection. Whether innate or acquired, immunity is conferred through many mechanisms by both specialized cells of the immune system such as macrophages, T cells, and B cells, and also by many nonimmunologic cells such as epithelial and endothelial cells. The importance of any one mechanism in host defense varies considerably with the site of infection, type of invading pathogen, host genetics, and various other environmental factors.

The core attributes of the immune system are its rapid response, diversity of effectors and their redundancy, coordination of effectors, high specificity, and the ability to "learn" through memory.[12] It is critical to recognize that each core attribute of immunity depends on the high availability of nutrients. Thus, poor qualitative and quantitative availability of micro- and macronutrients substantially compromises the most fundamental features of immune function.

Innate Immunity

Innate immunity refers to immune functions that are not modulated by previous exposure to a pathogen.[7] Characteristic of this first line of defense are rapid response and broad specificity but limited efficacy. The most basic of these effectors is the barrier of the skin, epithelial surfaces, and mucosa, followed by the flushing effects of secretory fluids such as tears and mucus. Certain enzymes and proteins may also be present in secretory fluids that may suppress bacterial or viral replication. These include lysozyme, lactoferrin, RNases, and proteins of the complement system that can lyse bacteria and infected cells. In addition, cells present in secretory fluids and blood, such as macrophages and neutrophils, can engulf and destroy organisms by using scavenging receptors that recognize a broad range of microbes. If stimulated by factors such as bacterial cell wall components or cytokines, these cells may also secrete oxygen and nitrogen radicals that nonspecifically react with and neutralize microbes. The febrile response constitutes another relatively nonspecific form of protection and may directly limit the growth of microbes and increase the efficiency of the other effectors of innate immunity. As innate immunity becomes activated during the early phase of infection, certain physiologic responses occur, such as sequestration of certain nutrients from the bloodstream and production of some microbicidal molecules. This is known as the acute-phase response. Although this may have targeted and beneficial effects in helping to control infections, the acute phase response is costly in terms of body nutrients that are expended, destroyed, or lost.[3]

Adaptive Immunity

Adaptive immunity is divided into two basic forms: cell-mediated and humoral (also referred to as antibody-mediated) immunity (Figure 1).[7] The former is governed by T cells (so named because they develop in the thymus gland) and the latter by B cells (in reference to their original discovery in an organ called the bursa, which is found in birds). Both cell types utilize receptors—the T cell receptor for T cells and antibody molecule for B cells—on their surfaces that recognize structures or shapes (i.e., antigens) unique to molecules of particular infectious organisms. When young T and B cells develop from precursors in the bone marrow, each expresses a unique receptor produced by random associations of specialized DNA

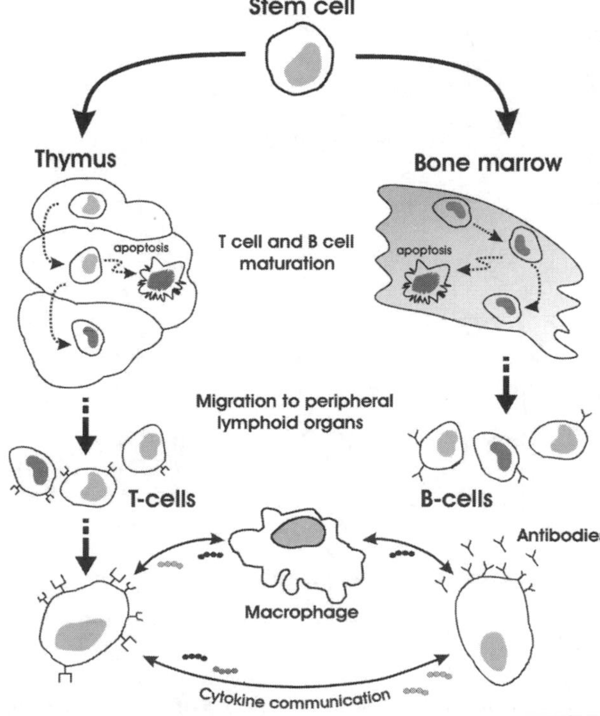

Figure 1. Schema for human T-cell and B-cell immunity.

segments within the cell. As the cells undergo a delicate process of maturation, only those having the appropriate receptors successfully migrate to the peripheral lymph nodes and enter the pool of naive cells (i.e., never stimulated by antigen) waiting to respond to an infection. This multitude of cells, each searching for the matching antigen for its receptor, forms the core of adaptive immunity. The process of generating this diversity is nutritionally and energetically expensive because most young T and B cells do not survive maturation or never find an antigen, and thus undergo a process of programmed cell death known as apoptosis.

Once in the periphery (Figure 2), if receptors on a cell recognize with sufficient affinity a foreign substance or pathogen (cognitive phase), the cell becomes activated and replicates many times (activation phase). This phenomenon is known as clonal expansion and is the primary means by which the body rapidly creates sufficient numbers of cells specialized to contend with a specific infection. Again, this process requires a large pool of readily available nutrients. These activated and replicating cells may have certain functions (effector phase), such as lysing infected cells, secretion of immunomodulators (cytokines), or producing antibody molecules that help to eliminate infectious agents. After clonal expansion and elimination of the pathogen, many cells die through apoptosis when their role is complete, but some go on to become memory cells. These provide a more rapid response in case of reinfection with the same or antigenically related pathogen. The specific functions of T cells and B cells are governed by the specific factors secreted by them once they are activated; these functions are discussed in detail below.

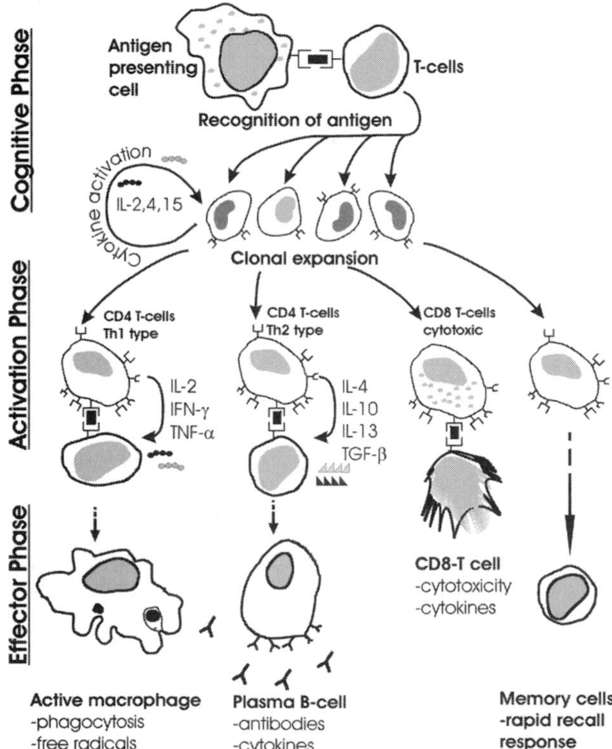

Figure 2. Schema for the three phases of the T-cell response and subsequent interaction with B cells and macrophages during the immune response. IL, interleukin; IFN-γ, interferon-γ; TNF-α, tumor necrosis factor-α; TGF-β, transforming growth factor-β; Th1, T helper type 1; Th2, T helper type 2.

T cells are divided into two main subclasses: CD8 and CD4. The CD8 T cells function as cytotoxic cells able to recognize and kill other cells infected with intracellular pathogens such as viruses. CD4 cells function by secreting immunomodulatory cytokines that can promote T-cell growth (interleukin-2 [IL-2], IL-15), facilitate antibody production by B cells (IL-4, IL-13), or activate microbicidal functions of macrophages (interferon-γ, tumor necrosis factor-α [TNF-α]). These CD4 T cells are frequently referred to as T helper (Th) cells. There is some evidence for segregated production of certain types of cytokines within two CD4 T-cell subsets referred to as Th1 and Th2. Th1 cells appear to produce cytokines that promote the function of macrophages (interferon-γ, TNF-α), whereas Th2 cells produce cytokines that may deactivate macrophages (IL-10, transforming growth factor-β) and promote antibody production by B cells (IL-4, IL-13). The balance between Th1- and Th2-type activities is therefore an important coordinated feature within the immune system.

B-cell function is mediated by the types of antibodies produced. The main types of antibody molecules or immunoglobulins (Ig) are IgM, IgA, IgG1, IgG2, IgG3, and IgG4. They are referred to as isotypes because the antigen recognition function of each is identical, but other parts differ and confer abilities to interact with various components of the immune system. For example, IgM, the first isotype to be produced after activation of B cells, forms complexes with antigens that can easily be engulfed by macrophages and also interacts well with complement to lyse cells or pathogens. IgA is secreted and is the primary antibody found in secreted body fluids. The various IgG isotypes can be recognized by macrophages and neutrophils so that these cells can more effectively engulf and destroy objects recognized by IgG. Therefore, nutrient deficiencies that perturb antibody production and isotype selection will result in dysregulated immunity. Examples of this can be seen in the effects of specific nutrients, described below.

Nutritional Modulation of Immune Function

Protein-Energy Malnutrition

The first effects of malnutrition on immune function were studied in children experiencing protein-energy malnutrition (PEM). Indeed, it is increasingly recognized that childhood, or prenatal, malnutrition may permanently impair the immature immune system at birth and infancy. At any age, it is clear that multiple aspects of immune function are adversely affected.[3,5] The epithelial integrity of malnourished persons was reduced, rendering them more susceptible to invasive organisms. Several studies also documented reduction in neutrophil activity. With respect to adaptive immunity, there were reductions in the number of circulating T and B cells, accompanied by a loss of T-cell function and a reduction in antibody responses.[5,13] Inadequate supply of amino acids can also dysregulate antioxidant status and impair cytokine regulation.[17] Recently, a cytokine-like protein known as leptin was discovered that influences immune function and is modulated by nutritional status. The further study of leptin is likely to shed light on the mechanisms linking nutrition and immune function.[17]

As mentioned above, one of the deleterious effects of PEM is increased susceptibility to infection, which leads to a generalized increase in inflammatory mediators via activation of the acute-phase response and further loss of nutrients.[3] The importance of this is underscored by the results from studies providing a combination of amino acids, fatty acids, and nucleotides to patients hospitalized due to injury or infection. A recent meta-analysis suggests that while such therapies may not reduce mortality, they can decrease length of hospital stay and requirements for ventilation and cause patients to experience lower infection rates. Interestingly, the heterogeneity in these studies also suggests an interaction between each patient's genotype and the response to nutritional therapy.[18] There is a need for additional research in this area to identify the potential to tailor individual diets.

Vitamin A

The discovery in the early 1920s of vitamin A as an anti-infective therapy was recently reviewed.[19] In general, vitamin A is one of the central nutrients influencing immune function, and its effects have been reviewed elsewhere.[20-22] Vitamin A deficiency compromises the integrity of mucosal epithelia and causes loss of microvilli and mucin in the small intestine.[20,23] It also is central in the development and differentiation of neutrophils, monocytes, lymphocytes, and many other immunologic cells. Vitamin A deficiency can selectively reduce CD4 T lymphocytes in lymphoid tissues and peripheral blood,[24] and may promote apoptosis, resulting in premature loss of cell populations such as neutrophils from the blood. Activation of T cells and B cells also appears to require vitamin A. Evidence suggests that vitamin A deficiency dysregulates the Th1-Th2 balance by favoring Th1 activation.[25] A recent study in humans indicates that vitamin A deficiency may favor the overall production of Th1 cytokines but also impairs the Th1 response of cells following direct stimulation.[26] Perhaps associated with this effect is the observation that qualitatively different antibody isotypes may be produced during vitamin A deficiency.[24] Indeed, recent evidence indicates that retinoic acid, a metabolite of vitamin A, regulates factors required for Ig isotype switching and development of certain B cells into IgG-expressing cells.[27]

Zinc

Zinc is also one of the most crucial nutrients for adequate immune function. The effects of zinc on immune function have been extensively reviewed.[28-30] Even subclinical zinc deficiency has a profound effect on immune status. T- and B-cell production is compromised in the thymus and bone marrow because of an increase in apoptosis in precursors of these cells.[31] Interestingly, production of cells of the neutrophil and macrophage lineages appears to be less affected, although function may be compromised, thereby preserving some level of innate immunity.[30] Given that cells of the immune system require a large number of enzymes that need zinc to function, it is not surprising that zinc deficiency has profound effects on immune function. Lymphocytes become less responsive to cytokine activation, and microbicidal ability of macrophages and neutrophils is suppressed.[32] It has also been demonstrated that experimentally induced zinc deficiency in humans results in an imbalance between Th1 and Th2 cell subpopulations such that Th1 function is selectively suppressed.[33] However, there are also reports from survey data indicating that zinc deficiency decreases Th2 responses as well.[26] A better understanding of the molecular and cellular changes due to inadequate zinc will most likely lead to development therapies influencing a variety of immunologic and physiologic functions.

Other Nutrients

Other nutrients can significantly modulate immune function. Presented below is a brief description of the effects of certain specific nutrients due to their emerging or historical importance in nutrition and immune function. For a more comprehensive review of these and other nutrients in nutrition and disease, the reader is referred to recent reviews.[13,16]

Selenium

Although the role of selenium has not been completely elucidated, adequate selenium availability is important during infection.[34-36] Selenium deficiency in animals results in marked suppression of lymphocyte activation and an increase in oxygen radical production by neutrophils. Selenium is a crucial component of glutathione peroxidase, an important antioxidant enzyme. For this reason, selenium may be important for cells that produce free radicals or are exposed to substantial oxidative stress, such as macrophages and neutrophils. Some studies have suggested that selenium can protect macrophages and other cells from prooxidants.

One of the most interesting aspects of the interaction of selenium and infection relates to Keshan disease. This virus-related cardiomyopathy is endemic in some parts of China and has been controlled in recent years by selenium supplementation. To explore the mechanism of this effect, scientists studied a selenium-deficient mouse model of Coxsackie-virus-induced myocarditis. Unexpectedly, it was observed that selenium deficiency allowed a normally benign infection to become virulent and enhanced myocardial damage. Of greatest interest was that the virus isolated from the deficient mice had been transformed to a more virulent form. A number of factors appear to be involved, including changes in the viral genome and a lack of antioxidant activity.[37]

Fatty Acids

Several types of fatty acids have been found to have immunologic effects. Polyunsaturated fatty acids (PUFAs) are generally categorized as the n-6 series (primarily vegetable oils) and the n-3 series (fish oils and certain vegetable oils such as linseed). Depending on the type of PUFA in the diet, immune and other cells produce different quantities and types of prostaglandins that have different effects on the immune response. Diets rich in n-3 PUFAs tend to inhibit macrophage and other cell functions, whereas those rich in n-6 PUFAs tend to enhance certain immune functions and can promote an inflammatory response. Thus, the ratio of n-6 to n-3 PUFAs may have an important influence on immune function. Another class of fatty acids, conjugated linoleic acids (CLAs), has strong effects on both the innate and adaptive immune systems.[38] In animal models, immune-induced wasting and lymphocyte proliferation can be attenuated by CLAs, and the inflammatory cytokines TNF-α and IL-6 can be downregulated. Interestingly, different isomers of CLA exert distinct effects on specific T-cell populations and immunoglobulin subclasses. The understanding of the mechanism by which CLAs and PUFAs affect immune function will aid in the development of nutritionally based therapies against infectious diseases, inflammatory disorders, and allergies.

Vitamins E and C

Vitamin E is an important fat-soluble antioxidant, and its effects are reviewed extensively in Chapter 45 of this book and elsewhere.[39] Deficiency in vitamin E impairs B- and T-cell-mediated immunity. Vitamin E acts in part by reducing prostaglandin synthesis and by preventing the oxidation of PUFAs in cell membranes.[40] Trials in healthy elderly people showed that supplementation with vitamin E improves specific antibody production in response to vaccination.[41] A reduction in the incidence of infections was also observed. Vitamin E is one of the few nutrients for which higher-than-recommended doses can further enhance certain immune functions, at least temporarily. The optimal dose of vitamin E for stimulating immune function has not been determined.

Vitamin C is a water-soluble antioxidant found in body fluids rather than in cellular membranes. It complements and synergizes with effects of other antioxidants, such as vitamin E, by regenerating the reduced preoxidized forms. Vitamin C is important in the function of phagocytes, and the failure of these cells to perform normally may contribute to the impairment of the response to infection that is seen in vitamin C deficiency. It should, however, be mentioned that there is little evidence to support the widely held belief that vitamin C protects against the common cold.

Vitamin B_6

Studies in the 1940s first established that vitamin B_6 deficiency can impair immune function.[13] The vitamin is essential for a wide variety of reactions necessary for the synthesis and metabolism of amino acids. The effect on immune function is not surprising given that antibodies and cytokines, as well as other proteins, are made up of amino acids. Animal and human studies demonstrate that vitamin B_6 deficiency impairs lymphocyte growth and maturation, and both antibody production and T-cell activity are impaired.

Iron

Iron is one of the most critical elements for health, and it has been demonstrated to have effects on immune function. Iron deficiency compromises humoral and cellular immunity and results in reductions in peripheral T cells and atrophy of the thymus.[42] However, there is a growing body of evidence for adverse effects of too much iron.[43] Iron treatment can lead to acute exacerbations of infection, most notably malaria. In a recent randomized trial in Tanzania, preschool children who received iron and folic acid supplements were 12% (95% CI 2–23, $P = 0.02$) more likely to die or need treatment in a hospital for an adverse event. In addition, there was a nonsignificant 15% (95% CI = 7, $P = 0.19$) increase in mortality.[44] Recent discovery of the peptide known as hepcidin has shed new light on the link between iron and immune function.[45] Hepcidin is produced by hepatocytes and is a critical regulator of iron metabolism due to increased or decreased total body iron, inflammation, and anemia. Hepcidin inhibits the efflux of iron from cells such as enterocytes, hepatocytes, and macrophages. This decreases intestinal iron absorption and decreases iron levels in the blood. This shift of iron from the circulation to cellular stores makes it less available to pathogens. In addition to hepcidin, recent discoveries indicate immunomodulatory effects of non-transferrin-bound iron.[46] Specifically, non-transferrin-bound iron increased the expression of adhesion molecules, intercellular adhesion molecule-1 (ICAM-1), vascular cell adhesion molecule-1 (VCAM-1), and E-selectin, thereby indicating a role in inflammation-mediated processes. Thus, the effects of both hepcidin and non-transferrin-bound iron are consistent with the notion that too much iron is deleterious. Ongoing studies of the interactions between iron, immune function, and disease are likely to be critical for global public health programs in which blanket iron supplementation or fortification is routinely advocated to reduce anemia.

Summary

A general summary of nutritional deficiencies and their effects on immune function are presented in Table 1 and schematically in Figure 3. Several features of Table 1 are notable. First, it is clear that any particular nutrient deficiency influences many facets of immune function. Second, each nutrient deficiency may preferentially influence certain effects of immune function while other aspects are unaffected. Third, many aspects of the effects

Table 1. Role of Selected Nutrients on General Immune Functions in Humans

	Humoral Immunity	Barrier and Epithelial Integrity	Cell-Mediated Immunity	T-cell Cytokine Production
Protein-energy malnutrition	X	X	X	X
Vitamin A	X	X	X	X
Zinc	X	X	X	X
Selenium			X	X
Polyunsaturated fatty acids			X	
Vitamin E	X		X	
Vitamin C			X	
Vitamin B-6	X	X	X	
Thiamin		X		
Iron	X		X	

of nutrient deficiencies are unknown. These effects illustrate the complexity of the interaction between nutrition and immune function. Given that individuals suffering from nutrient deficiencies are rarely deficient in only one nutrient and have different levels of deficiency in multiple nutrients, the ultimate influence of poor nutrition on specific immune functions is difficult to predict. Such individuals would experience dysregulated immunity and be less competent to adequately cope with infectious diseases. The second half of this chapter will explore in more detail the consequences of poor nutrition on infectious disease morbidity and mortality. An overview of the impact of infection on general nutritional status will also be presented so that the cycle of poor nutrition and infection is better understood.

Nutrition and Infection

As mentioned above, poor nutritional status has a profound effect on dysregulating the immune system. Several

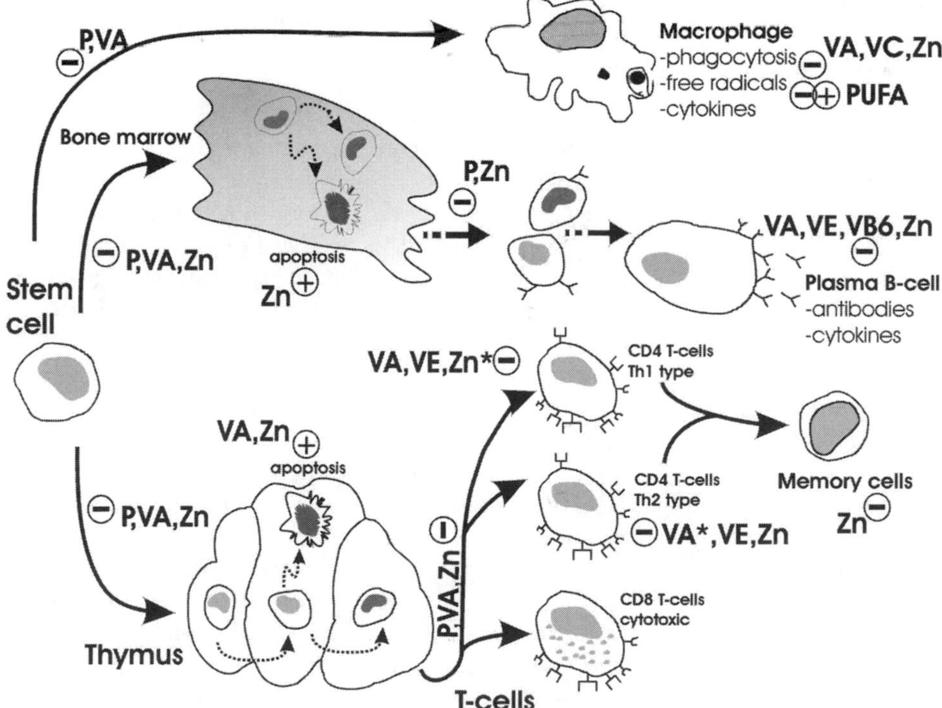

Figure 3. Specific sites of action of selected nutrient deficiencies on the immune response. (+), the deficiency has an enhancing effect on the function; (−), the deficiency has an inhibiting effect on the function; P, protein-energy malnutrition; PUFA, polyunsaturated fatty acids ([+/−] indicates that the impact depends on the ratio of n-6 to n-3 fatty acids in the diet); VA, vitamin A; VB6, vitamin B_6; VE, vitamin E; Zn, zinc; VA*, vitamin A has been shown in animal models to result in an overexpression of Th1-type cytokines such as interferon-γ, denoted as a possible preferential inhibition of the Th2 response; Zn*, zinc has been shown in experimental human Zn deficiency to preferentially inhibit Th1-type cytokines.

laboratory, animal, and epidemiologic field studies have also indicated that malnutrition or selective nutrient deficiencies influence the burden of infectious disease. Moreover, infections themselves result in loss of nutrients and poor nutritional status.

The following sections focus primarily on the relationship of PEM, vitamin A, and zinc status on morbidity and mortality from malaria, diarrhea, and respiratory infections. These represent the primary infectious threats to childhood health throughout the world. The effects on human immunodeficiency virus (HIV) and other infections are briefly presented, along with the effect of other nutrients if warranted. A central theme that emerges from this body of knowledge is that poor nutritional status and selective nutrient deficiencies have differential effects on the susceptibility to different infections. It is therefore not entirely valid to speak of nutrition and infection function in terms of increased or decreased susceptibility. Rather, one must specify the influence of a specific nutrient on selective pathophysiologic aspects of specific infectious diseases.

Malaria

Malaria is the most significant parasitic disease of human beings and remains a major cause of morbidity, anemia, and mortality worldwide. Malaria currently accounts for 200 million morbid episodes and 2 to 3 million deaths each year, estimates that have been increasing over the past three decades.[47] It has long been acknowledged that populations residing in malarious areas generally live under conditions leading to poor nutritional status. As described below, malaria itself is a substantial burden to the population and exacerbates poor nutritional status.

Effect of Malaria on Nutrition and Growth

Malaria can cause growth failure, particularly in young children, and is a contributing factor to malnutrition. Several early reports documented weight loss in young African children after a febrile malaria episode.[48-50] Two studies in The Gambia indicated that *Plasmodium falciparum* malaria was linked to lower weight gain and growth faltering, particularly in children below age 36 months.[51,52] However, in El Salvador no differences in weight or height were observed in areas with low or high transmission of *Plasmodium vivax*, a less malignant species of malaria.[53] In contrast, in Papua, New Guinea, there were more malnourished individuals in villages with high *P. falciparum* transmission intensity than in control villages with lower transmission.[54]

Studies of growth in children taking prophylactic doses of chloroquine provide more definitive evidence for the effects of malaria on growth. A controlled trial of pyrimethamine prophylaxis in Ghanaian 7-year-old children resulted in a small excess weight gain in those taking the drug.[55] Another 2-year study in Nigeria indicated that children given chloroquine prophylaxis from birth onward tended to have slightly greater height and weight.[56] Interestingly, only one child given chloroquine died from malnutrition compared with six such deaths in the control group. A large-scale malaria control program in northern Nigeria involving insecticide spraying and drug prophylaxis also resulted in small but significant changes in weight gain.[57] Similar control measures in Tanzania found no such effects in 2- to 18-month-old children.[58] However, in Kenya and Tanzania the use of bed nets for 1 year resulted in up to 25% fewer malnourished children, with the most pronounced effects in children 18 months of age.[59,60]

Effect of PEM

Before 1950, it was widely accepted that malnutrition led to greater susceptibility to malaria. Several reports before 1940 from Africa and southeast Asia stated that malaria was more frequent and severe in groups and individuals who were undernourished.[61,62] However, between 1954 and 1975, several studies from Africa promoted the notion that malnutrition was in fact protective for malaria.[63-65] Additional work in the early 1970s suggested that refeeding of famine victims in Niger and Sudan activated low-grade infections.[66,67] This led to the widespread misconception that malnourished children are protected against malaria infection, morbidity, and mortality.[68,69] Careful analysis of these works revealed that study populations comprised only clinic cases and malnourished children and that comparisons were made between those with and without malaria. Thus, in the absence of healthy community control subjects, one can only conclude that malaria is less exacerbated by malnutrition than other conditions.

In the past 10 years, more complete studies have evaluated malnutrition as a risk factor for malaria mortality in hospital admissions.[70-72] These studies indicate that malnourished patients are 1.3 to 3.5 times more likely to die or suffer permanent neurologic sequelae. Additional analyses confirm the greater effect of malnutrition on risk of death for diarrhea and pneumonia,[72] a finding that helps explain the spurious findings mentioned above. In addition, longitudinal studies indicate that malnutrition predisposes children to malarial illness.[73-75] A recent review examining the global burden of malaria confirmed that poor nutrition increased the severity of malaria episodes and led to greater deaths.[76] Thus, malnutrition clearly exacerbates malaria infection and morbidity and most likely increases the likelihood of mortality.

The famine or starvation situation is a special case, and it is consistently observed in humans and animals that refeeding an infected starved host reactivates low-grade infections. The implication is that antimalarial measures should be included during nutritional rehabilitation of famine victims.

Effect of Vitamin A

Early studies in vitamin-A-deficient rats and mice showed an increased susceptibility to malaria that was readily reversed by supplementation.[77,78] Cross-sectional studies in preschool children and adults reported inverse associations between plasma vitamin A levels and *P. falciparum* parasitemia.[79] One study observed that low baseline vitamin A status was associated with increased risk of parasitemia.[80] In addition, a study from Nigeria indicated that consumption of red palm oil may be associated with modest protection against malaria.[81] A substudy of a vitamin A trial in preschool children in Ghana reported no statistically significant effects of vitamin A on *P. falciparum* morbidity or mortality.[82] Another trial of vitamin A supplementation in children reported no effect on malaria parasitemia.[83] However, a controlled field trial in preschool children in Papua, New Guinea was carried out specifically to examine the effects of vitamin A on malaria morbidity, and reported a 30% reduction in clinical attacks of *P. falciparum* malaria.[84] The main effect was in children 12 to 36 months of age, who also harbored 68% fewer parasites in their blood and had 28% fewer enlarged spleens, a sign of malaria infection. Interestingly, vitamin A did not have an effect on more severe attacks of malaria accompanied by high levels of parasites in the blood. It has subsequently been demonstrated that vitamin A supplements can offset the adverse effect of malaria on growth.[83] In addition, there is suggestive evidence from clinical trials that vitamin A supplements may protect pregnant women against malaria[85] or reduce the severity of malaria when given as an adjunct to treatment.[86] However, these latter findings require additional validation. From a mechanistic standpoint, other studies indicate that vitamin A may potentiate immune-mediated killing of the parasite[87] or have a direct toxic effect on the parasite.[88]

Effect of Zinc

As mentioned earlier, zinc is essential for a variety of lymphocyte functions, many of which are implicated in resistance to malaria, including production of IgG, interferon-γ, and TNF-α and microbicidal activity of macrophages.[89] Cross-sectional studies in school-age children in Papua, New Guinea reported inverse associations between measures of zinc status and *P. falciparum* parasitemia.[90] In addition, a placebo-controlled trial of zinc supplementation in preschool children in The Gambia documented a 30% reduction in health center attendance due to *P. falciparum*, although this was not statistically significant.

A placebo-controlled trial of zinc supplementation for preschool children in Papua, New Guinea provides additional evidence for the role of zinc in malaria.[91] The study indicated that zinc supplementation reduced by 38% the frequency of health center attendance due to *P. falciparum* malaria. Moreover, a 69% reduction was observed for malaria episodes accompanied by high levels of parasitemia (i.e., >100,000 parasites/μL), suggesting that zinc may preferentially protect against more severe malaria episodes. A subsequent study in Burkina Faso did not observe a protective effect of daily zinc supplementation on *P. falciparum* attacks. However, the daily surveillance methodology that was used biased the study toward assessing impact on less severe malaria attacks.[92] A recently completed randomized trial in the Peruvian Amazon indicated that zinc supplementation reduced the frequency of clinical attacks due to *P. vivax*.[93] Additional information is needed to document the geographic regions and conditions of malaria transmission in which zinc might be effective.

Effect of Other Nutrients

Multiple studies have attempted to evaluate the benefit of iron supplementation in malaria-endemic areas. Some of these studies reported that iron supplementation increased the risk of developing or reactivating malarial illness,[66,94] whereas others reported no significant adverse effects.[95,96] To resolve this issue, a systematic review and meta-analysis of controlled trials of iron supplementation was conducted.[97] Iron supplementation resulted in a nonsignificant 9% increase in the risk of a malaria attack. For trials providing baseline data, the absolute increase in infection rates was 5.7%, which was nonsignificant. Iron supplements were also associated with a nonsignificant 12% increase in risk of spleen enlargement. Qualitative assessment of parasite density suggested a tendency toward higher levels in those receiving iron. The data indicate that prophylactic iron supplementation was associated with increases in certain malariometric indexes. However, these tended to be relatively small effects and were often nonsignificant. In contrast, improvements in hematologic status after iron supplementation were substantial and anemia dropped by 50%. However, as mentioned above, a recently published study from Tanzania indicated that daily oral iron supplementation at currently recommended doses resulted in an 11% (95% CI 1–23, $P = 0.03$) increased risk of hospitalization and a nonsignificant 15% (95% CI 7–41, $P = 0.19$) increase in mortality.[44] These data are consistent with other recent studies indicating adverse effects of iron supplementation on *P. vivax*.[93,98] Thus, routine supplementation with iron in preschool children in areas with malaria can result in an increased risk of severe illness and death. As such, current guidelines for universal supplementation with iron may need to be revisited.

Several of the B vitamins can influence the course of malaria in humans.[99] These include folic acid, riboflavin, and thiamine. Of greatest interest is that riboflavin deficiency is associated with greater resistance against malaria. This is possibly linked to riboflavin's role as an essential factor for glutathione peroxidase, an antioxidative enzyme. It has been proposed that riboflavin deficiency promotes an oxidative environment leading to destruction of the parasite. In contrast, poor thiamine status is associated with greater risk of severe malaria and also simple clinical malaria.[100]

Vitamin E deficiency in animals is associated with protection against malaria infection.[99] As discussed above, the proposed explanation is that the absence of antioxidants makes the parasite more vulnerable to damage by oxygen radicals produced by the immune system. The relevance of this to human malaria remains unknown.

These data indicate that although antioxidant vitamins may exacerbate malaria under some conditions, it is difficult to predict the effect of a nutrient on malaria based on its antioxidant properties alone. In addition, data are lacking for the effects of antioxidant nutrients in humans.

Diarrheal Disease

Diarrheal diseases occur most frequently in developing countries in which poverty, malnutrition, and poor sanitation are prevalent. Reports from the early 1960s of increased prevalence of diarrhea in malnourished children confirmed the long-suspected link between nutritional status and diarrheal disease.[101] Subsequent clinical and epidemiologic studies clearly indicated that diarrhea is exacerbated by malnutrition as defined by anthropometry or deficiencies in micronutrients such as vitamin A and zinc.[102-104] In addition, as detailed below, diarrhea adversely influences nutritional status through poor appetite, malabsorption, loss of nutrients through the gut, and the acute-phase response.

Effect of Diarrheal Disease on Nutrition and Growth

Multiple studies have documented the negative effect of diarrhea, primarily on weight but also on growth, of children during or after an episode of acute diarrhea.[105-107] Faltering of weight gain varied from 10% to 20% in populations with a lower prevalence of malnutrition[105,108] to as much as 70% to 80% in those with a high prevalence of malnutrition.[106,109] As might be expected, the degree of faltering is inversely proportional to the duration of the diarrheal episode. Persistent diarrhea, approximately 3% to 20% of all diarrheal episodes, strongly affects growth[110,111] and increases the risk of mortality.[112] Interestingly, the presence of asymptomatic gastrointestinal pathogens such as *Cryptosporidium parvum* can also adversely affect growth.[113]

The effect of diarrhea on growth in children is due to several factors, including reduced appetite, poor nutrient absorption, and altered feeding patterns. Reductions in dietary intake during diarrhea are well documented[114] and can be as much as 15% to 20%.[115] Moreover, illness can reduce intestinal absorption by direct enterocyte and crypt cell destruction by the pathogen or its toxins, the immune response of the patient, reduction of transit time, and increased fecal losses.[116] Diarrhea may also increase intestinal permeability,[117] which can lead to increases in excretion of sugars, micronutrients such as zinc and copper,[118] and vitamins.[119] During shigellosis, substantial amounts of protein are lost in the stool.[120]

Interestingly, the effects of diarrhea are reduced in breast-fed infants and in children consuming adequate and high-quality diets or food supplements.[121,122] This highlights the need for diets adequate in both protein content and energy density for children with diarrhea and in the convalescent period after diarrhea.

Effect of PEM

As mentioned, early studies indicated a greater prevalence of diarrheal diseases in malnourished children.[151,101,105,108] This is due largely to increased duration of diarrheal illness.[123] The duration of episodes caused by *Shigella* and enterotoxigenic *Escherichia coli* is particularly affected, being up to 3-fold longer. Undernutrition also predisposes children to persistent diarrhea.[124] Other studies indicate that the incidence of diarrhea can be elevated 1.5- to 2.0-fold in malnourished populations[103,125-127] and that the rate of stool output in poorly nourished children is increased.[128]

Given the effects of poor nutrition on morbidity, it is not surprising that diarrheal mortality is potentiated by poor nutritional status. Studies from India and Bangladesh documented that malnourished children are 14- to 24-fold more likely to suffer hospital-based acute diarrheal fatality and post-discharge follow-up fatality.[129,130] The risk of dying from diarrheal diseases is proportional to the degree of malnutrition. A review of six prospective studies showed a progressive increase in mortality with deteriorating nutritional status, as indicated by weight for age.[131] In the Philippines, a large prospective study concluded that the risk of mortality increased 1.6 times per unit decrease in weight for age Z-score.[132] In conclusion, childhood malnutrition is consistently associated with increased risk of death for both acute and persistent diarrhea.

Effect of Vitamin A

A meta-analysis of multiple clinical trials has indicated that vitamin A supplementation can reduce overall mortality by 23% in children 6 months to 5 years of age.[133] Because diarrhea is a major cause of mortality worldwide, it was of interest to determine whether diarrhea mortality was affected. Data from mortality trials in which cause was determined showed that supplementation with vitamin A reduced diarrheal mortality by 35% to 50%.[134-137] However, a more complex relationship emerged from analysis of community-based morbidity trials. In Ghana, supplemented children had a lower incidence of diarrheal episodes with dehydration or with high numbers of liquid stools, resulting in 17% fewer clinic visits and 38% fewer hospitalizations.[137,138] Additional work from Brazil indicated that vitamin A supplements preferentially reduced diarrheal episodes with high numbers of liquid stools per day.[139] Careful examination of vitamin A supplementation studies concluded that there was no effect on diarrhea incidence.[133] The overall interpretation of this body of data is that vitamin A supplementation reduces the severity of diarrhea and associated complications, including mortality, but does not reduce incidence.

Because vitamin A supplementation significantly reduced diarrhea mortality, several studies examined the effects of vitamin A administration as an adjunct to case management of diarrhea. Generally, vitamin A had limited benefit regarding duration or severity[140] except for patients with clinical signs of vitamin A deficiency or malnutrition or for non-breast-fed infants.[141,142] In contrast, a controlled trial in Bangladeshi children suggested that vitamin A supplementation may shorten the course of acute shigellosis.[143]

As expected from the effect of diarrhea episodes on general nutritional status, diarrhea itself predisposes people to vitamin A deficiency.[144,145] Several studies have shown that children with acute and persistent diarrhea have a strong association with xerophthalmia or low serum retinol levels. Decreased serum retinol levels in children with acute diarrhea may be partially explained by increased urinary losses of retinol[146] from impaired renal reabsorption of retinol-binding protein during fever.[147]

Effect of Zinc

Zinc is a potent modulator of the immune response and is critical to normal functioning of all cells. It is therefore not surprising that a strong relationship exists among dietary zinc intake, zinc status, and diarrheal disease. Data from several recent field studies suggest that subclinical zinc deficiency represents one of the most deleterious nutritional disorders in developing countries.

In India, low serum zinc levels were associated with an increased incidence of severe diarrhea.[148] A subsequent community-based, controlled trial in Indian children showed that daily zinc supplementation reduced diarrheal incidence by up to 26% and prevalence by 35%.[31] Similar trends were seen in the prevention of persistent diarrhea by 14% and dysentery by 21%.[149] Generally, these effects were most marked in boys, children with low serum zinc levels, and children over 11 months of age. A study in Guatemala also observed a 22% reduced incidence of acute and persistent diarrhea, mainly in boys.[150] Original data from similar studies in Mexico, Peru, Vietnam, and Papua, New Guinea were pooled and analyzed with the results from India and Guatemala. This analysis indicated that zinc supplementation reduced the diarrheal incidence by 18% and prevalence by 25%.[151] Trends toward reduction of persistent diarrhea and dysentery were also observed. Sex- or age-dependent effects were not prominent.

Trials of prophylactic zinc supplementation have also shown benefits in very young infants. In Brazil, an 8-week course of daily zinc supplementation to low-birth-weight full-term infants decreased diarrheal prevalence by 28%.[152] In India, small-for-gestational-age infants up to age 9 months had a significantly lower incidence of diarrhea, improved weight gain, and, most importantly, a 68% decrease in mortality.[153] This last study indicates the strong potential role of zinc supplementation in reducing overall childhood mortality. Several studies are under way to examine the impact of zinc on childhood mortality.

Zinc has also been examined for its role as an adjunct for treating diarrhea. An initial pilot study of Indian children with acute diarrhea showed a 9% reduction in duration after zinc supplementation. The effect was more pronounced in children with low zinc levels in the rectal mucosa.[154] In a controlled, community-based study in India, children with an acute diarrheal episode who received oral zinc had a 23% faster recovery and, if zinc was given within 3 days of onset of the episode, were 39% less likely to experience more than 1 week of diarrhea.[155] Reductions in the number of watery stools were also noted. Similar findings were observed in a study in Bangladesh.[156] Strong effects of zinc supplementation were also found in the treatment of persistent diarrhea. The study in Bangladesh showed a 33% reduction of duration, with supplemented children being more able to conserve weight and maintain serum zinc levels.[156] Analysis of pooled data from these trials and others indicated that children given zinc supplements during an acute diarrheal episode recovered 15% faster and had 20% fewer episodes of longer than 1 week.[157] For persistent diarrhea, the pooled analysis indicated that zinc supplements led to 29% faster recovery and 49% lower rates of treatment failure.[157] These data indicate that improved zinc intake, through supplementation programs or other means, could have a very significant impact on reducing diarrheal morbidity, and possibly mortality, worldwide.[158]

In 2001, as a result of this body of evidence, a joint World Health Organization/United Nations Children's Fund Task Force recommended the use of zinc in the treatment of diarrhea. It is also recommended as part of standard case management in persistent diarrhea and in those with severe malnutrition. Subsequent results from an intriguing study in Bangladesh indicated that field implementation of diarrheal treatment that included zinc supplementation reduced subsequent childhood mortality by 50%.[159] Although promising, further evidence is required to justify the use of zinc in the treatment of other diseases such as pneumonia and malaria. Improved dietary intake through food fortification or selection of zinc-rich cultivars may provide other ways of controlling zinc deficiency.

Other Nutrients

Other nutrients may also play a role in diarrheal disease. Selenium, an essential trace element, is needed in cells to metabolize hydrogen peroxide and protect against other oxidants. Selenium requirements are greater in infants and children, and its concentration in human milk is affected by maternal intake.[160] In an experimental swine dysentery model, selenium supplementation was associated with improved clinical response and weight gain during recovery.[161] Deficiency of copper, another essential micronutrient, has been associated with persistent diarrhea that resolves after supplementation.[162,163] The relevance of copper deficiency to diarrheal disease burden worldwide remains unclear. Other nutrients may also be important. In India, consumption of short-chain fatty acids by patients with diarrhea enhanced absorption of sodium and water from the large bowel and improved colonic mucosal function.[164] One short-chain fatty acid in particular, butyrate, improved colonic blood flow healing after colonic anastomosis.[165] Nucleotides are another group of nutrients that may affect diarrhea. A multicenter, controlled trial in Spanish infants showed that nucleotide-supplemented formula given during the first 6 months of life reduced the incidence of diarrhea by 36% and also lessened the duration and severity.[166] Reduction in the incidence and prevalence of diarrhea was also observed in a controlled study in Chilean children given nucleotide-fortified infant formula.[167] Although the mechanism of this effect is unknown, it is clear that repair of extensively damaged intestinal mucosa and an adequate immune response require a sufficient supply of nucleotides. The addition of nucleotides to the diet may therefore increase the recovery from diarrhea.[168]

Respiratory Infections

Acute lower respiratory diseases are one of the most important disease burdens of infants and young children in developing countries. Similar to diarrheal disease, no single infectious agent is responsible for respiratory diseases. Causative organisms include viral and bacterial pathogens. As seen for malaria and diarrheal disease, nutrition is a major factor affecting morbidity and mortality from respiratory infections.

Effect of Acute Respiratory Infections on Nutrition

Relatively few studies have examined the effect of acute upper or lower respiratory diseases on nutrition and growth. Studies in Brazil,[169] Guatemala,[170] Papua, New Guinea,[171] and the Philippines[172] confirm that gains in weight or height were reduced during and after episodes of acute lower respiratory infection. Acute respiratory illnesses have been associated with reduced appetite and up to a 20% reduction in food intake.[173,174] Thus, acute lower respiratory illnesses adversely affect the nutritional status of children.

Effect of PEM

Although a link between malnutrition and respiratory infections has long been suspected, the relationship has only recently been critically examined.[175] Field studies using symptom-based diagnosis in the Philippines,[176] Bangladesh,[177,178] and India[179] indicate that malnourished children are nearly twice as likely to experience an acute lower respiratory infection. However, a study in Guatemala did not find this association. Studies of clinical or radiographic pneumonia carried out in The Gambia,[72] Brazil,[169] and Chile[180] also indicate that undernutrition is a key risk factor for hospitalization for pneumonia. Others report increased severity of symptoms,[181] bacteremia, and other complications.[182] These reports suggest that malnutrition is a key risk factor for pneumonia mortality. A large-scale study in the Philippines documented a 1.7-fold increased mortality risk for per unit decrease in weight-for-age Z-score,[132] and in The Gambia, pneumonia fatality rates were substantially higher in malnourished patients.[72] Moreover, malnourished children who recovered from pneumonia in the hospital had a three times greater chance of dying after returning home than did normal survivors.[183] Thus, poor nutritional status is associated with increased risk for acute respiratory disease and an associated risk of mortality from pneumonia.

Effect of Vitamin A

Respiratory infections have been linked to increased risk of vitamin A deficiency and xerophthalmia, but the association between low serum retinol levels and pneumonia may be explained by the acute-phase response to infection, during which the synthesis of retinol-binding protein is attenuated and vitamin A is lost in the urine. Still, some field studies have reported vitamin A deficiency as a risk factor for subsequent respiratory disease in preschool children.[184,185] However, in carefully controlled prospective field trials of vitamin A supplementation, no reductions were reported in mortality or morbidity associated with respiratory diseases.[186]

Vitamin A supplementation was also examined as an adjunctive treatment for pneumonia.[141,187,188] These trials did not show a benefit on the duration of illness or incidence of adverse outcomes. However, a study in Peru indicated that high-dose vitamin A administration to children hospitalized with pneumonia resulted in more severe disease than in children given placebo.[189] These studies indicate that vitamin A supplementation has little, if any, role in the prevention or therapy of pneumonia. This conclusion has recently been affirmed by systematic reviews of the literature[190,191]

Effect of Zinc

As is the case for malaria and diarrhea, there is emerging evidence for a role of zinc in the prevention of respiratory infections, including pneumonia.[192] Considerable reported evidence has indicated that poor zinc status substantially increases the risk of respiratory infections and complications. In an Indian urban slum, children with low plasma zinc levels were 3.5-fold more likely to experience respiratory infections than children with normal zinc levels.[148] In Vietnam, a study in growth-retarded children indicated that zinc supplementation led to an approximately 2.5-fold reduction in the incidence of respiratory infections.[193] In India, daily zinc supplements reduced the incidence of acute lower respiratory infections in infants and preschool children during a 6-month period.[194] In contrast, community-based trials in Guatemala[150] and Mexico[195] did not reveal significant effects of zinc supplementation on the incidence of respiratory infection in young infants or preschool children. Pooled data from these studies and others showed that zinc supplementation was clearly associated with a 38% reduced incidence of pneumonia.[151] In the last 5 years, community-based, controlled trials in India[196] and Bangladesh[197] indicated that routine daily or weekly zinc supplementation reduced the incidence of pneumonia by 26% and 17%, respectively. The latter study also reported a reduction in mortality. Thus, prophylactic zinc supplementation has the potential to reduce the incidence and possibly the mortality of acute respiratory infections. The use of zinc as an adjunct therapy for case management of pneumonia has also been recently evaluated. One trial in Bangladesh indicated that zinc reduced the duration of severe pneumonia by 30%.[198] However, another carried out in India showed no additional benefit of zinc given as an adjunct to treatment.[199] While there is some indication that adjunctive therapy may help, additional information is needed to confirm the effect and conditions of efficacy.

Studies have also examined the influence of zinc supplementation as therapy for the common cold.[200] Some randomized, double-blind, placebo-controlled trials showed reductions in the duration of symptoms of the common cold,[201,202] whereas others did not.[203,204] Although zinc lozenges may have some potential for ameliorating the common cold in some persons and conditions, the effective formulation and dose remain unclear. Zinc lozenges are also associated with greater adverse effects in general, with bad taste and nausea as prominent symptoms.[200]

Other Nutrients

Selenium may play an important role in acute lower respiratory infections, and deficiency may increase the risk of pneumonia in premature and malnourished children. Severely malnourished children may suffer from very low plasma selenium concentrations and low erythrocyte and plasma glutathione peroxidase activity, which may predispose them to the development of serious infections.[205] Critically ill patients with low plasma selenium concentration were three times more likely to acquire ventilator-associated pneumonia or suffer organ system failure and mortality.[206] In a recent double-blind, controlled trial in Chinese children hospitalized with pneumonia or bronchiolitis associated with respiratory syncytial virus, selenium supplements accelerated the recovery rate from signs of respiratory distress.[207] In severely burned patients, a double-blind, placebo-controlled trial of selenium supplementation in combination with copper and zinc reduced bronchopneumonia and led to shorter hospital stays.[208] Thus, selenium supplementation may reduce the morbidity and mortality of acute respiratory diseases in humans. Vitamin D, calcium, or both may also play a role in susceptibility of children to pneumonia and other respiratory infections. In a case-control study conducted in Ethiopia, children with clinical or radiologic evidence of rickets had a 13-fold increase in the risk of pneumonia compared with children without rickets.[209] Continued study of the interactions between respiratory infections and nutrition may lead to new interventions or therapies. For example, a recently discovered protein called Gfi1 is a zinc finger protein that can specifically limit the inflammatory immune response of alveolar macrophages of the lung, thereby limiting the adverse effects of inflammatory cytokines such as TNF-α, IL-1, and IL-6.[210]

Important Nutritional Interactions with Other Infectious Diseases

Measles

Trials in developing countries have demonstrated significant decreases in measles-associated pneumonia and mortality in children given vitamin A supplements compared with children given a placebo.[24] The benefits of vitamin A for measles are not limited to those with overt or subclinical deficiency. When children in US hospitals were treated with vitamin A for severe measles, the illness was less severe and of shorter duration. The mechanism is unclear and may involve some pharmacologic action. An immune mechanism may also be involved because vitamin-A-treated measles patients have increased numbers of lymphocytes and measles-specific antibodies.[24]

HIV and AIDS

There is evidence that nutritional status may be an important determinant of survival in individuals infected with HIV, the virus that causes AIDS.[16] In the later stages of the disease, severe malnutrition is common, and wasting is one of the most prominent characteristics of advanced disease. Although nutritional factors are not likely to be the most important determinants of the disease, they may influence initial susceptibility to HIV infection. The nutritional deficiencies observed in HIV-infected individuals, especially deficiencies of vitamins A, B_6, and B_{12}, have been associated with deficits in immune function (lower counts of Th cells) and accelerated disease progression. Recent research indicates that selenium deficiency may be an important predictor of decreased survival in AIDS patients. Further studies are indicated.[13,16,211]

Recent results from randomized trials in men and nonpregnant women have demonstrated the benefits of vitamins B, C, and E on the immune status of HIV-infected individuals.[212] In Thailand, supplementation with multivitamins led to delayed progression of HIV as assessed by CD4 counts and clinical indicators.[213] In Tanzania, a trial of multivitamin supplementation delayed the progression of HIV disease in women and delayed the initiation of antiretroviral therapy.[214] Similarly, a multivitamin supplementation of pregnant and lactating women reduced morbidity in their infants.[215] However, among HIV-infected pregnant women, vitamin A supplements increased the risk of mother-to-child transmission. However, it should be noted that vitamin A supplements were beneficial in reducing morbidity and mortality in HIV-infected children. Observational studies have yielded conflicting results on the role of zinc status in HIV disease progression.[216,217] This led to concern that zinc supplementation may hasten HIV disease progression. However, a recent trial indicated that zinc supplementation to HIV-infected children improved health and did not influence viral load.[218] For adults and children, more research is warranted on the role of nutrients on health among HIV-infected individuals.

Several other issues concerning nutrition, infection, and immune function are important but are beyond the scope of this chapter. These include other infectious diseases such as tuberculosis and helminth infections. Likewise, the interaction between overnutrition or obesity, infection, and immunity is important, along with the relationship between nutrition and cancer. The reader is referred to other recently published and comprehensive reviews of these topics for additional information.[13,16]

Conclusion

This chapter has attempted to describe the relationships among nutritional status, immune function, and morbidity and mortality from infectious disease. One of the main themes underlying these relationships is that nutritional status is a predominant factor influencing immune function and infectious disease. In addition, it is clear that infection adversely affects nutritional status. More importantly, however, is that the relationship between nutrition and infection is complex. Thus, it is not adequate to discuss poor nutrition simply as having a suppressive effect on immune status or increasing the disease burden of an infection. Rather, the nature of the nutritional deficiency and specific immune functions required for resistance to certain infections must be specifically delineated.

In this context, the example of vitamin A is illustrative. Vitamin A supplementation of deficient populations reduces the severity and mortality but not the incidence of diarrheal disease. In contrast, vitamin A supplementation appears to reduce the incidence of moderately severe episodes of malaria, but may have little effect on malaria mortality. In the same populations, however, vitamin A appears to have little if any effect on respiratory disease or mortality, but has a profound effect on reducing measles mortality. On the other hand, the effects of zinc supplementation in deficiency populations is somewhat more consistent with relatively similar effects on malaria, diarrhea, and respiratory disease. However, qualitative differences are apparent in the effects of zinc on these infections as well.

Such differences in the effect of a nutrient on immune function or infectious disease might be expected because of the diverse metabolic roles played by different nutrients. Unfortunately, considerable gaps in knowledge remain regarding the physiologic links between the cellular effects of nutrients and the clinical outcomes. The mechanisms underlying the effect of any nutrient on mortality remain obscure. It is assumed that such effects may be immunologically mediated, but specific evidence for this is lacking.

Given that the primary effect of various forms of malnutrition is dysregulation of immune function, it is worth considering if overall systemic homeostasis is perturbed due to malnutrition. Thus, not only would immune competence be affected, but the ability of the host to endure the physiologic challenge of illness would be diminished, thereby resulting in increased mortality. If so, then single-point measurements such as blood levels of some factor, cell counts, or anthropometry would be relatively insensitive markers of such dysregulation. Conversely, measurement of the robustness of homeostatic processes in response to challenge would be more sensitive. For example, measuring the kinetics of a glucose-tolerance test, onset of an inflammatory response, changes in antibody production, kinetics of cell populations, or dynamics of gene expression may reveal associations with malnutrition that are more closely associated with clinical outcomes. Thus, to better understand the effects of malnutrition on health, a systems approach may be needed wherein the interactions of the parts are the focus, rather than the parts themselves. This may reveal systemic adaptations in response to malnutrition that confer both advantages and disadvantages for survival. Clearly, additional work is needed to expand and complement what has already been discovered regarding nutrition, immune function, and physiology. In the years to come, the emerging sciences of nutrigenomics and proteomics promise to provide considerable insight into the role of nutrition on the immune system and health.

From the public health perspective, considerable progress has been made on the identification of potentially effective dietary interventions in the prevention, and in some cases, treatment of infectious diseases. The use of nutrients such as zinc, vitamin A, selenium, vitamin E, nucleotides, and others have opened new avenues for research in nutrition and disease control. There is a need now to evaluate the implementation of these effective interventions within the public health context. These advances may go beyond the immediate benefit of reducing the burden of illness and improve the quality of life through enhanced development of the human potential.

References

1. Silverstein AM. *A History of Immunology.* San Diego: Academic Press; 1989; 422 pp.
2. Scrimshaw NS, Taylor CE, Gordon JE. *Interactions of Nutrition and Infection.* Geneva: World Health Organization; 1968.
3. Beisel WR. Infection induced malnutrition—from cholera to cytokines. Am J Clin Nutr. 1995;62: 813–819

4. Prasad AS, Cavdar AO, Brewer GJ, Aggatt PJ. *Zinc Deficiency in Human Subjects*. New York: Alan R. Liss; 1983; 284 pp.
5. Chandra RK. Nutrition and immunity. Lessons from the past and new insights into the future. Am J Clin Nutr. 1991;53:1087–1101.
6. Hurley LS. Nutrients and genes: interactions in development. Nutr Rev. 1969;27:3–6.
7. Beisel WR. Single nutrients and immunity. Am J Clin Nutr. 1982;35(suppl):417–469.
8. Bryce J, Boschi-Pinto C, Shibuya K, Black RE, for the WHO Child Health Epidemiology Group. WHO estimates of the causes of death in children. Lancet. 2005;365:1147–1152.
9. Caulfield LE, de Onis M, Blossner M, Black RE. Undernutrition as an underlying cause of child deaths associated with diarrhea, pneumonia, malaria, and measles. Am J Clin Nutr. 2004;80: 193–198.
10. Rice AL, Sacco L, Hyder A, Black RE. Malnutrition as an underlying cause of childhood deaths associated with infectious diseases in developing countries. Bull World Health Organ. 2000;78: 1207–1221.
11. Black RE. Zinc deficiency, infectious disease and mortality in the developing world. J Nutr. 2003; 133(5 Suppl 1):1485S–1489S.
12. Benjamini E, Coico R, Sunshine G. *Immunology: A Short Course*. 4th ed. New York: John Wiley & Sons; 1996; 498 pp.
13. Gershwin ME, German JB, Keen CL, eds. *Nutrition and Immunology: Principles and Practice*. Totawa, NJ: Humana Press; 1999; 520 pp.
14. Bhaskaram P. Micronutrient malnutrition, infection, and immunity: an overview. Nutr Rev. 2002; 60:S40–S45.
15. Gershwin ME, Nestel P, Keen CL. *Handbook of Nutrition and Immunity*. Totowa, NJ: Humana Press; 2004; 365 pp.
16. Semba RD, ed. *Nutrition and Health in Developing Countries*. Totowa, NJ: Humana Press; 2001; 568 pp.
17. Cunningham-Rundles S, McNeeley DF, Moon A. Mechanisms of nutrient modulation of the immune response. J Allergy Clin Immunol. 2005;115: 1119–1129.
18. Grimble RF. Nutritional modulation of immune function. Proc Nutr Soc. 2001;60:389–397.
19. Semba RD. Vitamin A as "anti-infective" therapy, 1920–1940. J Nutr. 1999;129:783–791.
20. Semba RD. The role of vitamin A and related retinoids in immune function. Nutr Rev. 1998;56: S38–S48.
21. Stephensen CB. Vitamin A, infection, and immune function. Annu Rev Nutr. 2001;21:167–192.
22. Villamor E, Fawzi WW. Effects of vitamin A supplementation on immune responses and correlation with clinical outcomes. Clin Microbiol Rev. 2005; 18:446–464.
23. Rojanapo W, Lamb AJ, Olson JA. The prevalence, metabolism and migration of goblet cells in rat intestine following the induction of rapid, synchronous vitamin A deficiency. J Nutr. 1980;110: 178–188.
24. Semba RD. Vitamin A, immunity, and infection. Clin Infect Dis. 1994;19:489–499.
25. Cantorna MT, Nashold FE, Hayes CE. In vitamin A deficiency multiple mechanisms establish a regulatory T helper cell imbalance with excess Th1 and insufficient Th2 function. J Immunol. 1994;152: 1515–1522.
26. Wieringa FT, Dijkhuizen MA, West CE, van der Ven-Jongekrijg J, van der Meer JW, Muhilal. Reduced production of immunoregulatory cytokines in vitamin A- and zinc-deficient Indonesian infants. Eur J Clin Nutr. 2004;58:1498–1504.
27. Chen Q, Ross AC. Vitamin A and immune function: retinoic acid modulates population dynamics in antigen receptor and CD38-stimulated splenic B cells. Proc Natl Acad Sci U S A. 2005;102: 14142–14149.
28. Shankar AH, Prasad AS. Zinc and immune function: the biological basis of altered resistance to infection. Am J Clin Nutr. 1998;68:447S–463S.
29. Fischer Walker C, Black RE. Zinc and the risk for infectious disease. Annu Rev Nutr. 2004;24: 255–275.
30. Fraker PJ, King LE. Reprogramming of the immune system during zinc deficiency. Annu Rev Nutr. 2004;24:277–298.
31. Fraker P, Telford W. Regulation of apoptotic events by zinc. In: Berdanier C, ed. *Nutrition and Gene Expression*. Boca Raton, Fl: CRC Press; 1996; 189–208.
32. Fraker PJ, King LE, Laakko T, Vollmer TL. The dynamic link between the integrity of the immune system and zinc status. J Nutr. 2000;130(5S Suppl): 1399S–1406S.
33. Prasad AS. Effects of zinc deficiency on Th1 and Th2 cytokine shifts. J Infect Dis. 2000;182: S62–S68.
34. McKenzie RC, Rafferty TS, Beckett GJ. Selenium: an essential element for immune function. Immunol Today. 1998;19:342–345.
35. Arthur JR, McKenzie RC, Beckett GJ. Selenium in the immune system. J Nutr. 2003;133(5 Suppl 1):1457S–1459S.
36. Rayman MP. The importance of selenium to human health. Lancet. 2000;356:233–241.
37. Beck MA. Selenium and host defence towards viruses. Proc Nutr Soc. 1999;58:707–711.
38. O'Shea M, Bassaganya-Riera J, Mohede IC. Immunomodulatory properties of conjugated linoleic

acid. Am J Clin Nutr. 2004;79(6 Suppl): 1199S–1206S.

39. Meydani SN, Han SN, Wu D. Vitamin E and immune response in the aged: molecular mechanisms and clinical implications. Immunol Rev. 2005;205: 269–284.
40. Meydani SN, Meydani M, Verdon CP, Shapiro AA, Blumberg JB, Hayes KC. Vitamin E supplementation suppresses prostaglandin E1(2) synthesis and enhances the immune response of aged mice. Mech Ageing Dev. 1986;34:191–201.
41. Meydani SN, Meydani M., Blumberg JB, et al. Vitamin E supplementation and in vivo immune response in healthy elderly subjects. A randomized controlled trial. JAMA. 1997;277:1380–1386.
42. Bowlus CL. The role of iron in T cell development and autoimmunity. Autoimmun Rev. 2003;2: 73–78.
43. Oppenheimer SJ. Iron and its relation to immunity and infectious disease. J. Nutr. 2001; 131:616S–633S.
44. Sazawal S, Black RE, Ramsan M, et al. Effects of routine prophylactic supplementation with iron and folic acid on admission to hospital and mortality in preschool children in a high malaria transmission setting: community-based, randomised, placebo-controlled trial. Lancet. 2006;367:133–143.
45. Vyoral D, Petrak J. Hepcidin: a direct link between iron metabolism and immunity. Int J Biochem Cell Biol. 2005;37:1768–1773.
46. Kartikasari AE, Georgiou NA, Visseren FL, van Kats-Renaud H, Sweder van Asbeck B, Marx JJ. Endothelial activation and induction of monocyte adhesion by nontransferrin-bound iron present in human sera. FASEB J. 2006;20:353–355.
47. Guinovart C, Navia MM, Tanner M, Alonso PL. Malaria: burden of disease. Curr Mol Med. 2006; 6:137–140.
48. Garnham PCC. Malarial immunity in Africans: effects in infancy and early childhood. Am J Trop Med Hyg. 1949;43:47–61.
49. Bruce-Chwatt LJ. Malaria in African infants and effect on growth and development in children in southern Nigeria. Ann Trop Med Parasitol. 1952; 46:173–200.
50. Frood JDL, Whitehead RG, Coward WA. Relationship between pattern of infection and development of hypoalbuminaemia and hypo-lipoproteinaemia in rural Ugandan children. Lancet. 1971; 2:1047–1049.
51. Rowland MGM, Cole TJ, Whitehead RG. A quantitative study into the role of infection in determining nutritional status in Gambian village children. Br J Nutr. 1977;37:441–450.
52. Marsden PD. The Sukuta Project: a longitudinal study of health in Gambian children from birth to 18 months of age. Trans R Soc Trop Med Hyg. 1964;58:455–489.
53. Faich GA, Mason J. The prevalence and relationships of malaria, anemia, and malnutrition in a coastal area of El Salvador. Am J Trop Med Hyg. 1975;24:161–167.
54. Sharp PT, Harvey P. Malaria and growth stunting in young children of the highlands of Papua New Guinea. Papua New Guinea Med J. 1980;23: 132–140.
55. Colbourne MJ. The effect of malaria suppression in a group of Accra school children. Trans R Soc Trop Med Hyg. 1955;49:356–369.
56. Bradley-Moore AM, Greenwood BM, Bradley AK, Kirkwood BR, Gilles HM. Malaria chemoprophylaxis with chloroquine in young Nigerian children. III. Its effect on nutrition. Ann Trop Med Parasitol. 1985;79:575–584.
57. Molineaux L, Gramiccia G. *The Garki Project*. Geneva: World Health Organization; 1980.
58. Draper KC, Draper CC. Observations on the growth of African infants with special reference to the effects of malaria control. J Trop Med Hyg. 1960;63:165–171.
59. Snow RW, Molyneux CS, Njeru EK, et al. The effects of malaria control on nutritional status in infancy. Acta Trop. 1997;65:1–10
60. Shiff C, Checkley W, Winch P, Premji Z, Minjas J, Lubega P. Changes in weight gain and anaemia attributable to malaria in Tanzanian children living under holoendemic conditions. Trans R Soc Trop Med Hyg. 1996;90:262–265.
61. Gill CA. *The Genesis of Epidemics and the Natural History of Disease: An Introduction to the Science of Epidemiology*. London: Bailliere, Tindall, and Cox; 1928.
62. Williams CD. Clinical malaria in children. Lancet. 1940;1:441–443.
63. Edington GM. Cerebral malaria in the Gold Coast African: four autopsy reports. Ann Trop Med Parasitol. 1954;48:300–306.
64. Hendrickse RG. Interactions of nutrition and infection: experience in Nigeria. In: Wolstenhome GEW, O'Connor M, eds. *Nutrition and Infection*. Boston: Little, Brown; 1967; 98–111.
65. Hendrickse RG, Hasan AH, Olumide LO, Akinkunmi A. Malaria in early childhood: an investigation of five hundred seriously ill children in whom a "clinical" diagnosis of malaria was made on admission to the children's emergency room at University College Hospital, Ibadan. Ann Trop Med Parasitol. 1971;65:1–20.
66. Murray MJ, Murray AB, Murray MB, Murray CJ. The adverse effect of iron repletion on the course of certain infections. Br Med J. 1978;2:1113–1115.

67. Murray MJ, Murray AB, Murray NJ, Murray MB. Diet and cerebral malaria: the effect of famine and refeeding. Am J Clin Nutr. 1978;31:57–61.
68. Latham MC. Needed research on the interactions of certain parasitic diseases and nutrition in humans. Rev Infect Dis. 1982;4:896–900.
69. McGregor IA. Malaria and nutrition. In: Wernsdorfer WH, McGregor IA, eds. *Malaria: Principles and Practice of Malariology*. London: Churchill Livingstone; 1988; 753–767.
70. Randriamiharisoa FA, Razanamparany NJD, Ramialimanana V, Razanamparany MS. [Epidemiological data on children hospitalized with malaria from 1983 to 1992]. Arch Inst Pasteur Madagascar. 1993;60:38–42.
71. Olumese PE, Sodeinde O, Ademowo OG, Walker O. Protein energy malnutrition and cerebral malaria in Nigerian children. J Trop Pediatr. 1997;43: 217–219.
72. Man WD, Weber M, Palmer A, et al. Nutritional status of children admitted to hospital with different diseases and its relationship to outcome in The Gambia, West Africa. Trop Med Int Health. 1998; 3:678–686.
73. Tanner M, Burnier E, Mayombana C, et al. Longitudinal study on the health status of children in a rural Tanzanian community: parasitoses and nutrition following control measures against intestinal parasites. Acta Trop. 1987;44:137–174.
74. Williams TN, Maitland K, Phelps L, et al. Plasmodium vivax: a cause of malnutrition in young children. QJM. 1997;90:751–757.
75. Friedman JF, Kwena AM, Mirel LB, et al. Malaria and nutritional status among pre-school children: results from cross-sectional surveys in western Kenya. Am J Trop Med Hyg. 2005;73:698–704.
76. Caulfield LE, Richard SA, Black RE. Undernutrition as an underlying cause of malaria morbidity and mortality in children less than five years old. Am J Trop Med Hyg. 2004;71(2 Suppl):55–63.
77. Krishnan S, Krishnan AD, Mustafa AS, Talwar GP, Ramalingaswami V. Effect of vitamin A and undernutrition on the susceptibility of rodents to a malarial parasite Plasmodium berghei. J Nutr. 1976; 106:784–791.
78. Stoltzfus RJ, Jalal F, Harvey PWJ, Nesheim MC. Interactions between vitamin A deficiency and Plasmodium berghei infection in the rat. J Nutr. 1989; 119:2030–2037.
79. Shankar AH. Nutritional modulation of malaria morbidity and mortality. J Infect Dis. 2000; 182(suppl):S37–S53.
80. Sturchler D, Tanner M, Hanck A, et al. A longitudinal study on relations of retinol with parasitic infections and the immune response in children of Kikwawila village, Tanzania. Acta Trop. 1987;44: 213–227.
81. Cooper KA, Adelekan DA, Esimai AO, Northrop-Clewes CA, Thurnham DI. Lack of influence of red palm oil on severity of malaria infection in preschool Nigerian children. Trans R Soc Trop Med Hyg. 2002;96:216–223.
82. Binka FN, Ross DA, Morris SS, et al. Vitamin A supplementation and childhood malaria in northern Ghana. Am J Clin Nutr. 1995;61:853–859.
83. Villamor E, Mbise R, Spiegelman D, et al. Vitamin A supplements ameliorate the adverse effect of HIV-1, malaria, and diarrheal infections on child growth. Pediatrics. 2002;109:E6.
84. Shankar AH, Genton B, Semba RD, et al. Effect of vitamin A supplementation on morbidity due to Plasmodium falciparum in young children in Papua New Guinea: a randomised trial. Lancet. 1999;354: 203–209.
85. Cox SE, Staalsoe T, Arthur P, et al. Maternal vitamin A supplementation and immunity to malaria in pregnancy in Ghanaian primigravids. Trop Med Int Health. 2005;10:1286–1297.
86. Varandas L, Julien M, Gomes A, et al. A randomised, double-blind, placebo-controlled clinical trial of vitamin A in severe malaria in hospitalised Mozambican children. Ann Trop Paediatr. 2001;21: 211–222.
87. Serghides L, Kain KC. Mechanism of protection induced by vitamin A in falciparum malaria. Lancet. 2002;359:1404–1406.
88. Hamzah J, Skinner-Adams TS, Davis TM. In vitro antimalarial activity of retinoids and the influence of selective retinoic acid receptor antagonists. Acta Trop. 2003;87:345–353.
89. Good MF, Kaslow DC, Miller LH. Pathways and strategies for developing a malaria blood-stage vaccine. Annu Rev Immunol. 1998;16:57–87.
90. Gibson RS, Heywood A, Yaman C, Sohlstrom A, Thompson LU, Heywood P. Growth in children from the Wosera subdistrict, Papua New Guinea, in relation to energy and protein intakes and zinc status. Am J Clin Nutr. 1991;53:782–789.
91. Shankar AH, Genton B, Baisor M, et al. The influence of zinc supplementation on morbidity due to Plasmodium falciparum: a randomized trial in preschool children in Papua New Guinea. Am J Trop Med Hyg. 2000;62:663–669.
92. Muller O, Becher H, van Zweeden AB, et al. Effect of zinc supplementation on malaria and other causes of morbidity in west African children: randomised double blind placebo controlled trial. BMJ. 2001; 322:1567–1572.
93. Richard SA, Zavaleta N, Caulfield LE, et al. Zinc and iron supplementation and malaria, diarrhea, and respiratory infections in children in the Peruvian Amazon. Am J Trop Med Hyg. 2006; in press.
94. Smith AW, Hendrickse RG, Harrison C, Hayes RJ, Greenwood BM. The effects on malaria of

treatment of iron-deficiency anaemia with oral iron in Gambian children. Ann Trop Paediatr. 1989;9: 17–23.

95. Harvey PWJ, Heywood PF, Nesheim MC, et al. The effect of iron therapy on malarial infection in Papua New Guinean school children. Am J Trop Med Hyg. 1989;40:12–18.
96. Menendez C, Kahigwa E, Hirt R, et al. Randomised placebo-controlled trial of iron supplementation and malaria chemoprophylaxis for prevention of severe anaemia and malaria in Tanzanian infants. Lancet. 1997;350:844–850.
97. International Nutritional Anemia Consultative Group. *Safety of Iron Supplementation Programs in Malaria-endemic Regions*. Washington, DC: International Life Sciences Institute Press; 1999.
98. Nacher M, McGready R, Stepniewska K, et al. Haematinic treatment of anaemia increases the risk of Plasmodium vivax malaria in pregnancy. Trans R Soc Trop Med Hyg. 2003;97:273–276.
99. Shankar AH. Nutritional modulation of malaria morbidity and mortality. J Infect Dis. 2000; 182(suppl 1):S37–S53.
100. Krishna S, Taylor AM, Supanaranond W, et al. Thiamine deficiency and malaria in adults from southeast Asia. Lancet. 1999;353:546–549.
101. Gordon JE, Behar M, Scrimshaw NS. Acute diarrhoeal disease in less developed countries. 1. An epidemiological basis for control. Bull World Health Organ. 1964;31:1–7.
102. Chen LC, Scrimshaw NS, eds. *Diarrhea and Malnutrition: Interactions, Mechanisms, and Interventions*. New York: Plenum Press; 1983; 318 pp.
103. Schorling JB, McAuliffe JF, de Souza MA, Guerrant RL. Malnutrition is associated with increased diarrhoea incidence and duration among children in an urban Brazilian slum. Int J Epidemiol. 1990; 19:728–735.
104. Palmer DL, Koster FT, Alam AKMJ, Islam MR. Nutritional status: a determinant of severity of diarrhea in patients with cholera. J Infect Dis. 1976; 134:8–14.
105. Martorell R, Habicht JP, Yarbrough C, Lechtig A, Klein RE, Western KA. Acute morbidity and physical growth in rural Guatemalan children. Am J Dis Child. 1975;129:1296–1301.
106. Rowland MGM, Rowland SGL, Cole TJ. Impact of infection on the growth of children from 0 to 2 years in an urban West African community. Am J Clin Nutr. 1988;47:134–138.
107. Bhandari N, Sazawal S, Clemens JD, Kashyap DK, Dhingra U, Bhan MK. Association between diarrheal duration and nutritional decline: implications for an empirically validated definition of persistent diarrhea. Indian J Pediatr. 1994;61:559–566.
108. Condon-Paoloni D, Cravioto J, Johnston FE, De Licardie ER, Scholl TO. Morbidity and growth of infants and young children in a rural Mexican village. Am J Public Health. 1977;67:651–656.
109. Zumrawi FY, Dimond H, Waterlow JC. Effects of infection on growth in Sudanese children. Hum Nutr Clin Nutr. 1987;41:453–461.
110. Black RE. Persistent diarrhea in children of developing countries. Pediatr Infect Dis. 1993;12: 751–761.
111. Baqui AH, Sack RB, Black RE, Chowdhury HR, Yunus M, Siddique AK. Cell-mediated immune deficiency and malnutrition are independent risk factors for persistent diarrhea in Bangladeshi children. Am J Clin Nutr. 1993;58:543–548.
112. Fauveau V, Henry FJ, Briend A, Yunus M, Chakraborty J. Persistent diarrhea as a cause of childhood mortality in rural Bangladesh. Acta Paediatr Suppl. 1992;381:12–14.
113. Checkley W, Gilman RH, Epstein LD, et al. Asymptomatic and symptomatic cryptosporidiosis: their acute effect on weight gain in Peruvian children. Am J Epidemiol. 1997;145:156–163.
114. Brown KH, Stallings RY, Creed de Kanashiro HC, Lopez de Romana G, Black RE. Effects of common illnesses on infants' energy intakes from breast milk and other foods during longitudinal community-based studies in Huascar (Lima), Peru. Am J Clin Nutr. 1990;52:1005–1013.
115. Martorell R, Yarbrough C, Yarbrough S, Klein RE. The impact of ordinary illnesses on the dietary intakes of malnourished children. Am J Clin Nutr. 1980;33:345–350.
116. O'Loughlin EV, Scott RB, Gall DG. Pathophysiology of infectious diarrhea: changes in intestinal structure and function. J Pediatr Gastroenterol Nutr. 1991;12:5–20.
117. Lunn PG, Northrup-Clewes CA, Downes RM. Intestinal permeability, mucosal injury, and growth faltering in Gambian infants. Lancet. 1991;338: 907–910.
118. Castillo-Duran C, Vial P, Uauy R. Trace mineral balance during acute diarrhea in infants. J Pediatr. 1988;113:452–457.
119. Paerregaard A, Ellett K, Krasilnikoff PA. Vitamin B12 and folic acid absorption and hematological status in children with postenteritis enteropathy. J Pediatr Gastroenterol Nutr. 1990;11:351–355.
120. Black RE, Brown KH, Becker S, Alim AR, Huq I. Longitudinal studies of infectious diseases and physical growth of children in rural Bangladesh. II. Incidence of diarrhea and association with known pathogens. Am J Epidemiol. 1982;115:315–324.
121. Marquis GS, Habicht JP, Lanata CF, Black RE, Rasmussen KM. Breast milk or animal-product foods improve linear growth of Peruvian toddlers consuming marginal diets. Am J Clin Nutr. 1997; 66:1102–1109.
122. Rivera J, Martorell R, Lutter CK. Interaction of

dietary intake and diarrheal disease in child growth. Arch Latinoam Nutr. 1989;39:292–307.
123. Chen LC, Huq E, Huffman SL. A prospective study of the risk of diarrheal diseases according to the nutritional status of children. Am J Epidemiol. 1981;114:284–292.
124. Deivanayagam N, Mala N, Ashok TP, Ratnam SR, Sankaranarayanan VS. Risk factors for persistent diarrhea among children under 2 years of age. Case control study. Indian Pediatr. 1993;30:177–185.
125. Guerrant RL, Schorling JB, McAuliffe JF, de Souza MA. Diarrhea as a cause and an effect of malnutrition: diarrhea prevents catch-up growth and malnutrition increases diarrhea frequency and duration. Am J Trop Med Hyg. 1992;47:28–35.
126. El Samani FZ, Willett WC, Ware JH. Predictors of simple diarrhoea in children under 5 years: a study of a Sudanese rural community. Soc Sci Med. 1989;29:1065–1070.
127. Lindtjorn B, Alemu T, Bjorvatn B. Nutritional status and risk of infection among Ethiopian children. J Trop Pediatr. 1993;39:76–82.
128. Black RE, Merson MH, Eusof A, Huq I, Pollard R. Nutritional status, body size and severity of diarrhoea associated with rotavirus or enterotoxigenic Escherichia coli. Am J Trop Med Hyg. 1984;87: 83–89.
129. Ryder RW, Reeves WC, Sack RB. Risk factors for fatal childhood diarrhea: a case-control study from two remote Panamanian islands. Am J Epidemiol. 1985;121:605–610.
130. Roy SKI, Chowdhury AK, Rahaman MM. Excess mortality among children discharged from hospital after treatment for diarrhoea in rural Bangladesh. Br Med J. 1983;287:1097–1099.
131. Pelletier DL, Frongillo EA Jr, Habicht JP Epidemiologic evidence for a potentiating effect of malnutrition on child mortality. Am J Public Health. 1993;83:1130–1133.
132. Yoon PW, Black RE, Moulton LH, Becker S. The effect of malnutrition on the risk of diarrheal and respiratory mortality in children <2 y of age in Cebu, Philippines. Am J Clin Nutr. 1997;65: 1070–1077.
133. Beaton GH, Martorell R, L Abbe KA, et al, eds. *Effectiveness of Vitamin A Supplementation in the Control of Young Child Morbidity and Mortality in Developing Countries.* Final Report to the Canadian International Development Agency. Toronto: University of Toronto; 1992.
134. Rahmathullah L, Underwood BA, Thulasiraj RD, et al. Reduced mortality among children in Southern India receiving a small weekly dose of vitamin A. N Engl J Med. 1990;323:929–935.
135. West KP Jr, Pokhrel RP, Katz J, et al. Efficacy of vitamin A in reducing preschool child mortality in Nepal. Lancet. 1991;338:67–71.
136. Daulaire NMP, Starbuck ES, Houston RM, Church MS, Stukel TA, Pandey MR. Childhood mortality after a high dose of vitamin A in a high risk population. BMJ. 1992;304:207–210.
137. Ghana VAST Study Team. Vitamin A supplementation in northern Ghana: effects on clinic attendances, hospital admissions, and child mortality. Lancet. 1993;342:7–12.
138. Arthur P, Kirkwood B, Ross D, et al. Impact of vitamin A supplementation on childhood morbidity in northern Ghana. Lancet. 1992;339:361–362.
139. Barreto ML, Santos LMP, Assis AMO, et al. Effect of vitamin A supplementation on diarrhoea and acute lower-respiratory-tract infections in young children in Brazil. Lancet. 1994;344:228–231.
140. Henning B, Stewart K, Zaman K, Alam AN, Brown KH, Black RE. Lack of therapeutic efficacy of vitamin A for non-cholera, watery diarrhoea in Bangladeshi children. Eur J Clin Nutr. 1992;46: 437–443.
141. Donnen P, Dramaix M, Brasseur D, Bitwe R, Vertongen F, Hennart P. Randomized placebo-controlled clinical trial of the effect of a single high dose or daily low dose of vitamin A on the morbidity of hospitalized, malnourished children. Am J Clin Nutr. 1998;68:1254–1260.
142. Bhandari N, Bahl R, Sazawal S, Bhan MK. Breast-feeding status alters the effect of vitamin A treatment during acute diarrhea in children. J Nutr. 1997;127:59–63.
143. Hossain S, Biswas R, Kabir I, et al. Single dose vitamin A treatment in acute shigellosis in Bangladeshi children: randomised double blind controlled trial. BMJ. 1998;316:422–426.
144. Sommer A, Tarwotjo I, Katz J. Increased risk of xerophthalmia following diarrhea and respiratory disease. Am J Clin Nutr. 1987;45:977–980.
145. Salazar-Lindo E, Salazar M, Alvarez JO. Association of diarrhea and low serum retimil in Peruvian children. Am J Clin Nutr. 1993;58:110–113.
146. Alvarez JO, Salazar-Lindo E, Kohatsu J, Miranda P, Stephensen CB. Urinary excretion of retinol in children with acute diarrhea. Am J Clin Nutr. 1995; 61:1273–1276.
147. Mitra AK, Alvarez JO, Wahed MA, Fuchs GJ, Stephensen CB. Predictors of serum retinol in children with shigellosis. Am J Clin Nutr. 1998;68: 1088–1094.
148. Bahl R, Bhandari N, Hambidge KM, Bhan MK. Plasma zinc as a predictor of diarrheal and respiratory morbidity in children in an urban slum setting. Am J Clin Nutr. 1998;68(suppl):414S–417S.
149. Sazawal S, Black RE, Bhan MK, et al. Zinc supplementation reduces the incidence of persistent diarrhea and dysentery among low socioeconomic children in India. J Nutr. 1996;126:443–450.
150. Ruel MT, Rivera JA, Santizo MC, Lonnerdal B,

Brown KH. Impact of zinc supplementation on morbidity from diarrhea and respiratory infections among rural Guatemalan children. Pediatrics. 1997; 99:808–813.

151. Bhutta ZA, Black RE, Brown KH, et al, for the Zinc Investigators' Collaborative Group. Prevention of diarrhea and pneumonia by zinc supplementation in children in developing countries: pooled analysis of randomized controlled trials. J Pediatr. 1999;135:689–697.
152. Lira PI, Ashworth A, Morris SS. Effect of zinc supplementation on the morbidity, immune function, and growth of low-birth-weight, full term infants in northeast Brazil. Am J Clin Nutr. 1998; 68(suppl):418S–424S.
153. Sazawal S, Black RE, Menon VP, et al. Effect of zinc and mineral supplementation in small for gestational age infants on growth and mortality. FASEB J. 1999;13:A376.
154. Sachdev HPS, Mittal NK, Mittal SK, Yadav HS. A controlled trial on utility of oral zinc supplementation in acute dehydrating diarrhea in infants. J Pediatr Gastroenterol Nutr. 1988;7:877–881.
155. Sazawal S, Black RE, Bhan MK, Bhandari N, Sinha A, Jalla S. Zinc supplementation in young children with acute diarrhea in India. N Engl J Med. 1995; 333:839–844.
156. Roy SK, Tomkins AM, Akramuzzaman SM, et al. Randomised controlled trial of zinc supplementation in malnourished Bangladeshi children with acute diarrhoea. Arch Dis Child. 1997;77:196–200.
157. Bhutta ZA, Bird SM, Black RE, et al. Therapeutic effects of oral zinc in acute and persistent diarrhea in children in developing countries: pooled analysis of randomized controlled trials. Am J Clin Nutr. 2000;72:1516–1522.
158. Penny ME, Lanata CF. Zinc in the management of diarrhea in young children. N Engl J Med. 1995; 333:873–874.
159. Baqui AH, Black RE, El Arifeen S, et al. Effect of zinc supplementation started during diarrhoea on morbidity and mortality in Bangladeshi children: community randomised trial. BMJ. 2002;325: 1059–1065.
160. Bedwal RS, Nair N, Sharma MP, Mathur RS. Selenium—its biological perspectives. Med Hypotheses. 1993;41:150–159.
161. Teige J, Tollersrud S, Lund A, Larsen HL. Swine dysentery: the influence of dietary vitamin E and selenium on the clinical and pathological effects of Treponema hyodysenteriae infection in pigs. Res Vet Sci. 1982;32:95–100.
162. Cordano A, Baertl JM, Graham CG. Copper deficiency in infancy. Pediatrics. 1964;34:324–326.
163. Cordano A. Clinical manifestations of nutritional copper deficiency in infants and children. Am J Clin Nutr. 1998;67(suppl):1012S–1016S.
164. Ramakrishna BS, Mathan VI. Colonic dysfunction in acute diarrhoea: the role of luminal short chain fatty acids. Gut. 1993;34:1215–1218.
165. Velazquez OC, Lederer HM, Rombeau JL. Butyrate and the colonocyte. Production, absorption, metabolism, and therapeutic implications. Adv Exp Med Biol. 1997;427:123–134.
166. Lama More RA, Gil-Alberdi Gonzalez B. [Effect of nucleotides as dietary supplement on diarrhea in healthy infants]. An Esp Pediatr. 1998;48: 371–375.
167. Brunser O, Espinoza J, Araya M, Cruchet S, Gil A. Effect of dietary nucleotide supplementation on diarrhoeal disease in infants. Acta Paediatr. 1994; 83:188–191.
168. Leleiko NS, Walsh MJ. Dietary purine nucleotides and the gastrointestinal tract. Nutrition. 1995;11: 725–730.
169. Victora CG, Barms FC, Kirkwood BR, Vaughan JP. Pneumonia, diarrhoea and growth in the first 4 years of life. A longitudinal study of 5914 Brazilian children. Am J Clin Nutr. 1990;52:391–396.
170. Cruz JR, Pareja G, de Fernandez A, Peralta F, Caceres P, Cano F. Epidemiology of acute respiratory tract infections among Guatemalan ambulatory preschool children. Rev Infect Dis. 1990;12(Suppl 8): S1029–S1034.
171. Smith TA, Lehmann D, Coakley C, Spooner V, Alpers MP. Relationships between growth and acute lower-respiratory infections in children aged less than 5 y in a highland population of Papua New Guinea. Am J Clin Nutr. 1991;53:963–970.
172. Adair L, Popkin BM, Van Derslice J, et al. Growth dynamics during the first two years of life: a prospective study in the Philippines. Eur J Clin Nutr. 1993;47:42–51.
173. Pereira SM, Begum A The influence of illnesses on the food intake of young children. Int J Epidemiol. 1987;16:445–450.
174. Brown KH, Sanchez-Grinan M, Perez F, Peerson JM, Ganoza L, Stern JS. Effects of dietary energy density and feeding frequency on total daily energy intakes by recovering malnourished children. Am J Clin Nutr. 1995;62:13–18.
175. Bale JR. Creation of a research program to determine the etiology and epidemiology of acute respiratory tract infection among children in developing countries. Rev Infect Dis. 1990;12(Suppl 8): S861–S866.
176. Tupasi TE, Lucero MG, Magdangal DM, et al. Etiology of acute lower respiratory tract infection in children from Alabang, Metro Manila. Rev Infect Dis. 1990;12(Suppl 8):S929–S939.
177. Zaman K, Baqui AH, Yunus M, et al. Association between nutritional status, cell-mediated immune status and acute lower respiratory infections in Bangladeshi children. Eur J Clin Nutr. 1996;50: 309–314.

178. Rahman MM, Rahman AM. Prevalence of acute respiratory tract infection and its risk factors in under five children. Bangladesh Med Res Couric Bull. 1997:23:47–50.
179. Deb SK. Acute respiratory disease survey in Tripura in case of children below five years of age. J Indian Med Assoc. 1998;96:111–116.
180. Atalah E. Bustos P, Gomez E. Infantile malnutrition: social cost or respiratory and digestive pathology. Arch Latinoam Nutr. 1983;33:395–408.
181. James JW. Longitudinal study of the morbidity of diarrheal and respiratory infections in malnourished children. Am J Clin Nutr. 1972;25:690–694.
182. Johnson WB, Aderele WI, Gbadero DA. Host factors and acute lower respiratory infections in preschool children. J Trop Pediatr. 1992;38:132–136.
183. West TE, Goetghebuer T, Milligan P, Mulholland EK, Weber MW. Long-term morbidity and mortality following hypoxaemic lower respiratory tract infection in Gambian children. Bull World Health Organ. 1999;77:144–148.
184. Sommer A, Katz J, Tarwotjo I. Increased risk of respiratory disease and diarrhea in children with preexisting mild vitamin A deficiency. Am J Clin Nutr. 1984;40:1090–1095.
185. Bloem MW, Wedel M, Egger RJ, et al. Mild vitamin A deficiency and risk of respiratory tract diseases and diarrhea in preschool and schoolchildren in northeastern Thailand. Am J Epidemiol. 1990; 131:332–339.
186. Vitamin A and Pneumonia Working Group. Potential interventions for the prevention of childhood pneumonia in developing countries: a meta-analysis of data from field trials to assess the impact of vitamin A supplementation on pneumonia morbidity and mortality. Bull World Health Organ. 1995;73: 609–619.
187. Nacul LC, Kirkwood BR, Arthur P, Morris SS, Magalhaes M, Fink MC. Randomized, double blind, placebo controlled clinical trial of efficacy of vitamin A treatment in non-measles childhood pneumonia. BMJ. 1997;315:505–510.
188. Rodriguez A, Hamer DH, Rivera J, et al. Effects of moderate doses of vitamin A as an adjunct to the treatment of pneumonia in underweight and normal weight children: a randomized, double-blind, placebo-controlled trial. Am J Clin Nutr. 2005;82: 1090–1096.
189. Stephensen CB, Franchi LM, Hernandez H, Campos M, Gilman RH, Alvarez JO. Adverse effects of high-dose vitamin A supplements in children hospitalized with pneumonia. Pediatrics 1998; 101:E3
190. Huiming Y, Chaomin W, Meng M. Vitamin A for treating measles in children. Cochrane Database Syst Rev. 2005;(4):CD001479.
191. Brown N, Roberts C. Vitamin A for acute respiratory infection in developing countries: a meta-analysis. Acta Paediatr. 2004;93:1437–1442.
192. Hambidge M, Krebs N. Zinc, diarrhea, and pneumonia. J Pediatr. 1999;135:661–664.
193. Ninh NX, Thissen JP, Collette L, Gerard G, Khoi HH, Ketelslegers JM. Zinc supplementation increases growth and circulating insulin-like growth factor I (IFG-I) in growth-retarded Vietnamese children. Am J Clin Nutr. 1996;63:514–519.
194. Sazawal S, Black RE, Jalla S, Mazumdar S, Sinha A, Bhan MK. Zinc supplementation reduces the incidence of acute lower respiratory infections in infants and preschool children: a double-blind, controlled trial. Pediatrics. 1998;102:1–5.
195. Rosado JL, Lopez P, Muñoz E, Martinez H, Allen LH. Zinc supplementation reduced morbidity, but neither zinc nor iron supplementation affected growth or body composition of Mexican preschoolers. Am J Clin Nutr. 1997;65:13–19.
196. Bhandari N, Bahl R, Taneja S, et al. Effect of routine zinc supplementation on pneumonia in children aged 6 months to 3 years: randomised controlled trial in an urban slum. BMJ. 2002;324: 1358–1362.
197. Brooks WA, Santosham M, Naheed A, et al. Effect of weekly zinc supplements on incidence of pneumonia and diarrhoea in children younger than 2 years in an urban, low-income population in Bangladesh: randomised controlled trial. Lancet. 2005; 366:999–1004.
198. Brooks WA, Yunus M, Santosham M, et al. Zinc for severe pneumonia in very young children: double-blind placebo-controlled trial. Lancet. 2004;363:1683–1688.
199. Mahalanabis D, Chowdhury A, Jana S, et al. Zinc supplementation as adjunct therapy in children with measles accompanied by pneumonia: a double-blind, randomized controlled trial. Am J Clin Nutr. 2002;76:604–607.
200. Macknin ML. Zinc lozenges for the common cold. Cleveland Clin J Med. 1999;66:27–32.
201. Eby GA, Davis DR, Halcomb WW. Reduction in duration of common colds by zinc gluconate lozenges in a double-blind study. Antimicrob Agents Chemother. 1984;25:20–24.
202. Mossad SB, Macknin ML, Medendom SV, Mason P. Zinc gluconate lozenges for treating the common cold. A randomized, double-blind, placebo-controlled study. Arch Intern Med. 1996;125: 81–88.
203. Douglas RM, Miles HB, Moore BW, Ryan P, Pinnock CB. Failure of effervescent zinc acetate lozenges to alter the course of upper respiratory tract infections in Australian adults. Antimicrob Agents Chemother. 1987;31:1263–1265.
204. Farr BM, Conner EM, Betts RF, Oleske J, Min-

nefor A, Gwaltney JM Jr. Two randomized controlled trials of zinc gluconate lozenge therapy of experimentally induced rhinovirus colds. Antimicrob Agents Chemother. 1987;31:1183–1187.
205. Thomas AG, Miller V, Shenkin A, Fell GS, Taylor F. Selenium and glutathione peroxidase status in paediatric health and gastrointestinal disease. J Pediatr Gastroenterol Nutr. 1994;19:213–219.
206. Forceville X, Vitoux D, Gauzit R, Combes A, Lahilaire P, Chappuis P. Selenium, systemic immune response syndrome, sepsis, and outcome in critically ill patients. Crit Care Med. 1998;26:1536–1544.
207. Liu X, Yin S, Li G. [Effects of selenium supplement on acute lower respiratory tract infection caused by respiratory syncytial virus]. Chung Bus Yu Fang I Hsueh Tsa Chih. 1997;31:358–361.
208. Berger MM, Spertini F, Shenkin A, et al. Trace element supplementation modulates pulmonary infection rates after major bums: a double-blind, placebo-controlled trial. Am J Clin Nutr. 1998;68: 365–371.
209. Muhe L, Tilahun M, Lulseged S, et al. Etiology of pneumonia, sepsis and meningitis in infants younger than three months of age in Ethiopia. Pediatr Infect Dis. 1999;18(10 suppl):S56–S61.
210. Jin J, Zeng H, Schmid KW, Toetsch M, Uhlig S, Moroy T. The zinc finger protein Gfi1 acts upstream of TNF to attenuate endotoxin-mediated inflammatory responses in the lung. Eur J Immunol. 2006;36:421–430.
211. Lanzillotti JS, Tang AM. Micronutrients and HIV disease: a review pre- and post-HAART. Nutr Clin Care. 2005;8:16–23.
212. Fawzi W. Micronutrients and human immunodeficiency virus type 1 disease progression among adults and children. Clin Infect Dis. 2003;37(Suppl 2): S112–S116.
213. Jiamton S, Pepin J, Suttent R, et al. A randomized trial of the impact of multiple micronutrient supplementation on mortality among HIV-infected individuals living in Bangkok. AIDS. 2003;17: 2461–2469.
214. Fawzi WW, Msamanga GI, Spiegelman D, et al. A randomized trial of multivitamin supplements and HIV disease progression and mortality. N Engl J Med. 2004;351:23–32.
215. Fawzi WW, Msamanga GI, Wei R, et al. Effect of providing vitamin supplements to human immunodeficiency virus-infected, lactating mothers on the child's morbidity and CD4+ cell counts. Clin Infect Dis. 2003;36:1053–1062.
216. Kupka R, Fawzi W. Zinc nutrition and HIV infection. Nutr Rev. 2002;60:69–79.
217. Villamor E, Aboud S, Koulinska IN, et al. Zinc supplementation to HIV-1-infected pregnant women: Effects on maternal anthropometry, viral load, and early mother-to-child transmission. Eur J Clin Nutr. 2006 Feb 1 Epub.
218. Bobat R, Coovadia H, Stephen C, et al. Safety and efficacy of zinc supplementation for children with HIV-1 infection in South Africa: a randomised double-blind placebo-controlled trial. Lancet. 2005;366:1862–1867.

47 Food Allergy

Steve L. Taylor and Susan L. Hefle

Centuries ago, Lucretius stated "What is food to one is bitter poison to another." Food allergies and sensitivities can be collectively referred to as "individualistic adverse reactions to foods" because these illnesses affect only certain individuals within the population. Although these diseases are often grouped together under the general heading of "food allergy," a variety of different types of illnesses are involved. The existence of several different types of adverse reactions to foods with varied symptomology, severity, prevalence, and causative factors is not recognized by some physicians. Consumers are even more likely to be confused regarding the definition and classification of adverse reactions to foods. Consumers perceive that "food allergies" are common,[1] but many self-diagnosed cases of "food allergy" incorrectly associate foods with a particular malady or ascribe various mild forms of postprandial eating discomfort to this category of illness.

Classification

Table 1 provides a classification scheme for the different types of illnesses that are known to occur in association with food ingestion that only involve certain individuals in the population. Two major groups of individualistic adverse reactions to foods are known: true food allergies and food intolerances. The true food allergies involve abnormal immunologic mechanisms, whereas the food intolerances do not. Knowing and recognizing the difference between immunologic food allergies and nonimmunologic food intolerances is crucial. Intolerances can usually be controlled by limiting the amount of the food or food ingredient that is eaten. In contrast, total avoidance is essential with true food allergies.

A food allergy is an abnormal immunologic response to a food or food component, usually a naturally occurring protein.[2] Two different types of abnormal immunologic responses are known to occur. Immediate hypersensitivity reactions are antibody mediated, whereas delayed hypersensitivity reactions are cell mediated.

In contrast, food intolerances do not involve abnormal responses of the immune system.[2] Three major categories of food intolerances are recognized: anaphylactoid reactions, metabolic food disorders, and food idiosyncrasies.

Immunoglobulin-E-Mediated Food Allergy

Mechanism. Immediate hypersensitivity reactions are mediated by allergen-specific immunoglobulin (Ig)E antibodies (Figure 1). In IgE-mediated food allergies, allergen-specific IgE antibodies are produced by B cells in response to the immunologic stimulus created by exposure of the immune system to the allergen.[3] Food allergens are usually naturally occurring proteins present in the food.[4] The allergen-specific IgE antibodies bind to the surfaces of mast cells in the tissues and basophils in the blood. This is the sensitization phase of the allergic response. The sensitization phase is asymptomatic. On

Table 1. Classification of Individualistic Adverse Reactions to Foods

- True Food Allergies
  - Antibody-Mediated Food Allergies
    - Immunoglobulin E-mediated food allergies (e.g., peanut, cow's milk)
    - Exercise-associated food allergies
  - Cell-Mediated Food Allergies
    - Celiac disease
    - Other types of delayed hypersensitivity
- Food Intolerances
  - Anaphylactoid Reactions
  - Metabolic Food Disorders
    - Lactose intolerance
  - Idiosyncratic Reactions
    - Sulfite-induced asthma

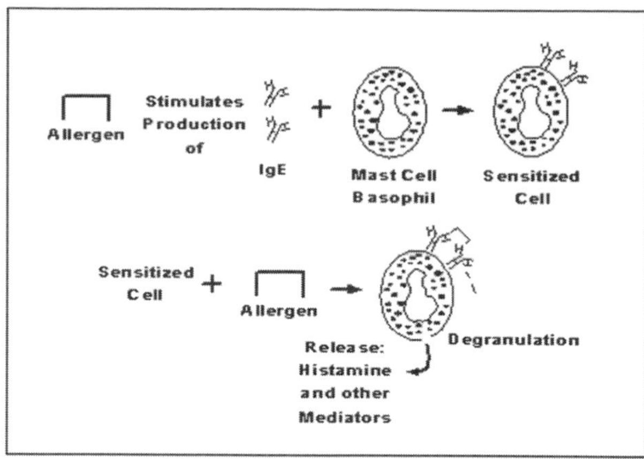

Figure 1. Mechanism of immunoglobulin-E-mediated food allergy.

subsequent exposure to the specific allergen, the allergen cross-links two of the IgE antibodies affixed to the surfaces of mast cells or basophils. This interaction triggers the disruption of the mast cell or basophil membrane and the release of a variety of potent, physiologically active mediators into the bloodstream and tissues. The granules within mast cells and basophils contain many of the important mediators of the allergic reaction. These potent mediators are actually responsible for the symptoms of immediate hypersensitivity reactions. Histamine is perhaps the most important of the mediators released from mast cells and basophils in an allergic reaction. Histamine can elicit inflammation, pruritus, and contraction of the smooth muscles in the blood vessels, gastrointestinal tract, and respiratory tract.[2] Other important mediators include various leukotrienes and prostaglandins. The leukotrienes are associated with some of the symptoms that develop more slowly in IgE-mediated food allergies, such as late-phase asthmatic reactions. This same type of IgE-mediated reaction is also responsible for allergic reactions to other environmental substances such as pollens, mold spores, animal danders, and bee venoms; only the source of the allergen is different.

During the sensitization phase, an individual forms allergen-specific IgE antibodies after exposure to a specific food protein. However, even among individuals predisposed to allergies, exposure to food proteins does not usually result in the formation of IgE antibodies. In healthy individuals, exposure to a food protein in the gastrointestinal tract results in oral tolerance through either the formation of protein-specific IgG, IgM, or IgA antibodies or no immunologic response whatsoever (clonal anergy).[5] Heredity and other physiologic factors are important in predisposing individuals to the development of IgE-mediated allergies—including food allergies.[6] Studies with monozygotic and dizygotic twins demonstrate that genetics is an extremely important parameter and that identical twins may even inherit the likelihood of responding to the same allergenic food (e.g., peanuts).[7,8] Approximately 65% of patients with clinically documented allergy have first-degree relatives with allergic disease.[6] Conditions that increase the permeability of the small intestinal mucosa to proteins such as viral gastroenteritis, premature birth, and cystic fibrosis also seem to increase the risk of development of food allergy.

Symptoms. The onset time for these reactions ranges from a few minutes to several hours after the consumption of the offending food. IgE-mediated food allergies involve numerous symptoms ranging from mild and annoying to severe and life-threatening (Table 2). No individual with IgE-mediated food allergy experiences all of the symptoms noted in Table 2. Furthermore, the symptoms are not necessarily consistent from one episode to another for an individual. The nature and severity of symptoms can also vary as a result of the amount of the offending food that has been ingested and the length of time since the previous exposure. An individual who experiences only mild symptoms on ingestion of a specific food (e.g., oral pruritus) may develop more serious manifestations on subsequent occasions, especially if avoidance of the offending food is not routinely practiced.

Gastrointestinal symptoms and cutaneous symptoms are among the more common manifestations of IgE-mediated food allergies. Respiratory symptoms are less commonly encountered but can be severe and life-threatening. Mild respiratory symptoms such as rhinitis and rhinoconjunctivitis are more likely to be encountered with exposure to environmental allergens such as directly inhaled airborne pollens or animal danders. However, respiratory reactions associated with food allergies can occasionally be severe (asthma and laryngeal edema). Those few food-allergic individuals who experience severe respiratory reactions in connection with the inadvertent ingestion of the offending food are most likely to be at risk for life-threatening episodes.[9] Of the many symptoms involved in IgE-mediated food allergies, systemic anaphylaxis is the most severe manifestation. Systemic anaphylaxis, also sometimes referred to as anaphylactic shock, involves multiple organ systems and numerous symptoms.

Table 2. Symptoms Associated with Immunoglobulin-E-Mediated Food Allergy

Gastrointestinal:	Nausea Vomiting Diarrhea Abdominal cramping
Cutaneous:	Urticaria Dermatitis or eczema Angioedema Pruritis
Respiratory:	Rhinitis Asthma Laryngeal edema
Generalized:	Anaphylactic shock

The symptoms can involve the gastrointestinal tract, respiratory tract, skin, and cardiovascular system. Death can occur from severe hypotension coupled with respiratory and cardiovascular complications. Anaphylactic shock is the most common cause of death in the occasional fatalities associated with IgE-mediated food allergies.[9,10] The number of deaths occurring from IgE-mediated food allergies is not recorded in most countries, but more than 100 deaths are thought to occur in the United States each year.[11]

Prevalence. The overall prevalence of IgE-mediated food allergies for all age groups is likely in the range of 3.5% to 4.0% in the United States. Few epidemiologic investigations involving clinical confirmation of IgE-mediated food allergies have been conducted using representative groups of adults. Most clinical investigations on the prevalence of IgE-mediated food allergies among adults have involved groups of patients seen at allergy clinics. Such selected groups of adults are unlikely to represent the entire population, and the prevalence rates for these groups are likely to be higher than for the general population. A large-scale epidemiologic investigation of the prevalence of IgE-mediated food allergy was conducted in The Netherlands.[12] This study revealed that although more than 10% of Dutch adults believed that they had adverse reactions to foods, the prevalence of these reactions was approximately 2% when clinical histories were confirmed by blinded food challenges.[12] The prevalence rate for IgE-mediated food allergies among infants and young children is well known and is likely considerably higher than that for adults.[13] Clinical trials among groups of unselected infants suggest that the prevalence of IgE-mediated food allergies is in the range of 4% to 8%.[14,15] Despite the lack of clinical epidemiologic trials among adults, recent surveys conducted in both the United States and England indicate that the self-perceived prevalence of peanut allergy alone is 0.5% to 0.6% among all age groups.[16,17] Surveys in the United States of the self-perceived prevalence of tree nut, fish, and crustacean (shellfish) allergies indicate that 0.5%, 0.4%, and 1.9%, respectively, believe that they have these particular food allergies.[16,18] These surveys did not include clinical investigations to confirm that peanut, tree nut, fish, or shellfish allergies truly existed in these individuals. Because these food allergies are often rather profound, overestimates associated with reliance on self-diagnosis are probably minimal. If the prevalence of these four food allergies is estimated at 3.4% and the prevalence of all food allergies among infants is 4% to 8%, then an overall estimate for IgE-mediated food allergies of 3.5% to 4.0% seems reasonable.

Natural History. Many food-allergic infants outgrow their allergies within a few months to several years after the onset.[19] Allergies to certain foods, such as cow's milk, are more commonly outgrown then are allergies to certain other foods such as peanut. Allergies to peanuts were considered to be a lifelong affliction until recently, when clinical researchers demonstrated that peanut allergy, especially when acquired very early in life, can be outgrown.[20] The mechanisms involved in the loss of sensitivity to specific foods are not precisely known, but the development of immunologic tolerance is definitely involved.[5]

Prevention of Sensitization. IgE-mediated food allergies are most likely to develop in high-risk infants, those born to parents with histories of allergic disease of any type (e.g., pollens, mold spores, animal danders, bee venoms, food). Preventing the development of food allergies in such infants has been a subject of great interest. Various strategies have been investigated. Restricting the mother's diet during pregnancy (excluding commonly allergenic foods such as peanuts) does not seem to help prevent allergy in the infant.[21] These observations suggest that sensitization does not occur in utero. Breastfeeding for extended periods of time seems to delay but may not prevent the development of IgE-mediated food allergies,[22] and infants can be sensitized to allergenic foods through exposure to the allergens in breast milk.[23] Apparently, allergenic food proteins can resist digestion, be absorbed at least to a small extent from the small intestine, and be secreted in breast milk, leading to sensitization. The exclusion of certain commonly allergenic foods from the maternal diet during the lactation period will help to prevent sensitization through breast milk. The elimination of peanuts from the diet of lactating women with high-risk infants is often recommended, but milk and eggs are usually considered to be too important nutritionally to exclude from the diets of lactating women. The use of probiotics during lactation may also help to lessen the likelihood of allergic sensitization.[24] Hypoallergenic infant formula may also prevent the development of food allergies in high-risk infants,[25] although these formulas are more often used to prevent reactions after sensitization has already occurred. The use of partial whey hydrolysate formula has been advocated because the partial hydrolysate is more likely to prevent sensitization than a formula based on whole milk.[26] High-risk infants may still develop food allergies once solid foods are introduced into the diet.[22]

Common Allergenic Foods and Food Ingredients. Eight foods or food groups—milk, eggs, fish, shellfish (e.g., shrimp, crab, lobster), peanuts, soybeans, tree nuts (e.g., walnuts, almonds, hazelnuts), and wheat—are responsible for the majority of IgE-mediated food allergies worldwide,[27] but regional differences exist. Examples of food allergies that occur more frequently in certain parts of the world than in others would include celery allergy in Europe,[28] sesame seed allergy in several areas of the world,[29,30] and buckwheat allergy in Japan.[31] These regional differences are likely related to food preferences in those areas, and sometimes to coexistent pollen allergies (e.g., celery allergy in individuals sensitized to mugwort pollen). Beyond the eight major foods or food groups, more than 160 other foods have been documented to cause IgE-mediated food allergies.[32] Because food allergens are proteins, any food that contains protein is likely to elicit allergic sensitization on at least rare occasions. The eight most commonly allergenic foods or food groups contain comparatively high amounts of protein and are commonly consumed in the diet. However, several other commonly consumed foods with high protein contents, such as beef, pork, chicken, and turkey, are rarely allergenic.

Ingredients derived from the commonly allergenic foods will also be allergenic if they contain sufficient residual protein from the source material. The most common questions concerning food ingredients involve edible oils, protein hydrolysates, lecithin, flavors, gelatin, spices, and colors. The Food Allergen Labeling and Consumer Protection Act of 2004 mandates source labeling of ingredients derived from commonly allergenic sources, with a few exceptions (highly refined oils and ingredients that become exempt through notifications or petitions that must be approved by the US Food and Drug Administration).

When the processing of edible oils includes hot solvent extraction with bleaching and deodorizing, virtually all of the protein is removed from the source material. Clinical challenge trials have shown that highly refined oils from peanut, soybean, and sunflower seeds are safe for ingestion by individuals allergic to the source material.[33] Oils from other sources, such as sesame seeds and tree nuts, may receive less processing and contain allergenic residues.[30,34] Cold-pressed oils may also contain allergenic residues.[35]

Protein hydrolysates are often obtained from commonly allergenic sources: soybean, wheat, milk, and peanuts. Several processes, including acid hydrolysis and enzymatic hydrolysis, are used to obtain these hydrolysates. The degree of hydrolysis of the proteins in hydrolysates varies according to the functional use, source, and method. If the proteins are only partially hydrolyzed, they are likely to retain their allergenicity. If they are extensively hydrolyzed, they may be safe for most individuals allergic to the source material. However, even extensively hydrolyzed casein in hypoallergenic infant formula has triggered allergic reactions in some infants extremely sensitive to milk.[25] However, infant formulas based on partial whey hydrolysates are even more likely to elicit allergic reactions in infants allergic to milk.[36]

Lecithin can be derived from soybean, egg, rice, or sunflower seeds, although soybean is by far the most common source. Commercial soy lecithin contains trace residues of soy proteins. The soy protein residues in lecithin include IgE-binding proteins,[37] but the levels may be insufficient to elicit allergic reactions in most soybean-allergic individuals. Many soybean-allergic individuals do not avoid lecithin.

Most flavoring formulations do not contain protein, and few formulations contain any components derived from allergenic sources.[38] Flavoring has caused allergic reactions, especially in meat products in which flavors can have dual functions and thus be present in higher amounts.[39]

Gelatin is most frequently derived from beef and pork and is generally not considered allergenic when ingested. Gelatin can also be derived from fish, but fish gelatin is unlikely to elicit reactions in fish-allergic individuals.[40]

Spices are rare causes of allergic reactions,[41] but have occasionally been implicated. Avoidance of specific spices in the diet can be difficult.

None of the colorants used in foods is derived from commonly allergenic sources. However, the natural colorants carmine and annatto contain protein residues, and both have been implicated in rare allergic reactions.[42]

Many other food ingredients are derived from commonly allergenic sources, for example; phytosterols, vitamin E, and isoflavones from soybean; lactose, butter acid, and butter esters from milk; and isinglass and fish oil from fish. The Food Allergen Labeling and Consumer Protection Act of 2004 and similar legislation or regulation in other countries mandate the source labeling of all of these ingredients. Many of these ingredients are not known to pose hazards to individuals allergic to the source food, although clinical evidence of the lack of allergenicity is typically not available. Source labeling of these ingredients will further restrict the dietary choices for food-allergic consumers.

Food Allergens. Food allergens are almost always naturally occurring proteins.[4] Foods contain hundreds of thousands of different proteins, and only a small percentage are known allergens. The major allergens have been identified, purified, and characterized for most of the commonly allergenic foods.[4,43] Multiple allergenic proteins exist in some commonly allergenic foods. Foods may contain both major and minor allergens. Major allergens are defined as proteins that bind to serum IgE antibodies from more than 50% of patients with a specific food allergy. For example, milk contains three major allergens: casein, β-lactoglobulin, and α-lactalbumin.[44] These also happen to be the major milk proteins. Milk may also contain several minor allergens (e.g., bovine serum albumin), although the level of evidence for clinical relevance is less convincing for these minor allergens.[45] Peanuts contain at least three major allergens:[4] *Ara h* 1, *Ara h* 2, and *Ara h* 3. Peanuts also contain numerous minor allergens.[46] In contrast, codfish (*Gad c* 1), Brazil nut (*Ber e* 1), and shrimp (*Pen a* 1) contain primarily one major allergenic protein.[4]

Effect of Processing on Allergenicity. Allergenic food proteins are remarkably stable under food-processing conditions.[33] As noted earlier, proteins can be removed from products derived from allergenic sources; the highly refined edible oils are the best example. Most allergenic food proteins are quite stable to heat, so that typical heat-processing conditions do not affect the allergenicity of the resulting products.[33] Some exceptions are certain fruit and vegetable allergens that are sensitive to heat[47];

fish allergens may be destroyed by canning but not other heat processes.[48] Food allergens also tend to be resistant to proteolysis,[49] which allows them to survive digestive processes and arrive in the intestine in immunologically active form. The resistance to proteolysis means that these allergens may survive, in whole or in part, the acid and enzymatic hydrolysis methods used to prepare protein hydrolysates.[33]

Treatment. Avoidance diets are the most reliable means for preventing allergic reactions to foods.[50] For example, people who are allergic to peanuts should simply avoid peanuts in all forms. Pharmacologic approaches (epinephrine and antihistamines) are available for treating the symptoms of an allergic reaction.[51] New therapies are under development and show some promise, including anti-IgE immunotherapy[52] and vaccines that might cure specific food allergies, but at present, avoidance diets remain the only strategy for prevention of allergic reactions to foods.

Threshold Doses. Practical experience demonstrates that exposure to trace levels of the offending food can elicit adverse reactions. Anecdotal reports suggest that reactions could occur from exposure to the small quantities by using shared utensils or containers, kissing the lips of someone who has eaten the offending food, or opening packages of or inhaling vapors from the offending food. Although these situations are not well documented, the amount of the offending food that would be ingested from such occurrences would be quite low. Other episodes have been more thoroughly documented. Allergic reactions have occurred to peanut protein in sunflower seed butter prepared on equipment used for peanut butter,[53] milk protein in sorbet manufactured with equipment also used for ice cream,[54] and milk protein in "Tofutti" manufactured with equipment also used for ice cream.[39] Although complete avoidance must be maintained, threshold doses do exist below which allergic individuals will not experience adverse reactions.[55,56] Threshold doses are likely in the low-milligram range for the most sensitive individuals, and are variable over several orders of magnitude among individuals allergic to any specific food. The possibility that the threshold doses vary from one allergenic food to another remains to be determined.

Cross-reactions. In the construction of safe and effective avoidance diets, questions often arise regarding the need to avoid closely related foods. For some foods, cross-reactions do seem to occur with closely related foods. For example, shrimp-allergic individuals will also typically be sensitive to other crustaceans such as crab and lobster.[57] Similarly, cross-reactions commonly occur between different species of avian eggs,[58] and between milk from cows and that from goats.[59] In contrast, some peanut-allergic individuals are allergic to other legumes such as soybean,[60] but this is not common. Clinical hypersensitivity to one legume, such as peanuts or soybeans, does not warrant exclusion of the entire legume family from the diet unless allergy to each individual legume is confirmed by clinical challenge trials.[61]

Cross-reactions are also known to occur between certain types of pollens and foods. Examples would include ragweed pollen and melons, mugwort pollen and celery, mugwort pollen and hazelnut, and birch pollen and various foods, including carrots, apples, hazelnuts, and potatoes.[4] Cross-reactions are also known to occur between allergies to natural rubber latex and banana, chestnut, avocado, and kiwi, among others.[62]

Impact of Agricultural Biotechnology. Concerns have arisen regarding the possible allergenicity of foods developed through agricultural biotechnology.[63] Genetic modifications result in the transfer of one or more genes from one biologic source to another. These genes code for specific proteins. Because food allergens are usually proteins, these novel proteins could be or could become allergens. Millions of proteins exist in nature, including many in foods, and only a small percentage are allergens, so the probability of transferring a protein with allergenic potential into a transgenic food is small. Several decision-tree strategies have been developed to assess the likelihood of allergenicity of these novel proteins from genetically modified foods.[63] Certainly, the probability of transferring an allergen is enhanced if the gene is derived from a known allergenic source. The reliability of allergy-assessment strategies was documented with the discovery[64] that a gene from Brazil nuts cloned into soybeans to enhance the methionine content of soybeans coded for the major allergen from Brazil nuts, *Ber e* 1; commercialization of that transgenic variety of soybeans was immediately halted.

Oral Allergy Syndrome. Oral allergy syndrome is one of the more common and mildest forms of IgE-mediated food allergy.[65] In this syndrome, ingestion of the offending foods (often fresh fruits and vegetables) elicits mild oropharyngeal symptoms: pruritus, urticaria, and angioedema. Fresh fruits and vegetables contain comparatively low quantities of protein, but oral allergy syndrome is an IgE-mediated response involving reactions to specific proteins.[65] Apparently, the allergens in these fresh fruits and vegetables are rapidly digested by the proteases of the gastrointestinal tract,[33] and systemic reactions are rarely encountered. The allergens are also apparently heat labile,[33] because heat-processing eliminates their effects. Individuals with oral allergy syndrome are initially sensitized to one or more environmental pollens, frequently birch pollen or mugwort pollen.[65] Once sensitized to the pollen allergens, these individuals are reactive to proteins that exist in foods that cross-react with these allergens.

Exercise-induced Food Allergies. Exercise-induced food allergies are a subset of the immediate hypersensitivity reactions to foods. They involve allergen-specific IgE antibodies, but occur only when the food is eaten just before exercise.[66] Numerous foods have been implicated, including shellfish, wheat, celery, and peach. The symptoms are as individualistic and variable as those for other food allergies. Exercise-induced allergies can also exist without any role for food intake.[66] The mechanism of this illness is not well understood except for the involvement of IgE antibodies. With the recent national emphasis on increased physical activity, reports of this condition could increase.

Cell-mediated Allergy

Delayed hypersensitivities are cell-mediated allergic reactions and involve tissue-bound T lymphocytes that are sensitized to a specific foodborne substance that triggers the reaction.[2] These reactions often result in localized tissue inflammation. In such reactions, symptoms begin to appear 6 to 24 hours after consumption of the offending food.

Celiac Disease. Celiac disease, also known as celiac sprue, nontropical sprue, or gluten-sensitive enteropathy, is a malabsorption syndrome occurring in sensitive individuals after the consumption of wheat, rye, barley, triticale, spelt, and kamut.[2,67] Celiac disease is characterized by mucosal damage in the small intestine resulting from consumption of the offending grains or protein-containing products derived from those grains.[67] This mucosal damage leads to nutrient malabsorption. The loss of absorptive function, along with the ongoing inflammatory process, results in diarrhea, bloating, weight loss, anemia, bone pain, chronic fatigue, weakness, muscle cramps, and, in children, failure to gain weight and growth retardation.[2] Evidence suggests that intraepithelial T cells in the small intestine are involved in the inflammatory mechanism occurring with celiac disease;[68] however, the precise role of the intestinal T cells in celiac disease remains to be defined.

Celiac disease is an inherited trait, although its inheritance is complex.[2] It occurs in approximately 5% of first-degree relatives of patients with celiac disease, and approximately 75% of monozygotic twin pairs are concordant for it.[69] Histocompatibility locus antigen (HLA) class II genes are the major genes associated with celiac disease, but concordance for celiac disease is only 25% to 40% in siblings who are identical for one or both HLA haplotypes. Thus, genes outside of the HLA locus likely have some as-yet-undefined role in disease susceptibility.

The exact prevalence of celiac disease is a matter of some debate. Prevalence estimates from different parts of the world are complicated by the use of different diagnostic approaches. Celiac disease seems to be latent or asymptomatic in some individuals whose symptoms only appear occasionally.[67,70] The prevalence of celiac disease seems to be highest in certain European regions and in Australia,[71] occurring in approximately 1 out of every 250 people. Even within European populations, considerable variability is observed in the prevalence of celiac disease.[71] In the United States, symptomatic celiac disease occurs in approximately 1 out of every 3000 individuals,[2] but 1 in every 133 individuals may be at risk for the development of symptoms.[72]

Celiac disease is associated with the ingestion of gliadin from wheat and related prolamin proteins from other grains.[2] The prolamin fraction of wheat is known as gluten; thus, celiac disease is sometimes called gluten-sensitive enteropathy. A defect in mucosal processing of gliadin in patients with celiac disease provokes the generation of toxic peptides that contribute to the abnormal T-cell response and the subsequent inflammatory reaction.[68] The mechanism involved in celiac disease and the exact role of gliadin remain to be determined.

The tolerance for wheat, rye, barley, and related grains among those with celiac disease is unknown. Clearly, the threshold dose may vary from one individual to another, because in latent forms of celiac disease, normal dietary quantities of the offending grains seem to cause little problem. Many people with celiac disease attempt to avoid all sources of these grains, including a wide variety of common food ingredients derived from them.[73] Most of these individuals also avoid oats, although the role of oats in the elicitation of celiac disease was refuted.[74] Because oats are often contaminated with wheat in commerce, some caution may still be necessary. Although evidence is scant, spelt and kamut, which are basically varieties of wheat, are likely to trigger celiac disease in susceptible individuals.

The risk of death as a direct result of celiac disease is low,[67,75] but individuals who have celiac disease for prolonged periods are at increased risk for the development of T-cell lymphoma.[2,67] Patients with celiac disease also are more likely to have various other autoimmune diseases, including dermatitis herpetiformis, thyroid diseases, Addison's disease, pernicious anemia, autoimmune thrombocytopenia, sarcoidosis, insulin-dependent diabetes mellitus, and IgA nephropathy.[67,76]

Food Intolerances

In contrast to true food allergies, food intolerances involve one of several non-immunologic mechanisms. The distinction between food allergies and intolerances is important with respect to treatment and mechanism. Individuals with various types of food intolerances are typically able to tolerate some amount of the offending substance in their diet. In contrast, the threshold doses for the offending food with true food allergies are small. Thus, the management of food intolerances is much easier. With a few very notable exceptions, little research has been conducted on food intolerances. In many cases, the cause-and-effect relationship between ingestion of the offending food or food ingredient and the adverse reaction has not been carefully established.

Anaphylactoid Reactions. Anaphylactoid reactions are a non-IgE-mediated release of mediators from mast cells and basophils.[2] Because the same mediators are involved as in true IgE-mediated food allergies, the symptoms are similar. Although anaphylactoid reactions are documented with adverse reactions to drugs, no proof exists that anaphylactoid reactions occur with foods.

Metabolic Food Disorders. Metabolic food disorders occur as the result of genetically determined metabolic deficiencies that either affect the ability to metabolize a specific substance in foods or heighten sensitivity to a particular foodborne chemical.[2] Lactose intolerance is an example of a metabolic food disorder.[2]

Lactose intolerance is associated with a deficiency of the enzyme β-galactosidase (lactase) in the intestinal tract that leads to an inability to metabolize lactose from milk and other dairy products.[77] The symptoms of lactose intolerance are mild, confined to the gastrointestinal tract, and include abdominal discomfort, flatulence, and frothy diarrhea.[77] Lactose intolerance affects a large number of people worldwide, with a frequency as high as 60% to 90% among blacks, Native Americans, Hispanics, Asians, Jews, and Arabs.[2] In contrast, the prevalence among North-American whites is approximately 6% to 12%.[2] The usual treatment for lactose intolerance is the avoidance of dairy products containing lactose, but lactose-intolerant individuals can tolerate some lactose in their diets,[2] and most have virtually no symptoms on consumption of the amount of lactose in 235 mL (1 cup) of milk.[2] In addition, some dairy products (e.g., yogurt and acidophilus milk) are better tolerated than others, apparently because they contain bacteria with β-galactosidase.[2] Thus, lactose intolerance is a manageable condition.

Food Idiosyncrasies. Food idiosyncrasies are adverse reactions to foods or food ingredients that occur through unknown mechanisms. The best example of an idiosyncratic reaction is sulfite-induced asthma.[78] Cause and effect is well established for sulfite-induced asthma, but has not been well established in other types of food idiosyncrasies. Psychosomatic illnesses are also included in this category.

Sulfites are common food additives that also occur naturally in certain foods, especially fermented foods, usually in small amounts.[78] Although asthma is the only well-established symptom associated with sulfite sensitivity, only a small percentage of asthmatics are sulfite sensitive.[78] Individuals with severe asthma who require steroids for control of symptoms are the primary risk group for sulfite sensitivity, but only approximately 5% of these are sulfite sensitive.[78] Sulfite-induced asthma can be severe, and deaths have been documented.[78] Sulfites added to foods must be declared on product labels, so avoidance diets are reasonably easy to develop.[78] Sulfite-sensitive individuals with asthma can tolerate the ingestion of small quantities of sulfites, especially when they are incorporated into certain types of foods.[79] Although sulfite-induced asthma poses a considerable risk to sensitive individuals, this condition is manageable once it is recognized.

Many of the other idiosyncratic reactions also involve various food additives. Examples include tartrazine (a commonly used food colorant also known as F;D&C Yellow no. 5) in asthma and/or chronic urticaria, other food colors in chronic urticaria; monosodium glutamate (a commonly used flavor enhancer) in asthma and monosodium glutamate symptom complex; and aspartame in migraine headache and urticaria.[80] Although tartrazine has been implicated in the elicitation of asthma and chronic urticaria for several decades, criticisms have arisen regarding the design of the clinical studies.[80] Both asthma and chronic urticaria are chronic conditions that are likely to flare at unpredicted times in susceptible individuals, many of whom take various medications continually to control symptoms. In the clinical studies, medications were withdrawn from the patients for variable periods before the challenges, which were often not blinded. When the symptoms were exacerbated, the investigators concluded that tartrazine was responsible. However, the alternative explanation might be that the symptoms flared simply because critical medications were withdrawn. In studies in which some of the medications were continued, tartrazine challenges had no effect on similar patients.[80]

Monosodium glutamate symptom complex, a mild subjective illness, has not been confirmed by double-blind, placebo-controlled food challenges,[80,81] and a national panel concluded that the role of monosodium glutamate in the elicitation of the complex was not proven, especially at doses less than 3 g.[81] Monosodium glutamate has also been implicated as a causative factor in asthma, but the clinical studies linking the two are subject to the same criticisms as mentioned for tartrazine.[80]

Conclusion

Food allergies and intolerances affect a small but significant portion of the population. Symptoms can range from mildly annoying to severe and life-threatening. The true food allergies present the biggest risk because symptoms can occasionally be severe and the threshold dose of the offending food required to provoke a reaction is small. The only management strategy for individuals with food allergies and intolerances is the specific avoidance of the allergen. Construction of safe and effective avoidance diets can be difficult for individuals with true food allergies.

References

1. Sloan AE, Powers ME. A perspective on popular perceptions of adverse reactions to foods. J Allergy Clin Immunol. 1986;78:127–133.
2. Taylor SL, Hefle SL. Food allergies and other food sensitivities. Food Technol. 2001;55(9):68–83.
3. Mekori YA. Introduction to allergic disease. Crit Rev Food Sci Nutr. 1996;36:S1–S18.
4. Bohle B, Swoboda I, Spitzauer S, et al. Food antigens: structure and function. In: Metcalfe DD, Sampson HA, Simon RA, eds. *Food Allergy: Adverse Reactions to Foods and Food Additives, 3rd ed.* Malden, MA: Blackwell Publishing; 2003:38–50.

5. Strobel S. Oral tolerance: immune responses to food antigens. In: Metcalfe DD, Sampson HA, Simon RA, eds. *Food Allergy: Adverse Reactions to Foods and Food Additives, 2nd ed.* Boston: Blackwell Science; 1997:107–135.
6. Chandra RK. Food allergy: setting the theme. In: Chandra RK, ed. *Food Allergy.* St. John's, Newfoundland: Nutrition Research Education Foundation; 1987:3–5.
7. Lack G, Fox DES, Golding J. The role of the uterine environment in the pathogenesis of peanut allergy. J Allergy Clin Immunol. 1999;103:S95.
8. Sicherer SH, Furlong TJ, Maes HH, et al. Genetics of peanut allergy: twin study. J Allergy Clin Immunol. 2000;106:53–56.
9. Sampson HA, Mendelson L, Rosen J. Fatal and near-fatal anaphylactic reactions to foods in children and adolescents. N Engl J Med. 1992;327:380–384.
10. Yunginger JW, Sweeney KG, Sturner WQ, et al. Fatal food-induced anaphylaxis. J Am Med Assoc. 1988;260:1450–1452.
11. Burks AW, Sampson HA. Anaphylaxis and food allergy. In: Metcalfe DD, Sampson HA, Simon RA, eds. *Food Allergy: Adverse Reactions to Foods and Food Additives, 3rd ed.* Malden, MA: Blackwell Publishing; 2003:192–205.
12. Neistijl Jansen JJ, Kardinaal AFM, Huijbers G, et al. Prevalence of food allergy and intolerance in the adult Dutch population. J Allergy Clin Immunol. 1994;93:446–456.
13. Sampson HA. Food allergy. Curr Opinion Immunol. 1990;2:542–547.
14. Bock SA, Lee WY, Remigio L, et al. Studies of hyper-sensitivity reactions to foods in infants and children. J Allergy Clin Immunol. 1978;62:327–334.
15. Sampson HA. Update on food allergy. J Allergy Clin Immunol. 2004;113:805–819.
16. Sicherer SH, Munoz-Furlong A, Burks AW, et al. Prevalence of peanut and tree nut allergy in the U.S. determined by a random digit dial telephone survey. J Allergy Clin Immunol. 1999;103:559–562.
17. Emmett SE, Angus FJ, Fry JS, et al. Perceived prevalence of peanut allergy in Great Britain and its association with other atopic conditions and with peanut allergy in other household members. Allergy. 1999; 54:380–385.
18. Sicherer SH, Munoz-Furlong A, Sampson HA. Prevalence of seafood allergy in the United States by a random telephone survey. J Allergy Clin Immunol. 2004;114:159–165.
19. Sampson HA. Epidemiology of food allergy. Pediatr Allergy Immunol. 1996;7(Suppl. 9):42–50.
20. Slolnick H, Conover Walker MK, Barnes-Koerner C, et al. The natural history of peanut allergy. J Allergy Clin Immunol. 2001;107:367–374.
21. Wood RA. Natural history and prevention of food hypersensitivity. In: Metcalfe DD, Sampson HA, Simon RA, eds. *Food Allergy: Adverse Reactions to Foods and Food Additives, 3rd ed.* Malden, MA: Blackwell Publishing; 2003:425–437.
22. Zeiger RS, Heller S. The development and prediction of atopy in high-risk children: follow-up at seven years in a prospective randomized study of combined maternal and infant food allergy avoidance. J Allergy Clin Immunol. 1995;95:1179–1190.
23. Van Asperen PP, Kemp AS, Mellis CM. Immediate food hypersensitivity reactions on the first known exposure to food. Arch Dis Child. 1983;58:253–256.
24. Kirjavainen PV, Apostolou E, Salminen SJ, et al. New aspects of probiotics: a novel approach in the management of food allergy. Allergy. 1999;54: 909–915.
25. Businco L, Dreborg S, Einarsson R, et al. Hydrolysed cow's milk formulae. Allergenicity and use in treatment and prevention. An ESPACI position paper. Pediatr Allergy Immunol. 1993;4:101–111.
26. Vandenplas Y, Hauser B, Van den Borre C, et al. The long-term effect of a partial whey hydrolysate formula on the prophylaxis of atopic disease. Eur J Pediatr. 1995;154:488–494.
27. Food and Agricultural Organization of the United Nations. Report of the FAO Technical Consultation on Food Allergies. Rome, Italy, November 13–14, 1995.
28. Wuthrich B, Stager J, Johannson SGO. Celery allergy associated with birch and mugwort pollenosis. Allergy. 1990;45:566–571.
29. Sporik R, Hill D. Allergy to peanuts, nuts, and sesame seed in Australian children. Br Med J. 1996; 313:1477–1478.
30. Kanny G, de Hauteclocque C, Moneret-Vautrin DA. Sesame seed and sesame seed oil contain masked allergens of growing importance. Allergy. 1996;51: 952–957.
31. Ebisawa M, Ikematsu K, Imai T, Tachimoto H. Food allergy in Japan. Allergy Clin Immunol Int. 2003; 15:214–217.
32. Hefle SL, Nordlee JA, Taylor SL. Allergenic foods. Crit Rev Food Sci Nutr. 1996;36:S69–S89.
33. Taylor SL, Lehrer SB. Principles and characteristics of food allergens. Crit Rev Food Sci Nutr. 1996;36: S91–S118.
34. Teuber SS, Brown RL, Haapanen LAD. Allergenicity of gourmet nut oils processed by different methods. J Allergy Clin Immunol. 1997;99: 502–507.
35. Hoffman DR, Collins-Williams C. Cold-pressed peanut oils may contain peanut allergen. J Allergy Clin Immunol. 1994;93:801–802.
36. Businco L, Cantani A, Longhi M, et al. Anaphylactic reactions to a cow milk whey protein hydrolysate (Alfa-Re Nestle) in infants with cow's milk allergy. Ann Allergy. 1989;62:333–335.
37. Muller U, Weber W, Hoffmann A, et al. Commer-

cial soybean lecithins: a source of hidden allergens? Z Lebensm Unter Forsch. 1998;207:341–351.
38. Taylor SL, Dormedy ES. The role of flavoring substances in food allergy and intolerance. Adv Food Nutr Res. 1998;42:1–44.
39. Gern JE, Yang E, Evrard HM, et al. Allergic reactions to milk-contaminated "non-dairy" products. N Engl J Med. 1991;324:976–979.
40. Hansen TK, Poulsen LK, Skov P, et al. A randomized, double-blind, placebo-controlled oral challenge study to evaluate the allergenicity of commercial, food-grade fish gelatin. Food Chem Toxicol. 2004; 42:2037–2044.
41. Niinimaki A, Bjorksten F, Puukka M, et al. Spice allergy: results of skin prick tests and RAST with spice extracts. Allergy. 1989;44:60–65.
42. Lucas CD, Taylor SL, Hallagan JB. The role of natural color additives in food allergy. In: Taylor SL, ed. *Advances in Food and Nutrition Research, Vol. 43.* New York: Academic Press; 2001:195–216.
43. Taylor SL, Hefle SL. Foods as allergens. In: Brostoff J, Challacombe SJ, eds. *Food Allergy and Intolerance, 2nd ed.* London: Saunders; 2002:403–412.
44. Wal JM. Cows' milk proteins/allergens. Ann Allergy Asthma Immunol. 2002;89(Suppl):3–10.
45. Baldo BA. Milk allergies. Aust J Dairy Technol. 1984;39:120–128.
46. Bannon GA, Besler M, Hefle SL, et al. Peanut (*Arachis hypogaea*). Internet Symp Food Allergens. 2000; 2:87–122.
47. Jankiewicz A, Baltes W, Bogl K, et al. Influence of food processing on the immunochemical stability of celery allergens. J Sci Food Agric. 1997;75:357–370.
48. Bernhisel-Broadbent J, Strause D, Sampson HA. Fish hypersensitivity. II. Clinical relevance of altered fish allergenicity caused by various preparation methods. J Allergy Clin Immunol. 1992;90:622–629.
49. Bannon GA, Goodman RE, Leach JN, et al. Digestive stability in the context of assessing the potential allergenicity of food proteins. Comments Toxicol. 2002;8:271–275.
50. Taylor SL, Hefle SL, Munoz-Furlong A. Food allergies and avoidance diets. Nutr Today. 199;34:15–22.
51. Furukawa CT. Nondietary management of food allergy. In: Chiaramonte LT, Schneider AT, Lifshitz F, eds. *Food Allergy: A Practical Approach to Diagnosis and Management.* New York: Marcel Dekker, 1988: 365–375.
52. Leung DYM, Sampson HA, Yunginger JW, et al. Effect of anti-IgE therapy in patients with peanut allergy. N Engl J Med. 2003;348:986–993.
53. Yunginger JW, Gauerke MB, Jones RT, et al. Use of radioimmunoassay to determine the nature, quantity and source of allergenic contamination of sunflower butter. J Food Pro. 1983;46:625–628.
54. Laoprasert N, Wallen ND, Jones RT, et al. Anaphylaxis in a milk-allergic child following ingestion of lemon sorbet containing trace quantities of milk. J Food Prot. 1998;61:1522–1524.
55. Taylor SL, Hefle SL, Bindslev-Jensen C, et al. Factors affecting determination of threshold doses for allergenic foods: how much is too much? J Allergy Clin Immunol. 2002;109:24–30.
56. Morisset M, Moneret-Vautrin DA, Kanny G, et al. Thresholds of clinical reactivity to milk, egg, peanut and sesame in immunoglobulin E-dependent allergies: evaluation by double-blind and single-blind placebo-controlled oral challenges. Clin Exp Allergy. 2003;33:1046–1051.
57. Daul CB, Morgan JE, Lehrer SB. Hypersensitivity reactions to crustacea and mollusks. Clin Rev Allergy. 1993;11:201–222.
58. Langeland T. A clinical and immunological study of allergy to hen's egg white. VI. Occurrence of proteins cross-reacting with allergens in hen's egg white as studied in egg white from turkey, duck, goose, seagull, and in hen egg yolk, and hen and chicken sera and flesh. Allergy. 1983;39:339–412.
59. Bernard H, Creminon C, Negroni L, et al. IgE cross-reactivity with caseins from different species in humans allergic to cows' milk. Food Agric Immunol. 1999;11:101–111.
60. Herian AM, Taylor SL, Bush RK. Identification of soybean allergens by immunoblotting with sera from soy-allergic adults. Int Arch Allergy Appl Immunol. 1990;92:193–198.
61. Bernhisel-Broadbent J, Sampson HA. Cross-allergenicity in the legume botanical family in children with food hypersensitivity. J Allergy Clin Immunol. 1989;83:435–440.
62. Blanco C, Carrillo T, Castillo R, et al. Latex allergy: clinical features and cross-reactivity with fruits. Ann Allergy. 1994;73:309–314.
63. Goodman RE, Hefle SL, Taylor SL, van Ree R. Assessing genetically modified crops to minimize the risk of increased food allergy: a review. Int Arch Allergy Immunol. 2005;137:153–166.
64. Nordlee JA, Taylor SL, Townsend JA, et al. Identification of Brazil nut allergen in transgenic soybeans. N Engl J Med. 1996;334:688–692.
65. Pastorello E, Ortolani C. Oral allergy syndrome. In: Metcalfe DD, Sampson HA, Simon RA, eds. *Food Allergy: Adverse Reactions to Foods and Food Additives, 3rd ed.* Malden, MA: Blackwell Publishing; 2003: 169–182.
66. O'Connor ME, Schocket AL. Exercise- and pressure-induced syndromes. In: Metcalfe DD, Sampson HA, Simon RA, eds. *Food Allergy: Adverse Reactions to Foods and Food Additives, 3rd ed.* Malden, MA: Blackwell Publishing; 2003:262–269.
67. Murray JA. Gluten-sensitive enteropathy. In: Metcalfe DD, Sampson HA, Simon RA, eds. *Food Allergy: Adverse Reactions to Foods and Food Additives,*

3rd ed. Malden, MA: Blackwell Publishing; 2003: 242–261.
68. Maiuri L, Picarella A, Boirivant M, et al. Definition of the initial immunologic modifications upon in vitro gliadin challenge in the small intestine of celiac patients. Gastroenterology. 1996;110:1368–1378.
69. Holtmeier W, Rowell DL, Nyberg A, et al. Distinct δ T cell receptor repertoires in monozygotic twins concordant for coeliac disease. Clin Exp Immunol. 1997;107:148–157.
70. Duggan JM. Recent developments in our understanding of adult coeliac disease. Med J Aust. 1997; 166:312–315.
71. Logan RFA. Descriptive epidemiology of celiac disease. In: Branksi D, Rozen P, Kagnoff MF, eds. *Gluten-Sensitive Enteropathy, Frontiers in Gastrointestinal Research, Vol 19.* Basel: Karger; 1992:1–14.
72. Fasano A, Berti I, Gerarduzzi T, et al. Prevalence of celiac disease in at-risk and not-at-risk groups in the United States. Arch Int Med. 2001;163:286–292.
73. Inman-Felton AE. Overview of gluten sensitive enteropathy (celiac sprue). J Am Diet Assoc. 1999;99: 352–362.
74. Janatuinen EK, Pikkarainen PH, Kemppainen TA, et al. A comparison of diets with and without oats in adults with celiac disease. N Engl J Med. 1995; 333:1033–1037.
75. Corrao G, Corazza GR, Bagnardi V, et al. Mortality in patients with celiac disease and their relatives: a cohort study. Lancet. 2001;358:356–361.
76. Troncone R, Greco L, Auricchio S. Gluten-sensitive enteropathy. Pediatr Clin North Am. 1996;43:355–373.
77. Suarez FL, Savaiano DA. Diet, genetics, and lactose intolerance. Food Technol. 1997;51(3):74–76.
78. Taylor SL, Bush RK, Nordlee JA. Sulfites. In: Metcalfe DD, Sampson HA, Simon RA, eds. *Food Allergies: Adverse Reactions to Foods and Food Additives, 3rd ed.* Boston: Blackwell Scientific; 2003:324–341.
79. Taylor SL, Bush RK, Selner JC, et al. Sensitivity to sulfited foods among sulfite-sensitive asthmatics. J Allergy Clin Immunol. 1988;81:1159–1167.
80. Bush RK, Taylor SL, Hefle SL. Adverse reactions to food and drug additives. In: Adkinson NF, Bochner BS, Yunginger JW, Holgate ST, Busse WW, Simons FER, eds. *Allergy Principles and Practice, Vol. 2, 6th ed.* St. Louis: Mosby; 2003: 1645–1663.
81. Raiten DJ, Talbot JM, Fisher KD, eds. *Analysis of Adverse Reactions to Monosodium Glutamate (MSG).* Bethesda MD: Life Sciences Research Office, Federation of American Societies for Experimental Biology; 1995.

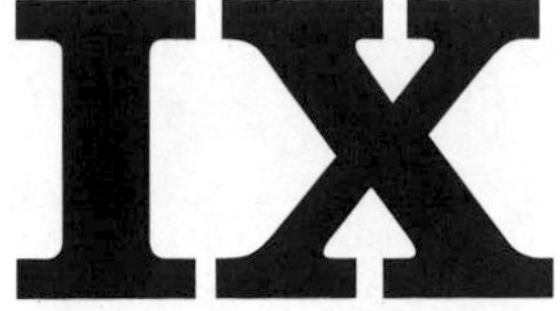

Nutrition and Chronic Diseases

48

Obesity as a Health Issue

Edward Saltzman

Introduction

Obesity results in multiple comorbid conditions, increased mortality rates, diminished quality of life, and increased health care costs. The growing worldwide prevalence of obesity, coupled with its far-reaching adverse effects, has placed it in the public health spotlight. Recognition of the importance of identifying and, ultimately, preventing obesity has stimulated declaration of global standards for classifying body weight, although controversy still exists regarding modification of the classification in adults based on ethnic background or age and the classification of childhood and adolescent obesity. Despite increased public awareness, obesity prevalence has continued to rise, and successful strategies for prevention and long-term treatment of obesity remain elusive. However, these issues are now being addressed in the arenas of government, industry, public health, and medical care.

Definitions and Classification

The adverse effects of obesity are the result of excess body fat.[1] Outside of the research environment, methods to accurately measure body fat in diverse populations are either not widely available, impractical in field or clinical settings, or are prohibitively expensive. Measures of body composition that are potentially useful at the population and clinical levels include anthropometry and bioelectrical impedance. However, both of these techniques are limited by interobserver variability, can be influenced by several factors, including hydration status and acute or chronic illness, and require reference standards that are age, gender, and ethnicity specific. Even if accurate population data for body fat were available, large studies relating the relationship between body fat and health outcomes are lacking. The majority of research efforts linking obesity to adverse outcomes have used surrogates of adiposity, such as the body mass index (BMI) or weight for height.

Body Mass Index

Current body weight classification is based on the BMI, defined as weight in kilograms divided by height in meters squared (kg/m^2), according to the classification scheme of the World Health Organization[2] and adopted by the National Institutes of Health[3] (Table 1). The rationale for the use of the BMI is that it is correlated with body fat, as well as its ease of calculation in field and clinical settings. Although BMI serves as a surrogate for body fat, more importantly, it serves to predict health risk. In diverse populations, elevated BMI is associated with risk of mortality[4] and a wide spectrum of diseases.[5] For public health purposes, BMI allows classification of the proportion of a population at risk for adverse outcomes and allows assessment of prevention and intervention programs.[6] At the clinical level, BMI is interpreted with other clinical data to assess nutritional status, health risk, and eligibility for various treatments of overweight and undernutrition.

Although BMI generally correlates well with body fat, several factors influence this relationship, including gender, age, race, and ethnic background. A single BMI classification for the entire adult age range does not reflect the increase in fat mass and loss of lean mass over the adult lifespan, even if weight remained stable. Differences among ethnic groups and with aging in the relationship between BMI and body composition, as well as the relationship between BMI and health outcomes, have raised concern about a single global BMI classification scheme. At a specific BMI, body fat and disease risk are higher in several Asian populations than in Caucasians. A World Health Organization panel did not recommend changes in BMI classification for Asian or other higher-risk populations, but defined BMI action points along the spectrum of BMI that could be

Table 1. Classification of Body Weight by Body Mass Index (BMI)

Classification	BMI (kg/m²)	Class	Disease Risk Waist Circumference (inches)	
			≤40 (men) ≤35 (women)	>40 (men) >35 (women)
Underweight	<18.5			
Normal	18.5–24.9			
Overweight	25.0–29.9		Increased	High
Obesity	30.0–34.9	I	High	Very high
	35.0–39.9	II	Very high	Very high
		III	Extremely high	Extremely high

From NHLBI Obesity Education Initiative Expert Panel on the Identification Evaluation and Treatment of Overweight and Obesity in Adults. Clinical guidelines on the identification, evaluation, and treatment of overweight and obesity in adults—the evidence report. Obes Res. 1998;6(Suppl 2):51S–209S.

adopted internally by specific populations and countries (Figure 1).

Central Fat Distribution

Central obesity is associated with risk for type 2 diabetes mellitus, dyslipidemia, hypertension, the metabolic syndrome, and coronary heart disease (CHD).[7,8] Central obesity confers risk independent of BMI and, in some populations, better predicts health risk and mortality than BMI.[9] The health risk imposed by central body fat appears to result from visceral fat accumulation, although a pathogenic role for subcutaneous fat has also been suggested.[10] Central fat distribution is classified by a single measurement of waist circumference (Table 1), which better predicts visceral fat than the waist-to-hip ratio.[11] Sagittal diameter has also been found to predict visceral fat and, in some investigations, has been better associated with metabolic disorders than waist circumference.[11] The relationships between waist circumference, intra-abdominal fat, and health outcomes also vary with age, ethnicity, and BMI; however, like BMI, refinement of waist circumference cutoffs within BMI categories or by ethnicity or age has not yet been widely accepted.

Prevalence

The prevalence of obesity has increased substantially in the United States and in many other countries over the last several decades. As illustrated in Figure 2, the National Health and Nutrition Examination Surveys data show that in US adults the prevalence of overweight has remained stable, whereas the prevalence of obesity has increased to 30%.[12] Although obesity prevalence varies considerably with gender, age, ethnicity, socioeconomic status, and educational level, prevalence has increased within categories of each of these variables.[13] A cause for concern is the increase in Class III, or extreme obesity, which increased in prevalence from less than 1% to 4.9% over the past 4 decades.

Waist circumference has also increased in US adults in the last 4 decades, with an overall increase from 1960 to 1962 and 1999 to 2000 of 10 cm in men and 17 cm in women. Significant increases were also observed within each category of BMI[14]; because waist circumference increases with BMI, observed increases within BMI categories, reflect at least in part, the increases in average BMI within these categories.

Etiology

Obesity ultimately results from an imbalance between energy intake and expenditure, and it is commonly stated that excess intake of energy-dense and high-fat food combined with low levels of physical activity have resulted in the present obesity epidemic. However, evidence for the etiological factors contributing to the marked increases

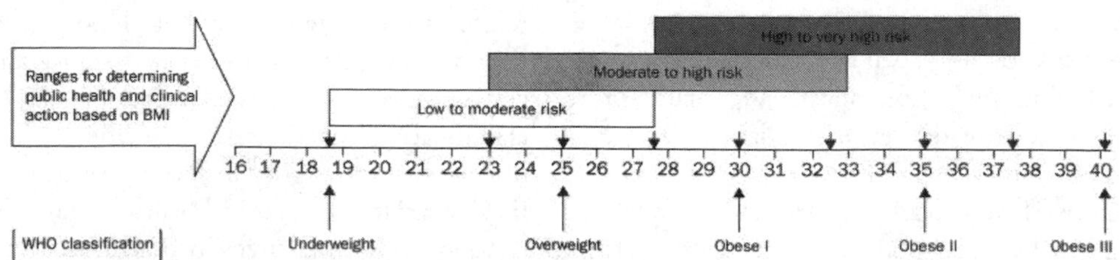

Figure 1. World Health Organization Classification of body-mass index (BMI) and Public Health Action Points. (From WHO Expert Consultation, 2004[6]; copyright 2004 with permission from Elsevier.)

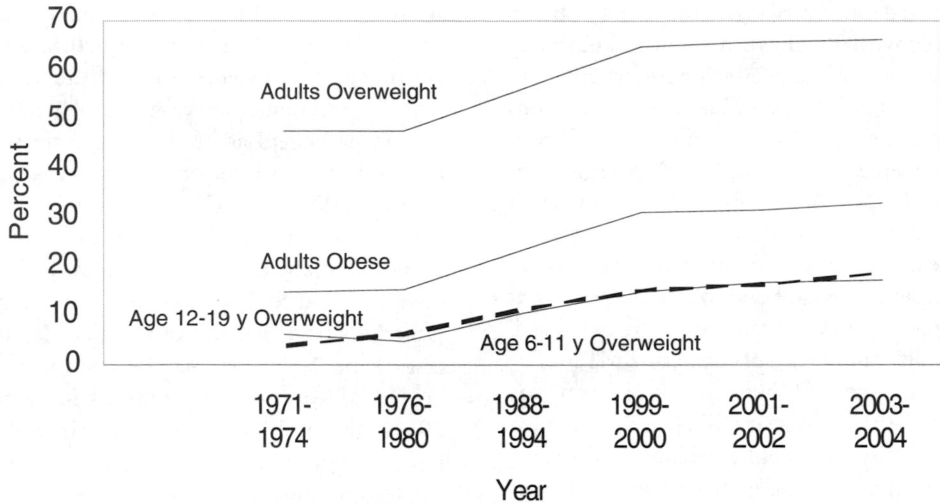

Figure 2. Trends in US overweight and obesity. Redrawn from data from the Centers for Disease Control and Prevention, National Center for Health Statistics, and National Health and Nutrition Examination Surveys.

in obesity prevalence over the last several decades remains a matter of debate and speculation.

Energy intake, as well as the per capita food energy supply, has increased in the United States and in other developed nations in the last 3 decades.[15] In the National Health and Nutrition Examination Surveys, from 1976 to 1980 and 1999 to 2000, average daily intake increased by 179 kcal for men and by 355 kcal for women.[16] Factors proposed to have contributed to increased energy intake include a greater proportion of food eaten outside of the home,[17] larger portion sizes,[18] sugar-sweetened beverage consumption,[19] and snacking.[18] In children and adolescents, proposed factors include fast food intake,[20] intake of sweetened soft drinks (which has increased while consumption of low-fat milk and water has declined),[21] availability of energy-dense snack and fast foods at school, and food advertising on television and in electronic or print media.[22] Preferential intake of energy-dense foods high in sugar or fat may be facilitated by their relatively lower cost in comparison to healthier choices and the perceived value of "supersizing."[15]

Decreases in energy expended on activities of daily living, in the workplace, and with recreational activities have been proposed as contributors to increases in obesity. In support of this, in 2003, 16% of US adults reported no leisure-time physical activity, and 46% reported a minimum of 30 minutes of moderate activity on most days.[23] However, between 1989 and 1996, the 32% reporting no leisure-time physical activity decreased by half, from 32% to 16%,[24] at a time in which obesity prevalence increased. Weight gain has been associated with time spent watching television or participating in sedentary behaviors in adults and children.[25,26] However, not all lines of evidence support declines in physical activity as a factor leading to the rise in obesity. Walking as a mode of transportation has actually modestly increased in the last decade,[27] as has the proportion of adults engaged in some degree of leisure-time activity, as noted above. Furthermore, advances in energy-saving technology at home and in the workplace have generally predated increases in obesity prevalence by several decades, and advances in the last 2 decades are relatively small in contrast to previous decades.[15]

Understanding of the genetic bases of obesity has dramatically grown in the last decade. Despite the description of rare single-gene defects that result in extreme obesity, and the identification of at least 600 genes, polymorphisms, and genetic markers associated with obesity,[28] the genetic basis of common overweight or obesity remains unclear. Future developments are likely to identify genes to serve as targets for interventions, gene-diet interactions that may facilitate the prevention or treatment of overweight, and methods to better match individuals with appropriate prevention or treatment strategies.

Mortality and Morbidity

Mortality

Most observational studies have found a J- or U-shaped relationship between BMI and mortality. Increased mortality risk associated with BMI ≥30 kg/m^2 has been observed for all-cause mortality and for mortality due to cardiovascular disease and certain cancers.[4,29-32] In general, the overall relative risk (RR) of mortality due to obesity in comparison to the BMI category with lowest mortality is in the range of 1 to 2.[29] In a recent meta-analysis of 26 observational studies with follow-up of over 3 to 36 years, McGee et al.[31] reported that the RR of all-cause mortality in men and women with BMI ≥30 kg/m^2 was 1.27 and 1.2, with slightly higher RR for mortality due to coronary heart disease (men 1.5; women 1.4).

BMI in the overweight range has inconsistently been associated with increased mortality. Flegal et al[33] recently calculated the relative risk of mortality and excess deaths due to underweight, overweight, and obesity in the National Health and Nutrition Examination Surveys I, II, and III data sets. Mortality risk for BMI ≥35 kg/m^2 was consistently increased, but overweight and Class I obesity were not associated with significantly increased mortality risks. The inconsistency of the overweight-mortality relationship may be due in part to the influence of populations for whom the BMI associated with minimal mortality in some studies exceeded 25 kg/m^2, such as African Americans and the elderly.[4,34] Although mortality increases with BMI in all ethnic groups, there is a relatively smaller increase in African Americans compared with Caucasians, which is, at least partially due to the greater risk at lower BMI. When absolute mortality rates are examined, increases in mortality along the spectrum of BMI for African Americans are evident.[34] Increasing age also appears to mitigate the influence of obesity, likely due to the increased overall mortality rate in older persons. In the Cancer Prevention Study II, increased RR of mortality was found for ages 30 to 64, 65 to 74, and ≥75, but in those over age 75, the increase in RR was about one-half that of the younger groups.

Morbidity

Obesity adversely affects virtually every organ system and is associated with diminished quality of life and discrimination (Table 2). Generally, risks for comorbidities such as type 2 diabetes mellitus, dyslipidemia, cardiomyopathy, and sleep apnea are related to both duration of and degree of obesity. The adverse health effects of obesity result from metabolic actions of adipose tissue or from the mechanical effect of excess weight. Metabolic actions include liberation of free fatty acids that cause insulin resistance[35] and production of inflammatory cytokines and prothrombotic factors. Structural effects of obesity are manifest by osteoarthritis of the knee and hip, back pain, and accumulation of fat in the neck, which contributes to pathogenesis of obstructive sleep apnea. Specific comorbidities of interest are discussed below.

Table 2. Health Effects of Obesity

Cardiovascular	**Genitourinary**
Coronary heart disease	Urinary incontinence
Stroke	Proteinuria
Congestive heart failure	**Cancer**
Cardiomyopathy	Breast
Left ventricular hypertrophy	Colon
Sudden death	Endometrium
Deep vein thrombosis	Esophagus
Pulmonary	Gastric cardia
Asthma	Gallbladder
Obstructive sleep apnea	**Musculoskeletal**
Pulmonary embolus	Osteoarthritis
Obesity hypoventilation syndrome	Back pain
Endocrine	Gout
Type 2 diabetes	**Neurological/Senses**
Dyslipidemia	Pseudotumor cerebri
Metabolic syndrome	Macular degeneration
Infertility	
Gastrointestinal	
Gastroesophageal reflux	
Gallstones	
Nonalcoholic fatty liver disease	

Type 2 Diabetes. Obesity, central fat distribution, and weight gain[36,37] contribute to the risk for type 2 diabetes. In US adults with type 2 diabetes, 85% are overweight or obese, and 55% are obese.[16] An estimated 14.4% of US adults have diabetes or impaired fasting glucose. Because type 2 diabetes may be asymptomatic or result in only mild symptoms for months to years, an estimated 29% of those with the disease remain undiagnosed.[38] The health implications are substantial, given that diabetes is the leading cause of chronic kidney disease and acquired blindness and also contributes to cardiovascular risk by hyperglycemia and by promoting dyslipidemia and hypertension.

Cardiovascular Disease. Obesity and central body fat distribution are associated with increased risk for multiple types of cardiovascular disease, including CHD,[7,30,39,40] cardiomyopathy,[41] congestive heart failure,[42] hypertension,[43] sudden death,[44] and stroke.[45] Obesity increases CHD and stroke risk by promoting traditional risk factors such as hypertension, dyslipidemia, and diabetes, but elevated risk remains after adjustment for these factors, suggesting that obesity is a risk factor for CHD independent of traditional risks.[46] In the Framingham Heart Study and in the Cancer Prevention Study II, overall risks for incident CHD and for CHD mortality associated with obesity were increased two-fold to three-fold compared with those with lower BMI.[4,39] Increased risk of CHD mortality has also been observed in those who were obese as adolescents, regardless of adult weight,[47] and in those who gained weight in adulthood.

Mechanisms relating inflammatory mediators to cardiovascular disease pathogenesis include increases of hepatic production of fibrinogen, induction of insulin resistance, and stimulation of endothelial release of adhesion molecules.[48] BMI and body fat are also associated with hemostatic factors that may increase the risk for CHD, including platelet activation, fibrinogen, Von Willebrand factor, factor VII, factor VIII, and the primary inhibitor of fibrinolysis, plasminogen activator inhibitor 1.[1,49] Another proposed marker of CHD risk, impaired endothelial function, is associated with obesity.[50]

Obstructive Sleep Apnea. The prevalence of obstructive sleep apnea in obese patients is estimated to be 12% to 40%,[51] although the actual prevalence varies considerably between clinical surveys and population studies. Obstructive sleep apnea is likely the most underdiagnosed weight-related comorbidity, and it has been estimated in middle-aged adults that up to 93% of women and 82% of men with treatable obstructive sleep apnea are undiagnosed.[52] In a series of patients evaluated before weight loss surgery, and who were previously undiagnosed with obstructive sleep apnea and underwent overnight polysomnography, obstructive sleep apnea was diagnosed in 35% to 88%.[53,54] Obstructive sleep apnea is associated with daytime fatigue, diminished quality of life, traffic accidents,[55] hypertension, cardiac arrhythmias, transient cardiac ischemia, congestive heart failure, and increased risk of sudden death.[56]

Venous Thromboembolic Disease. Obesity is an independent risk factor for deep vein thrombosis and pulmonary embolism in free-living ambulatory persons[57,58] and in hospitalized medical and surgical patients.[59,60] Additional risk factors associated with obesity for venous thromboembolic disease include abdominal fat distribution,[58] venous insufficiency, obesity hypoventilation syndrome or severe sleep apnea, and chronic heart failure. A preliminary investigation also suggests that the obesity-associated increase in prothrombotic factors may contribute to venous thromboembolic disease in obese persons.[61]

Cancer. Obesity increases risk for developing and dying from cancer of the breast (in postmenopausal women), colon, endometrium, esophagus, stomach, liver, kidney, and other organs.[32,62] For most of these neoplasms, the relative risk of incident cancer and cancer mortality associated with obesity is in the range of 1.2 to 2.0, and, for some cancers, a dose-response relationship exists, in which the heaviest subjects had substantially higher risks.[32,62] It has been estimated that 3% of cancers in the United States may be attributable to obesity,[63] whereas estimates are similar for European men and are estimated to be 6% for European women.[64] Further, overweight and obesity have been estimated to account for 14% of cancer mortality in men and 20% in women.

In postmenopausal women, obesity, central fat distribution, and adult weight gain are associated with increased breast cancer risk,[62,65,66] as well as with breast cancer recurrence and mortality.[32] Obesity appears to be associated with a decreased risk of breast cancer in premenopausal women,[62,65] although central fat distribution in premenopausal women may increase risk.[66] Obese women are less likely to undergo mammographic screening,[67] and tumors are diagnosed at advanced stages in obese women compared with leaner women.[68] Proposed mechanisms linking obesity to breast cancer include endogenous estrogen production by body fat, hyperinsulinemia, and alterations in insulin-like growth factor 1 and its binding proteins. Cancer of the endometrium may also be promoted by circulating estrogens produced by excess body fat. The risk of endometrial cancer incidence and mortality is increased in obesity two-fold to four-fold, and it has been estimated that obesity contributes to 39% of endometrial cancer.[64]

Colon cancer incidence[62,69] and mortality[32] are associated with obesity and central fat distribution, with the obesity-related risks greater for men than for women. Proposed mechanisms linking obesity, especially central obesity, to colon cancer are hyperinsulinemia, insulin resistance, insulin-like growth factors, and tumor growth stimulated by leptin.

Obesity is associated with increased risk for adenocarcinoma of the esophagus but not squamous cell carcinoma.[70] In addition, a more modest increased risk is observed for cancer of the gastric cardia.[70] A plausible link between obesity and these cancers is gastroesophageal reflux promoted by obesity, but thus far, conclusive evidence for this association is lacking.[70]

Hepatobiliary Disease. Obesity increases risk for nonalcoholic fatty liver disease, which represents a spectrum ranging from steatosis (fatty infiltration of the liver) to the more inflammatory nonalcoholic steatohepatitis to fibrosis and then to cirrhosis. Nonalcoholic fatty liver disease is estimated to occur in 10% to 24% of the population worldwide[71] and has been found in 30% to 100% in a series of obese adults.[71] Up to 25% of patients with nonalcoholic steatohepatitis may progress to cirrhosis.[72] Nonalcoholic fatty liver disease associated with obesity or diabetes also contributes to treatment failure and progression of liver disease in those with chronic hepatitis C infection.[73]

Musculoskeletal Disease. Obesity is a major risk factor for osteoarthritis of the knee. When highest and lowest BMI tertiles of cross-sectional studies were examined, women in the highest tertiles had a two-fold to seven-fold increased risk of knee osteoarthritis.[74] Evidence linking obesity with hip osteoarthritis is somewhat weaker than for that of the knee, with an overall two-fold increased risk.[75] osteoarthritis is a common cause of disability in older persons, who report more frequent functional limitations when osteoarthritis not is accompanied by obesity. In the US National Health Interview Survey, those with disability of the lower extremities were 2.4 times more likely to be obese than those without this disability.[76]

Psychosocial Issues

In addition to traditional medical comorbidities, obesity is also associated with diminished quality of life, social stigmatization, discrimination, reduced rates of marriage, and body image dissatisfaction. Although depression has been believed to be associated with obesity, only those with BMI $\geq$ 35 kg/m^2 have been found to have an increased prevalence of major depression.[77] The psychosocial consequences of obesity may be perceived by patients as far worse than any medical comorbidity. Obese persons face discrimination in interpersonal relations and in the workplace. Health-related quality of life (HRQL) is impaired in adults as well as children.[78,79] HRQL impairment appears to be more significant in clinical populations or in those presenting for obesity treatment, than in population surveys or general school populations of children, suggesting that HRQL is a motivating factor in seeking medical attention. Domains of HRQL most affected by obesity include vitality, physical functioning, and bodily pain (especially knee and back pain).[78]

Overweight in adolescence and adulthood is associated

with lower education levels, lower socioeconomic status, increased rates of poverty, and increased likelihood of never having been employed.[80,81] Many of these issues and other social issues, such as the likelihood of marrying or having a partner, have been more consistently observed in women than in men[80,81] and vary between ethnic groups as well.

Health Care and Other Costs

The economic cost of obesity includes health care costs and costs due to disability and absenteeism from work.[82,83] Health care costs increase in proportion to degree of obesity for those who are presently obese,[84] and Medicare expenditures are increased for older persons who were obese when younger.[85] US health care costs attributable to obesity-related conditions in 2000 exceeded $11 billion,[84] which is almost twice those for healthy-weight adults. The proportion of total medical costs in the United States attributable to obesity is estimated to be 5% to 7%, approximately half of which is borne by Medicare and Medicaid.[15]

Childhood Obesity

Like obesity in adults, obesity in children and adolescents has dramatically increased in the last several decades. Two current schemes are used to classify body weight in children ages 2 to 18. In the United States, overweight is defined as BMI ≥ 95th percentile for age and gender, whereas BMI ≥ 85th to 94.9th percentile is designated as at risk for overweight; the Centers for Disease Control and Prevention growth charts for 2000 serve as standards.[86] The International Obesity Task Force of the World Health Organization has defined childhood overweight and obesity by using the adult standards of BMI of 25 and 30 kg/m^2, respectively, at age 18 and regressing backwards to identify the associated BMI at earlier ages.[87] In the United States, prevalence of overweight among ages 2 to 18 has increased two to three times since the mid-1970s (Figure 2), and is now 16.5%.[12] Marked differences among ethnic groups and genders emerge with increasing age through childhood and adolescence.[12] Also, the degree of overweight (the extent to which weight surpasses the 95th percentile) is increasing at a rate greater than the prevalence of childhood obesity.[88] Significant increases in obesity prevalence have also been reported for children and adolescents in many other industrialized and developing nations.[89]

Childhood and adolescent overweight is associated with many of the same comorbid conditions as that in adults, including glucose intolerance and type 2 diabetes, dyslipidemia, hypertension, obstructive sleep apnea and nonalcoholic fatty liver disease, and others more specific to the child's age. Clinical manifestation of end organ damage, such as CHD, however, may not be apparent for decades. In contrast, type 2 diabetes, previously a disease almost exclusively limited to adults, is now being reported in obese children and adolescents. Population data regarding diabetes among children and adolescents are incomplete, and surveys vary widely in prevalence and incidence among the population studied (e.g., in populations at high risk, such as Native Americans, compared with lower-risk Caucasians). In a clinical series of multi-ethnic children attending an obesity treatment clinic, 25% of children were glucose intolerant and 4% of adolescents had diabetes.[90] Psychosocial problems associated with overweight or obesity in children and adolescents include social isolation, teasing, bullying, low self-esteem, and diminished HRQL.[79,91]

Obesity in childhood may increase the risk for adulthood obesity and disease. The ability of childhood BMI to predict adult BMI is greatest for older children or adolescents, for children with greater BMI, and for children with at least one obese parent.[92] BMI exceeding the 95th percentile at age 13 is associated with a ≥50% probability of adult obesity.[92] In terms of the association between childhood obesity and adult morbidity, many, but not all, studies suggest an increased risk of cardiovascular risk factors and mortality in adults who were obese as children or adolescents.[93,94] The degree to which this phenomenon is due to the persistence of obesity into adulthood, however, remains an issue of debate, because some trials assessing the relationship between childhood BMI and adult health outcomes did not control for adult BMI.[92]

Prevention

Prevention of unhealthy weight gain has become an international public health priority. Although some trials to date have been successful in changing dietary and physical activity behaviors, inconsistent prevention of weight gain has been reported in trials conducted with adults (conducted at the level of the family, community, and workplace) and with children (conducted at the level of the family, community, and in schools).[95,96] A framework for structuring and assessing interventions has been published by the International Obesity Task Force[97] and the Institute of Medicine.[98] Proposed interventions target individuals, schools, the food and advertising industry, community organizations, and local, state, and federal government agencies. Some interventions target prenatal and postnatal periods of the life cycle believed to be critical for the development of obesity, for example, promotion of infant breast-feeding. For children, interventions to modify dietary patterns (increase fruit, vegetables, and whole grains; and decrease sweets, snacks, and high-fat foods) are targeted at school meal programs, changing the contents and prices of snack bars and vending machines, instituting policies regarding foods sold in schools, promoting nutrition education, and regulating food advertisements directed at children and adolescents.[99] Interventions directed at adults include mandatory nutrition labeling of foods eaten out of the home, taxing or subsidizing specific classes of foods, and encouraging intake of specific foods by policy changes to public assistance programs.[99] Strategies to increase physical activity include limits on "screen time" (time spent watching television or at the computer), the provision of more frequent and more intense physical activity in schools, and providing a safe environment for physical activity.

Treatment

Treatment for obesity includes dietary, physical activity, behavioral, pharmacological, and surgical interventions. Although research has focused on the efficacy and safety of each of these modalities, effective weight control requires dietary and physical activity components that are reinforced, enhanced, and maintained by behavioral strategies. Pharmacological and surgical options are adjuncts that further facilitate or improve upon lifestyle measures. Although a detailed review of obesity treatment is beyond the scope of this discussion, several recent systematic reviews are available.[100-102]

Dietary treatments are classified into low-calorie diets ($\geq$ 800 kcal/d) and very-low-calorie diets (<800 kcal/d). General low-calorie diet recommendations are to reduce intake by approximately 500 kcal/d from maintenance requirements to achieve a weight loss of 0.5 to 1 kg/wk.[3] In trials of low-calorie diets lasting 3 to 12 months, average weight loss has been 8% of initial weight.[3] Recent trials examining the relative efficacy of low-carbohydrate diets compared with low-fat diets demonstrated that lower-carbohydrate diets may effect greater weight loss at 6 months, but at 1 year there is no significant difference.[103,104] Very-low-calorie diets result in weight loss that is approximately double that observed with low-calorie diets, but require more intensive medical monitoring. Long-term weight control following very-low-calorie diets has been reported to be no better than with low-calorie diets,[3] although some investigators have found that long-term weight loss after very-low-calorie diets exceeds that with low-calorie diets.[105] Long-term weight loss after very-low-calorie diets appears to be best in those who lose greater amounts of weight while on a very-low-calorie diet and who maintain participation in dietary, exercise, and behavioral interventions.[105]

Increasing physical activity without concomitant decreases in energy intake is unlikely to result in significant weight loss unless the energy cost of activity is substantial and intake remains stable. However, physical activity contributes to weight loss, enhances self-efficacy, and is associated with reduced morbidity incidence, severity, and mortality.[106] Substantial physical activity (over 30 min/d of vigorous activity or over 1 h/d of moderate activity) appears to be an important component of maintenance of lost weight.[107]

Drugs for treatment of obesity act on the central nervous system to suppress appetite or increase satiation, in the gut to inhibit the absorption of dietary fat, and in the periphery to increase thermogenesis. Drug treatment is indicated for those with BMI $\geq$ 30 kg/m^2 or for those with BMI $\geq$ 27 kg/m^2 with weight-related comorbidity. Drug treatment is associated with weight losses of 3 to 6 kg beyond placebo after treatment for 1 year.[101] An alternative, but perhaps equally important, way of assessing efficacy of drug treatment is by the proportion of those who are able to reduce weight. Drug treatment has been shown to increase the number of responders to lifestyle interventions and to increase the numbers of those able to achieve 10% or greater losses of initial weight.[108]

Surgical treatment of obesity consists of procedures that restrict food intake, such as the adjustable laparoscopic gastric band or the older vertical banded gastroplasty, or those that combine varying degrees of malabsorption with restriction, such as the gastric bypass and the more malabsorptive biliopancreatic diversion. Surgery is indicated in those with BMI $\geq$ 40 kg/m^2 or with BMI $\geq$ 35 kg/m^2 with weight-related comorbidities. Surgery results in losses of 20% to 40% of initial weight, with the more malabsorptive procedures resulting in a greater loss.[109] Long-term results in cohorts without substantial attrition are scarce, but a 5- to 10-year follow-up suggests that the majority of patients have maintained significant weight losses.

Effects of Obesity Treatment on Comorbid Conditions

Loss of 5% to 10% of initial weight has been associated with improvements in diabetes, hypertension, dyslipidemia, sleep apnea, and other conditions.[3] In addition, short-term weight loss results in reduced levels of inflammatory markers and improvement in prothrombotic factors and endothelial function.[49,50,110] Lifestyle interventions in those with impaired glucose tolerance have demonstrated that modest degrees of weight loss combined with increases in physical activity prevent progression to frank diabetes.[111,112] Although approximately 80% of those who lose weight are unable to maintain losses of at least 10%,[113] persistent benefits occur in blood glucose and cardiovascular risk factors following weight loss interventions; persistent benefits are more likely to occur in those who maintain at least some lost weight or had elevations in risk factors before weight loss.[100,114] Surgically induced weight loss has resulted in high rates of amelioration or resolution of many comorbidities, including diabetes, hypertension, cardiomyopathy, dyslipidemia, sleep apnea, and quality of life.[102]

Whether intentional weight loss results in decreased mortality remains a topic of debate. Several,[115-119] but not all,[120-122] investigations have demonstrated that intentional weight loss in those with diabetes and other conditions is associated with reduced mortality rates. Interestingly, in one investigation, those reporting an intention to reduce weight experienced reduced mortality regardless of whether weight was actually lost.[116] With gastric bypass surgery, survival beyond 1 year after surgery has recently been shown to improve.[123]

Conclusion

The rise in obesity prevalence in children and adults portends serious health and economic consequences. Much of weight-related comorbidity is underdiagnosed or undertreated, further worsening long-term health outcomes and quality of life. Although attention has been most focused on treatment of obesity and its comorbidities, long-term weight control is far from optimal. The more recent focus on prevention is clearly needed, but how to enact population-level changes and how to fund such changes remain daunting challenges.

References

1. De Lorenzo F, Mukherjee M, Kadziola Z, et al. Association of overall adiposity rather than body mass index with lipids and procoagulant factors. Thromb Haemost. 1998;80:603–606.
2. World Health Organization. *Physical Status: The Use and Interpretation of Anthropometry.* Geneva: World Health Organization; 1995.
3. NHLBI Obesity Education Initiative Expert Panel on the Identification Evaluation and Treatment of Overweight and Obesity in Adults. Clinical guidelines on the identification, evaluation, and treatment of overweight and obesity in adults—the evidence report. Obes Res. 1998;6(Suppl 2): 51S–209S.
4. Calle EE, Thun MJ, Petrelli JM, et al. Body-mass index and mortality in a prospective cohort of U.S. adults. N Engl J Med. 1999;341:1097–1105.
5. Must A, Spadano J, Coakley EH, et al. The disease burden associated with overweight and obesity. JAMA. 1999;282:1523–1529.
6. W. H. O. Expert Consultation. Appropriate body-mass index for Asian populations and its implications for policy and intervention strategies. Lancet. 2004;363(9403):157–163.
7. Rexrode KM, Carey VJ, Hennekens CH, et al. Abdominal adiposity and coronary heart disease in women. JAMA. 1998;280:1843–1848.
8. Folsom AR, Kushi LH, Anderson KE, et al. Associations of general and abdominal obesity with multiple health outcomes in older women: the Iowa Women's Health Study. Arch Int Med. 2000;160: 2117–2128.
9. Janssen I, Katzmarzyk PT, Ross R. Waist circumference and not body mass index explains obesity-related health risk. Am J Clin Nutr. 2004;79: 379–384.
10. Frayn KN. Visceral fat and insulin resistance—causative or correlative? Br J Nutr. 2000; 83(Suppl 1):S71–S77.
11. Valsamakis G, Chetty R, Anwar A, et al. Association of simple anthropometric measures of obesity with visceral fat and the metabolic syndrome in male Caucasian and Indo-Asian subjects. Diabet Med. 2004;21:1339–1345.
12. Hedley AA, Ogden CL, Johnson CL, et al. Prevalence of overweight and obesity among US children, adolescents, and adults, 1999–2002. JAMA. 2004; 291:2847–2850.
13. Baskin ML, Ard J, Franklin F, et al. Prevalence of obesity in the United States. Obes Rev. 2005;6:5–7.
14. Okosun IS, Chandra KM, Boev A, et al. Abdominal adiposity in U.S. adults: prevalence and trends, 1960–2000. Prev Med. 2004;39:197–206.
15. Finkelstein EA, Ruhm CJ, Kosa KM. Economic causes and consequences of obesity. Annu Rev Public Health. 2005;26:239–257.
16. Centers for Disease Control and Prevention. Prevalence of overweight and obesity among adults with diagnosed diabetes—United States, 1988–1994 and 1999–2002. MMWR Morb Mortal Wkly Rep. 2004;53:1066–1068.
17. McCrory MA, Fuss PJ, Hays NP, et al. Overeating in America: association between restaurant food consumption and body fatness in healthy adult men and women ages 19 to 80. Obes Res. 1999;7: 564–571.
18. Nielsen SJ, Popkin BM. Patterns and trends in food portion sizes, 1977–1998. JAMA. 2003;289: 450–453.
19. Schulze MB, Manson JE, Ludwig DS, et al. Sugar-sweetened beverages, weight gain, and incidence of type 2 diabetes in young and middle-aged women. JAMA. 2004;292:927–934.
20. Ebbeling CB, Sinclair KB, Pereira MA, et al. Compensation for energy intake from fast food among overweight and lean adolescents. JAMA. 2004;291: 2828–2833.
21. Ludwig DS, Peterson KE, Gortmaker SL. Relation between consumption of sugar-sweetened drinks and childhood obesity: a prospective, observational analysis. Lancet. 2001;357:505–508.
22. Lobstein T, Dibb S. Evidence of a possible link between obesogenic food advertising and child overweight. Obes Rev. 2005;6:203–208.
23. Centers for Disease Control and Prevention. Adult participation in recommended levels of physical activity—United States, 2001 and 2003. MMWR Morb Mortal Wkly Rep. 2005;54:1208–1212.
24. Prevalence of no leisure-time physical activity—35 states and the District of Columbia, 1988–2002. MMWR Morb Mortal Wkly Rep. 2004;53(4): 82–86.
25. Hu FB, Li TY, Colditz GA, et al. Television watching and other sedentary behaviors in relation to risk of obesity and type 2 diabetes mellitus in women. JAMA. 2003;289:1785–1791.

26. Gortmaker SL, Must A, Sobol AM, et al. Television viewing as a cause of increasing obesity among children in the United States, 1986–1990. Arch Pediatr Adolesc Med. 1996;150:356–362.
27. Ham SA, Macera CA, Lindley C. Trends in walking for transportation in the United States, 1995 and 2001. Prev Chronic Dis. 2005;2:A14.
28. Perusse L, Rankinen T, Zuberi A, et al. The human obesity gene map: the 2004 update. Obes Res. 2005; 13:381–490.
29. Flegal KM, Williamson DF, Pamuk ER, et al. Estimating deaths attributable to obesity in the United States. Am J Public Health. 2004;94:1486–1489.
30. Manson JE, Willett WC, Stampfer MJ, et al. Body weight and mortality among women. N Engl J Med. 1995;333:677–685.
31. McGee DL: Diverse Populations Collaboration. Body mass index and mortality: a meta-analysis based on person-level data from twenty-six observational studies. Ann Epidemiol. 2005;15:87–97.
32. Calle EE, Rodriguez C, Walker-Thurmond K, et al. Overweight, obesity, and mortality from cancer in a prospectively studied cohort of U.S. adults. N Engl J Med. 2003;348:1625–1638.
33. Flegal KM, Graubard BI, Williamson DF, et al. Excess deaths associated with underweight, overweight, and obesity. JAMA. 2005;293:1861–1867.
34. Stevens J. Obesity and mortality in African-Americans. Nutr Rev. 2000;58:346–353.
35. Roden M, Price TB, Perseghin G, et al. Mechanism of free fatty acid-induced insulin resistance in humans. J Clin Invest. 1996;7:2859–2865.
36. Haffner S, Katz M, Dunn J. Increased upper body and overall adiposity is associated with decreased sex hormone binding globulin in postmenopausal women. Int J Obes. 1991;15:471–478.
37. Koh-Banerjee P, Wang Y, Hu FB, et al. Changes in body weight and body fat distribution as risk factors for clinical diabetes in US men. Am J Epidemiol. 2004;159:1150–1159.
38. Centers for Disease Control and Prevention. Prevalence of diabetes and impaired fasting glucose in adults—United States. MMWR Morb Mortal Wkly Rep. 2003;52:833–837.
39. Hubert HB, Feinleib M, McNamara PM, et al. Obesity as an independent risk factor for cardiovascular disease: A 26-year follow-up of participants in the Framingham Heart Study. Circulation. 1983; 67:968–977.
40. Rimm EB, Stampfer MJ, Giovannucci E, et al. Body size and fat distribution as predictors of coronary heart disease among middle-aged and older US men. Am J Epidemiol. 1995;141:1117–1127.
41. Alpert MA. Obesity cardiomyopathy: pathophysiology and evolution of the clinical syndrome. Am J Med Sci. 2001;321:225–236.
42. Kenchaiah S, Evans JC, Levy D, et al. Obesity and the risk of heart failure. N Engl J Med. 2002;347: 305–313.
43. Huang Z, Willett WC, Manson JE, et al. Body weight, weight change, and risk for hypertension in women. Ann Intern Med. 1998;128:81–88.
44. Messerli F, Soria F. Ventricular dysrhythmias, left ventricular hypertrophy, and sudden death. Cardiovasc Drugs Ther. 1994;8:557–563.
45. Rexrode KM, Hennekens CH, Willett WC, et al. A prospective study of body mass index, weight change, and risk of stroke in women. JAMA. 1997; 277:1539–1545.
46. Eckel RH, Krauss RM. American Heart Association call to action: obesity as a major risk factor for coronary heart disease. Circulation. 1998;97: 2099–2100.
47. Must A, Jacques PF, Dallal GE, et al. Long-term morbidity and mortality of overweight adolescents. A follow-up of the Harvard Growth Study of 1922 to 1935. N Engl J Med. 1992;327:1350–1355.
48. Yudkin JS, Kumari M, Humphries SE, et al. Inflammation, obesity, stress and coronary heart disease: is interleukin-6 the link? Atherosclerosis. 2000;148:209–214.
49. Davi G, Guagnano MT, Ciabattoni G, et al. Platelet activation in obese women: role of inflammation and oxidant stress. JAMA. 2002;288:2008–2014.
50. Raitakari M, Ilvonen T, Ahotupa M, et al. Weight reduction with very-low-caloric diet and endothelial function in overweight adults: role of plasma glucose. Arterioscler Thromb Vasc Biol. 2004;24: 124–128.
51. O'Keeffe T, Patterson EJ. Evidence supporting routine polysomnography before bariatric surgery. Obes Res. 2004;14:23–26.
52. Young T, Evans L, Finn L, et al. Estimation of the clinically diagnosed proportion of sleep apnea syndrome in middle-aged men and women. Sleep. 1997;20:705–706.
53. Frey WC, Pilcher J. Obstructive sleep-related breathing disorders in patients evaluated for bariatric surgery. Obes Surg. 2003;13:676–683.
54. van Kralingen KW, de Kanter W, de Groot GH, et al. Assessment of sleep complaints and sleep-disordered breathing in a consecutive series of obese patients. Respiration. 1999;66:312–316.
55. Teran-Santos J, Jimenez-Gomez A, Cordero-Guevara J, et al. The association between sleep apnea and the risk of traffic accidents. N Engl J Med. 1999;340(11):847–851.
56. Shamsuzzaman AS, Gersh BJ, Somers VK. Obstructive sleep apnea: implications for cardiac and vascular disease. JAMA. 2003;290:1906–1914.
57. Goldhaber SZ, Grodstein F, Stampfer MJ, et al. A prospective study of risk factors for pulmonary embolism in women. JAMA. 1997;277:642–645.

58. Hansson PO, Eriksson H, Welin L, et al. Smoking and abdominal obesity: risk factors for venous thromboembolism among middle-aged men: "the study of men born in 1913." Arch Intern Med. 1999;159:1886–1890.
59. Blaszyk H, Bjornsson J. Factor V leiden and morbid obesity in fatal postoperative pulmonary embolism. Arch Surg. 2000;135:1410–1413.
60. Cohen AT, Alikhan R, Arcelus JI, et al. Assessment of venous thromboembolism risk and the benefits of thromboprophylaxis in medical patients. Thromb Haemost. 2005;94:750–759.
61. Abdollahi M, Cushman M, Rosendaal FR. Obesity: risk of venous thrombosis and the interaction with coagulation factor levels and oral contraceptive use. Thromb Haemost. 2003;89:493–498.
62. Bianchini F, Kaaks R, Vainio H. Overweight, obesity, and cancer risk. Lancet Oncol. 2002;3: 565–574.
63. Polednak AP. Trends in incidence rates for obesity-associated cancers in the US. Cancer Detect Prev. 2003;27:415–421.
64. Bergstrom A, Pisani P, Tenet V, et al. Overweight as an avoidable cause of cancer in Europe. Int J Cancer. 2001;91:421–430.
65. Huang Z, Hankinson SE, Colditz GA, et al. Dual effects of weight and weight gain on breast cancer risk. JAMA. 1997;278:1407–1411.
66. Harvie M, Hooper L, Howell AH. Central obesity and breast cancer risk: a systematic review. Obes Rev. 2003;4:157–173.
67. Wee CC, McCarthy EP, Davis RB, et al. Screening for cervical and breast cancer: is obesity an unrecognized barrier to preventive care? Ann Intern Med. 2000;132:697–704.
68. Cui Y, Whiteman MK, Flaws JA, et al. Body mass and stage of breast cancer at diagnosis. Int J Cancer. 2002;98:279–283.
69. Giovannucci E, Ascherio A, Rimm EB, et al. Physical activity, obesity, and risk for colon cancer and adenoma in men. Ann Intern Med. 1995;122: 327–334.
70. Hampel H, Abraham NS, El-Serag HB. Meta-analysis: obesity and the risk for gastroesophageal reflux disease and its complications. Ann Intern Med. 2005;143:199–211.
71. Angulo P, Lindor KD. Treatment of non-alcoholic steatohepatitis. Best Pract Res Clin Gastroenterol. 2002;16:797–810.
72. Scheen AJ, Luyckx FH. Obesity and liver disease. Best Pract Res Clin Endocrinol Metab. 2002;16: 703–716.
73. Bressler BL, Guindi M, Tomlinson G, et al. High body mass index is an independent risk factor for nonresponse to antiviral treatment in chronic hepatitis C. Hepatology. 2003;38:639–644.
74. Wluka A, Flavia F, Spector T. Obesity, arthritis, and gout. In: Bray GS, Bouchard C, eds. *Handbook of Obesity,* 2nd ed. New York: Marcel Dekker; 2004; 953–966.
75. Lievense AM, Bierma-Zeinstra SM, Verhagen AP, et al. Influence of obesity on the development of osteoarthritis of the hip: a systematic review. Rheumatology. 2002;41:1155–1162.
76. Weil E, Wachterman M, McCarthy EP, et al. Obesity among adults with disabling conditions. JAMA. 2002;288:1265–1268.
77. Onyike CU, Crum RM, Lee HB, et al. Is obesity associated with major depression? Results from the Third National Health and Nutrition Examination Survey. Am J Epidemiol. 2003;158:1139–1147.
78. Fontaine KR, Barofsky I. Obesity and health-related quality of life. Obes Rev. 2001;2:173–182.
79. Williams J, Wake M, Hesketh K, et al. Health-related quality of life of overweight and obese children. JAMA. 2005;293:70–76.
80. Gortmaker SL, Must A, Perrin JM, et al. Social and economic consequences of overweight in adolescence and young adulthood. N Engl J Med. 1993; 329:1008–1012.
81. Viner RM, Cole TJ. Adult socioeconomic, educational, social, and psychological outcomes of childhood obesity: a national birth cohort study. Br Med J. 2005;330:1354.
82. Bungum T, Satterwhite M, Jackson AW, et al. The relationship of body mass index, medical costs, and job absenteeism. Am J Health Behav. 2003;27: 456–462.
83. Finkelstein E, Fiebelkorn C, Wang G. The costs of obesity among full-time employees. Am J Health Promot. 2005;20:45–51.
84. Arterburn DE, Maciejewski ML, Tsevat J. Impact of morbid obesity on medical expenditures in adults. Int J Obes. 2005;29:334–339.
85. Daviglus ML, Liu K, Yan LL, et al. Relation of body mass index in young adulthood and middle age to Medicare expenditures in older age. JAMA. 2004;292:2743–2749.
86. Kuczmarski RJ, Ogden CL, Guo SS, et al. 2000 CDC Growth Charts for the United States: methods and development. Vital Health Stat 11. 2002; 246:1–190.
87. Cole TJ, Bellizzi MC, Flegal KM, et al. Establishing a standard definition for child overweight and obesity worldwide: international survey. Br Med J. 2000;320:1240–1243.
88. Jolliffe D. Extent of overweight among US children and adolescents from 1971 to 2000. Int J Obes. 2004;28:4–9.
89. Popkin BM, Gordon-Larsen P. The nutrition transition: worldwide obesity dynamics and their determinants. Int J Obes. 2004;28(Suppl 3):S2–S9.

90. Sinha R, Fisch G, Teague B, et al. Prevalence of impaired glucose tolerance among children and adolescents with marked obesity. N Engl J Med. 2002; 346:802–810.
91. Janssen I, Craig WM, Boyce WF, et al. Associations between overweight and obesity with bullying behaviors in school-aged children. Pediatrics. 2004; 113:1187–1194.
92. Whitlock EP, Williams SB, Gold R, et al. Screening and interventions for childhood overweight: a summary of evidence for the US Preventive Services Task Force. Pediatrics. 2005;116:e125–e144.
93. Must A, Strauss RS. Risks and consequences of childhood and adolescent obesity. Int J Obes. 1999; 23(Suppl 2):S2–S11.
94. Berenson GS, Srinivasan SR. Emergence of obesity and cardiovascular risk for coronary artery disease: the Bogalusa Heart Study. Prev Cardiol. 2001;4: 116–121.
95. Hardeman W, Griffin S, Johnston M, et al. Interventions to prevent weight gain: a systematic review of psychological models and behaviour change methods. Int J Obes. 2000;24:131–143.
96. Summerbell CD, Waters E, Edmunds LD, et al. Interventions for preventing obesity in children. Cochrane Database Syst Rev. 2005:CD001871.
97. Swinburn B, Gill T, Kumanyika S. Obesity prevention: a proposed framework for translating evidence into action. Obes Rev. 2005;6:23–33.
98. Koplan JP, Liverman CT, Kraak VI. Preventing childhood obesity: health in the balance: executive summary. J Am Diet Assoc. 2005;105:131–138.
99. Finkelstein E, French S, Variyam JN, et al. Pros and cons of proposed interventions to promote healthy eating. Am J Prev Med. 2004;27(3 Suppl):163–167.
100. Douketis JD, Macie C, Thabane L, et al. Systematic review of long-term weight loss studies in obese adults: clinical significance and applicability to clinical practice. Int J Obes. 2005;29:1153–1167.
101. Li Z, Maglione M, Tu W, et al. Meta-analysis: pharmacologic treatment of obesity. Ann Intern Med. 2005;142:532–546.
102. Maggard MA, Shugarman LR, Suttorp M, et al. Meta-analysis: surgical treatment of obesity. Ann Intern Med. 2005;142:547–559.
103. Foster GD, Wyatt HR, Hill JO, et al. A randomized trial of a low-carbohydrate diet for obesity. N Engl J Med. 2003;348:2082–2090.
104. Stern L, Iqbal N, Seshadri P, et al. The effects of low-carbohydrate versus conventional weight loss diets in severely obese adults: one-year follow-up of a randomized trial. Ann Intern Med. 2004;140: 778–785.
105. Saris WH. Very-low-calorie diets and sustained weight loss. Obes Res. 2001;9:295S–301S.
106. Blair SN, Brodney S. Effects of physical inactivity and obesity on morbidity and mortality: current evidence and research issues. Med Sci Sports Exerc. 1999;31:S646–S662.
107. Schoeller DA, Shay K, Kushner RF. How much physical activity is needed to minimize weight gain in previously obese women? Am J Clin Nutr. 1997; 66:551–556.
108. Padwal R, Li SK, Lau DC. Long-term pharmacotherapy for obesity and overweight. Cochrane Database Syst Rev. 2004;3:CD004094.
109. Brolin R. Bariatric surgery and long-term control of morbid obesity. JAMA. 2002;228:2793–2796.
110. Esposito K, Pontillo A, Di Palo C, et al. Effect of weight loss and lifestyle changes on vascular inflammatory markers in obese women: a randomized trial. JAMA. 2003;289:1799–1804.
111. Tuomilehto J, Lindstrom J, Eriksson JG, et al. Prevention of type 2 diabetes mellitus by changes in lifestyle among subjects with impaired glucose tolerance. N Engl J Med. 2001;344:1343–1350.
112. Knowler WC, Barrett-Connor E, Fowler SE, et al. Reduction in the incidence of type 2 diabetes with lifestyle intervention or metformin. N Engl J Med. 2002;346:393–403.
113. Wing RR, Phelan S. Long-term weight loss maintenance. Am J Clin Nutr. 2005;82:222S–225S.
114. National Task Force on the Prevention and Treatment of Obesity. Overweight, obesity, and health risk. National Task Force on the Prevention and Treatment of Obesity. Arch Intern Med. 2000;160: 898–904.
115. Williamson DF, Thompson TJ, Thun M, et al. Intentional weight loss and mortality among overweight individuals with diabetes. Diabetes Care. 2000;23:1499–1504.
116. Gregg EW, Gerzoff RB, Thompson TJ, et al. Intentional weight loss and death in overweight and obese U.S. adults 35 years of age and older. Ann Intern Med. 2003;138:383–389.
117. Williamson DF, Pamuk E, Thun M, et al. Prospective study of intentional weight loss and mortality in overweight white men aged 40–64 years. Am J Epidemiol. 1999;149:491–503.
118. Williamson DF, Pamuk E, Thun M, et al. Prospective study of intentional weight loss and mortality in never-smoking overweight US white women aged 40–64 years. Am J Epidemiol. 1995;141:1128–1141.
119. Wannamethee SG, Shaper AG, Lennon L. Reasons for intentional weight loss, unintentional weight loss, and mortality in older men. Arch Intern Med. 2005;165:1035–1040.
120. Diehr P, Bild DE, Harris TB, et al. Body mass

index and mortality in nonsmoking older adults: the Cardiovascular Health Study. Am J Public Health. 1998;88:623–629.
121. Yaari S, Goldbourt U. Voluntary and involuntary weight loss: associations with long term mortality in 9,228 middle-aged and elderly men. Am J Epidemiol. 1998;148:546–555.
122. French SA, Folsom AR, Jeffery RW, et al. Prospective study of intentionality of weight loss and mortality in older women: the Iowa Women's Health Study. Am J Epidemiol. 1999;149:504–514.
123. Flum DR, Dellinger EP. Impact of gastric bypass operation on survival: a population-based analysis. J Am Coll Surg. 2004;199:543–551.

49
Atherosclerotic Cardiovascular Disease

Heather I. Katcher, Peter J. Gillies, and
Penny M. Kris-Etherton

Introduction

Nutrition has assumed a prominent role for both the prevention and treatment of cardiovascular disease (CVD). There have been many new developments in the field since the last edition of *Present Knowledge in Nutrition*. These advances offer great promise for recommending dietary patterns that prevent or halt the progression—or even induce the regression—of established CVD. Collectively, these new advances in nutrition research offer the potential to lower risk of CVD to an extent not imagined 10 years ago. The new developments in nutrition encompass: identifying dietary patterns that can therapeutically target an expanding number of CVD risk factors, increasing our understanding of how specific foods and under-studied nutrients affect CVD risk, and gaining a better understanding of nutrient-gene interactions to elucidate the genetic basis for differences in diet responsiveness.

With respect to the effects of diet on risk factors for CVD, recent research has shown that different dietary patterns can lower LDL cholesterol (LDL) and blood pressure as much as drug therapy.[1,2] In addition, there is exciting evidence that demonstrates the effects of diet on important new risk factors for CVD, including C-reactive protein and other markers of inflammation, cellular adhesion molecules, oxidative stress, and endothelial function. Relative to functional foods and under-studied nutrients, contemporary nutrition research has advanced our understanding of the role of a growing number of foods and nutrients such as omega-3 fatty acids and trans fatty acids, on CVD risk, resulting in health claims and qualified health claims for different foods and dietary recommendations for fatty acids. Research developments in nutrigenomics (the study of nutrient-gene interactions) have provided insight into how individuals differ in their response to diets that vary in nutrient profile. As advances are made, this will eventually provide tools for conducting genetic screens to provide personalized nutrition guidance for individuals to reduce risk of CVD well beyond what is achievable presently.

Because diet affects many CVD and other chronic disease risk factors, it is evident that it plays a central role in health and disease. The broad diversity of dietary patterns provides a basis to develop innovative new approaches that target multiple risk factors for many chronic diseases. Identifying optimal dietary patterns for individuals that maximally benefit CVD risk status is a long-sought goal. The objective of this chapter is to review new developments in the field of cardiovascular nutrition. Specifically, we will discuss the pathobiology of CVD and the points where nutrition regulates its development and progression. In addition, we will discuss the role of individual nutrients, with an emphasis on omega-3 and trans fatty acids, and the effects of cardioprotective dietary patterns on CVD risk. Lastly, we will discuss our present understanding of how genotype determines response to different dietary patterns and, consequently, CVD risk.

Pathogenesis of Coronary Heart Disease

CVDs include diseases of the heart and blood vessels, including stroke. Coronary heart disease (CHD) is the most common CVD, accounting for approximately 53% of deaths from CVD in the United States.[3] CHD is caused by atherosclerosis, the narrowing of the coronary arteries due to fatty buildups of plaque, but the term

CHD encompasses any disease of the coronary arteries and resulting complications such as chest pain and heart attack. The understanding of the pathogenesis of CHD has enabled researchers to study the effects of various nutrients and foods on metabolic pathways and to identify dietary components that influence cardiovascular health.

The understanding of the pathogenesis of CHD has evolved from a disorder of lipid accumulation to a condition of chronic inflammation in the arteries.[4] Inflammatory events characterize the pathophysiology of atherosclerosis at every stage; immune cells infiltrate early atherosclerotic lesions, their effector molecules accelerate the progression of these lesions, and activation of inflammation can elicit acute coronary syndromes.[5] In addition, the likelihood of acute coronary syndrome is determined by the degree of inflammatory activity and associated plaque instability rather than the extent of arterial constriction.[6] In fact, in many cases, there is less than a 50% blockage of the artery at the time of a heart attack.[7] Plaque rupture and thrombosis leading to an acute coronary syndrome can be due to: a) erosion of the endothelial cells, which exposes thrombotic factors; b) disruption of microvessels in the plaque, which can lead to hemorrhage or thrombosis in the plaque, causing rupture; or c) weakening and degradation of the fibrous cap, leading to rupture.[7] Each of these processes is accelerated by a state of inflammation. Currently, traditional risk factors and dietary and pharmaceutical treatments are being re-evaluated for their effects on inflammatory markers and processes.

C-reactive protein is an acute-phase protein that increases during systemic inflammation. It is perhaps the most widely studied inflammatory biomarker. Blood levels of C-reactive protein predict future coronary events in individuals without CHD, as well as recurrent ischemia and death in individuals with stable and unstable angina and those who present with an acute coronary syndrome or myocardial infarction.[8] C-reactive protein is a robust CVD risk factor because it adds prognostic information at all LDL levels and at all Framingham risk scores (Figure 1).[9] In addition, C-reactive protein is an easily assessed risk factor because it has a long half-life (18–20 hours), does not have a circadian cycle, has a standardized assay, and has accepted normal ranges and screening guidelines from the American Heart Association (AHA) and Centers for Disease Control (CDC).[10] C-reactive protein is also a reliable biomarker irrespective of sex, age, blood pressure, lipid levels, and smoking status. The primary function of C-reactive protein is not established, but it may play a role in atherosclerosis by increasing adhesion molecule expression, inhibiting nitric oxide synthase, and enhancing LDL uptake by macrophages.[11]

Role of Omega-3 Fatty Acids in the Prevention of CVD

There is a robust database from epidemiological and clinical trials demonstrating that omega-3 fatty acids reduce the risk of death from CVD[12] Recent studies have added to our understanding of the effects that omega-3 fatty acids from plant and marine sources have on CVD risk. This has resulted in the release of dietary guidance from many worldwide nutrition organizations that eicosapentaenoic acid (EPA) plus docosahexaenoic acid (DHA) should be consumed for those with or at risk for CVD.

Marine Sources of Omega-3 Fatty Acids

Fish and fish oil are rich sources of long-chain omega-3 fatty acids, especially EPA and DHA. To date, the association between fish consumption and CHD mortality has been studied in over 220,000 individuals followed for an average of 11.8 years.[13] Compared with individuals who rarely eat fish, the reduction in risk of death from CHD is 38% for individuals who consume the most fish (≥5 times a week).[13] It is estimated that each 20 g/d increase in fish intake is related to a 7% lower risk of

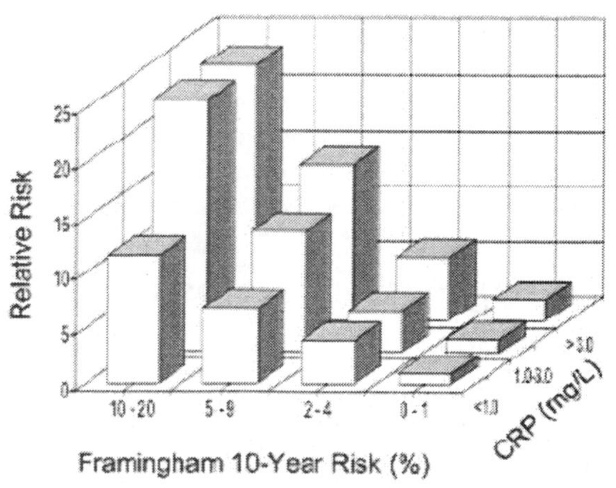

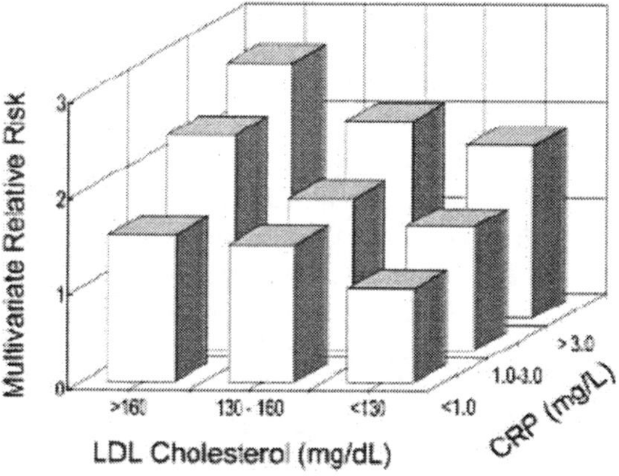

Figure 1. C-reactive protein provides prognostic information at all levels of low-density lipoprotein (LDL) cholesterol and at all levels of the Framingham Risk Score. (Adapted with permission from Ridker et al.[9]; copyright 2002 The Massachusetts Medical Society. All rights reserved.)

CHD mortality.[13] Individuals who consume five or more servings of fish per week also have the greatest reduction in risk of stroke (approximately 31% lower risk) compared with those who eat fish less than once a month.[14] However, intake of even 1 to 3 servings of fish per month is associated with a significant reduction in risk of CHD mortality (11%) and stroke (9%).[13,14]

In a recent analysis, the percentage of EPA + DHA in the membranes of red blood cells, referred to as the "omega-3 index," was also an independent predictor of mortality from CHD and sudden cardiac death.[15] This index correlates well with the amount of EPA + DHA levels in the heart before and after supplementation with fish oil in cardiac transplant patients,[16] which makes it a useful surrogate marker of cardiac EPA + DHA levels. Studies are currently being carried out to evaluate the clinical relevance of the omega-3 index and determine the dose-response relationship between intake of various omega-3 fatty acids, the omega-3 index, and clinical outcome variables.

In randomized clinical trials, the intake of omega-3 fatty acids from fish and fish oil results in a marked reduction in CVD mortality and sudden death in patients who have previously had a heart attack. The largest of these studies are the Diet and Reinfarction Trial (DART) and the Gruppo Italiano por lo Studio della Streptochinasi nell'Infarto Miocardico (GISSI) study. In the DART study, 2033 men recovering from a heart attack received dietary advice to: a) reduce fat intake and increase the ratio of polyunsaturated to saturated fat in their diet; (b) increase fatty fish intake to at least two servings a week (200–400 g); or c) increase cereal fiber intake.[17] In two years, men who had been advised to eat fish had a 29% reduction in all-cause mortality, whereas no significant reduction in death was seen in the other dietary treatment groups. Similar protective effects were seen in the GISSI trial, the largest prospective randomized, controlled trial on the effects of omega-3 fatty acids for secondary prevention of CHD. In this study, 11,324 patients surviving a recent heart attack were randomized to receive 850 mg/d of omega-3 fatty acid ethyl esters (EPA and DHA), 300 mg/d of vitamin E, both vitamin E and omega-3 fatty acids, or neither treatment.[18] After 3.5 years, individuals taking 850 mg/d omega-3 fatty acids had a 45% reduction in sudden death and a 35% reduction in death from CHD compared with individuals receiving a placebo. These benefits were apparent within 4 months of treatment.[19] As promising as these studies are, they leave a number of key questions unanswered, such as the relative importance of EPA versus DHA and the role of these fatty acids in a primary prevention setting.

The Japanese EPA Lipid Intervention Study addressed these questions in a large-scale, randomized, controlled study involving EPA-ethyl ester and a statin.[20] In this study, 18,645 subjects (mean age 61 years, 31% male) were randomized to 10 mg/d pravastatin or 5 mg/d simvastatin (control group) or the same statin doses with 1800 mg/d of highly purified EPA. At baseline, about 15% of subjects had diabetes, 36% were hypertensive, and 20% had coronary artery disease. After more than 4.5 years of follow-up, the primary end point of major coronary events, defined as sudden cardiac death, heart attack, unstable angina, and coronary artery bypass graft/percutaneous coronary intervention, was significantly reduced by 19% in the EPA plus statin group compared with the statin-only group (2.8% vs. 3.5% of patients had an event).[21] A similar, but insignificant, trend occurred in the 14,981 subjects with no history of coronary artery disease: 1.4% among those treated with a statin plus EPA versus 1.7% in the control group experienced one of these events, representing an 18% reduction in risk.

Although the majority of clinical trial evidence demonstrates that intake of omega-3 fatty acids from fish or fish oil is effective in the secondary prevention of CHD, not all studies have shown a protective effect. In a recent clinical trial, 3114 men under age 70 taking nitrates or another treatment for angina were: a) advised to eat two portions of oily fish each week or take three fish oil capsules daily; b) advised to eat more fruits, vegetables, and oats; c) given both types of dietary advice; or d) given no specific dietary advice.[22] At 3 to 9 years follow-up, there was no benefit of increased fish intake on mortality; in fact, men who ate more fish had an even higher risk of cardiac death (11.5% vs. 9%). One reason proposed to explain this finding is that individuals in the fish group may have made detrimental diet and lifestyle changes because they thought they were protected by their increased intake of omega-3 fatty acids.[22] The authors also speculated that it was possible that the patients' medications adversely interacted with the fish or fish oil, though no evidence was found of any adverse effects.

Plant-Derived Sources of Omega-3 Fatty Acids

Plant-derived omega-3 fatty acids are present as α-linolenic acid (ALA) in flaxseed, canola oil, and some nuts, beans, and green leafy vegetables. In five of seven epidemiological studies, the intake of ALA or the presence of ALA in the blood and tissues was inversely associated with prevalence of CHD and cardiovascular events. The two largest of these studies are the Health Professional Follow-up Study and the Nurses' Health Study. In the Health Professional Follow-up study, 45,722 males between the ages of 40 to 75 were followed for 14 years. Each 1 g/d increase in ALA intake was associated with a 47% lower risk of CHD incidence among men with little or no EPA + DHA intake (<100 mg/d).[23] However, among men with a higher EPA + DHA intake (≥100 mg/d), ALA intake was not associated with CHD risk. In the 18-year follow-up of the Nurses' Health Study, which followed 76,723 registered nurses who were between 30 and 55 years of age at baseline, women in the two highest quintiles of ALA intake (median 1.16

and 1.39 g/d) had a 38% to 40% reduction in risk of sudden cardiac death compared with women in the lowest quintile (median 0.66g/d).[24] There was no relationship between ALA intake and other types of fatal CHD or nonfatal myocardial infarction. Overall, data from epidemiological studies suggest that 1.5 to 3 g/d ALA is protective against CVD, but this observation needs to be tested in randomized, controlled clinical trials.

To date, two clinical trials have evaluated the effects of a diet high in ALA on cardiac events and mortality, but neither is conclusive.[25] The Lyon Diet Heart Study reported a dramatic reduction in cardiac death and nonfatal myocardial infarction after increasing intake of ALA,[26] but it cannot be certain that these benefits were from ALA, because individuals in this study also made serveral other dietary changes that may have had health benefits (e.g., increasing intake of monounsaturated fatty acids, fruits, and vegetables and reducing intake of saturated fat). The other study was performed in 1968 by Natvig et al.[27] In this study, 13,578 men between the ages of 50 and 59 were randomized to 10 g linseed (flaxseed) oil/d providing 5.5 g/d ALA or a sunflower oil placebo.[27] Men were followed for 1 year, and no difference was seen in cardiovascular end points between groups. However, there was a low death rate in this study (0.4%), which may have made it difficult to detect a difference in a short period of time.

In summary, epidemiological evidence supports a role of ALA in CVD risk reduction, but clinical trials are needed to confirm a causative relationship and to determine the optimal intake for CVD prevention. It is not known if ALA itself is cardioprotective or if the health benefits from ALA are due to its conversion to long-chain omega-3 fatty acids. Although ALA can be elongated and desaturated to EPA, this only occurs to a modest extent in humans; the rate of conversion is approximately 7%.[28] The conversion of ALA to DHA is typically less than 5% in humans[29] and may be as low as 1%.[28] Therefore, ALA may have effects on CVD risk that are not mediated by EPA and/or DHA.

Mechanisms by Which Omega-3 Fatty Acids Reduce Risk of CVD

Reduction in Arrhythmias

The protective effects of omega-3 fatty acids were initially thought to be due to their anti-aggregatory, antithrombotic properties. However, current evidence suggests that the primary effect of omega-3 fatty acids is to reduce susceptibility to cardiac arrhythmias, which are disorders of the regular rhythmic beating of the heart. Particular attention has focused on ventricular fibrillation, the most common cause of sudden death in people with heart problems. Ventricular fibrillation is a condition in which the heart's electrical activity becomes disordered

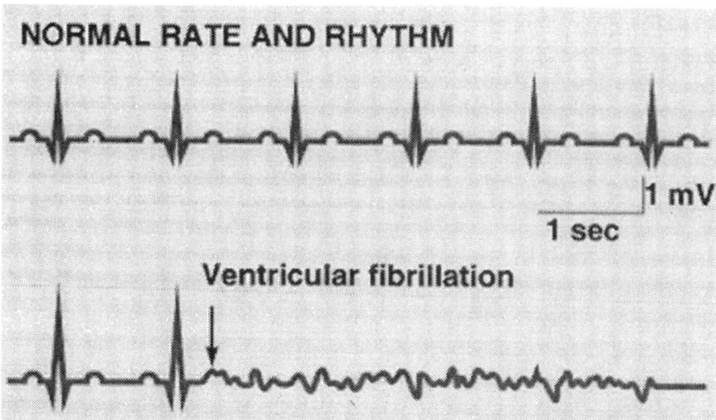

Figure 2. Comparison of an illustration of an electrocardiogram (ECG) reading from a healthy heart with a heart experiencing ventricular fibrillation. (From Sherwood 2005[36]; used with permission from Brooks/Cole, a division of Thomson Learning.)

(Figure 2). When this happens, the heart's lower chambers contract in a rapid, unsynchronized way and the heart pumps little or no blood. Omega-3 fatty acids prevent drug-induced arrhythmias in cultured myocardial cells, and a high intake of omega-3 fatty acids significantly reduces the risk of ventricular fibrillation during acute ischemia in long-term feeding studies in rats.[30] Intravenous infusion of fish oil or ALA to dogs reduced the risk of ventricular fibrillation by approximately 75% when a myocardial infarction was surgically induced.[31] In hearts isolated from rabbits and subjected to ischemia and reperfusion, ventricular fibrillation occurred during ischemia in 33% of hearts from rabbits fed a regular diet without flaxseed, whereas no ventricular fibrillation occurred in hearts from rabbits fed a regular diet with 10% flaxseed.[32] In humans, ischemic heart disease patients with an implantable cardioverter defibrillator that had the lowest serum phospholipid omega-3 fatty acid content had six times more treated ventricular fibrillation and ventricular tachycardia events than patients with the highest omega-3 fatty acid content.[33]

Clinical trials on omega-3 fatty acid supplementation to prevent arrhythmias have just begun. There have been two studies in humans with implantable cardioverter defibrillators, and thus far results have been conflicting. The first clinical trial to show direct experimental evidence that omega-3 fatty acids can increase myocardial electrical stability was by Schrepf et al. in 2004.[34] In this small pilot study, 10 patients with implanted cardioverter defibrillators who were experiencing multiple episodes of sustained ventricular tachycardia were enrolled. At baseline, ventricular tachycardia was inducible in 7 out of 10 patients, and immediately after intravenous infusion of omega 3 fatty acids (3.8 g EPA + DHA), ventricular tachycardia could not be induced in 5 of the 7 susceptible patients. Shortly after that study was published, a randomized, double-blind, placebo-controlled trial of fish oil supplementation in 200 patients with implantable cardioverter defibrillators was reported.[35] Patients qualified for the study if they had had a recent episode of sustained ventricular tachycardia or ventricular fibrillation, and were randomized to receive 1.8 g/d fish oil or placebo. In the 2-year study period, omega-3 supplementation had no overall effect on the incidence of ventricular tachycardia or ventricular fibrillation. In the subset of patients that had an episode of sustained ventricular tachycardia prior to enrollment, there was a significantly greater number of patients with ventricular tachycardia or ventricular fibrillation events compared with individuals in the control group, suggesting that fish oil could be pro-arrhythmic in this population.[35] However, there was no increase in the risk of death for participants taking fish oil. Of the 14 deaths during the study period, four were in the fish oil group and 10 were in the placebo group. Based on these studies, many scientists are recommending that people with an implantable defibrillator and a history of ventricular tachycardia or ventricular fibrillation should not take fish oil supplements.

Effects on Serum Lipids

The effects of omega-3 fatty acids on the synthesis, secretion, and metabolism of lipoproteins are well documented, and the biological mechanisms underlying their effects are increasingly being understood at the molecular level.[37] In patients with hypertriglyceridemia, omega-3 fatty acids lower triglycerides in a dose-dependent manner by inhibiting the synthesis of very-low-density lipoprotein cholesterol (VLDL) and triglycerides in the liver.[38] Two to four grams of EPA + DHA per day can lower triglycerides 20% to 40%.[39] The triglyceride-lowering effect is greater in hypertriglyceridemic versus normotriglyceridemic subjects.[40] Studies suggest that EPA and DHA are similarly effective in lowering serum triglycerides.[41,42] It should be noted that the triglyceride-lowering effect of omega-3 fatty acids is sometimes accompanied by an increase in serum cholesterol. Overall, randomized trials have found that the intake of omega-3 fatty acids increases total cholesterol 0% to 6%, increases LDL 10 mg/dL or less, increases high-density lipoprotein cholesterol (HDL) 3 to 5 mg/dL, and decreases triglycerides 10% to 25% in normotriglyceridemic subjects and 10% to 30% in hypertriglyceridemic subjects.[43]

Effects on Blood Pressure

Omega-3 fatty acids have a small, dose-related hypotensive effect in patients with hypertension, and little to no effect in normotensive individuals. In an analysis of 36 randomized trials in which patients took an average of 4.1 g/d EPA + DHA, the reduction in blood pressure was 2.1 and 1.6 mmHg for systolic and diastolic blood pressure, respectively.[44] Blood pressure effects tended to be greater in populations that were older (>45 years) and in hypertensive populations (BP $\geq$ 140/90 mmHg).[44]

Slowed Progression or Stabilization of Atherosclerotic Plaques

Omega-3 fatty acids may slow the progression of atherosclerosis and stabilize atherosclerotic plaque. Omega-3 fatty acids in the diet decrease atherosclerosis in a variety of animal models.[45] Also, a recent study in patients with advanced carotid atherosclerosis reported a stabilizing effect of omega-3 fatty acids on atherosclerotic plaque. Participants awaiting carotid endarterectomy (surgical removal of carotid plaque) were randomized to receive six capsules per day containing 1 g fish oil, 1 g sunflower oil, or 1 g of a control oil, in addition to 1 mg α-tocopherol.[46] Participants took the capsules until the date of their surgery (range 7–189 days). Researchers found that in the group that was supplemented with fish oil, omega-3 fatty acids readily incorporated themselves into atherosclerotic plaques, making the plaques more likely to have a thick fibrous cap and have less inflammatory infiltrate, and thus less prone to rupture. In contrast, there was no effect of the sunflower or control oil capsules on plaque fatty acid composition or plaque stability.

Anti-Inflammatory Effects

Several lines of evidence suggest that omega-3 fatty acids have anti-inflammatory properties, the mechanisms of which are the subject of ongoing investigations. One hypothesis holds that the omega-3 fatty acids EPA and DHA compete with the omega-6 fatty acid arachidonic acid for enzymatic conversion to eicosanoid hormones.[47] An increased intake of omega-3 fatty acids favors the production of thromboxane A_3, which is relatively inactive, over the production of thromboxane A_2, a potent vasoconstrictor and platelet aggregator. There also is an increase in omega-3 derived leukotriene B_5, which is relatively inactive, and a reduction in arachidonic acid-derived leukotriene B_4, a potent chemotactic factor for leukocytes.

There is a growing body of evidence that various marine-derived omega-3 fatty acids reduce oxidative stress, inhibit endothelial cell activation, and reduce the production of inflammatory cytokines such as tumor necrosis factor-α, interleukin 1, and interleukin 6 in vitro[48] and in vivo.[47] With respect to inflammatory biomarkers, it is noteworthy that the intake of omega-3 fatty acids is associated with lower C-reactive protein.[49,50] The specific omega-3 fatty acids and underlying biology that mediate this effect remain to be elucidated.

A new hypothesis proposes that EPA is metabolized to a novel class of lipid mediators called "resolvins" (for "resolution phase interaction products") that interact with a G-protein-coupled receptor ChemR23.[51] A striking feature of resolvins is their ability to attenuate the inflammatory process at concentrations in the low-nanomolar range. Although proof of this principle has been established in a murine model of inflammatory bowel disease, the extension of the resolvin hypothesis to other disease states, particularly atherosclerosis, and the transition of this new biology to humans await further investigation.

Effect of Trans Fatty Acids on CVD Risk

Production of partially hydrogenated fats containing trans fatty acids began in the 1960s as a low-cost alternative to saturated animal fats, and became commonly used in deep-fat frying, baking, and spreads. However, by the 1990s, convincing epidemiological and clinical studies showed that trans fatty acids adversely affect blood lipids and are associated with increased cardiovascular risk.[52] In fact, trans fatty acids were shown to have the most unfavorable effects on blood lipids of all dietary fatty acids, including saturated fats. Saturated and trans fats raise LDL to a similar extent; however, compared with saturated fat, trans fats lower HDL. In effect, the LDL to HDL cholesterol ratio with a trans fatty acid-enriched diet is nearly double that of a diet with an equivalent amount of saturated fat.[52] As depicted in Figure 3, a 2% increase in trans fatty acids raises the ratio of LDL to HDL cholesterol 0.1 unit. This is equivalent to a 53% increase in risk of CHD.[52]

In prospective studies, a higher intake of trans fatty acids was correlated with CHD incidence, providing further evidence that trans fat intake is related to cardiovascular risk.[62,63] Trans fat intake is also associated with increased levels of inflammatory markers and impaired endothelial function in cross-sectional and clinical studies.[64-66] The adverse effects of trans fats have led to consumer demand to remove them from the food supply. Beginning in 2006, manufacturers of conventional foods and some dietary supplements in the United States are required by the Food and Drug Administration (FDA) to list all non-conjugated trans fats on the nutrition facts panel, which will help consumers to reduce consumption of foods that may increase their risk of CHD. Conjugated trans fatty acids are found naturally in foods derived from ruminant animals, and are not required to be listed with trans fats on the food label. These naturally occurring fatty acids include vaccenic acid and conjugated linoleic acid, which have been shown to have anti-cancer, anti-atherogenic, anti-adipogenic, anti-diabetogenic, and anti-inflammatory properties in cell and animal models and in humans.[67] The specific effects of these fatty acids are currently under investigation.

Metabolic Syndrome

As the focus of CVD prevention has gravitated toward early intervention, the National Cholesterol Education Program (NCEP) Adult Treatment Panel (ATP) III introduced the clinical condition of metabolic syndrome into its guidelines and presented criteria for diagnosis and instructions for treatment.[68] According to NCEP guidelines, metabolic syndrome is diagnosed by the presence of any three of the following five conditions: low HDL, elevated triglycerides, high blood pressure, increased abdominal obesity, and elevated fasting glucose (Table 1). Each of these criteria are independent risk factors for CVD and, when clustered together, increase the risk of heart disease, stroke, and type 2 diabetes. The specific cutoffs for these criteria, however, are still being debated.[69] Several other risk factors have also been proposed to be components of the syndrome, including the presence of small, dense LDL and elevated plasminogen activator inhibitor-1 and C-reactive protein.

Metabolic syndrome is associated with a two-fold greater risk of developing CVD and a five-fold greater risk of type 2 diabetes.[71] It is highly prevalent, affecting approximately 27% of adults age 20 and over in the United States, and prevalence increases with age and body weight.[72] Insulin resistance is believed to be at the heart

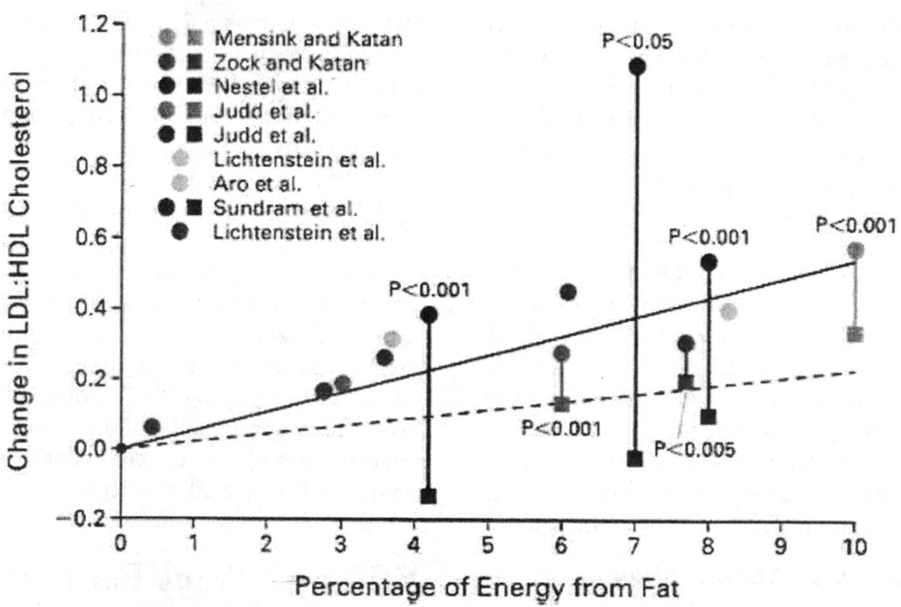

Figure 3. Results of randomized clinical trials[53-61] of the effects of a diet high in trans fatty acids (circles) or saturated fatty acids (squares) on the ratio of LDL to HDL cholesterol. A diet with isocaloric amounts of cis fatty acids was used as the comparison group. The solid line indicates the best-fit regression for trans fatty acids. The dashed line indicates the best-fit regression for saturated fatty acids. (Adapted with permission from Ascherio et al.[52]; copyright 1999 The Massachusetts Medical Society. All rights reserved.)

Table 1. Criteria for Clinical Diagnosis of Metabolic Syndrome*

Measure (any 3 of 5 constitute diagnosis of metabolic syndrome)	Categorical Cutpoints
Elevated waist circumference†	≥102 cm in men ≥88 cm in women
Elevated triglycerides	≥150 mg/dL (1.7 mmol/L) or on drug treatment for elevated triglycerides
Reduced HDL-C	<40 mg/dL (0.9 mmol/L) in men <50 mg/dL (1.1 mmol/L) in women or on drug treatment for reduced HDL-C
Elevated blood pressure	≥130 mm Hg systolic blood pressure or ≥85 mm Hg diastolic blood pressure or on antihypertensive drug treatment in a patient with a history of hypertension
Elevated tasting glucose	≥100 mg/dL or on drug treatment for elevated glucose

*The diagnosis of metabolic syndrome is made when three or more of these risk factors are present.
†Lower waist circumference cut point (e.g., ≥90 cm [35 inches] in men and ≥80 cm [31 inches] in women) appears to be appropriate for Asian Americans.
Used with permission from Grundy et al., 2005.[70]

of the syndrome, and people in affluent societies are primarily affected. Because metabolic syndrome generally does not occur in the absence of obesity and physical inactivity, the first-line clinical therapy to treat metabolic syndrome is lifestyle modification, which includes improvements to diet and exercise habits and behavioral changes. Exercise involves at least 30 minutes of physical activity 5 days per week. Behavioral modification consists of stress management, meal planning, reducing portion size, reading food labels, self-monitoring, and setting achievable goals. Dietary changes include limiting intake of saturated fats, cholesterol, and simple sugars, and increasing consumption of fruits, vegetables, and whole grains.[73]

Lifestyle intervention has been shown to be very effective in reducing the development of metabolic syndrome in subjects with impaired glucose tolerance,[74] and in decreasing the prevalence in subjects with existing metabolic syndrome.[75] The Diabetes Prevention Program, an intensive lifestyle intervention program, was designed to achieve and maintain a 7% weight loss with 150 minutes of exercise per week and a low saturated fat and cholesterol diet with about 25% of calories from fat. The lifestyle intervention resulted in a 41% reduction in the incidence of metabolic syndrome compared with the placebo group, and a 17% reduction in the metformin group.[74] In the study by Esposito et al.,[75] 40 out of 90 patients in the intervention group had metabolic syndrome, compared with 78 out of 90 patients in the control group at the 2-year follow-up. In this study, the intervention group followed a Mediterranean-style diet with foods rich in monounsaturated fatty acids, polyunsaturated fatty acids, and fiber, with 28% of calories from fat and an accompanying physical activity program (an increase in physical activity of about 60%); the control group followed a prudent diet with under 30% of calories from fat and also increased physical activity by about 60%.[75] Body weight decreased more in the intervention group (−4 kg) than in the control group (−1.2 kg). Collectively, lifestyle interventions that result in significant weight loss are effective in decreasing metabolic syndrome. Moreover, the importance of individualizing diet therapy for individuals at risk for or with metabolic syndrome is evident based on the current studies reported.[74,75] Thus, tailoring diet therapy for metabolic syndrome that leads to weight loss is expected to achieve the greatest success therapeutically.

Prevention and Treatment of CVD with Diet

Functional Foods

The health benefits of foods extend beyond their macro- and micronutrient content. They also have bioactive components, nutrients or non-nutrients that are thought to elicit cardioprotective effects. Such foods are referred to as functional foods[76] and include unmodified whole foods such as fruits, vegetables, and whole grains, and foods that have been fortified to enhance the level of a specific nutrient or food component that has been associated with the prevention or treatment of a disease or other clinical condition (Table 2). Examples of fortified foods include calcium-fortified orange juice, fiber-supplemented snack bars, folate-enriched cereals, and stanol- or sterol ester-enhanced foods such as margarine, yogurt, snack bars, and orange juice.

Diets that use functional foods for the management of dyslipidemia are scientifically grounded in the paradigm that what we know from medical pharmacology can often be turned into nutritional pharmacology to elicit health benefits. There are only a limited number of sites of biological intervention capable of bringing about clinically meaningful changes in lipid and lipoprotein metabolism; thus, it is not surprising that drugs and nutrients tend to overlap in their sites of action (Figure 4). In contrast to drugs that are designed to target a specific site and to do so in a powerful way, cardioprotective nutrients and bioactives tend to operate at multiple sites and in

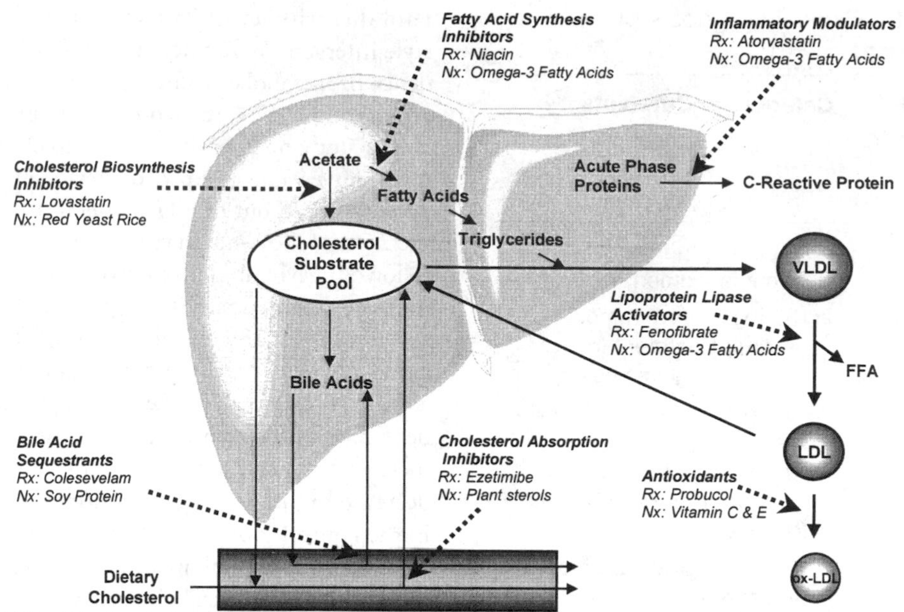

Figure 4. Effects of dietary bioactives and drugs on lipid and lipoprotein metabolism. Rx, approved pharmaceutical agent; Nx, nutrient or food bioactive. The overlap of nutrients and drugs at common points of metabolic regulation is noteworthy.

Table 2. Examples of Functional Foods, their Bioactive Components, and Recommended Amounts

Functional Food	Bioactive Component	Potential Benefit	Recommended Amounts
Whole oats	Beta-glucan, soluble fiber	Lowers total and LDL cholesterol	3 g/d
Soy	Proteins and flavonoids	Lowers total and LDL cholesterol	25 g/d
Flaxseed	Omega-3 fatty acids	Reduces risk of CVD	Not determined
Fish	Omega-3 fatty acids	Reduces risk of CVD	0.5–1.8 g EPA + DHA/d
Garlic	Organosulfur compounds	Lowers total and LDL cholesterol	600–900 mg/d (supplement) or 1 fresh clove
Black tea	Polyphenols	Reduces risk of CVD	Not determined
Stanol/sterol-fortified foods	Plant stanols and sterols	Lowers total and LDL cholesterol	1.7 g/d stanols, 1.3 g/d sterols
Psyllium	Soluble fiber	Lowers total and LDL cholesterol	1 g/d
Nuts	Unsaturated fatty acids, vitamin E	Reduces risk of CVD	1.5 oz/d
Cocoa	Flavanols	Reduces inflammation, LDL oxidation, and improves platelet function	Not determined
Walnuts	Polyunsaturated fatty acids, alpha-linolenic acid	Reduces risk of CVD	1.5 oz/d
Whole grains	Soluble fiber, folate, antioxidants	Reduces risk of CVD	At least 3 oz-equivalents/d
Olive oil	Monounsaturated fatty acids, phenolic compounds	Reduces risk of CVD	2 tablespoons (23 g/d)
Red wine and grapes	Resveratrol	Reduces platelet aggregation	8–16 oz/d

CVD, cardiovascular disease; LDL, low-density lipoprotein.
Adapted with permission from Hasler et al.,[76] copyright 2004 with permission from The American Dietetic Association.

small but additive ways to bring about clinically meaningful changes. An advantage of nutritional pharmacology is the potential to circumvent the side effects commonly associated with drugs.

Current dietary advice integrates the health benefits of nutrients and functional foods into a comprehensive total diet plan. This means that instead of offering guidance to achieve specific levels of certain nutrients or focusing on a particular food or meal, dietitians give specific instructions on how to modify one's total diet for optimum health.[77] Since the ideal diet for the treatment of CVD is not yet known, we present the primary diets under investigation for patients with or at risk of CVD.

Diets for the Prevention of CVD

Therapeutic Lifestyle Changes Diet

The Therapeutic Lifestyle Changes (TLC) diet was introduced by the NCEP ATP III and is endorsed by the American Heart Association to reduce CVD risk in people with elevated LDL or metabolic syndrome.[68] The TLC diet replaces the Step II diet (<30% fat, <7% saturated fat, <200 mg cholesterol) and emphasizes the importance of a healthy dietary pattern that is low in saturated fat and trans-fat and rich in fruits, vegetables, whole grains, fat-free and low-fat dairy products, and lean meat, fish, and poultry (Table 3). The primary target of the TLC diet is LDL (Table 4).

Table 3. Nutrient Composition of the Theraputic Lifestyle Changes (TLC) Diet

Nutrient	Recommended Intake
Saturated fat*	<7% of total calories
Polyunsaturated fat	Up to 10% of total calories
Monounsaturated fat	Up to 20% of total calories
Total fat	25%–35% of total calories
Carbohydrate†	50%–60% of total calories
Fiber	20–30 g/d
Protein	Approximately 15% of total calories
Cholesterol	<200 mg/d
Total calories‡	Balance energy intake and expenditure to maintain desirable body weight/ prevent weight gain

* *Trans* fatty acids are another low-density lipoprotein-raising fat that should be kept at a low intake.
† Carbohydrates should be derived predominantly from foods rich in complex carbohydrates including grains, especially whole grains, fruits, and vegetables.
‡ Daily energy expenditure should include at least moderate physical activity (contributing approximately 200 kcal/d).
Used with permission from the Executive Summary of The National Cholesterol Education Program (NCEP) Expert Panel on Detection, Evaluation, and Treatment of High Blood Cholesterol in Adults (Adult Treatment Panel III), 2001.[68]

Table 4. Approximate and Cumulative LDL Cholesterol Reduction Achievable by the TLC Diet

Dietary Component	Dietary Change	Approximate LDL Reduction
Major		
Saturated fat	<7% of calories	8%–10%
Dietary cholesterol	<200 mg/d	3%–5%
Weight reduction	Lose 10 lbs	5%–8%
Other LDL-Lowering Options		
Viscous fiber	5–10 g/d	3%–5%
Plant sterol/stanol esters	2 g/d	6%–15%
Cumulative Estimate		20%–30%

LDL, low-density lipoprotein.
Used with permission from Third Report of the National Cholesterol Education Program (NCEP) Expert Panel on Detection, Evaluation, and Treatment of High Blood Cholesterol in Adults (Adult Treatment Panel III), 2002.[78]

Since it is now known that a low-fat, high-carbohydrate diet can lead to an atherogenic lipid profile characterized by reduced HDL, elevated triglycerides, and small, dense LDL, the NCEP revised recommendations for total fat intake from less than 30% of total energy intake to 25% to 35% to allow for an increased intake of unsaturated fat in place of carbohydrates in persons with metabolic syndrome or diabetes.[78] A total fat intake above 35% is not recommended since it is associated with excess saturated fat and possibly higher caloric intake. Due to the strong relationship between obesity and CVD, ATP III recommends that individuals balance their energy intake and expenditure to maintain a desirable body weight and prevent weight gain. Daily energy expenditure should include at least moderate physical activity (contributing about 200 kcal/d). The TLC diet also includes the option of adding 10 to 25 g/d of viscous (soluble) fiber, 2 g/d of plant-derived sterols or stanols, and the use of soy protein as a replacement for some animal products, all of which independently reduce LDL.

Portfolio Diet

The portfolio diet aims to achieve maximal LDL reduction through diet by including four functional foods known to reduce LDL with a plant-based diet that is very low in both cholesterol and saturated fat.[79] Similar to the TLC diet, LDL is the primary target of treatment based on observational and experimental evidence in animal, clinical, genetic, and population studies showing a strong causal relationship between elevated LDL and CHD. The four dietary components of the portfolio diet are soy protein, nuts (almonds), viscous fibers, and plant sterols, each of which reduce LDL 4% to 7%. Each is also permitted by the FDA to carry a health claim/qualified health claim that they reduce CVD risk (Table 5).

Researchers hypothesized that the inclusion of these components in the diet would have an additive effect on LDL reduction. In a recent trial, 34 hyperlipidemic men and women underwent three 1-month treatments in random order: 1) a very-low-saturated fat control diet; 2) the same diet plus 20 mg lovastatin (a 3-hydroxy-3-methylglutaryl coenzyme A reductase inhibitor); and 3) a portfolio diet high in plant sterols, soy protein, almonds, and viscous fiber. All foods and medications were provided except for fresh fruits and vegetables. The portfolio diet was as effective as the statin in reducing LDL: both reduced LDL approximately 30%.[2] In subjects with C-reactive protein below the 75th percentile (≤3.5 mg/L), the portfolio diet and statin significantly reduced C-reactive protein 24% and 16%, respectively.[80] The preliminary results from these studies suggest that a diet that combines several cholesterol-lowering foods is an effective, non-pharmacologic method of reducing LDL in individuals at increased risk of CVD.

Table 5. Health Claims/Qualified Health Claim Approved by the US Food and Drug Administration for Components of the Portfolio Diet

Dietary Component	FDA Approved Health Claims/ Qualified Health Claim
Soluble fiber	Diets low in saturated fat and cholesterol and rich in fruits, vegetables, and grain products that contain some types of dietary fiber, particularly soluble fiber, may reduce the risk of heart disease, a disease associated with many factors.
Nuts*	Eating 1.5 ounces per day of most nuts as part of a diet low in saturated fat and cholesterol may reduce the risk of heart disease.
Soy protein	Diets low in saturated fat and cholesterol that include 25 g of soy protein a day may reduce the risk of heart disease.
Plant sterol esters	Foods containing at least 0.65 g per serving of plant sterols, eaten twice a day with meals for a daily total intake of at least 1.3 g, as part of a diet low in saturated fat and cholesterol, may reduce the risk of heart disease.
Plant stanol esters	Foods containg at least 1.7 g per serving of plant stanol esters, eaten twice a day with meals for a total daily intake of at least 3.4 g, as part of a diet low in saturated fat and cholesterol, may reduce the risk of heart disease.

* Qualified health claim.

Mediterranean Diet

The landmark Seven Countries Study in the 1950s was the first to report that certain Mediterranean populations had a low prevalence of CHD and low serum cholesterol despite consumption of a higher-fat diet (33%–40% of calories from fat).[81] Subsequent studies have shown that adherence to a Mediterranean diet reduces cardiovascular mortality.[82-84] The common dietary characteristics of Mediterranean countries with a low incidence of CVD include an abundance of fruits and vegetables, fish, and nuts, moderate amounts of wine, and olive oil as the main source of dietary fat. This dietary pattern also includes low to moderate consumption of milk and dairy, mostly in the form of cheese, and little intake of red meat.

The Lyon Diet Heart Study illustrates the potential for a Mediterranean diet to reduce risk of CVD. In this study, men and women who previously had a myocardial infarction had 70% reduced all-cause mortality following adherence to a Mediterranean diet for 46 months, compared with participants following a standard low-fat diet.[26] Regarding CVD risk factors, a compilation of 27 well-controlled trials lasting from 3 to 8 weeks showed that both a low-fat diet and the Mediterranean diet lower total and LDL cholesterol, but a low-fat diet reduces HDL proportionately more than it decreases LDL and increases triglycerides (Figure 5). In contrast, adherence to a Mediterranean diet does not adversely affect triglycerides (Figure 5), and it decreases the LDL to HDL cholesterol ratio. In summary, the Mediterranean diet appears to reduce cardiovascular mortality and may be preferential to a low-fat diet because it reduces total and LDL cholesterol, lowers the LDL to HDL cholesterol ratio, and does not adversely affect triglycerides.

Dietary Approaches to Stop Hypertension (DASH) Diet

DASH Study. Hypertension increases risk of CHD and adverse cardiovascular events by approximately two- to three-fold.[86] However, until the DASH diet, the only non-pharmaceutical treatments for hypertension were salt reduction, weight management, and moderation of alcohol consumption.[87] The DASH diet is high in fruits and vegetables, low-fat dairy, whole grains, poultry, fish, and nuts, and low in fat, sweets, and sugary beverages (Table 6). In the DASH trial, 459 men and women whose systolic blood pressure was less than 160 mmHg and whose diastolic blood pressure was between 80 and 95 mmHg had reductions in blood pressure occur within 2 weeks of

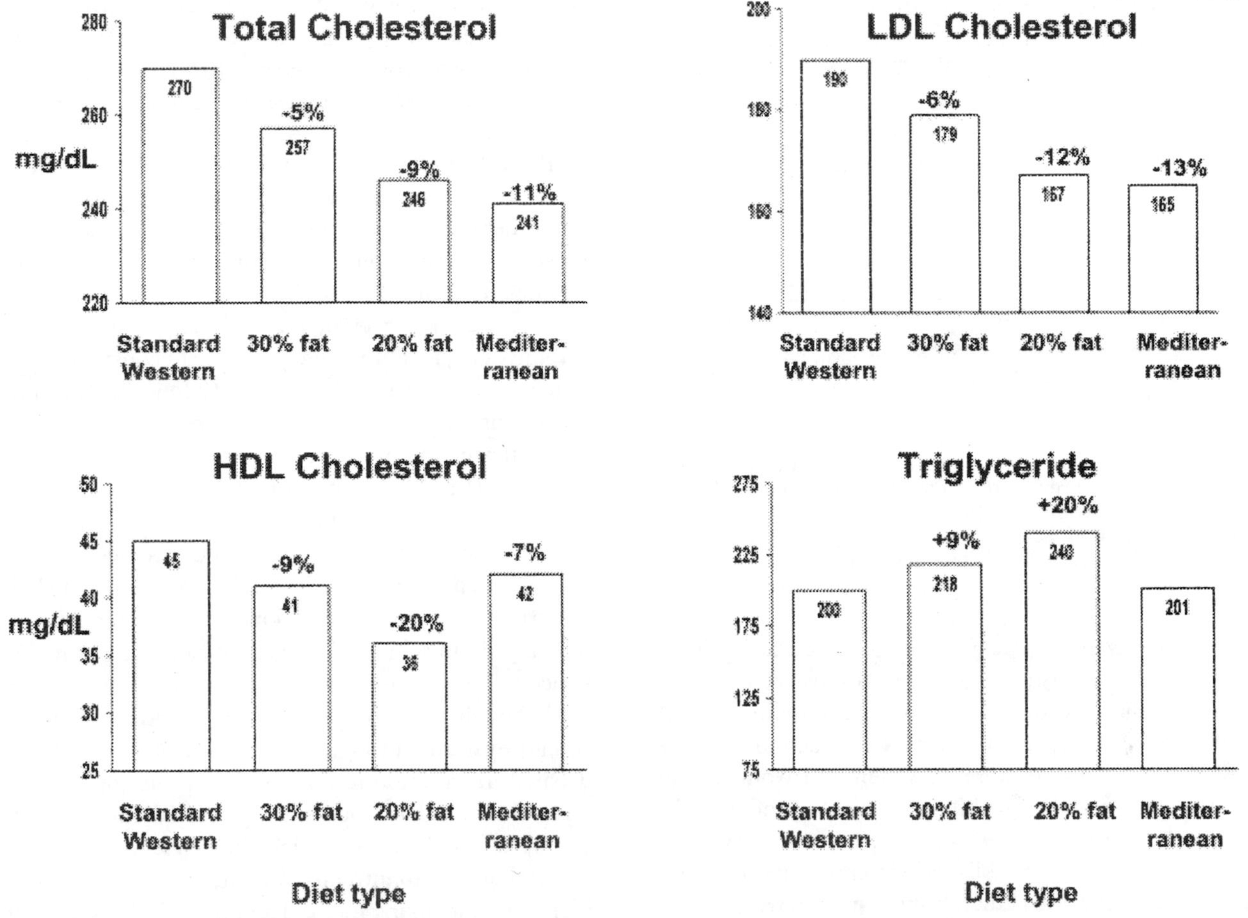

Figure 5. Predicted changes in plasma cholesterol and triglyceride concentrations caused by four types of diet treatment: 1) a standard Western diet, 2) a diet with 30% fat (step 1), 3) a 20% low-fat diet, and 4) the Mediterranean diet. The standard Western and Mediterranean diets have 38% fat. (From Sacks and Katan[85] copyright 2002 with permission from Excerpta Medica.)

starting the DASH diet. These reductions were comparable to reductions typically seen with hypertensive drugs.[1] The DASH diet also significantly lowered total, LDL, and HDL cholesterol without significantly affecting triglyceride concentrations.[88] Relative to the control diet, the DASH diet decreased total cholesterol 13.7 mg/dL, LDL 10.7 mg/dL, and HDL 3.7 mg/dL, with no change in triglycerides or body weight.[88]

Table 6. Composition of the Dietary Approaches to Stop Hypertension (DASH) Diet.[89]

Food Group	Daily Servings
Grains and grain products	7–8
Vegetables	4–5
Fruits	4–5
Low-fat or fat-free dairy	2–3
Meat, poultry, and fish	2 or less
Nuts, seeds, and dry beans	4–5 per week
Fats and oils	2–3
Sweets	5 per week

DASH-Sodium Study. To explore the effect of sodium restriction combined with the DASH diet and a typical American diet, the DASH sodium trial subsequently compared the two meal plans at sodium levels of 1500, 2400, and 3300 mg/d in 412 men and women whose blood pressure exceeded 120/80 mmHg.[90] Reducing dietary sodium lowered blood pressure for both eating plans; however, at each sodium level blood pressure was lower on the DASH eating plan than on the typical American diet (Figure 6).[90] Total, LDL, and HDL cholesterol were also lower at each sodium level on the DASH diet compared with the typical American diet, though these effects were not statistically significant.[91] However, within each diet, sodium intake did not significantly affect serum total cholesterol, LDL, HDL, or triglycerides.

PREMIER Study. Since all foods were provided in the DASH trials, the PREMIER study tested the DASH eating plan under free-living conditions for 6 months.[92] Food was not provided, and researchers compared blood pressure response in three groups: 1) advice only: partici-

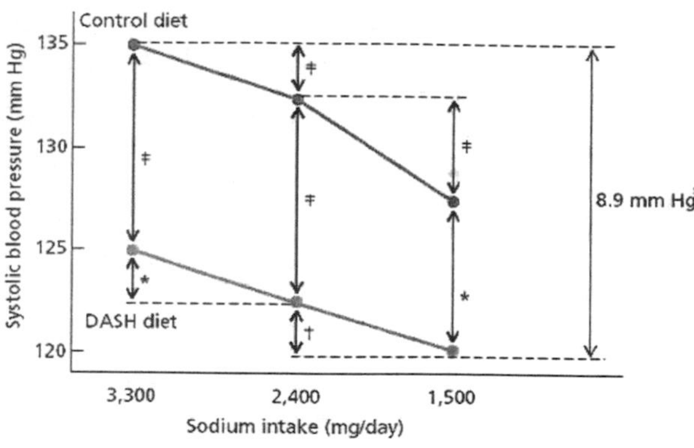

*$P < .05$; †$P < .01$; ‡$P < .001$

Figure 6. Reduction in systolic blood pressure in the DASH-Sodium study. Participants were randomized to a control diet or the DASH diet; within each group, each participant rotated through three sodium intake levels (3300, 2400, and 1500 mg/d). (Adapted with permission from Sacks et al.[31]; copyright 2001 The Massachusetts Medical Society. All rights reserved.)

pants were given a single counseling session and printed handouts; 2) established recommendations: subjects participated in 18 sessions of behavioral counseling; and 3) established recommendations plus instructions for the DASH diet. Subjects were 810 men and women with systolic blood pressure of 120 to 159 mmHg and diastolic blood pressure of 80 to 95 mmHg. In this study, both groups receiving the established recommendations, with and without the DASH diet, lost substantial weight (5–6 kg). The effects attributed to the DASH diet were less than in previous studies and were not significantly different from the established recommendation group. However, hypertension was best controlled in the established recommendations plus DASH group; 77% of participants with stage 1 hypertension ended the study with blood pressure lower than 140/90 mmHg. Also, unlike the other treatment groups, participants in only the DASH plus established recommendations group had a significant increase in insulin sensitivity.[93] In summary, it appears that the DASH diet is feasible under free-living conditions and is effective in reducing blood pressure and total and LDL cholesterol in individuals with and without hypertension.

Low Glycemic Index Diet

The glycemic index is a ranking of carbohydrate-containing foods according to their 2-hour blood glucose response compared with a standard, usually glucose or white bread. A food's glycemic index is an estimate of its relative postprandial glycemic response. Postprandial hyperglycemia is an important risk factor for CVD; an elevated 2-hour blood glucose level following an oral glucose tolerance test is associated with increased all-cause and CVD mortality in individuals with and without diabetes.[94,95] It is hypothesized that a diet emphasizing low-glycemic index foods will minimize postprandial glucose levels, which may reduce CVD risk. In epidemiological studies, individuals who consume diets with the highest glycemic index have a greater risk of CHD compared with those who consume diets with the lowest glycemic index.[96] They also have a greater incidence of metabolic syndrome.[97]

Regarding CVD risk factors, studies that have compared a low-glycemic index diet with a high-glycemic index diet in general report a significant reduction in total cholesterol, a small but non-significant decrease in LDL, and no effect on HDL or triglyceride levels.[98] In most of these studies, body weight, energy intake, and fat, protein, carbohydrate, and fiber intake were held constant. In randomized clinical trials, the effects of a low-glycemic index diet on insulin sensitivity vary, with some studies showing a significant improvement and others showing no such improvement.[99] Low-glycemic index meals enhance satiety and reduce total energy intake at the next meal,[95] and in a recent study, energy expenditure decreased less following an energy-restricted, low-glycemic load diet compared with an isocaloric, low-fat diet, which may potentially aid in achieving weight loss and weight maintenance.[100]

Although the concept of glycemic index is relatively straightforward and logical, its clinical usefulness is still debated. In addition to only having a minimal effect on glycemic control and lipids, the glycemic index of a food can be affected by its particle size, ripeness, degree of processing, macronutrient content, variety, and type of preparation (cooking method and time).[99] In some cases, the glycemic index of foods is counterintuitive. For example, dairy, fruit, and chocolate have high levels of simple sugars but have a low glycemic index due to their fat and fructose content. Additionally, foods with a low glycemic index can have a high glycemic response if eaten in large quantities.[101] Thus, if the concept of glycemic index were to be used in clinical practice, it would best be used in conjunction with other dietary strategies such as portion control and reduction of dietary carbohydrate and saturated fat.[102]

Moderate Carbohydrate Restriction

The OmniHeart study compared a diet that was very similar to the DASH diet with diets that shifted 10% of calories from carbohydrate to either protein or unsaturated fat. The study diet had 58% of calories from carbohydrate (compared with 55% in the DASH diet) and 15% of calories from protein (compared with 18% in the DASH diet). All food was provided during this trial of 164 adults with prehypertension or hypertension. All three diets lowered systolic blood pressure by 8.2 to 9.5 mmHg and LDL by 11.6 to 14.2 mg/dL. However, the high-protein diet further reduced systolic blood pressure 1.4 mmHg, LDL 3.3 mg/dL, and HDL 1.4 mg/dL. Compared with the carbohydrate-rich diet, the unsaturated fat diet further reduced systolic blood pressure by 1.3 mmHg overall and raised HDL 1.1 mg/dL.[103] In summary, all three diets appear to reduce overall heart disease risk by lowering blood pressure and improving cholesterol levels. However, these results suggest that the substitution of carbohydrate with protein or unsaturated fat may have additional benefits on blood pressure and/or cholesterol levels.

Low-Carbohydrate Diet

Low-carbohydrate diets such as the Atkins Diet have recently risen in popularity as a means of rapid weight loss. Low-carbohydrate diets have generally less than 50 g of carbohydrate per day or less than 10% of energy from carbohydrate.[104] As a result, these diets are generally high in protein and fat (most frequently derived from animal and marine food sources). Calorie restriction is not a feature of this diet because it occurs naturally due to the appetite-suppressing effects associated with ketosis, as well as the limited selection of food choices. Professional organizations have cautioned against the use of low-carbohydrate diets because they "restrict foods that provide essential nutrients and don't provide the variety of foods needed to meet nutritional needs."[105]

Several randomized, controlled clinical trials have compared low-carbohydrate diets with low-fat diets in adults, and all have reported a 4- to 6-kg greater weight loss in the low-carbohydrate group at 6 months.[106-109] However, two of these studies followed participants for a year and found no significant weight loss compared with baseline from the low-carbohydrate diet at 12 months.[107,110] Despite a high intake of dietary fat on this diet (2 to 2.5 times the amount recommended by the AHA),[111] a low-carbohydrate weight-loss diet improves several cardiovascular risk factors. Low-carbohydrate diets consistently lower triglycerides and increase HDL (Figure 7), as well as reduce the percentage of small, dense LDL particles compared with a low-fat diet.[112] The magnitude of reduction in triglycerides on a low-carbohydrate diet is strongly related to baseline triglyceride levels, which can explain 79% of the variability in triglyceride response.[112] In addition, a low-carbohydrate diet frequently reduces fasting insulin[113,114] and C-reactive protein[115-116] and improves the postprandial lipid profile.[117] It is important to note that in almost all cases, total and LDL cholesterol are slightly higher after a low-carbohydrate diet than after a low-fat diet (Figure 7).[112] However, the increase in total cholesterol may be compensated for by a proportionately greater increase in HDL.[118] Overall, current research suggests that low-carbohydrate diets can be used safely for short-term weight loss without ad-

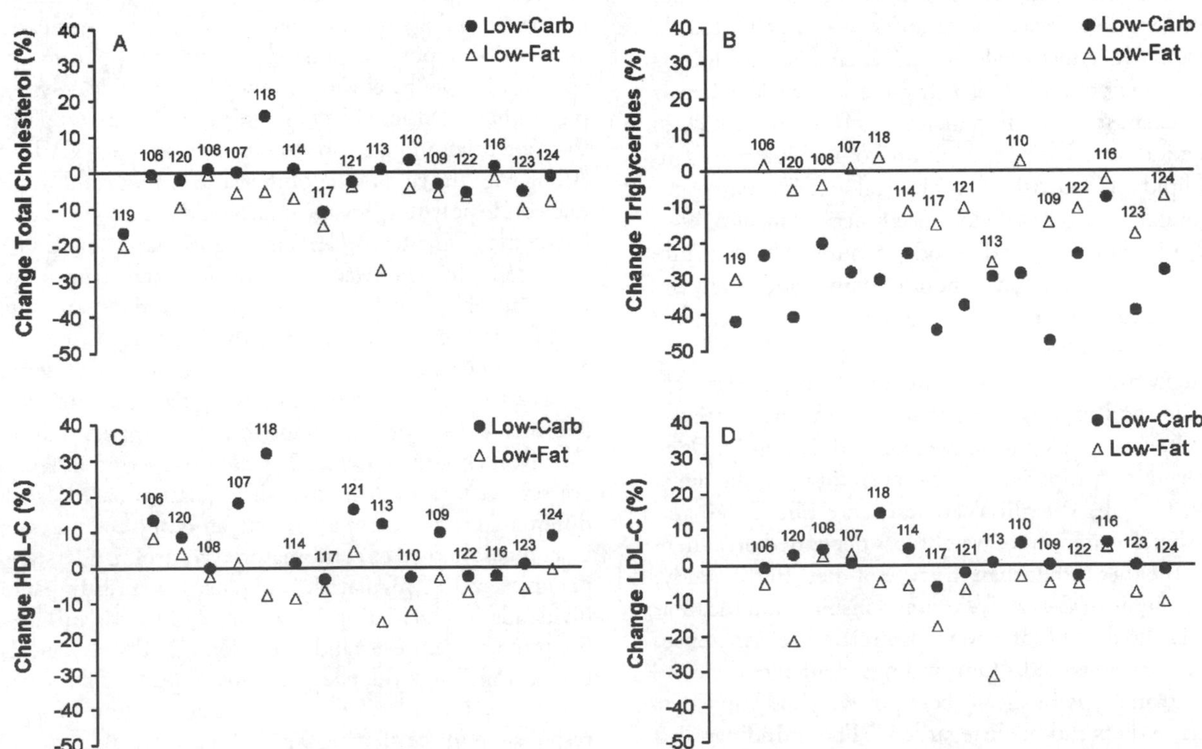

Figure 7. Relative changes in total cholesterol (A), triglycerides (B), HDL-C (C), and LDL-C (D) in prospective studies comparing very low carbohydrate diets and low-fat diets. Numbers correspond to studies in the reference list. (Adapted from Volek et al.[112] copyright 2005 with permission from the American Society for Nutritional Sciences.)

versely affecting cardiovascular risk factors; however, little is known about the long-term health effects of these diets.

Importance of Lifestyle Modification

Although diet plays a major role in CVD risk, it is important to adjust other modifiable risk factors for maximum CVD risk reduction. These risk factors include high blood pressure, physical inactivity, obesity, smoking, elevated cholesterol, and diabetes mellitus. In a recent study of 2339 men and women ages 70 to 90 from 11 European countries, a combination of a Mediterranean dietary pattern, moderate alcohol consumption, non-smoking status, and physical activity was associated with a mortality rate that was about one-third that of those with none or only one of these protective factors.[82] Likewise, adherence to similar healthy lifestyle practices was associated with an 83% reduction in the rate of CHD and a 91% reduction in diabetes in women in the Nurses' Health Study, and a 71% reduction in colon cancer in men in the Health Professionals Follow-up Study.[125] As these studies demonstrate, an overall healthy lifestyle is associated with a significant reduction in CVD risk.

Cardioprotective diets should include a physical activity component for maximum risk reduction. Physical inactivity is a major risk factor for CHD, associated with at least a two-fold increased risk compared with those who are active.[126] The benefits from integrating physical activity with diet modification are often greater than that achieved by diet alone. For example, a low saturated fat diet primarily reduces total and LDL cholesterol and has little to no effect on HDL or triglyceride levels, whereas aerobic exercise most often increases HDL and decreases triglyceride levels.[127] In addition to improvements in blood lipids, CVD risk from physical activity may occur by favorable changes in endothelial function, insulin resistance, inflammation, and blood pressure. The Institute of Medicine recommends 1 hour of daily, moderately intense physical activity, including aerobic and resistance exercise, for weight-independent health benefits.[128]

Equally important, if not more important, than selecting a diet and exercise plan that reduces cardiovascular risk is choosing one that can be followed. Recently, Dansinger et al.[124] compared the efficacy of four popular diets: Atkins, Ornish, Weight Watchers, and The Zone, and found that the amount of weight loss depended on adherence to the diet rather than the type of diet. In this study, improvements in C-reactive protein, insulin, and the total to HDL cholesterol ratio were also related to adherence. The authors remarked, "Our findings challenge the concept that one type of diet is best for everybody and that alternative diets can be disregarded." These findings also reflect the need to personalize one's diet based on food preferences, lifestyle, cardiovascular risk profile, and genetic makeup.

Understanding Cardiovascular Nutrition in a Molecular World

The human response to diet is incredibly complex and highly variable.[129] One of the frontiers of nutrition research is to understand this complexity using the powerful tools of molecular biology. When the data collection is undertaken on a global scale, this type of molecular nutrition is often referred to as nutritional genomics.[130,131] Within the field, two guiding concepts have gained prominence. First, there is nutrigenomics, in which the focus is on the global assessment of nutrient-gene interactions at the level of the transcriptome, proteome, and metabolome; second, there is nutrigenetics, in which the focus is on the impact of functional variations in gene structure (the simplest form being single-nucleotide polymorphisms) on the human response to diet. Whereas nutrigenomics provides a scientific basis for population-based dietary guidelines, nutrigenetics tailors this advice to the genetic background of the individual.

It may justly be said that cardiovascular nutrition has been a major beneficiary of both nutrigenomics and nutrigenetics. At one point in time, it was considered a major accomplishment just to characterize the impact of different fatty acids on serum lipids.[132] Now the highly variable response of humans to dietary fat is being put into molecular context as we begin to understand genetic variations in the various apolipoproteins that regulate lipoprotein metabolism.[133-134] The pace of progress is remarkable. Just as quickly as a new apolipoprotein is discovered (e.g., ApoA-V, a potent regulator of serum triglycerides[135]), molecular biology quickly follows with the identification of functional polymorphisms in the apolipoprotein,[136] and the apolipoprotein and its single-nucleotide polymorphisms become the subject of clinical studies investigating the potential impact on the progression of CVD.[137] Along with the cataloging of the various genes and single-nucleotide polymorphisms of fatty acid metabolism, there has come a greater understanding of the regulation of these genes by ligand-activated nuclear transcription factors. The ability of fatty acids to activate the peroxisome proliferator-activated receptor, the retinoid X receptor, and hepatocyte nuclear factor-4 allows these receptors to act as fatty acid biosensors and to regulate the trafficking and metabolism of fatty acids in a coordinated manner. Finally, it should be noted that even transcription factors are subject to a higher order of regulation based on the differential recruitment of co-activators and co-repressors in a process known as combinatorial control. Understanding this level of regulatory complexity is already paying dividends in elucidating how trans fatty acids influence lipoprotein synthesis and secretion.[138] There has also been compelling evidence that polyunsaturated fatty acids play a key role in regulating the transcription of genes responsible for conferring insulin and carbohydrate control of lipid synthesis.[139] Clearly, nutritional genomics promises to bring nutrition science into the mainstream of life science research.

Future Directions: Managing Dietary Guidance in an Ever-Changing World

Nutrition is a dynamic field, and new information about the role of diet in the prevention and treatment of CVD is being reported at a remarkable rate. Not unexpectedly, in some instances this process questions and even overturns popular or long-standing concepts and beliefs. For example, there have been nutrients and dietary patterns that were thought to be protective against CVD based on a seemingly robust database; however, subsequent studies have brought dietary recommendations predicated on this database into question. This scenario has unfolded with soy, antioxidants, and a low-fat dietary pattern.[140-142] With respect to soy protein, differences in processing techniques used to isolate the various soy proteins, as well as the amount evaluated may have contributed to the variability in cholesterol-lowering activity. Likewise, the lack of benefit observed in clinical trials evaluating the cardioprotective effects of antioxidants may reflect in part the antioxidant studied, the specific isomeric form of the antioxidant used (e.g., α-tocopherol vs. γ-tocopherol), the amount of antioxidant(s) used, or characteristics of the subject cohort studied (i.e., high-oxidative stress vs. low-antioxidant defense). A key issue that may underlie the unanticipated lack of benefit on risk of CVD from a low-fat dietary pattern in the Women's Health Initiative trial may relate to the lack of, or inconsistent, compliance to the experimental diets. Thus, although there is a general understanding of how diet modifies CVD risk, ever-present debates that bring new science to the forefront make it necessary to continually examine our hypotheses and, as appropriate, refine our dietary guidance.

In summary, impressive advances in our understanding of diet and CVD have occurred in the past decade. The application of molecular biology and genetics has given us a deeper understanding of the biological mechanisms of CVD. Consequently, we can now target many different pathways more aggressively, and do so depending on an individual's clinical profile. The ability to individualize lifestyle interventions may ultimately permit maximal CVD risk reduction to be achieved. The concept of dietary patterns and total lifestyle interventions have come to the forefront, enabling us to implement intensive primary and secondary interventions that simultaneously target multiple CVD risk factors. We now have a cornucopia of existing and new foods and lifestyle interventions that can be combined to achieve unprecedented CVD risk reduction. It is important to emphasize that while our advances in developing innovative science-based approaches for CVD risk reduction bodes well for the future, much remains to be done to effectively communicate this new science to consumers and health professionals. This is particularly true if we are to individualize diet plus lifestyle interventions as the path forward for achieving our goal of maximal reduction of CVD risk. This strategic approach should be a primary focus of the cardiovascular nutrition science community in the years ahead.

References

1. Appel LJ, Moore TJ, Obarzanek E, et al. A clinical trial of the effects of dietary patterns on blood pressure. DASH Collaborative Research Group. N Engl J Med. 1997;336:1117–1124.
2. Jenkins DJ, Kendall CW, Marchie A, et al. Direct comparison of a dietary portfolio of cholesterol-lowering foods with a statin in hypercholesterolemic participants. Am J Clin Nutr. 2005;81:380–387.
3. American Heart Association. Heart Disease and Stroke Statistics 2005 Update. Dallas, TX: AHA; 2005.
4. Ross R. Atherosclerosis—an inflammatory disease. N Engl J Med. 1999;340:115–126.
5. Hansson GK. Inflammation, atherosclerosis, and coronary artery disease. N Engl J Med. 2005;352: 1685–1695.
6. Mullenix PS, Andersen CA, Starnes BW. Atherosclerosis as inflammation. Ann Vasc Surg. 2005;19: 130–138.
7. Shishehbor MH, Bhatt DL. Inflammation and atherosclerosis. Curr Atheroscler Rep. 2004;6:131–139.
8. Ridker PM. Clinical application of C-reactive protein for cardiovascular disease detection and prevention. Circulation. 2003;107:363–369.
9. Ridker PM, Rifai N, Rose L, Buring JE, Cook NR. Comparison of C-reactive protein and low-density lipoprotein cholesterol levels in the prediction of first cardiovascular events. N Engl J Med. 2002; 347:1557–1565.
10. Libby P, Ridker PM. Inflammation and atherosclerosis: role of C-reactive protein in risk assessment. Am J Med. 2004;116(suppl 6A):9S–16S.
11. Labarrere CA, Zaloga GP. C-reactive protein: from innocent bystander to pivotal mediator of atherosclerosis. Am J Med. 2004;117:499–507.
12. Din JN, Newby DE, Flapan AD. Omega 3 fatty acids and cardiovascular disease—fishing for a natural treatment. BMJ. 2004;328:30–35.
13. He K, Song Y, Daviglus ML, et al. Accumulated evidence on fish consumption and coronary heart disease mortality: a meta-analysis of cohort studies. Circulation. 2004;109:2705–2711.
14. He K, Song Y, Daviglus ML, et al. Fish consumption and incidence of stroke: a meta-analysis of cohort studies. Stroke. 2004;35:1538–1542.
15. Harris WS, Von Schacky C. The omega-3 index: a new risk factor for death from coronary heart disease? Prev Med. 2004;39:212–220.
16. Harris WS, Sands SA, Windsor SL, et al. Omega-

3 fatty acids in cardiac biopsies from heart transplantation patients: correlation with erythrocytes and response to supplementation. Circulation. 2004;110:1645–1649.

17. Burr ML, Fehily AM, Gilbert JF, et al. Effects of changes in fat, fish, and fibre intakes on death and myocardial reinfarction: diet and reinfarction trial (DART). Lancet. 1989;2:757–761.
18. Dietary supplementation with n-3 polyunsaturated fatty acids and vitamin E after myocardial infarction: results of the GISSI-Prevenzione trial. Gruppo Italiano per lo Studio della Sopravvivenza nell'Infarto miocardico. Lancet. 1999;354:447–455.
19. Marchioli R, Barzi F, Bomba E, et al. Early protection against sudden death by n-3 polyunsaturated fatty acids after myocardial infarction: time-course analysis of the results of the Gruppo Italiano per lo Studio della Sopravvivenza nell'Infarto Miocardico (GISSI)-Prevenzione. Circulation. 2002;105: 1897–1903.
20. Yokoyama M, Origasa H. Effects of eicosapentaenoic acid on cardiovascular events in Japanese patients with hypercholesterolemia: rationale, design, and baseline characteristics of the Japan EPA Lipid Intervention Study (JELIS). Am Heart J. 2003;146: 613–620.
21. Yokoyama M. Effects of eicosapentaenoic acid (EPA) on major cardiovascular events in hypercholesteroemic patients: the Japan EPA Lipid Intervention Study (JELIS). Presented at the American Heart Association Scientific Sessions; November 13–16, 2005; Dallas, TX.
22. Burr ML, Ashfield-Watt PA, Dunstan FD, et al. Lack of benefit of dietary advice to men with angina: results of a controlled trial. Eur J Clin Nutr. 2003; 57:193–200.
23. Mozaffarian D, Ascherio A, Hu FB, et al. Interplay between different polyunsaturated fatty acids and risk of coronary heart disease in men. Circulation. 2005;111:157–164.
24. Albert CM, Oh K, Whang W, et al. Dietary alpha-linolenic acid intake and risk of sudden cardiac death and coronary heart disease. Circulation. 2005; 112:3232–3238.
25. Harris WS. Alpha-linolenic acid: a gift from the land? Circulation. 2005;111:2872–2874.
26. de Lorgeril M, Salen P, Martin JL, Monjaud I, Delaye J, Mamelle N. Mediterranean diet, traditional risk factors, and the rate of cardiovascular complications after myocardial infarction: final report of the Lyon Diet Heart Study. Circulation. 1999;99:779–785.
27. Natvig H, Borchgrevink CF, Dedichen J, Owren PA, Schiotz EH, Westlund K. A controlled trial of the effect of linolenic acid on incidence of coronary heart disease. The Norwegian vegetable oil experiment of 1965–66. Scand J Clin Lab Invest Suppl. 1968;105:1–20.
28. Goyens PL, Spilker ME, Zock PL, Katan MB, Mensink RP. Compartmental modeling to quantify alpha-linolenic acid conversion after longer term intake of multiple tracer boluses. J Lipid Res. 2005; 46:1474–1483.
29. Brenna JT. Efficiency of conversion of alpha-linolenic acid to long chain n-3 fatty acids in man. Curr Opin Clin Nutr Metab Care. 2002;5:127–132.
30. Leaf A, Kang JX, Xiao YF, Billman GE. Clinical prevention of sudden cardiac death by n-3 polyunsaturated fatty acids and mechanism of prevention of arrhythmias by n-3 fish oils. Circulation. 2003; 107:2646–2652.
31. Billman GE, Kang JX, Leaf A. Prevention of sudden cardiac death by dietary pure omega-3 polyunsaturated fatty acids in dogs. Circulation. 1999;99: 2452–2457.
32. Ander BP, Weber AR, Rampersad PP, Gilchrist JS, Pierce GN, Lukas A. Dietary flaxseed protects against ventricular fibrillation induced by ischemia-reperfusion in normal and hypercholesterolemic rabbits. J Nutr. 2004;134:3250–3256.
33. Christensen JH, Riahi S, Schmidt EB, et al. n-3 Fatty acids and ventricular arrhythmias in patients with ischaemic heart disease and implantable cardioverter defibrillators. Europace. 2005;7:338–344.
34. Schrepf R, Limmert T, Claus Weber P, Theisen K, Sellmayer A. Immediate effects of n-3 fatty acid infusion on the induction of sustained ventricular tachycardia. Lancet. 2004;363:1441–1442.
35. Raitt MH, Connor WE, Morris C, et al. Fish oil supplementation and risk of ventricular tachycardia and ventricular fibrillation in patients with implantable defibrillators: a randomized controlled trial. JAMA. 2005;293:2884–2891.
36. Sherwood L. Human Physiology: From Cells to Systems. 5th ed. Pacific Grove, CA: Brooks Cole; 2004.
37. Fernandez ML, West KL. Mechanisms by which dietary fatty acids modulate plasma lipids. J Nutr. 2005;135:2075–2078.
38. Nestel PJ. Fish oil and cardiovascular disease: lipids and arterial function. Am J Clin Nutr. 2000;71: 228S–231S.
39. Kris-Etherton PM, Harris WS, Appel LJ. Omega-3 fatty acids and cardiovascular disease: new recommendations from the American Heart Association. Arterioscler Thromb Vasc Biol. 2003;23:151–152.
40. Harris WS. n-3 fatty acids and serum lipoproteins: human studies. Am J Clin Nutr. 1997;65: 1645S–1654S.
41. Grimsgaard S, Bonaa KH, Hansen JB, Nordoy A. Highly purified eicosapentaenoic acid and docosahexaenoic acid in humans have similar triacylglyc-

erol-lowering effects but divergent effects on serum fatty acids. Am J Clin Nutr. 1997;66:649–659.
42. Mori TA, Burke V, Puddey IB, et al. Purified eicosapentaenoic and docosahexaenoic acids have differential effects on serum lipids and lipoproteins, LDL particle size, glucose, and insulin in mildly hyperlipidemic men. Am J Clin Nutr. 2000;71:1085–1094.
43. Wang C, Lichtenstein A, Balk E, Kupelnick B, DeVine D, Lawrence A, Lau J. Effects of Omega-3 Fatty Acids on Cardiovascular Disease. Evidence Report/Technology Assessment No. 94 (Prepared by Tufts-New England Medical Center Evidence-based Practice Center, under Contract No. 290-02-0022). AHRQ Publication No. 04-E009-2. Rockville, MD: Agency for Healthcare Research and Quality; 2004.
44. Geleijnse JM, Giltay EJ, Grobbee DE, Donders AR, Kok FJ. Blood pressure response to fish oil supplementation: metaregression analysis of randomized trials. J Hypertens. 2002;20:1493–1499.
45. Calder PC. n-3 Fatty acids and cardiovascular disease: evidence explained and mechanisms explored. Clin Sci (Lond). 2004;107:1–11.
46. Thies F, Garry JM, Yaqoob P, et al. Association of n-3 polyunsaturated fatty acids with stability of atherosclerotic plaques: a randomised controlled trial. Lancet. 2003;361:477–485.
47. Mori TA, Beilin LJ. Omega-3 fatty acids and inflammation. Curr Atheroscler Rep. 2004;6:461–467.
48. Zhao G, Etherton TD, Martin KR, et al. Anti-inflammatory effects of polyunsaturated fatty acids in THP-1 cells. Biochem Biophys Res Commun. 2005;336:909–917.
49. Zampelas A, Panagiotakos DB, Pitsavos C, et al. Fish consumption among healthy adults is associated with decreased levels of inflammatory markers related to cardiovascular disease: the ATTICA study. J Am Coll Cardiol. 2005;46:120–124.
50. Lopez-Garcia E, Schulze MB, Manson JE, et al. Consumption of (n-3) fatty acids is related to plasma biomarkers of inflammation and endothelial activation in women. J Nutr. 2004;134:1806–1811.
51. Arita M, Yoshida M, Hong S, et al. Resolvin E1, an endogenous lipid mediator derived from omega-3 eicosapentaenoic acid, protects against 2,4,6-trinitrobenzene sulfonic acid-induced colitis. Proc Natl Acad Sci U S A. 2005;102:7671–7676.
52. Ascherio A, Katan MB, Zock PL, Stampfer MJ, Willett WC. Trans fatty acids and coronary heart disease. N Engl J Med. 1999;340:1994–1998.
53. Mensink RP, Katan MB. Effect of dietary trans fatty acids on high-density and low-density lipoprotein cholesterol levels in healthy subjects. N Engl J Med. 1990;323:439–445.
54. Zock PL, Katan MB. Hydrogenation alternatives: effects of trans fatty acids and stearic acid versus linoleic acid on serum lipids and lipoproteins in humans. J Lipid Res. 1992;33:399–410.
55. Nestel P, Noakes M, Belling B, et al. Plasma lipoprotein lipid and Lp[a] changes with substitution of elaidic acid for oleic acid in the diet. J Lipid Res. 1992;33:1029–1036.
56. Judd JT, Clevidence BA, Muesing RA, Wittes J, Sunkin ME, Podczasy JJ. Dietary trans fatty acids: effects on plasma lipids and lipoproteins of healthy men and women. Am J Clin Nutr. 1994;59:861–868.
57. Judd JT, Baer D, Clevidence B. Blood lipid and lipoprotein modifying effects of trans monounsaturated fatty acids compared to carbohydrate, oleic acid, stearic acid, and C 12:0–16:0 saturated fatty acids in men fed controlled diets [abstract]. FASEB J. 1998;12:A229.
58. Lichtenstein AH, Ausman LM, Carrasco W, Jenner JL, Ordovas JM, Schaefer EJ. Hydrogenation impairs the hypolipidemic effect of corn oil in humans. Hydrogenation, trans fatty acids, and plasma lipids. Arterioscler Thromb. 1993;13:154–161.
59. Aro A, Jauhiainen M, Partanen R, Salminen I, Mutanen M. Stearic acid, trans fatty acids, and dairy fat: effects on serum and lipoprotein lipids, apolipoproteins, lipoprotein(a), and lipid transfer proteins in healthy subjects. Am J Clin Nutr. 1997;65:1419–1426.
60. Sundram K, Ismail A, Hayes KC, Jeyamalar R, Pathmanathan R. Trans (elaidic) fatty acids adversely affect the lipoprotein profile relative to specific saturated fatty acids in humans. J Nutr. 1997;127:514S–520S.
61. Lichtenstein AH, Ausman LM, Jalbert SM, Schaefer EJ. Effects of different forms of dietary hydrogenated fats on serum lipoprotein cholesterol levels. N Engl J Med. 1999;340:1933–1940.
62. Oh K, Hu FB, Manson JE, Stampfer MJ, Willett WC. Dietary fat intake and risk of coronary heart disease in women: 20 years of follow-up of the nurses' health study. Am J Epidemiol. 2005;161:672–679.
63. Oomen CM, Ocke MC, Feskens EJ, van Erp-Baart MA, Kok FJ, Kromhout D. Association between trans fatty acid intake and 10-year risk of coronary heart disease in the Zutphen Elderly Study: a prospective population-based study. Lancet. 2001;357:746–751.
64. de Roos NM, Schouten EG, Katan MB. Trans fatty acids, HDL-cholesterol, and cardiovascular disease. Effects of dietary changes on vascular reactivity. Eur J Med Res. 2003;8:355–357.
65. Lopez-Garcia E, Schulze MB, Meigs JB, et al. Consumption of trans fatty acids is related to plasma biomarkers of inflammation and endothelial dysfunction. J Nutr. 2005;135:562–566.

66. Mozaffarian D, Pischon T, Hankinson SE, et al. Dietary intake of trans fatty acids and systemic inflammation in women. Am J Clin Nutr. 2004;79:606–612.
67. Wahle KW, Heys SD, Rotondo D. Conjugated linoleic acids: are they beneficial or detrimental to health? Prog Lipid Res. 2004;43:553–587.
68. Executive Summary of The Third Report of The National Cholesterol Education Program (NCEP) Expert Panel on Detection, Evaluation, and Treatment of High Blood Cholesterol in Adults (Adult Treatment Panel III). JAMA. 2001;285:2486–2497.
69. Kahn R, Buse J, Ferrannini E, Stern M. The metabolic syndrome: time for a critical appraisal: joint statement from the American Diabetes Association and the European Association for the Study of Diabetes. Diabetes Care. 2005;28:2289–2304.
70. Grundy SM, Cleeman JI, Daniels SR, et al. Diagnosis and management of the metabolic syndrome. An American Heart Association/National Heart, Lung, and Blood Institute scientific statement. Circulation. 2005;112:2735–2752.
71. Grundy SM. Obesity, metabolic syndrome, and cardiovascular disease. J Clin Endocrinol Metab. 2004;89:2595–2600.
72. Ford ES, Giles WH, Mokdad AH. Increasing prevalence of the metabolic syndrome among u.s. Adults. Diabetes Care. 2004;27:2444–2449.
73. Pritchett AM, Foreyt JP, Mann DL. Treatment of the metabolic syndrome: the impact of lifestyle modification. Curr Atheroscler Rep. 2005;7:95–102.
74. Orchard TJ, Temprosa M, Goldberg R, et al. The effect of metformin and intensive lifestyle intervention on the metabolic syndrome: the Diabetes Prevention Program randomized trial. Ann Intern Med. 2005;142:611–619.
75. Esposito K, Marfella R, Ciotola M, et al. Effect of a mediterranean-style diet on endothelial dysfunction and markers of vascular inflammation in the metabolic syndrome: a randomized trial. JAMA. 2004;292:1440–1446.
76. Hasler CM, Bloch AS, Thomson CA, Enrione E, Manning C. Position of the American Dietetic Association: Functional foods. J Am Diet Assoc. 2004;104:814–826.
77. Freeland-Graves J, Nitzke S. Position of the American Dietetic Association: total diet *approach to communicating food and nutrition information. J Am Diet Assoc. 2002;102:100–108.
78. Third Report of the National Cholesterol Education Program (NCEP) Expert Panel on Detection, Evaluation, and Treatment of High Blood Cholesterol in Adults (Adult Treatment Panel III) final report. Circulation. 2002;106:3143–3421.
79. Kendall CW, Jenkins DJ. A dietary portfolio: maximal reduction of low-density lipoprotein cholesterol with diet. Curr Atheroscler Rep. 2004;6:492–498.
80. Jenkins DJ, Kendall CW, Marchie A, et al. Direct comparison of dietary portfolio vs statin on C-reactive protein. Eur J Clin Nutr. 2005;59:851–860.
81. Keys A. Coronary heart disease in seven countries. Circulation 1970;41 (suppl):1–211.
82. Knoops KT, de Groot LC, Kromhout D, et al. Mediterranean diet, lifestyle factors, and 10-year mortality in elderly European men and women: the HALE project. JAMA 2004;292:1433–9.
83. Trichopoulou A, Costacou T, Bamia C, Trichopoulos D. Adherence to a Mediterranean diet and survival in a Greek population. N Engl J Med. 2003;348:2599–2608.
84. Trichopoulou A, Orfanos P, Norat T, et al. Modified Mediterranean diet and survival: EPIC-elderly prospective cohort study. BMJ. 2005;330:991.
85. Sacks FM, Katan M. Randomized clinical trials on the effects of dietary fat and carbohydrate on plasma lipoproteins and cardiovascular disease. Am J Med. 2002;113(suppl 9B):13S–24S.
86. Padwal R, Straus SE, McAlister FA. Evidence based management of hypertension. Cardiovascular risk factors and their effects on the decision to treat hypertension: evidence based review. BMJ. 2001;322:977–980.
87. Karanja N, Erlinger TP, Pao-Hwa L, Miller ER 3rd, Bray GA. The DASH diet for high blood pressure: from clinical trial to dinner table. Cleve Clin J Med. 2004;71:745–753.
88. Obarzanek E, Sacks FM, Vollmer WM, et al. Effects on blood lipids of a blood pressure-lowering diet: the Dietary Approaches to Stop Hypertension (DASH) Trial. Am J Clin Nutr. 2001;74:80–89.
89. National Heart Lung and Blood Institute. Facts About the DASH Eating Plan. Available online at: http://www.nhlbi.nih.gov/health/public/heart/hbp/dash/new_dash.pdf. Accessed January 12, 2006.
90. Sacks FM, Svetkey LP, Vollmer WM, et al. Effects on blood pressure of reduced dietary sodium and the Dietary Approaches to Stop Hypertension (DASH) diet. DASH-Sodium Collaborative Research Group. N Engl J Med. 2001;344:3–10.
91. Harsha DW, Sacks FM, Obarzanek E, et al. Effect of dietary sodium intake on blood lipids: results from the DASH-sodium trial. Hypertension. 2004;43:393–398.
92. Appel LJ, Champagne CM, Harsha DW, et al. Effects of comprehensive lifestyle modification on blood pressure control: main results of the PREMIER clinical trial. JAMA. 2003;289:2083–2093.
93. Ard JD, Grambow SC, Liu D, Slentz CA, Kraus WE, Svetkey LP. The effect of the PREMIER interventions on insulin sensitivity. Diabetes Care. 2004;27:340–347.

94. Glucose tolerance and mortality: comparison of WHO and American Diabetes Association diagnostic criteria. The DECODE study group. European Diabetes Epidemiology Group. Diabetes Epidemiology: Collaborative analysis Of Diagnostic criteria in Europe. Lancet. 1999;354:617–621.
95. Dickinson S, Brand-Miller J. Glycemic index, postprandial glycemia and cardiovascular disease. Curr Opin Lipidol. 2005;16:69–75.
96. Liu S, Willett WC, Stampfer MJ, et al. A prospective study of dietary glycemic load, carbohydrate intake, and risk of coronary heart disease in US women. Am J Clin Nutr. 2000;71:1455–1461.
97. McKeown NM, Meigs JB, Liu S, Saltzman E, Wilson PW, Jacques PF. Carbohydrate nutrition, insulin resistance, and the prevalence of the metabolic syndrome in the Framingham Offspring Cohort. Diabetes Care. 2004;27:538–546.
98. Opperman AM, Venter CS, Oosthuizen W, Thompson RL, Vorster HH. Meta-analysis of the health effects of using the glycaemic index in meal-planning. Br J Nutr. 2004;92:367–381.
99. Pi-Sunyer FX. Glycemic index and disease. Am J Clin Nutr. 2002;76:290S–298S.
100. Pereira MA, Swain J, Goldfine AB, Rifai N, Ludwig DS. Effects of a low-glycemic load diet on resting energy expenditure and heart disease risk factors during weight loss. JAMA. 2004;292:2482–2490.
101. Franz MJ. The glycemic index: not the most effective nutrition therapy intervention. Diabetes Care. 2003;26:2466–2468.
102. Sheard NF, Clark NG, Brand-Miller JC, et al. Dietary carbohydrate (amount and type) in the prevention and management of diabetes: a statement by the american diabetes association. Diabetes Care. 2004;27:2266–2271.
103. Appel LJ, Sacks FM, Carey VJ, et al. Effects of protein, monounsaturated fat, and carbohydrate intake on blood pressure and serum lipids: results of the OmniHeart randomized trial. JAMA. 2005; 294:2455–2464.
104. Volek JS, Westman EC. Very-low-carbohydrate weight-loss diets revisited. Cleve Clin J Med. 2002; 69:849–853.
105. St Jeor ST, Howard BV, Prewitt TE, Bovee V, Bazzarre T, Eckel RH. Dietary protein and weight reduction: a statement for healthcare professionals from the Nutrition Committee of the Council on Nutrition, Physical Activity, and Metabolism of the American Heart Association. Circulation. 2001; 104:1869–1874.
106. Brehm BJ, Seeley RJ, Daniels SR, D'Alessio DA. A randomized trial comparing a very low carbohydrate diet and a calorie-restricted low fat diet on body weight and cardiovascular risk factors in healthy women. J Clin Endocrinol Metab. 2003;88: 1617–1623.
107. Foster GD, Wyatt HR, Hill JO, et al. A randomized trial of a low-carbohydrate diet for obesity. N Engl J Med. 2003;348:2082–2090.
108. Samaha FF, Iqbal N, Seshadri P, et al. A low-carbohydrate as compared with a low-fat diet in severe obesity. N Engl J Med. 2003;348:2074–2081.
109. Yancy WS, Jr., Olsen MK, Guyton JR, Bakst RP, Westman EC. A low-carbohydrate, ketogenic diet versus a low-fat diet to treat obesity and hyperlipidemia: a randomized, controlled trial. Ann Intern Med. 2004;140:769–777.
110. Stern L, Iqbal N, Seshadri P, et al. The effects of low-carbohydrate versus conventional weight loss diets in severely obese adults: one-year follow-up of a randomized trial. Ann Intern Med. 2004;140: 778–785.
111. Kappagoda CT, Hyson DA, Amsterdam EA. Low-carbohydrate-high-protein diets: is there a place for them in clinical cardiology? J Am Coll Cardiol. 2004;43:725–730.
112. Volek JS, Sharman MJ, Forsythe CE. Modification of lipoproteins by very low-carbohydrate diets. J Nutr. 2005;135:1339–1342.
113. Meckling KA, O'Sullivan C, Saari D. Comparison of a low-fat diet to a low-carbohydrate diet on weight loss, body composition, and risk factors for diabetes and cardiovascular disease in free-living, overweight men and women. J Clin Endocrinol Metab. 2004;89:2717–2723.
114. Volek JS, Sharman MJ, Gomez AL, et al. Comparison of a very low-carbohydrate and low-fat diet on fasting lipids, LDL subclasses, insulin resistance, and postprandial lipemic responses in overweight women. J Am Coll Nutr. 2004;23:177–184.
115. O'Brien KD, Brehm BJ, Seeley RJ, et al. Diet-induced weight loss is associated with decreases in plasma serum amyloid a and C-reactive protein independent of dietary macronutrient composition in obese subjects. J Clin Endocrinol Metab. 2005;90: 2244–2249.
116. Seshadri P, Iqbal N, Stern L, et al. A randomized study comparing the effects of a low-carbohydrate diet and a conventional diet on lipoprotein subfractions and C-reactive protein levels in patients with severe obesity. Am J Med. 2004;117:398–405.
117. Sharman MJ, Gomez AL, Kraemer WJ, Volek JS. Very low-carbohydrate and low-fat diets affect fasting lipids and postprandial lipemia differently in overweight men. J Nutr. 2004;134:880–885.
118. Volek JS, Sharman MJ, Gomez AL, Scheett TP, Kraemer WJ. An isoenergetic very low carbohydrate diet improves serum HDL cholesterol and triacylglycerol concentrations, the total cholesterol to HDL cholesterol ratio and postprandial pipemic responses compared with a low fat diet in normal weight, normolipidemic women. J Nutr. 2003;133: 2756–2761.

119. Rabast U, Kasper H, Schonborn J. Comparative studies in obese subjects fed carbohydrate-restricted and high carbohydrate 1,000-calorie formula diets. Nutr Metab. 1978;22:269–277.
120. Sondike SB, Copperman N, Jacobson MS. Effects of a low-carbohydrate diet on weight loss and cardiovascular risk factor in overweight adolescents. J Pediatr. 2003;142:253–258.
121. Brehm BJ, Spang SE, Lattin BL, Seeley RJ, Daniels SR, D'Alessio DA. The role of energy expenditure in the differential weight loss in obese women on low-fat and low-carbohydrate diets. J Clin Endocrinol Metab. 2005;90:1475–1482.
122. Aude YW, Agatston AS, Lopez-Jimenez F, et al. The national cholesterol education program diet vs a diet lower in carbohydrates and higher in protein and monounsaturated fat: a randomized trial. Arch Intern Med. 2004;164:2141–2146.
123. McAuley KA, Hopkins CM, Smith KJ, et al. Comparison of high-fat and high-protein diets with a high-carbohydrate diet in insulin-resistant obese women. Diabetologia. 2005;48:8–16.
124. Dansinger ML, Gleason JA, Griffith JL, Selker HP, Schaefer EJ. Comparison of the Atkins, Ornish, Weight Watchers, and Zone diets for weight loss and heart disease risk reduction: a randomized trial. JAMA. 2005;293:43–53.
125. Rimm EB, Stampfer MJ. Diet, lifestyle, and longevity—the next steps? JAMA. 2004;292:1490–1492.
126. Powell KE, Thompson PD, Caspersen CJ, Kendrick JS. Physical activity and the incidence of coronary heart disease. Annu Rev Public Health. 1987;8:253–287.
127. Varady KA, Jones PJ. Combination diet and exercise interventions for the treatment of dyslipidemia: an effective preliminary strategy to lower cholesterol levels? J Nutr. 2005;135:1829–1835.
128. Food and Nutrition Board, Institute of Medicine. Dietary Reference Intakes for Energy, Carbohydrate, Fiber, Fat, Fatty Acids, Cholesterol, Protein, and Amino Acids (Macronutrients). Washington, DC: National Academies Press; 2002. Available online at: http://www.nap.edu/books/0309085373/html. Accessed January 12, 2006.
129. Schaefer EJ. Lipoproteins, nutrition, and heart disease. Am J Clin Nutr. 2002;75:191–212.
130. Ordovas JM, Corella D. Nutritional genomics. Annu Rev Genomics Hum Genet. 2004;5:71–118.
131. van Ommen B, Stierum R. Nutrigenomics: exploiting systems biology in the nutrition and health arena. Curr Opin Biotechnol. 2002;13:517–521.
132. Mensink RP, Zock PL, Kester AD, Katan MB. Effects of dietary fatty acids and carbohydrates on the ratio of serum total to HDL cholesterol and on serum lipids and apolipoproteins: a meta-analysis of 60 controlled trials. Am J Clin Nutr. 2003;77:1146–1155.
133. Corella D, Ordovas JM. Single nucleotide polymorphisms that influence lipid metabolism: interaction with dietary factors. Annu Rev Nutr. 2005;25:341–390.
134. Masson LF, McNeill G, Avenell A. Genetic variation and the lipid response to dietary intervention: a systematic review. Am J Clin Nutr. 2003;77:1098–1111.
135. Pennacchio LA, Olivier M, Hubacek JA, et al. An apolipoprotein influencing triglycerides in humans and mice revealed by comparative sequencing. Science. 2001;294:169–173.
136. Pennacchio LA, Olivier M, Hubacek JA, Krauss RM, Rubin EM, Cohen JC. Two independent apolipoprotein A5 haplotypes influence human plasma triglyceride levels. Hum Mol Genet. 2002;11:3031–3038.
137. Talmud PJ, Martin S, Taskinen MR, et al. APOA5 gene variants, lipoprotein particle distribution, and progression of coronary heart disease: results from the LOCAT study. J Lipid Res. 2004;45:750–756.
138. Lin J, Yang R, Tarr PT, et al. Hyperlipidemic effects of dietary saturated fats mediated through PGC-1beta coactivation of SREBP. Cell. 2005;120:261–273.
139. Clarke SD. Polyunsaturated fatty acid regulation of gene transcription: a molecular mechanism to improve the metabolic syndrome. J Nutr. 2001;131:1129–1132.
140. Sacks FM, Lichtenstein A, Van Horn L, et al. Soy protein, isoflavones, and cardiovascular health: an American Heart Association Science Advisory for professionals from the Nutrition Committee. Circulation. 2006;113:1034–1044.
141. Kris-Etherton PM, Lichtenstein AH, Howard BV, et al. AHA science advisory: antioxidant vitamin supplements and cardiovascular disease. Circulation. 2004;110:637–641.
142. Howard BV, Van Horn L, Hsia J, et al. Low-fat dietary pattern and risk of cardiovascular disease. The Women's Health Initiative Randomized Controlled Dietary Modification Trial. JAMA. 2006;295:655–666.

50 Diabetes Mellitus

Judith Wylie-Rosett and Frank Vinicor

Introduction

Despite major advances in our understanding about and treatments for diabetes mellitus (DM), this multifaceted condition continues to pose major challenges to individuals, families, communities, and nations throughout the world. This chapter will first review basic concepts about DM; then discuss medical nutrition therapy (MNT) for those with extant DM, as well as new information regarding the prevention of type 2 DM; and conclude with important and interesting but still unresolved issues addressing nutrition and DM into the future.

An elevated blood glucose level remains the hallmark of DM. However, DM is actually a group of metabolic disorders resulting from impairment in insulin secretion, insulin action, or both.[1] Insulin facilitates glucose uptake and utilization and deposition of fat. Counterregulatory and other hormones (e.g., glucagon, growth hormone, epinephrine, cortisol, amylin, and GLP-1) decrease the cells' sensitivity to the effect of insulin and can also alter glucose metabolism.[2] Other emerging dimensions of the etiology and pathogenesis of DM include inflammation, vascular abnormalities, genetics, and beta-cell neogenesis and apoptosis.[3]

The goal of early diagnosis and treatment of DM is to restore normal metabolism in order to prevent short-term glucose perturbations, such as hyperglycemia and hypoglycemia, and longer-term microvascular, macrovascular, and neurologic complications.[1,4] Because DM involves overall dysregulation of fuel utilization, dyslipidemia is a common clinical comorbidity of DM, especially when the blood glucose level is elevated. DM involves an absolute or relative insulin deficiency, the latter primarily due to concomitant insulin resistance.[1] Causes of insulin resistance include obesity, genetic factors, aging, and some medications. Obesity, generally considered the major factor in the development of the metabolic precursors of DM, including insulin resistance and the so-called metabolic syndrome, reflects gene-nutrient interactions.[5] Understanding of gene-gene, gene-nutrient, and gene-nutrient-environment interactions can provide insights into the molecular basis of the metabolic dysregulation associated with DM.[5,6] This genetic heterogeneity is matched by clinical heterogeneity and the impact of various medications (e.g., steroids, novel antipsychotic agents).[7]

Present and Future Burden of DM

An estimated 20.8 million people in the United States have DM (14.6 million undiagnosed and 6.2 million diagnosed).[8] Age and body weight greatly affect the prevalence of DM.[8] Race and ethnicity also appear to be important factors in the prevalence of DM (although perhaps via age and/or body weight): the adult prevalence of DM is 13.1 million (8.7%) for non-Hispanic whites, 3.2 million (13.3%) for non-Hispanic blacks, 2.5 million (9.5%) for Hispanic/Latino Americans, and 99,500 (12.8%) for American Indians and Alaska Natives. The prevalence among Asian Americans and Pacific Islanders is not firmly established, but current data suggest that the rate is 1.5 to 2.0 times that of whites.[8]

The global prevalence of DM is expected to more than double between 2000 and 2030, from 171 million to 366 million.[9] Industrialization and a concomitant rise in obesity and sedentary lifestyles in developing countries likely contribute greatly to this rise in prevalence. As the global public health burden of DM increases, health economics and evidence-based decision making will determine resource allocation.[10]

Because of the growing public health burden of DM in the United States and throughout the world, three general approaches to reduce the burden of DM are being considered[11]: 1) primary prevention of DM in individuals at very high risk to ultimately develop this condition (controlling weight and physical activity); 2) secondary prevention: decreasing the onset and/or severity of DM complications (controlling metabolic disorders associated with DM); and 3) tertiary prevention: controlling and medically managing DM complications to reduce morbidity and mortality.[12]

Classification and Diagnosis of DM

Four basic types of DM are recognized: type 1 (formerly known as insulin-dependent or juvenile DM), type 2 (formerly known as non-insulin-dependent DM or adult-onset diabetes), gestational DM (hyperglycemia identified during pregnancy), and secondary diabetes (due to pancreatic damage or insulin resistance caused by other diseases or treatments).[1] According to the 1997 American Diabetes Association (ADA) diagnostic criteria,[1] DM is diagnosed on the basis of having a fasting plasma glucose level of at least 7.0 mmol/L (126 mg/dL) on two occasions; a random glucose level of at least 11.1 mmol/L (200 mg/dL) and symptoms of DM; or a 2-hour post-glucose challenge of at least 11.1 mmol/L (200 mg/dL). A fasting glucose level between 6.7 and 6.9 mmol/L (100–125 mg/dL) is considered impaired fasting glucose. Individuals who have impaired fasting glucose or impaired glucose tolerance (2-hour post-glucose challenge of 7.8–11 mmol/L [140–199 mg/dL]) are described as having prediabetes.[13]

In general, screening for undiagnosed diabetes occurs in settings where care is already occurring ("opportunistic screening") and for persons over the age of 45.[14] Risk factors other than prediabetes that would warrant screening at a younger age than 45 years and more frequently than every 3 years include obesity (Body Mass Index [BMI] of at least 30 kg/m^2), family history of diabetes (i.e., parent or sibling), dyslipidemia with a high-density lipoprotein cholesterol level of 0.90 mmol/L (35 mg/dL) or less and/or a triglyceride level of at least 2.82 mmol/L (250 mg/dL), blood pressure of 140/90 mmHg or greater, gestational diabetes or delivery of babies weighing more than 4.09 kg (9.0 lb), and being from an ethnic/racial group with a high prevalence of diabetes (e.g., Blacks, Asians, Native Americans, and Pacific Islanders).[1]

Type 1 DM

Individuals with type 1 DM represent 5% to 10% of known cases of diabetes.[1] Type 1 DM is characterized by severe insulin deficiency requiring exogenous insulin to prevent ketoacidosis, coma, and death. Onset usually occurs during childhood, adolescence, or early adulthood in lean individuals. However, type 1 DM can occur at any age, and almost half of new cases are diagnosed after 20 years of age.[15] The incidence of type 1 DM is higher in whites than in other ethnic and racial groups.

Type 1 DM is a T-cell-mediated autoimmune disease affecting the beta cells in the pancreatic islets of Langerhans. The etiology of type 1 DM probably involves a complex interaction of genetic and environmental factors. Viruses can trigger an autoimmune response or may directly damage the pancreatic beta cells, which presumably themselves become viewed as antigens. Aggregation of type 1 DM in families led to the identification of histocompatibility leukocyte antigen alleles as well as the presence of various serum autoantibodies before the onset of clinical disease.[16]

In considering the etiology of type 1 DM, it is important to distinguish between the onset of autoimmunity, which usually occurs years before the onset of hyperglycemia, and the onset of clinical disease.[16,17] Thus, viruses such as Coxsackie, mumps, and rubella may be associated with either phase. (Environmental toxins or "triggers" have received increased attention and are discussed at the end of this chapter in greater detail.)

As an example of how diet could be associated with type 1 DM, one hypothesis is that the enzyme glutamic acid decarboxylase is in bacteria on food and enters the body via the gastrointestinal system.[18] Theoretically, glutamic acid decarboxylase could be released from bacteria by enzymes of the small intestine and be recognized as foreign by the body's immune system. The beta cells of the pancreas, as an "innocent bystander" or secondarily, then become the target for immune attack in genetically at-risk individuals.[18] After the clinical onset of type 1 DM, an improvement in beta-cell function usually occurs with the initiation of insulin therapy; this is commonly referred to as a short-lived (6–12 months) honeymoon period.

In addressing primary prevention of type 1 DM, research is focusing on genetic linkage studies and antibody biomarkers in individuals at high risk for type 1 DM, with a focus on intensive insulin and other interventions such as immunosuppressive therapy to prevent the development or delay the onset of overt type 1 DM.[16]

Type 2 DM

Type 2 DM accounts for 90% to 95% of all cases of diabetes. Development of type 2 DM is associated with insulin resistance and inadequate pancreatic beta-cell compensatory insulin production.[1] Symptoms and signs associated with type 2 DM are often related to the presence of complications and include poor wound healing, blurred vision, recurrent gum or bladder infections, or changes in hand or foot sensation. Type 2 DM may be present for several years before a clinical diagnosis is made.[19] Many individuals are asymptomatic and their glucose elevation may be detected as the result of a routine blood test.

Cross-sectional and prospective studies indicate a wide variability in the prevalence of type 2 DM related to interaction between environment and genetic predisposition.[5,6] Many indigenous populations are lean and have low rates of type 2 DM, but the rates of DM and obesity dramatically increase with lifestyle or environmental changes.[8,9] Android fat distribution is associated with greater insulin resistance than gynoid fat distribution. Previously, a large waist-hip ratio had been considered a biomarker of insulin resistance, but current weight guidelines suggest use of an abdominal girth of at least 89 cm (35 in) in women and at least 102 cm (40 in) in men as an indicator of increased insulin resistance, hypertension, and dyslipidemia.[20] Insulin resistance increases with age, and the incidence of diabetes sharply rises in the elderly.[1]

Several factors may explain the pathogenesis of type 2 DM. In a few patients, genetic mutations appear to be associated with type 2 DM.[1,5] Linkage studies of families with maturity-onset DM of the young (MODY) have led to identification of several genetic mutations leading to this type of DM. A "thrifty genotype" that favors energy efficiency and could be maladaptive in an environment with an energy-dense food supply and low level of physical activity is another genetic concept being considered.[21] Finally, metabolic adaptations in the fetus of a malnourished and/or hyperglycemic mother may be associated with a "thrifty phenotype" in the newborn and subsequent insulin resistance and increased risk for type 2 DM.[22]

Gestational DM

Gestational DM is defined as "carbohydrate intolerance of variable severity with onset or first recognized during pregnancy."[1] The ADA recommends that a screening interview and assessment be conducted at the first prenatal visit, but glucose tolerance testing is not needed for low-risk women.[14] The criteria for being at low risk for gestational diabetes are having none of the following: at least 25 years of age; overweight or obese; family history of DM (i.e., first-degree relatives); history of abnormal glucose metabolism; history of poor obstetric outcome; or being from an ethnic or racial group with a high DM prevalence. Alternatively, women at high risk (marked obesity, personal history of gestational DM, glycosuria, or strong family history) should have glucose tolerance testing as soon as feasible. Women at moderate risk should have glucose testing between the 24th and 28th week of gestation.

Gestational DM may be diagnosed using either a 75 g or 100 g glucose load. Both the 75 g glucose load (2-hour test) and the 100 g glucose load diagnose diabetes on the basis of two abnormal values, and the criteria for abnormal glucose values include a fasting level of at least 5.3 mmol/L (95 mg/dL), a 1-hour level of at least 10.0 mmol/L (180 mg/dL), and a 2-hour level of at least 8.6 mmol/L (155 mg/dL). Gestational DM occurs more frequently in women from ethnic/racial groups at a higher risk for type 2 DM, in obese women, and in women with a family history of DM. Perhaps most importantly, it is now established that persons with gestational DM are at very high risk for subsequent DM after delivery, a risk that appears to be reduced by proper nutrition, activity, and possibly medication.[23]

Other Types of Diabetes

Other types of DM account for 1% to 5% of all cases of diabetes in the United States.[8] Disorders directly affecting the pancreas can secondarily cause DM.[1] DM can also be secondary to endocrinopathies leading to increased counterregulatory hormone production (e.g., acromegaly, Cushing's syndrome). Pharmacologic agents can also create insulin resistance or damage to the pancreatic beta cells. Steroids and novel antipsychotic medications that increase insulin resistance and visceral fat may increase insulin requirements beyond endogenous capacity.[1,7,8]

Prediabetes

Over the past 5 years, the term "prediabetes" has emerged, especially in the United States.[13] It represents a category of individuals who are at very high risk of progression to type 2 DM. Persons with impaired glucose tolerance and/or impaired fasting glucose are classified as having prediabetes.[1] An estimated 41 million adults in the United States over 40 years of age have prediabetes.[8] Efforts to reduce the subsequent public health burden of prediabetes focus on reducing the risk of progression to type 2 DM (see below).

Treatment of DM

The overall goal of therapy for DM is to normalize energy metabolism in order to prevent acute complications such as hyperglycemia and ketoacidosis while reducing the risk of hypoglycemia. Achieving normal carbohydrate, lipid, and protein metabolism will also reduce the risk of long-term complications, including microvascular, macrovascular, and neuropathic complications. Results from clinical trials in both type 1 and type 2 DM indicate that improving metabolic control (glycemia, blood pressure, and lipids) greatly reduces the development and progression rates for microvascular, macrovascular, and neuropathic complications.[24-28] The "ABCs of Diabetes" campaign is designed to increase awareness of the goals for metabolic control: A stands for the hemoglobin A1c test HbA1c (<7%), B for blood pressure (<130/80 mmHg), and C for low-density lipoprotein cholesterol (<100 mg/mL).[29]

Two studies deserve special recognition, each providing scientific and economic rationale for improved metabolic control. The Diabetes Control and Complications Trial (DCCT) was conducted in patients with type 1 DM to compare the effects of intensive versus conventional treatment of hyperglycemia.[24] Intensive treatment reduced the mean HbA1c from 9% to 7.2%, and greater attention to dietary strategies accounted for almost one fourth of the glycemic improvement.[30] The risk of development and progression of retinopathy, albuminuria, and neuropathy was reduced by between 50% and 75% over 8 years. Reduction in the risk of complications was linearly related to the reduction in HbA1c, indicating that risk reduction can be achieved by improving glycemic control, even if a perfect or normal metabolic state is not achieved.[30] These accomplishments, as well as efforts to attenuate the two- to three-fold increase in severe hypoglycemia and weight gain, were largely due to educational and nutritional strategies.[24,31] Most recently, longer-term follow-up of the DCCT cohort has documented a continued differential in the risk of microvascular[32] and macrovascular[33] complications, even though A1c levels in the two groups have been similar for approximately 8 years.

The United Kingdom Prospective Diabetes Study (UKPDS) examined the benefit of "metabolic control" (glucose and blood pressure) in patients newly diagnosed with type 2 DM.[26-28] Fundamentally, the UKPDS confirmed that the finding of the DCCT also applied to type 2 DM. There was a reduction in macrovascular and microvascular complications, and the best results were achieved in individuals who had both glucose and blood pressure control. Similarly, there was a clear dose-response relation between metabolic and blood pressure control and the risk of DM complications. In short, any improvement in diabetes regulation matters!

Medical Nutrition Therapy of Extant DM

For persons with DM, either type 1 or 2, management includes several modalities, such as a variety of pharmacologic agents, close personal and laboratory monitoring (e.g., self-blood glucose testing, A1c and renal function testing), and careful assessment by a variety of health professionals. All of these elements, integrated and coordinated, are essential in the management of DM and are beyond the scope of this update on the nutritional dimensions of diabetes. The reader is referred to ADA publications to review recommendations.[34] This section will focus on nutritional aspects for persons with DM.

The ADA's overall goal of nutrition recommendations is to achieve and maintain improvement in metabolic control to reduce the risk of acute and long-term diabetic complications. The process of determining nutritional recommendations, including standards of care, includes reviews by a multidisciplinary panel and annual publication (see clinical practice recommendations at http://www.diabetes.org). Periodically, additional expert nutrition panels conduct a more comprehensive technical literature review with a subsequent "scientific statement" to ensure that nutrition recommendations address relevant advances in nutrition knowledge related to DM and its complications.[35-39] Table 1 lists MNT strategies for each type of diabetes. Table 2 lists current general ADA nutrition recommendations.

Several additional aspects of MNT for persons with DM are important. First, one needs to distinguish between MNT and diabetes self-management training. Although there is and should be overlap, the intent of diabetes self-management training is to provide overall guidance related to all aspects of diabetes self-management and glycemic control. MNT is a more intensive and focused comprehensive nutrition therapy service that relies heavily on follow-up and provides repeated reinforcement to help change behavior.[40,41] Issues of who decides on the content of MNT, what the scientific review process is, who delivers this important therapeutic

Table 1. Medical Nutrition Therapy Implementation Strategies by Type of Diabetes Mellitus

Type 1

- Assess usual lifestyle, focusing on eating and physical activity habits.
- Plan insulin therapy to match insulin action to lifestyle.
- Monitor blood glucose levels while keeping lifestyle consistent.
- Adjust insulin and lifestyle to achieve blood glucose levels in the target range.
- Create algorithms for adjusting insulin for lifestyle flexibility and to correct blood glucose levels that are not in the target range.

Type 2

- If overweight, reduce calorie intake to achieve 5% to 10% weight loss.
- Increase physical activity.
- Monitor blood glucose approximately four times per day to assess pattern of glycemic control.
- If postprandial glucose level is high, spread food intake throughout the day (using five or six small meals/snacks rather than having fewer larger ones).
- Reduce and/or modify type of fat to achieve weight and lipid goals.

Gestational Diabetes

- Plan calorie intake to achieve desired weight gain based on desirable body weight.
- Balance carbohydrate intake throughout the day (usually 40–50% of calories).
- Monitor glucose approximately seven times per day; adjust intake to achieve glucose levels in target range.
- Add exogenous insulin if target glucose levels are not achieved by diet alone.

Secondary Diabetes

- Assess interrelationship between primary disease(s) and secondary diabetes to establish treatment priorities.
- Institute diabetes treatment as needed to avoid short-term and long-term complications.

Prediabetes (Impaired Fasting Glucose or Impaired Glucose Tolerance)

- If overweight, reduce calorie intake to achieve 5% to 10% weight loss.
- Increase physical activity.

Table 2. Current American Diabetes Association Nutrition Recommendations

- Achieve and maintain blood glucose as near to normal range as possible by balancing dietary intake and physical activity with each other and with any antidiabetic medications.
- Achieve and maintain optimal serum lipid levels.
- Provide adequate energy intake for achieving or maintaining a reasonable weight in adults, normal rate of growth and development in children and adolescents, and optimal nutrition during pregnancy and lactation or during recovery from catabolic illnesses.
- Prevent acute complications such as severe hypoglycemia or hyperglycemia.
- Prevent or treat long-term complications such as cardiovascular disease (including hypertension, dyslipidemia, and other risk factors), renal disease, and neuropathy (especially gastroparesis).
- Improve overall health through optimal nutrition

Data from UK Prospective Diabetes Study Group 1998.[26,27]

approach, and how economic considerations should affect decisions vary greatly by health system, culture, and country.[40,41]

Medical Nutrition Therapy for Type 1 DM

The focus of MNT is to assist in the achievement of metabolic normality if possible; with type 1 DM, this means coordinating nutrition approaches to insulin and physical activity, as well as moment-to-moment measures of blood glucose levels throughout the day with self-blood glucose monitoring. Multiple insulins are available (Table 3) and often are used in various combinations. A typical approach in terms of insulin use would be to inject a very-long-acting insulin in the morning to establish a constant basal amount of insulin, and supplement this basal insulin with injections of short-acting insulin before meals. Many other combinations exist. Thus, in terms of nutrition, the timing and content of meals need to be consistent as much as possible from day to day to keep the blood glucose as close to normal as possible over a 24-hour period. Added into the mix of various insulins and nutrition, physical activity is another important element influencing glucose control. Self-blood glucose monitoring, education, and experience allow the individual to learn how to keep all of this in balance.

The approaches to nutritional interventions used in the DCCT can be a powerful example of ideal nutrition counseling for patients with type 1 DM. Dietary behaviors associated with better glycemic control in the intensively treated group included adherence to an overall meal plan (timing and amount of carbohydrate), appropriate treatment of hypoglycemia (avoiding excessive consumption of carbohydrate to treat symptoms), prompt intervention for hyperglycemia (more insulin and/or less food), and consistent consumption of planned evening snacks.[31] Predictors of severe hypoglycemia requiring treatment included a history of impaired awareness of hypoglycemia or episodes of severe hypoglycemia, inconsistent food habits, and achieving a A1c level close to the normal range.[28] The mean level of weight gain in the intensively treated group was reduced by 50% after the intervention staff focused on strategies to control weight gain (e.g., avoiding excessive food consumption to prevent and treat hypoglycemia).[30]

The American Dietetic Association has developed and evaluated MNT for type 1 DM.[38] In the randomized field test, specific guidelines for nutrition counseling were used by dietitians with 24 patients, and results were com-

Table 3. Insulin Preparations: Onset, Peak, and Duration of Action

Insulins	Brand Name	Onset of Action	Peak Action	Duration of Action
Very Rapid Acting				
Insulin aspart analog	NovoLog			
Insulin lispro analog	Humalog	10–20 min	0.5–2.5 hours	3–5 hours
Regular insulin	Humulin R			
	Novolin R	30–40 min	2–4 hours	5–7 hours
Intermediate Acting				
NPH insulin	Humulin N			
	Novolin N	1–3 hours	4–10 hours	14–24 hours
Lente insulin	Humulin L	2–4 hours	4–15 hours	16–24 hours
Long Acting				
Ultralente insulin	Humulin U	3–4 hours	8–14 hours	18–24 hours
Insulin glargine	Lantus	1–2 hours	No peak	Approx. 24 hours

pared with those of 30 patients receiving "usual counseling" as the control treatment condition. The mean HbA1c in the guidelines-treated patient group was significantly reduced compared with the control group (1.0% vs. 0.3%).[38]

The process of intensifying type 1 DM management to improve glycemic control involves several stages and individualization of insulin, physical activity, monitoring, and nutrition therapy. The initial stage, usually lasting three or four visits, focuses on basic skills needed by newly diagnosed patients and those with little or no previous nutrition knowledge or a history of poor glycemic control. Nutrition counseling emphasizes consistency of carbohydrate intake and eating times. Blood glucose monitoring provides information about the patterns of response. Patients need to gain a basic understanding of the relationship between insulin action and lifestyle before moving on to more complex planning to achieve both better glycemic control and a more flexible lifestyle. An initial bolus dose of insulin is often estimated to provide one unit per 15 g carbohydrate. Gradually, algorithms are developed to adjust insulin for changes in carbohydrate intake or physical activity. After mastering insulin adjustment and supplementation, patients learn to adjust insulin for changes in food or activity using a ratio of carbohydrate intake to insulin dosage.

Medical Nutrition Therapy for Type 2 DM

Among efforts to establish normal metabolism to prevent longer-term DM complications, reducing cardiovascular risk is a primary goal for MNT and the overall management of type 2 DM.[4] Diet and exercise are considered to be the first step to achieve euglycemia, with focus often on the health risks associated with overweight and obesity. However, medical care standards and experience with type 2 DM indicates that to reduce both cardiovascular and microvascular risk, patients often must take five or more medications to achieve blood glucose, blood pressure, and cholesterol goals, as well as low-dose aspirin. Supporting the benefits of MNT, the amount of medication needed is likely to be less with a modest weight loss of 5% to 10% of body weight.[4,20,42] The impact of weight loss is most dramatically demonstrated by patients undergoing bariatric surgery, a procedure reserved for selected patients with type 2 DM and obesity. However, the effects of bariatric surgery appear to be largely independent of weight loss and may be due to changes in hormonal metabolism.[43]

Guidelines for MNT in type 2 DM, focusing particularly on controlling glycemia, dyslipidemia, and hypertension, have been validated and supported by a randomized clinical trial.[38] For hyperglycemia, there are four general types of oral agents: sulfonylureas (to stimulate insulin release), biguinides (to decrease hepatic glucose production), thiozolidindiones (to reduce insulin resistance), and α-glucosidase inhibitors (to decrease glucose absorption).[41] When lifestyle changes or MNT do not achieve euglycemia, combinations of these oral agents with or without concomitant insulin will optimize metabolic control. Likewise, for both hypertension and hyperlipidemia, a variety of agents exist and are increasingly being used in combination to treat type 2 DM (Table 4).[4] Thus, it is not surprising that many persons with type 2 DM are taking many medications on a daily basis.

Gestational DM

The goal of therapy in gestational DM is to achieve and maintain euglycemia to improve pregnancy outcomes; reduce risks to the fetus/baby, such as macrosomia and perinatal complications; and perhaps reduce chances of fetal malnutrition, with subsequent increased risk for adult chronic diseases.[23,44,45] Women with gestational DM actually have nutrition requirements similar to those of other pregnant women but are much more likely to also be overweight. The Fourth International Workshop/Conference on Gestational Diabetes Mellitus recommended the following caloric intake per kilogram of present pregnant weight: 167 kJ (40 kcal)/kg if less than 80% desirable body weight (DBW); 126 kJ (30kcal)/kg if 80% to 120% DBW; 100 kJ(24 kcal)/kg if 121% to 150% DBW; and 50 kJ (12 kcal)/kg if more than 150% DBW. A weight gain of 6.8 kg (15 lb) or less is recommended for women who are 150% or more DBW.[46] The recommendations addressed the effects of carbohydrate on the 1-hour postprandial glucose level, suggesting limiting carbohydrate to approximately 40% of energy intake and distribution intake into six feedings, with 10% to 15% for breakfast, 20% to 30% for lunch, 30% to 40% for dinner, and 10% for each of three between-meal snacks.[46]

Although experiences with the above approaches to MNT during pregnancy among persons with gestational DM have stood the test of time, most clinicians and investigators feel strongly that randomized, controlled trials are needed to establish more valid guidelines with respect to dietary composition (amounts and types of carbohydrates and fats), weight gain, and energy and carbohydrate restriction.

Diet and Nutrition Composition

Historical Overview

For all types of DM, issues of total calories and/or nutrition composition have been discussed for centuries. Historically, nutrition has been considered important in the management of DM, even though the specific recommendations for nutrition composition have varied widely. The first recommendation, from Papyrus Ebers in 1550 BC, focused on eating carbohydrate-containing foods. Restriction of carbohydrate-containing foods seemed to emerge in the 6th century AD. During the 17th and 18th centuries, recommendations varied from replacing sugar loss with a high-carbohydrate diet to eating meat and fat and avoiding carbohydrate. During the 19th and early

Table 4. Oral Antidiabetic Medications: Mechanism of Action and Side Effects

Medication Class and Mechanism of Action	Generic Name	Brand Name	Comments and Side Effects
Sulfonylureas			
Stimulate the pancreatic beta cell to produce more insulin	Chlorpropamide first-generation	Diabinese	Hypoglycemia risk, especially in the elderly.
	Tolazamide first-generation	Tolinase	Hypoglycemia risk.
	Glyburide second-generation	Micronase Diabeta Glynase Pres Tab	Hypoglycemic risk lower than first-generation sulfonylureas.
	Glipizide second-generation	Glucotrol Glucotrol XL	Take twice a day or once (XL). May cause hypoglycemia.
	Glimepiride third-generation	Amaryl	Take once a day.
Biguanides			
Reduce output of glucose from the liver	Metformin	Glucophage	Contraindicated in patients with congestive heart, renal, or liver problems. Check creatinine clearance if over 65 years of age.
Alpha Glucosidase Inhibitors			
Delay and block absorption of carbohydrate-containing foods	Acarbose Miglitol	Precose Glyset	May have side effects in the gastrointestinal tract
Thiazolidinediones			
Enhance insulin sensitivity	Rosiglitazone Pioglitazone	Avandia Actos	Fluid retention, which can lead to congestive heart failure in the elderly or other high-risk patients. Reduced effectiveness of birth control pills. Contraindicated in liver disease. Check liver enzymes on an ongoing basis.
Meglitinides			
Enhance insulin secretion in the presence of glucose	Repaglinide	Prandin	Some risk of hypoglycemia. Medication is taken when food is eaten because its action is dependent on the presence of glucose.

20th century, serious fasting and measured diabetic diets that limited carbohydrate were widely used. Simultaneously, some patients were actually treated with higher-carbohydrate diets that focused on potatoes or oatmeal. High carbohydrates became the preparatory diet for glucose tolerance tests to diagnose diabetes during the 1930s.

Since the 1950s, the ADA has used expert groups to develop recommendations and educational materials for the nutritional management of DM.[4,35] Initially, the focus was an "exchange system" for meal planning, with precalculated meal plans to achieve a macronutrient distribution of 20% protein, 40% fat, and 40% carbohydrate. Recommendations focused on achieving ideal body weight and avoiding simple sugars and individualization within this exchange system approach. Gradually, as cardiovascular complications became recognized as a large part of DM, recommendations focused on decreasing dietary fat and increasing carbohydrate consumption up to 60% of calories. By 1994, the ADA focused on individualization based on a dietitian's assessment, with no specific recommendations for the balance between total fat and carbohydrate intake.[4,35]

In considering the remarkable variation in nutrition recommendations over the past years and decades, greater scientific study and evidence-based recommendations are required to provide useful and validated recommendations.

Present Nutrition Recommendations

The approach for determining desirable macronutrient distribution among patients with DM is based on the Institute of Medicine Dietary Reference Intakes and on individual considerations with respect to body weight, metabolic control, concomitant conditions other than diabetes, diabetic complications, and food preferences.[47] MNT guidelines for the management of type 2 DM are in clinical trials.[48-50] For example, a recent study by Samaha et al. that compared very low carbohydrate with a ketosis induction to a low-fat diet included a subset of patients with type 2 DM.[51,52] After 6 and 12 months on the diet, the diabetic patients in the low-carbohydrate arm required fewer DM medications and tended to have better HbA1c levels than those in the low-fat arm.[49,53] More recent studies about various approaches to nutrition and weight loss are not only interesting on their own, but perhaps more importantly, indicate a commitment to greater scientific rigor in recommendations regarding various dietary approaches for chronic diseases, including DM.[54] For persons with DM, however, these studies must pay attention to more than just glycemic control; they must also address dsylipidemia and hypertension.

Specific Nutritional Components

Protein. Protein intake needs to be adequate for normal growth, development, and maintenance of body functions. Factors considered by the ADA in its recommendations included the adult Recommended Dietary Allowance for protein intake (0.8 g/kg body wt/d), or approximately 10% of total daily energy needs. (The average adult protein intake in the United States is approximately 20% of energy intake.[38,39]) The recommendations indicate that individuals who may need at least 20% of energy intake from protein include those in a catabolic state, those with growth needs (children, adolescents, and pregnant women), and individuals on very-low-energy diets to achieve weight loss.

Recommendations for protein intake in individuals with normal renal function are based on the review for Daily Recommended Intakes by the Institute of Medicine and are similar to recommendations for the general public.[4,47] However, the ADA recommends reducing protein intake to 0.6 g/kg body wt/d in selected patients to slow the rate of decline of glomerular filtration rate.[4,39]

Fat Macronutrients. Most observational and interventional studies indicate that total energy intake increases as the total and proportion of calories from fat rise. Higher fat intake is closely linked to overweight and obesity, and these conditions are related to the incidence of type 2 DM. Simultaneously, in considering the amount of fat in the diet, the satiety value of fat and controlling postprandial glycemic excursions must also be considered.[4,36,38] Finally, decreasing dietary fat and increasing carbohydrate intake can potentially worsen the dyslipidemia of type 2 DM by lowering high-density lipoprotein cholesterol levels and increasing the level of very-low-density lipoprotein cholesterol, triglyceride, and small, dense, low-density lipoprotein cholesterol particles—effects that can be ameliorated by weight loss.[38,47] Thus, one can appreciate the complexity of nutritional approaches to diabetes, especially in simultaneously balancing fat and carbohydrate intake.

Type of Fat. The ATP III guidelines classify most people with DM as being at high risk for cardiovascular disease within the next 10 years—that is, diabetes is a cardiovascular disease "risk factor equivalent."[55] Thus, the goals of treatment are lower than in the absence of diabetes: serum low-density lipoprotein level less than 70 mg/dL and dietary goals with less than 7% of calories from saturated fat and less than 200 mg cholesterol. Whether there are individuals with DM who are at lower risk for cardiovascular disease is controversial.[4,56] For prediabetes saturated fat should be restricted to no more than 10% of calories and dietary cholesterol intake to 300 mg/d.

Both monounsaturated and polyunsaturated fatty acids reduce low-density lipoprotein cholesterol levels, but they may differ with respect to their effect on high-density lipoprotein cholesterol levels. Reducing intake of total fat and saturated fatty acids in particular tends to further reduce a low high-density lipoprotein cholesterol level associated with insulin resistance and diabetes. However, weight loss may ameliorate this effect. In a meta-analysis of dietary intervention studies in patients with type 2 DM, Garg[57] reported that diets high in monounsaturated fats reduced the very-low-density lipoprotein cholesterol and triglyceride levels by 22% and 19% respectively and did not adversely affect body weight.

Hydrogenization of the cis-isomer of fatty acids in oils creates trans isomers that function like more saturated fatty acids in food products and potentially in the human body. Epidemiologic studies have linked "trans fatty acid" consumption to increased cardiovascular risk, but to date there are no intervention studies that specifically address the extent to which trans fatty acid intake may increase the risk of cardiovascular disease. Individuals with DM and/or other risk factors for cardiovascular disease should keep trans fatty acid intake as low as possible.[53]

Considerable interest exists in the intake of fish and omega-3 acids.[58] For example, the rates of diabetes and cardiovascular disease are lower in population groups with a high fish intake, perhaps because fatty acids from fish and other sources that have the double bond in the omega-3 position reduce triglyceride production.[59] A recent systematic review of clinical trials of fish oils conducted in patients with DM showed a 30% reduction in fasting triglyceride levels, a slight increase (approximately 2%) in low-density lipoprotein cholesterol, and no change in HbA1c levels.[59] Fasting glucose levels decreased in studies involving subjects with type 1 DM and tended to increase slightly in the studies involving subjects with type 2 DM. However, having DM should not be considered a contraindication to the use of omega-3 fatty acid supplements as a treatment option for hypertriglyceridemia.

Carbohydrates, Type of Carbohydrate, and Sweeteners. Postprandial hyperglycemia has become a major concern in the management of DM,[4,60] and there is considerable debate over the role of the amount and type of carbohydrate in obesity and diabetes.[61-64] The restriction of table sugar or sucrose is often used in an attempt to improve glycemic control. However, studies conducted in the 1970s and 1980s indicated that glycemic response to mono- and disaccharides did not result in higher postprandial glycemic response than polysaccharides.[35] Thus, the glycemic effect of carbohydrate-containing foods has been studied extensively and is the source of considerable debate with respect to its effects on glycemic control and weight.[35,36,61,62] The ADA's nutrition recommendations indicate that glycemic control was not contingent on restricting sucrose and suggested that the decision about sugar consumption should be based on overall nutrition considerations.[4,35,36] Nonetheless, consumption of large quantities of sugars (e.g., high-fructose corn syrup in soft drinks and other beverages) is a major source of excess calories.[61,63]

In further examining the effects of the amount and type of dietary carbohydrate in DM management, it has been documented that "intrinsic variables" can influence the degree of glucose excursions.[36] These intrinsic variables include the physical form of the food (i.e., juice vs. whole fruit, mashed potato vs. whole potato), ripeness, degree of processing, type of starch (i.e., amylose vs. amylopectin), style of preparation (e.g., cooking method and time, amount of heat or moisture used), and the specific type (e.g., fettucine vs. macaroni) or variety (e.g., long-grain rice vs. short-grain rice) of the food. Extrinsic variables that may influence glucose response include fasting or preprandial glucose level, degree of insulin resistance, and the macronutrient distribution.

The concept of "glycemic indexing" of food was developed to compare the effects of the quality of carbohydrate while keeping the amount of carbohydrate standardized. The estimated "glycemic load" of foods, meals, and dietary patterns is calculated by multiplying the glycemic index by the amount of carbohydrate in each food and then totaling all of the foods in a meal or dietary pattern. The role of the glycemic index and/or glycemic load is controversial,[65] although modifying the type as well as the amount of carbohydrate can improve glycemic control.[66]

Although fiber itself may complicate the interpretation of approaches using the glycemic index,[67] a dietary intake that contains 14 g fiber per 1000 kcal (recommended for the general public) is also recommended for people with DM.[35] To reach this goal, intake of legumes, fiber-rich grains, and whole fruits and vegetables often needs to be increased.[4]

In essence, given the many factors that can affect glucose metabolism, including those beyond nutrition per se (e.g., medicines, activity), it is often problematic to predict the exact plasma glucose response to specific carbohydrate-containing foods. Certainly, blood glucose self-monitoring and experience can help predict the glycemic effects of food products. Further, a variety of methods can be used to estimate the nutrient content of meals, including carbohydrate counting, the exchange system, and experience. To date, however, research has not demonstrated that one method of assessing the relationship between dietary carbohydrates and blood glucose is better than other methods. Still, with emerging evidence of the relations among postprandial glycemia and cardiovascular disease,[60] postprandial glucose levels are of increasing importance.

Several important dimensions of "carbohydrates and diabetes" deserve additional consideration. First, because DM complications are associated with tissue protein glycation and because heated foods containing sugar can also form glycation end products,[63,64] concern has been expressed about the possible role of these ingested glycated products in the pathogenesis of DM complications. Although only about 10% of ingested advanced glycation end products enter the circulation, they are excreted slowly, especially in patients with DM. However, considerably more research is needed to determine whether such dietary components can alter the risk of DM complications.

Second is the role of "carbohydrate substitutions." Fructose, mannitol, and sorbitol are often substituted for sucrose in "sugar-free" products. In experimental studies, these products can shift the balance from oxidation of fatty acids to esterification of fatty acids in the liver, which can in turn increase very-low-density lipoprotein synthesis.[35] Although the effects on serum lipids are inconsistent, susceptible individuals may have a worsening of dyslipidemia. These sweeteners appear to offer no documented advantage in the management of DM over other carbohydrate sources.

Third, reading the label on dietary products about carbohydrates can be confusing. Many food products list the "net" or "impact" carbohydrate on the front of the label, a value considerably lower than the "total" carbohydrate listed in the nutrient facts panel. Fiber or fiber plus the sugar alcohols is usually subtracted to obtain the net or impact carbohydrate value, but there is no standardization. If patients with DM use these products, monitoring is needed to determine the effects on blood glucose.[61]

Fourth is the possible role of sugar or fat replacers. "High-intensity sweeteners" are widely used as a replacement for various types of sugar in food and beverage products. Currently approved intense sweeteners include aspartame, saccharin, acesulfame K, and sucralose. Patients with DM use products containing these sweeteners to control energy and carbohydrate intake.[35] Fat replacers mimic one or more of the roles of fat in a food; they may be protein-based (usually from egg white or whey), carbohydrate-based (from modified starches, dextrins, or maltodextrins), or fat-based (from emulsifiers replacing triglycerides with mono- or disaccharides or from modification to achieve a partially absorbable or nonabsorbable fat). Patients with DM may encounter difficulty eating fat replacers if food products containing them are higher in energy density than the original product or when carbohydrate calculations are not adjusted.[35]

Fifth, alcohol consumption among persons with DM and the possible impact on both carbohydrate and fat metabolism need to be considered. In general, the recommendations with regard to alcohol intake are similar to those for the general public, and moderate intake (the equivalent of two or fewer drinks) does not have a major effect on metabolic control.[35] However, alcohol can inhibit hepatic glucose production and cause hypoglycemia if consumed without food in patients taking insulin or sulfonylureas. Conversely, consuming large amounts of alcohol can raise blood glucose levels, especially in the presence of severe insulin deficiency. Finally, alcohol intake should be avoided or severely limited by patients with pancreatitis, hypertriglyceridemia, neuropathy, myocardiopathy, or renal failure.

Micronutrients. The relations between DM and micronutrients are reciprocal: micronutrients can affect DM, and DM and its complications can alter the metabolism and impact of micronutrients. Poorly controlled diabetes can alter vitamin and mineral status, and micronutrients can affect glucose and overall energy homeostasis.[35]

Herbal and Other Supplements. Studies indicate that many patients with DM consume supplements and do not alert their health care professionals about this use.[68] Consultation regarding the use of supplements should help patients with DM evaluate the potential risks and benefits of these products.[69-74] One clinical study that evaluated the effects of a multivitamin supplement on quality of life and missed days of activity found some benefit for the subgroup with DM and those over 65 years of age.[70] Although antioxidant nutrients appear to play a role in reducing oxidative stress and possibly in insulin sensitivity, there is insufficient evidence at present to warrant making any specific recommendation about use of the substances in DM management.[4] This level of uncertainty has been raised by two large randomized, controlled trials that failed to demonstrate a positive impact of antioxidant vitamins on cardiovascular disease, including patients with DM.[75,76] A survey of providers of alternative therapies used in DM found that the 10 most commonly recommended nutrient supplements were biotin, vanadium, chromium, vitamin B_6, vitamin C, vitamin E, zinc, selenium, alpha-lipoic acid, and fructo-oligosaccharides, and the 10 most commonly recommended herbal supplements were gymnema, psyllium, fenugreek, bilberry, garlic, Chinese ginseng, dandelion, burdock, prickly pear cactus, and bitter melon.[71] Although these products may have some blood glucose-lowering effects, a patient's use of these products is not generally evaluated as part of his or her medical or dietary history. Having an open dialogue about the use of alternative therapies provides the opportunity to explore how they may interact with prescribed medications, either beneficially or harmfully.[71]

Some of these supplements have received more attention—in the laboratory, clinical world, and media—than others. Although some research suggests that chromium supplementation may improve insulin sensitivity and glucose metabolism in DM, research results are highly mixed. Limitations of the chromium studies to date include inadequate sample size, short duration, non-randomized design, lack of information about the pre-study chromium status of the study population, and different doses of chromium supplementation—all of which may account for the high variability of the findings.[72] Long-term clinical trials are needed to examine chromium in relation to DM using hard end-points (e.g., type 2 DM and cardiovascular disease) and metabolic parameters and to assess the safety of long-term chromium supplementation.[72]

Magnesium modulates glucose transport across cell membranes, and poorly controlled DM can induce hypomagnesemia by increasing urinary excretion, with possible increased insulin resistance.[35] The clinical usefulness of supplementation, usually by intake of magnesium-based antacids, for patients with type 2 DM and insulin resistance is, however, not established. As another example of the present disconnect between laboratory and clinical studies, in laboratory experiments, zinc and antioxidant requirements increase during wound healing,[35] but the need for supplementation for every patient postsurgery or with a foot ulcer remains to be confirmed.[4]

Other inorganic trace elements such as vanadium, copper, iron, potassium, sodium, and nickel may play an important role in the maintenance of normoglycemia by activating the beta cells of the pancreas. Sources of these elements are often contained in various alternative/complementary medications. For example, analysis of the mineral content of the leaves from four plants used in Asian traditional medicine (*Murraya koenigii*, *Mentha piperitae*, *Ocimum sanctum*, and *Aegle marmelos*) yielded moderate levels of copper, nickel, zinc, potassium, and sodium (which may account for the reported therapeutic benefit if the basic food supply is inadequate).[74] However, the need for this supplementation, should the nutrients in the dietary pattern recommended in the 2005 Dietary Guidelines be accomplished,[77] is not apparent among persons with DM based on more valid clinical studies.

The B vitamin group is a final category of "herbal supplements" to consider, particularly thiamin, riboflavin, niacin, and vitamin B_6, all of which are involved in glucose metabolism. Among persons with poorly controlled diabetes and polyuria associated with hyperglycemia, requirements may be altered by excess excretion in the urine. Ironically, nicotinic acid itself can worsen glycemic control when it is used to treat hyperlipidemia; however, uncontrolled studies suggest that it may also help to protect beta-cell function from autoimmune destruction. Folate and vitamin B_{12} levels play a role in homocysteine metabolism, and plasma levels of these nutrients are inversely related to homocysteine levels. In patients with type 2 DM, plasma homocysteine concentration is a significant predictor of cardiovascular events and death, perhaps due to worsening of endothelial dysfunction and/or structural vessel properties induced by oxidative stress.[78] Elevated fasting homocysteine levels appear to be a biomarker for subsequent development of type 2 DM in women.[79] However, to confirm that a particular measurement is actually a risk factor (vs. a risk marker), it is desirable that a randomized, controlled trial be conducted to show that the alteration in the compound being measured is associated with benefits to patients. Such clinical trials are being completed, and results do not indicate a relationship between homocysteine perturbations and subsequent stroke or myocardial infarctions.[80,81]

Prediabetes

There is convincing evidence that improved diabetes control—both secondary and tertiary prevention—can reduce long-term DM complications, and that MNT plays a very important role in normalization of blood glucose, blood pressure, and blood lipids. However, the dramatically increased prevalence of type 2 DM throughout the world portends a health care system becoming overwhelmed with "diabetes needs" despite the presence of validated scientific tools that can make a difference among patients with extant diabetes. Fortunately, over the past 5 to 6 years, studies have been conducted that establish the validity of efforts in primary prevention among those with prediabetes and the critical role of addressing obesity, overweight, and physical inactivity.[82-94]

The DaQing IGT and Diabetes Study provided preliminary evidence that diet and exercise interventions lowered the conversion to overt diabetes over the 6-year period.[85] The Finnish Diabetes Prevention Study (FDPS) in 577 individuals with impaired glucose tolerance achieved a 58% reduction in the incidence of type 2 DM with lifestyle interventions.[86-88] There were small but significant reductions in total cholesterol, triglyceride, and systolic blood pressure and a rise in high-density lipoprotein cholesterol in the lifestyle intervention arm but not in the control group, and PAI-1 levels fell significantly in the lifestyle group in proportion to weight reduction.[87] Studies from the FDPS of candidate genes affecting energy metabolism showed the importance of genetic polymorphism in defining responses to lifestyle interventions.[88]

The Diabetes Prevention Program, a randomized, controlled, clinical trial conducted in 3234 individuals with impaired glucose tolerance, showed that the incidence of diabetes could be reduced by 58% over a 3-year period with a 7% weight loss.[89-94] The 3-year reduction in diabetes incidence with weight loss was almost double the 31% reduction achieved with metformin, a medication that increases insulin sensitivity. Treatment effects did not differ by sex, race, or ethnic group. Unlike the lifestyle intervention, which was effective across the entire baseline body weight and fasting glucose ranges, metformin was ineffective in those with a BMI less than 30 kg/m^2 and minimally effective in those with a BMI less than 35 kg/m^2 or with a fasting glucose level of less than 110 mg/dL. As in the FDPS, insulin sensitivity improved in the lifestyle group, with a smaller increase in the metformin group, but did not change in the placebo group. Insulin secretion decreased in all groups, but was associated with improved beta-cell function only in the lifestyle group. The lifestyle intervention resulted in a lower prevalence and needed medical treatment of hypertension and dyslipidemia. The lifestyle intervention also lowered inflammatory biomarkers (CRP and PAI-1) associated with increased cardiovascular risk.[44] In the placebo group, of the participants who did not have the metabolic syndrome at baseline, 51% had developed it at the study's end. The lifestyle intervention reduced the prevalence by 33%; metformin reduced it by only 15%.

Using the Diabetes Prevention Program results compared with the placebo intervention, on average, the lifestyle intervention would delay the onset of diabetes by 11 years.[94] Expressed in terms of a lifetime, 83% of the placebo participants compared with 63% of the lifestyle participants would develop diabetes, amounting to a reduction in absolute risk for developing diabetes of 20% in the lifestyle group. The simulated lifetime cumulative incidence of microvascular and macrovascular complications and life expectancy indicated that compared with placebo, the lifestyle intervention would reduce the cumulative incidence of blindness by 39%, end-stage renal disease by 38%, amputation by 35%, stroke by 9%, and coronary heart disease by 8%, and would increase life expectancy by 0.5 years.[94] Compared with the placebo intervention, the lifestyle intervention cost per quality-adjusted life-years would be approximately $1100. For metformin, the cost per quality-adjusted life-year was calculated using costs of the generic form of the drug as $1800.

Both the Diabetes Prevention Program and FDPS asked participants to self-monitor their food intake.[86,87,91] In the Finnish study, participants were asked to complete 3-day food records four times per year; in the Diabetes Prevention Program, participants were asked to self-monitor their activity, food intake, calories, and fat grams daily during the first 24 weeks and then at least 1 week per month thereafter. In the Diabetes Prevention Program, the frequency of dietary self-monitoring was related to success at achieving both the physical activity goal and the weight loss goal. Moreover, participants who were 65 or older were more likely to complete self-monitoring records, report a lower percentage of calories from fat, and meet the activity and weight loss goals than those who were less than 45 years old.[91] Thus, it is not surprising that older participants had a greater (71%) risk reduction in the development of diabetes with lifestyle interventions.[48,92] Lifestyle coaches in the Diabetes Prevention Program taught the participants to use a problem-solving approach to manage high-risk situations (stress, vacations, eating out) and used a toolbox approach to deal with barriers to lifestyle change.

Thus, there is now convincing scientific and economic evidence that primary prevention of type 2 DM is both possible and cost-effective. However, in all studies to date, interventions were applied to individuals with a very high risk of developing DM—persons with prediabetes.[13] Whether such interventions would also be effective in persons who are overweight or obese or inactive, with a positive family history and so forth, but without prediabetes, is not yet established. Because most persons who develop type 2 DM emerge from the group with prediabetes[93] and because the size of the prediabetes population is quite large in the United States and probably throughout the world,[8,9] approaching the identification and preventive treatment of prediabetes remains the next great challenge for the medical and public health community.

Public Health Issues

Achieving population-level impact in the primary, secondary, and tertiary prevention of DM is a complex task. Addressing nutrition issues at all three levels requires collaborations involving a wide variety of partners to ensure an appropriate balance between efforts to prevent and treat DM complications and efforts to prevent the onset of DM. Clearly, factors beyond what occurs in a doctor's office have a dramatic impact on both preventive and management strategies for chronic diseases, including all types of DM. Insurance status, federal and state policies, opportunities for proper nutrition and activity at schools, reimbursement strategies, federal deficits: all these and other factors will have a significant impact on the individual health provider and/or patient in terms of how well DM can be prevented and/or treated. These typically are not issues that are discussed in the office, but they must be included in larger efforts to address all aspects of nutrition and diabetes.[95,96] The ability to capitalize on prevention opportunities requires a strong infrastructure to plan and support interventions, nurture partnerships, and monitor and evaluate progress. Much of the effort to date has targeted identifying individuals at risk for DM and also DM complications, and increasing public awareness of DM risks, especially in communities with populations at great risk for DM.

Many efforts within the voluntary, professional, academic, and private sectors address these challenges of DM. The National Diabetes Education Program, a partnership of the National Institutes of Health and the Centers for Disease Control and Prevention, tries to serve as a "coordinating entity" among more than 200 public and private organizations.[97] In addition, the Centers for Disease Control and Prevention's Division of Diabetes Translation is addressing community infrastructure and environmental issues to reduce the burden of DM, including public health surveillance systems for DM, applied translational research, state-based DM control programs, and public information.[98] The National Institutes of Health has also expanded the focus of research to address how environmental factors and community infrastructure are related to obesity and the risk of DM and other chronic illnesses. The ADA, an active member of the National Diabetes Education Program, is partnering with the American Cancer Society and the American Heart Association to provide unified public messages and recommendations that address the role of nutrition in reducing chronic disease burden.[99] With the growing awareness of the worldwide burden of DM, as well as the fact that scientific and economic studies, both in the care and prevention arenas, indicate that this burden does not have to occur, societal approaches need to be developed to complement clinical strategies to address DM in all of its complexities.[100]

Research Needs

There is considerable evidence on the effectiveness of MNT and the role of nutrition in preventing DM and in preventing and controlling complications. However, additional research is needed to address environmental factors related to the rapid rise in the prevalence of obesity and to develop effective techniques to reduce the obesity and physical inactivity epidemics—both of which are mutable (unlike age or race/ethnicity) and contribute to the increased prevalence of DM. Research is needed to examine how nutritional factors other than weight loss may affect the risk of developing DM.

Current research will yield additional evidence to assess the long-term effectiveness of weight-loss lifestyle interventions in preventing DM and the development of DM complications. MNT is not only an important component in the "ABCs" campaign to achieve goals for HbA1c, blood pressure, and cholesterol, but nutrition is also integral to current clinical trials addressing these risk factors.

Of particular practical need is a better understanding on how to both prevent and control weight gain. Evidence-based overweight and obesity guidelines were developed in 1998, and more recent research that addresses weight loss and DM prevention supports the overall approach in those guidelines.[11] The recommendations include a comprehensive assessment that includes measuring and evaluating relative body weight or body mass index (BMI), measuring body fat distribution (waist circumference as an index of visceral fat accumulation), evaluating overall risk status (for DM and related factors), and evaluating motivation to lose weight. Although weight is frequently measured, BMI evaluation is often not recorded, and few practice settings measure waist circumference and assess weight loss motivation. Research is needed to evaluate barriers to assessing weight, especially with respect to body fat distribution and motivation. The more recent DM prevention trials strongly support a 5% to 10% weight loss in 6 months with a comprehensive approach that combines dietary, physical activity, and behavioral interventions. Analysis from the Diabetes Prevention Program suggests that there may be a benefit of lifestyle changes even if no weight loss is achieved.[92,94,98]

The Look-AHEAD trial will determine the effects of weight loss on cardiovascular risks in individuals with type 2 DM.[101] Meal replacements, usually with a liquid formula, are of increasing interest and are being evaluated in this trial. A small, randomized trial of meal replacement in patients with type 2 DM found a greater weight loss using a liquid formula meal replacement approach than with individualized meal planning. However, previous research suggests that providing menus may be as effective as providing food.[101,102] Therefore, more research is needed to determine the extent to which being provided with a structure to avoid making food decisions facilitates achieving energy intake goals and weight loss. The short- and longer-term effects of these formulas on metabolic parameters are also of interest. To date, research on the metabolic effects has largely focused on ill patients. Meta-analyses were performed using 23 studies (784 patients) of liquid supplements (16 studies) and tube feeding (7 studies) to compare DM-specific with standard formulas.[101,102] Results indicated that the DM-specific formulas significantly reduced postprandial increases in blood glucose, peak blood glucose concentration, and glucose area under the curve (four trials showed a 35% lower area under the curve) compared with standard formulas. Individual studies reported a reduced requirement for insulin (26%–71% lower) and fewer acute complications with DM-specific versus standard nutritional formulas. However, there were no significant differences in high-density lipoprotein, total cholesterol, or triglyceride concentrations.[101,102]

Areas of Controversy and Uncertainty

Although broad research needs will require multiple methods of research ranging from studies in nutrition-gene interaction and effects on cell metabolism to studies that explore how community, state, national, and international policy may affect the prevalence of obesity and DM, a few aspects of both type 1 and 2 DM deserve particular attention because of the excitement, yet uncertainty, surrounding these topics.

Type 1 DM

The basic etiology of type 1 DM is not yet established: even if one assumes that an autoimmune mechanism is involved in progressive beta-cell destruction, the factor(s) initiating this autoimmunity is not clearly known.[16] Toxins or viral exposures have been suggested,[16] but more recently, the possibility of specific food ingredients at a critical time of life initiating autoimmunity has been explored. Two particular types of food are being investigated: cow's milk and cereal.

Over the past several years, interesting hypotheses have been proposed regarding whether the absence of breast-feeding and/or early exposure to infant formula (i.e., a cow's milk protein) might be involved in the initiation of type 1 autoimmunity.[16,103] Cross-sectional epidemiologic studies indicate a link between early introduction of cow's milk formula and the development of type 1 DM. Possible mechanisms suggested for this association include: 1) triggering autoantibody reactivity to the milk protein, and 2) almost by accident in an "innocent bystander" scenario in genetically susceptible individuals, a protein structure in the beta cell with great similarity to the cow's milk protein is recognized as foreign and thus attacked. Equally important may be the absence of the immunoprotection of breast-feeding.[104]

One ecologic study of the 37 world areas reporting a 3% yearly increase of type 1 DM evaluated DM incidence in relation to dietary patterns using the Food and Agriculture Organization's Food Balance Sheets.[17] The incidence of DM appeared to be related to the milk supply from 1961 to 2000. Several molecular, genetic, and clinical studies addressing the possible role of protein in cow's milk are ongoing, and a large-scale epidemiologic project called TRIGER is examining on a population basis a possible relation between cow's milk and type 1 DM.[105] Should a relationship be established, it may be relevant only in persons with genetic susceptibility to autoimmunity, and thus broader versus targeted recommendations for breast-feeding would need to be resolved.

Earlier studies suggested that exposure to certain food components might initiate later-onset autoimmunity conditions such as celiac disease from infant gluten exposure.[106] Likewise, the BABYDIAB and DAISY studies[107,108] suggested that there is a link between infant diet and the development of early autoimmunity against pancreatic beta cells. Further, the timing of this exposure (between 3 and 7 months) has been identified as a period of considerable vulnerability in the initiation of autoimmunity, particularly in so-called genetically high-risk individuals. However, as reviewed by Atkinson and Gale, substantial caution is appropriate in terms of any dramatic change in infant nutrition on a basis of these early studies.[109]

Type 2 DM

Nutrition and the Incidence of Type 2 DM. There have been numerous studies examining the role of various nutritional (or activity) factors and the incidence of type 2 DM. From the most general perspective, these studies can be divided into two categories: those that examine specific dietary components and the incidence of DM and those that focus on total calories/weight loss and DM. In the former category, such explicit dietary factors as total fat, nuts and peanut butter, fiber, coffee, etc. have been examined.[110-113] On the other hand, and especially within the framework of randomized, controlled trials in high-risk individuals with prediabetes, total caloric intake with associated weight loss and increased physical activity have been targeted.[85-95] The general tension between these two camps may reflect study design, statistical versus clinical significance, and issues such as relative versus absolute risk. In general, the studies that have identified specific food ingredients as related to type 2 DM incidence have been large observational studies that particularly address the statistical significance of relative risk as the determinant of importance.[111-113] The randomized trials that address total calories consumed along with accompanying increased physical activity address absolute risk and "numbers needed to treat" as indicators of public health importance.[85-95] By way of illustration, within a very large cohort study, even when results are adjusted for weight changes, activity, age, etc., individual dietary factors may be statistically significant when relative to a lowest quintile among study participants, and the highest group consuming a particular nutritional element will be seen as "statistically significant."[111-113] However, the overall contribution of that factor to the incidence of DM (i.e., the population attributable fraction of type 2 DM) may be very small, especially compared with overall calories consumed, weight changes, etc.[85-95] Thus, in terms of prevention of type 2 DM among a population, total calories consumed, body weight changes, and physical activity are likely to be much more important than any one specific dietary factor.

Metabolic Syndrome and Type 2 DM. During the past decade, the concept of the metabolic syndrome has swept through the academic, clinical, pharmacologic, and media worlds. In most major journals, associations of numerous conditions with the metabolic syndrome are made, epidemics of DM and cardiovascular disease are related to and presumably caused by the metabolic syndrome, and various nutritional and pharmacologic interventions are proposed. Although the basic linking pathophysiology of the metabolic syndrome has yet to be identified (if there is one), numerous definitions now exist, with the ATP III most frequently cited.[55,114] More recent studies have questioned the validity of the recommended definition, as well as the predictive power of the metabolic syndrome in the development of either type 2 DM or cardiovascular disease compared with other "prediction models/engines."[115-119] In the face of these and other uncertainties, major controversies and confusions have emerged among various prestigious voluntary professional organizations. Regarding type 2 DM and the metabolic syndrome, it would seem that there are many essential questions yet to be better understood and resolved before one can be confident that this syndrome has firm dimensions and well-understood characteristics. Acceptance of the metabolic syndrome as a "done deal" in terms of type 2 DM is at present highly premature.

Future Directions

Obesity, sedentary lifestyles, and demographic changes such as aging are the major factors associated with a worldwide increase in the prevalence of type 2 DM. The reported increases in the incidence of type 1 DM, especially at very young ages,[120] is not fully understood. Of interest is the relevancy of the so-called accelerator hypothesis, which if true could explain the increased number of patients with type 1 and 2 DM.[121,122]

The long-term goal of MNT in diabetes is to prevent and/or delay diabetic complications by restoring metabolism as close to normal as possible. The focus is on adjusting energy intake and expenditure to achieve a modest weight loss of approximately 10% and reducing the impact of cardiovascular risk factors such as hypertension and dyslipidemia. The distribution of macronutrient intake may vary based on a number of factors, including matching insulin to lifestyle in type 1 DM and reducing cardiovascular risk factors in type 2 DM. Assessing micronutrient status is needed for patients in poor control, with complications, or with other evidence of being at risk.

There is no one diabetic diet. MNT should be based on individual assessment and development of a treatment plan. Ideally, a registered dietitian who consults with the health care team and the patient assesses the patient's needs and develops an individualized treatment plan that considers overall health needs in addition to ameliorating the metabolic effects of DM and its complications. Clearly, nutrition has and will continue to have a major role among persons with established DM.

The importance of nutrition concepts and strategies has become even more important, given the solid and convincing evidence of the ability to prevent type 2 DM among those with so-called prediabetes. The risk for developing DM is closely linked to lifestyle and obesity. Thus, the next great challenge for many will be to convert the important primary prevention science into active, practical, and widely available behavioral programs. These efforts will require more than just traditional nutrition science; also they will require the involvement of public health, industry, government, and society at large.

References

1. American Diabetes Association Position Statement. (2006). Diagnosis and Classification of DM. Diabetes Care. 2006;29:S43–49. Available at: http://care.diabetesjournals.org/cgi/reprint/29/suppl_1/s43. Accessed March 13, 2006.
2. Matsumoto M, Accili D. The tangled path to glucose production. Nat Med. 2006;12:33–34.
3. Ramasamy R, Yan S, Schmidt A. The RAGE axis and endothelial dysfunction: maladaptive roles in the diabetic vasculature and beyond. Trends Cardiovas Med. 2005;15:237–243.
4. American Diabetes Association. Position Statement: standards of medical care in diabetes. Diabetes Care. 2006;28(suppl 1):S4–43. Available at: http://care.diabetesjournals.org/cgi/reprint/29/suppl_1/s4. Accessed March 13, 2006.
5. Roche HM, Phillips C, Gibney MJ. The metabolic syndrome: the crossroads of diet and genetics. Proc Nutr Soc. 2005;64:371–377.
6. Permutt MA, Wasson J, Cox N. Genetic epidemiology of diabetes. J Clin Invest. 2005;115:131–143.
7. American Diabetes Association; American Psychiatric Association; American Association of Clinical Endocrinologists; North American Association for the Study of Obesity. Consensus development conference on antipsychotic drugs and obesity and diabetes. Obes Res. 2004;12:362–368.
8. Centers for Disease Control. *National Diabetes Fact Sheet*. 2005. Available at: http://www.cdc.gov/diabetes/pubs/factsheet05.htm. Accessed Nov. 27, 2005.

9. Wild S, Roglic F, Green A, et al. Global prevalence of diabetes: estimated for the year 2000 and projections for 2030. Diabetes Care. 2004;27;1047–1053.
10. Darnton-Hill I, Nishida C, James WP. A life course approach to diet, nutrition and the prevention of chronic diseases. Public Health Nutr. 2004;7(1A): 101–121.
11. U.S. Department of Health and Human Services. *Diabetes Prevention and Control: A Public Health Imperative*. Available at: http://www.healthierus.gov/steps/summit/prevportfolio/strategies/reducing/diabetes/contents_diabetes.htm. Accessed Sept. 17, 2005.
12. Vinicor F. The public health burden of diabetes and the reality of limits. Diabetes Care. 1998;21(S3): 15–18.
13. Lefebvre P. Prediabetes, or what's in a name? Diab Med. 2005;31:519.
14. Simmons D, Thompson C, Engelgau M. Controlling the diabetes epidemic: how should we screen for undiagnosed diabetes and dysglycemia? Diab Med. 2005;22:207–212.
15. Gale E. Latent autoimmune diabetes in adults: a guide for the perplexed. Diabeteologia. 2005;48: 2195–2199.
16. Atkinson M. Thirty years of investigating the autoimmune basis for type 1 diabetes: why can't we prevent or reverse this disease? Diabetes. 2005;54: 1253–1263.
17. Muntoni S, Muntoni S. Epidemiological association between some dietary habits and the increasing incidence of type 1 diabetes worldwide. Ann Nutr Metab. 2005;50:11–19.
18. Mulder SJ. Bacteria of food and human intestine are the most possible sources of the gad-trigger of type 1 diabetes. Med Hypotheses. 2005;65: 308–311.
19. Harris M, Klein R, Welborn T, et al. Onset of NIDDM occurs at least 4–7 years before clinical diagnosis. Diabetes Care. 1992;15:815–819.
20. Obesity Education Initiative Expert Panel. *Clinical Guidelines on the Identification, Evaluation, and Treatment of Overweight and Obesity in Adults: The Evidence Report*. U.S. Department of Health and Human Services, Public Health Service, National Institutes of Health, National Heart Lung and Blood Institute, 1998. Available at: http://www.nhlbi.nih.gov/guidelines/obesity/ob_home.htm.
21. Prentice AM, Rayco-Solon P, Moore SE. Insight from the developing world: thrifty genotypes and thrifty phenotypes. Proc Nutr Soc. 2005;64: 153–161.
22. Bateson P, Barker D, Clutton-Brock T, et al. Developmental plasticity and human health. Nature. 2004;430:419–421.
23. Jovanovic L, Pettit D. Gestational diabetes mellitus. JAMA. 2004;286:2516–2518.
24. Diabetes Control and Complications Trial Research Group. The effect of intensive treatment of diabetes on the development and progression of long-term complications in insulin-dependent diabetes mellitus. N Engl J Med. 1993;329:977–986.
25. Eastman RC, Harris MI. Is there a glycemic threshold for mortality risk? Diabetes Care. 1998;21: 331–333.
26. UK Prospective Diabetes Study Group. Effect of intensive blood-glucose control with metformin on complications in overweight patients with type 2 diabetes (UKPDS 34). Lancet. 1998;352:8354–8365.
27. UK Prospective Diabetes Study Group. Tight blood pressure control and risk of macrovascular and microvascular complications in type 2 diabetes (UKPDS 38). Br Med J. 1998;317:703–713.
28. UK Prospective Diabetes Study Group. Intensive blood-glucose control with sulphonylureas or insulin compared to conventional treatment and risk of complications in patients with type 2 diabetes (UKPDS 33). Lancet. 1998;352:837–853.
29. National Diabetes Education Program (NDEP). *Four Steps to Diabetes Control: Know Your Diabetes ABCs*. Available at: http://www.ndep.nih.gov/diabetes/control/4Steps.htm#Step2
30. Diabetes Control and Complications Trial Research Group. Weight gain associated with intensive therapy in the Diabetes Control and Complications Trial. Diabetes Care. 1998;11:567–573.
31. Delehanty L, Halford BH. The role of diet behaviors in achieving improved glycemic control in intensively treated patients in the Diabetes Control and Complications Trial. Diabetes Care. 1993;16: 1453–1458.
32. Genuth S, Sun W, Cleary P, et al. Glycation and carboxymethyllysine levels in skin collagen predict the risk of future 10-year progression of diabetic retinopathy and nephropathy in the Diabetes Control and Complications Trial and epidemiology of diabetes interventions and complications participants with type 1 diabetes. Diabetes. 2005;54: 3103–3111.
33. Nathan D, Cleary P, Backlund J, et al. Intensive diabetes treatment and cardiovascular disease in patients with type 1 diabetes. N Engl J Med. 2005; 353:2643–2653.
34. American Diabetes Association. Clinical practice recommendations 2006. Diabetes Care. 2006; 29(S1):1–85.
35. Franz MJ, Bantle JP, Beebe CA, et al. Nutrition principles for the management of diabetes and related complications (technical review). Diabetes Care. 2002;17:490–518.
36. Sheard NF, Clark NG, Brand-Miller JC, et al. Dietary carbohydrate (amount and type) in the prevention and management of diabetes: a statement by

the American Diabetes Association. Diabetes Care. 2004;27:2266–2271.

37. American Diabetes Association, North American Association for the Study of Obesity, American Society for Clinical Nutrition. Weight management through lifestyle modification for the prevention and management of type 2 diabetes: rationale and strategies. Diabetes Care. 2004;27:2067–2073.
38. *Nutrition Practice Guidelines for Type 1 and Type 2 Diabetes Mellitus* [CD-ROM]. Chicago: American Dietetic Association, 2002.
39. American Diabetes Association. *Frequently asked Questions about Diabetes Self-Management and Medical Nutrition Therapy*. Available at: http://www.diabetes.org/for-health-professionals-and-scientists/recognition/dsmt-mntfaqs.jsp
40. American Dietetic Association and the American Association of Diabetes Educators. *Medicare Part B Referral Forms for Diabetes Self-Management Training and Medical Nutrition Therapy*. Available at: http://www.eatright.com/Public/Files/increasingaccesstodiabetescare(1).doc
41. American Diabetes Association. *Therapy for Diabetes Mellitus and Related Disorders*, 4th ed. Alexandria, VA: American Diabetes Association, 2004.
42. Norris SL, Zhang X, Avenell A, et al. Long-term effectiveness of lifestyle and behavioral weight loss interventions in adults with type 2 diabetes: a meta-analysis. Am J Med. 2004;117:762–774.
43. Buchwald H, Avidor Y, Braunwald E, et al. Bariatric surgery: a systematic review and meta-analysis. JAMA. 2004;292:1724–1737.
44. *Nutrition Practice Guidelines for Gestational Diabetes Mellitus.* Chicago: American Dietetic Association, 2002.
45. Gunderson EP. Gestational diabetes and nutritional recommendations. Curr Diab Rep. 2004;4: 377–386.
46. Jovanovic L American Diabetes Association's Fourth International Workshop/Conference on Gestational Diabetes: summary and discussion (therapeutic interventions) Diabetes Care. 1998; 21(Suppl 2):B131-B137.
47. Institute of Medicine. *Dietary Reference Intakes for Energy, Carbohydrate, Fiber, Fat, Fatty Acids, Cholesterol, Protein, and Amino Acids*. Washington DC: National Academy of Sciences Press, 2002.
48. Knowler WC, Barrett-Connor E, Fowler SE, et al. Diabetes Prevention Program Research Group. Reduction in the incidence of type 2 diabetes with lifestyle intervention or metformin. N Engl J Med. 2002;346:393–403.
49. Diabetes Prevention Program Research Group. Impact of intensive lifestyle and metformin therapy on cardiovascular disease risk factors in the Diabetes Prevention Program. Diabetes Care. 2005;28: 888–894.
50. Diabetes Prevention Program Research Group. Intensive lifestyle intervention or metformin on inflammation and coagulation in participants with impaired glucose tolerance. Diabetes. 2005;54: 1566–1572.
51. Samaha FF, Iqbal N, Seshadri P, et al. Low-carbohydrate as compared with a low-fat diet in severe obesity. N Engl J Med. 2003;348:2074–2081.
52. Stern L, Iqbal N, Seshadri P, et al. The effects of low-carbohydrate versus conventional weight loss diets in severely obese adults: one-year follow-up of a randomized trial. Ann Intern Med. 2004;140: 778–785.
53. Christiansen E, Schnider S, Palmvig B, et al. Intake of a diet high in trans monounsaturated fatty acids or saturated fatty acids. Effects on postprandial insulinemia and glycemia in obese patients with NIDDM. Diabetes Care. 1997;20:881–887.
54. Eckel, R. The dietary approach to obesity—is it the diet or the disorder? JAMA. 2005;293:96–97.
55. Executive summary of the third report of the National Cholesterol Education Program (NCEP) Expert Panel on Detection, Evaluation, and Treatment of High Blood Cholesterol in Adults (Adult Treatment Panel III). JAMA. 2001;285:2486–2497.
56. Vaccaro O, Eberly L, Neaton J, et al. Impact of diabetes and previous myocardial infarction on long-term survival. Arch Intern Med. 2004;164: 1438–1443.
57. Garg A. High-monounsaturated-fat diets for patients with diabetes mellitus: a meta-analysis. Am J Clin Nutr. 1998;67(Suppl 3):577S–582S.
58. Connor W. Will the dietary intake of fish prevent atherosclerosis in diabetic women? Am J Clin Nutr. 2004;80:535–536.
59. Nettleton JA, Katz R. n-3 long-chain polyunsaturated fatty acids in type 2 diabetes: a review 1. J Am Diet Assoc. 2005;105:428–440.
60. Tushuizen M, Diamant M, Heine R. Postprandial dysmetabolism and cardiovascular disease in type 2 diabetes. Postgrad Med J. 2005;81:1–6.
61. Wylie-Rosett J, Segal-Isaacson CJ, Segal-Isaacson A. Carbohydrates and increases in obesity: does the type of carbohydrate make a difference? Obes Res. 2004;12(Suppl 2):124S–129S.
62. Brand-Miller J, Hayne S, Petocz P, et al. Low-glycemic index diets in the management of diabetes: a meta-analysis of randomized controlled trials. Diabetes Care. 2003;26:2261–2267.
63. Howard BV, Wylie-Rosett J. Sugar and cardiovascular disease: A statement for healthcare professionals from the Committee on Nutrition of the Council on Nutrition, Physical Activity, and Metabolism of the American Heart Association. Circulation. 2002; 106:523–527.
64. Vlassara H, Cai W, Crandall J, et al. Inflammatory

mediators are induced by dietary glycotoxins, a major risk factor for diabetic angiopathy. Proc Natl Acad Sci USA. 2002;99:15596–15601.

65. Schulz M, Liese A, Mayer-Davis E, et al. Nutritional correlates of dietary glycaemic index: new aspects for a population perspective. Br J Nutr. 2005; 94:397–406.
66. Kripke C. Does a low glycemic index diet reduce CHD? Am Fam Physician. 2005;72:1224.
67. Pi-Sunyer X. Do glycemic index, glycemic load, and fiber play a role in insulin sensitivity, disposition index and type 2 diabetes? Diabetes Care. 2005;28: 2978–2979.
68. Venters J, Hunt A, Pope J, et al. Are patients with diabetes receiving the same message from dietitians and nurses? Diabetes Educator. 2004;30:293–300.
69. Liu JP, Zhang M, Wang WY, et al. Chinese herbal medicines for type 2 diabetes mellitus. Cochrane Database Syst Rev. 2004;(3):CD003642.
70. Barringer TA, Kirk JK, Santaniello AC, et al. Effect of a multivitamin and mineral supplement on infection and quality of life. A randomized, double-blind, placebo-controlled trial. Ann Intern Med. 2003;138:365–371.
71. Cicero AF, Derosa G, Gaddi A. What do herbalists suggest to diabetic patients in order to improve glycemic control? Evaluation of scientific evidence and potential risks. Acta Diabetol. 2004;41:91–98.
72. Cefalu WT, Hu FB. Role of chromium in human health and in diabetes. Diabetes Care. 2004;27: 2741–2751.
73. Schwartz JR, Marsh RG, Draelos ZD. Zinc and skin health: overview of physiology and pharmacology. Dermatol Surg. 2005;31(7 Pt 2):837–847.
74. Narendhirakannan RT, Subramanian S, Kandaswamy M. Mineral content of some medicinal plants used in the treatment of diabetes mellitus. Biol Trace Elem Res. 2005;103:109–115.
75. Lonn E, Bosch J, Yusuf S, et al. Effects of long-term vitamin E supplementation on cardiovascular events and cancer: a randomized controlled trial. JAMA. 2005;293:1338–1347.
76. Toole J, Malinow M, Chambliss L, et al. Lowering homocysteine in patients with ischemic stroke to prevent recurrent stroke, myocardial infarction, and heath: the Vitamin Intervention for Stroke Prevention (VISP) randomized controlled trial. JAMA. 2004;291:565–575.
77. U.S. Dept of Agriculture and Health and Human Services. *Dietary Guidelines Advisory Committee Report Dietary Guidelines for Americans 2005.* Available at: http://www.health.gov/dietaryguidelines/Default.htm. Accessed Jan. 14, 2005.
78. Huijberts MS, Becker A, Stehouwer CD. Homocysteine and vascular disease in diabetes: a double hit? Clin Chem Lab Med. 2005;43:993–1000.
79. Cho NH, Lim S, Jang HC, et al. Elevated homocysteine as a risk factor for the development of diabetes in women with a previous history of gestational DM: a 4-year prospective study. Diabetes Care. 2005;28:2750–2755.
80. Heart Outcomes Prevention Evaluation (HOPE) Investigators. Homocysteine lowering with folic acid and B vitamins in vascular disease. N Engl J Med. 2006 (e-pub ahead of print).
81. Bonaa K, Njolstad I, Ueland P, et al. Homocysteine lowering and cardiovascular events after acute myocardial infarction. N Engl J Med. 2006 (e-pub ahead of print).
82. Avenell A, Brown TJ, McGee MA, et al. What are the long-term benefits of weight reducing diets in adults? A systematic review of randomized controlled trials. J Hum Nutr Diet. 2004;17:317–335.
83. Anderson JW, Luan J, Hoie LH.Structured weight-loss programs: meta-analysis of weight loss at 24 weeks and assessment of effects of intervention intensity. Adv Ther. 2004;21:61–75.
84. Norris SL, Zhang X, Avenell A, et al. Long-term effectiveness of weight-loss interventions in adults with pre-diabetes: a review. Am J Prev Med. 2005; 28:126–139.
85. Pan XR, Li GW, Hu YH, et al. Effect of diet and exercise in preventing NIDDM in people with impaired glucose tolerance. The DaQing IGT and Diabetes Study. Diabetes Care. 1997;20:537–544.
86. Finnish Diabetes Prevention Study. Lifestyle intervention and 3-year results on diet and physical activity. Diabetes Care. 2003;26:3230–3236.
87. Uusitupa M, Lindi V, Louheranta A, et al. Long-term improvement in insulin sensitivity by changing lifestyles of people with impaired glucose tolerance: 4-year results from the Finnish Diabetes Prevention Study. Diabetes. 2003;52:2532–2538.
88. Uusitipa M. Gene–diet interaction in relation to the prevention of obesity and diabetes; evidence from the Finnish Diabetes Prevention Study. Nutr Metab Cardiovasc Dis. 2005;15:225–233.
89. Diabetes Prevention Program Research Group. A description of the lifestyle intervention. Diabetes Care. 2002;25:2165–2171.
90. Diabetes Prevention Program Research Group. The effect of metformin and intensive lifestyle intervention on the metabolic syndrome: the Diabetes Prevention Program randomized trial. Ann Intern Med. 2005;142:611–619.
91. Mayer-Davis EJ, Sparks KC, Hirsh K, et al. Dietary intake in the Diabetes Prevention Program cohort: baseline and 1-year post randomization. Ann Epidemiol. 2004;14:763–772.
92. Wing RR, Hamman RF, Bray GA, et al. Achieving weight and activity goals among Diabetes Prevention Program lifestyle participants. Obesity Res. 2004;2:1426–1434.
93. Centers for Disease Control and Prevention Primary Prevention Working Group. Primary prevention of type 2 DM by lifestyle intervention: implica-

tions for health policy. Ann Intern Med. 2004;140(S):951–957.

94. Wylie-Rosett J, Herman W, Goldberg R. Lifestyle intervention to prevent diabetes: intensive and cost effective. Curr Opin Lipid. 2006;17:37–44.
95. Jack L, Liburd L, Spencer T, et al. Understanding the environmental issues in diabetes self-management education research: a reexamination of 8 studies in community-based settings. Ann Intern Med. 2004;140(S):964–971.
96. Ogilvie D, Hamlet N. Obesity: the elephant in the corner. Br Med J. 2005;331:1545–1548.
97. National Diabetes Education Program. *Diabetes Prevention*. Available at: www.ndep.nih.gov/diabetes/prev/prevention.htm. Accessed Nov. 21, 2005.
98. Murphy D, Chapel T, Clark C. Moving diabetes care from science to practice: the evolution of the National Diabetes Prevention and Control Program. Ann Intern Med. 2004;140(S):978–984.
99. Eyre H, Kahn R, Robertson RM, et al. Preventing cancer, cardiovascular disease, and diabetes: a common agenda for the American Cancer Society, the American Diabetes Association, and the American Heart Association. Circulation. 2004;109:3244–3255.
100. Ebrahim S. Obesity, fat, and public health. Int J Epidemiol. 2006;35:1–2.
101. Ryan DH, Espeland MA, Foster GD, et al. Look AHEAD (Action for Health in Diabetes): design and methods for a clinical trial of weight loss for the prevention of cardiovascular disease in type 2 diabetes. Control Clin Trials. 2003;24:610.
102. Wing RR, Jeffery RW. Food provision as a strategy to promote weight loss. Obes Res. 2001;Suppl 4:271S–275S.
103. Vaarala O. Is type I diabetes a disease of the gut immune system triggered by cow's milk insulin? Adv Exp Med Biol. 2005;569:151–156.
104. Yoon J, Jun H. Autoimmune destruction of pancreatic beta cells. Am J Therapeutics. 2005;12:580–591.
105. Akerblom H, Virtanen S, Ilonen J, et al. Dietary manipulation of beta cell autoimmunity in infants at increased risk of type 1 diabetes: a pilot study. Diabetologia. 2005;48:829–837.
106. Farrell R. Infant gluten and celiac disease: too early, too late, too much too many questions. JAMA. 2005;293;2410–2412.
107. Ziegler A, Schmid S, Huber D, et al. Early infant feeding and risk of islet autoimmunity. JAMA. 2003;290:1721–1728.
108. Norris J, Barriga K, Klingensmith G, et al. Timing of initial cereal exposure in infancy and risk of islet immunity. JAMA. 2003;290:1713–1720.
109. Atkinson M, Gale E. Infant diets and type 1 diabetes: too early, too late or just to complicated? JAMA. 2003;290:1771–1772.
110. Freeman J. Health eating 101. Know your fats. Protect your heart by replacing harmful types with healthier ones. Diab Forecast. 2005;58:59–64.
111. Lovejoy J. The impact of nuts on diabetes and diabetes risk. Curr Diabetes Reports. 2005;5:379–384.
112. Murakami L, Okubo H, Sasaki S. Effect of dietary factors on incidence of type 2 diabetes: a systematic review of cohort studies. J Nut Sci Vitam. 2005;51:292–310.
113. Van Dam R, Hu F. Coffee consumption and risk of type 2 diabetes: a systematic review. JAMA. 2005;294:97–104.
114. Grundy SM, Cleeman JI, Merz CN, et al.; National Heart, Lung, and Blood Institute; American College of Cardiology Foundation; American Heart Association. Implications of recent clinical trials for the National Cholesterol Education Program Adult Treatment Panel III guidelines. Circulation. 2004;110:227–239.
115. Kahn R, Buse J, Ferrannini E, et al. The metabolic syndrome: time for a critical appraisal. Joint Statement from the ADA and the EASD. Diabetologia. 2005;48:1684–1699.
116. Greenland P. Critical questions about the metabolic syndrome. Circulation. 2005;112:3675–3676.
117. Stern M, Williams K, Gonzalez-Villalpando C, et al. Does the metabolic syndrome improve identification of individuals at risk of type 2 diabetes and/or cardiovascular disease? Diabetes Care. 2004;27:2676–2681.
118. Vinicor F, Bowman B. The metabolic syndrome: the emperor needs some consistent clothes [Response to Davidson and Alexander]. Diabetes Care. 2004;27:1243.
119. Zimmet P, Magliano D, Matsuzawa Y, et al. The metabolic syndrome: a global public health problem and a new definition. J Atheroscler Thromb. 2005;112:295–300.
120. Gale E. Spring harvest? Reflections on the rise of type 1 diabetes. Diabetologia. 2005;48:2445–2450.
121. Dabelea D, D'Agostino RB Jr, Mayer-Davis EJ, et al; SEARCH for Diabetes in Youth Study Group. Testing the accelerator hypothesis: body size, beta-cell function, and age at onset of type 1 (autoimmune) diabetes. Diabetes Care. 2006;29:290–294.
122. Wilkin T. Is the "accelerator hypothesis" worthy of our attention? Diabet Med. 2005;22:1458–1459.

51 Osteoporosis

Bess Dawson-Hughes

Osteoporosis is a prevalent condition involving both low mass and architectural deterioration of bone that lead to bone fragility and enhanced fracture risk. These changes can be assessed indirectly by bone mineral density (BMD) measurements. In 1994, the World Health Organization established the following definitions based on bone mass measurements at any site.[1] Normal is defined as BMD no lower than 1 standard deviation (SD) below the mean for young white women (T score > -1). Low bone mass or osteopenia is defined as BMD between 1 and 2.5 SD below the same reference mean (T score between -1 and -2.5). Osteoporosis is defined as BMD more than 2.5 SD below the reference mean (T score < -2.5). By using data from the Third National Health and Nutrition Examination Survey, Looker et al.[2] found that among women after menopause, 21% of white women, 16% of Mexican-American women, and 10% of African-American women in the United States had osteoporosis. In that analysis, another 38% of postmenopausal women in these groups had low bone mass. In the same survey, 8.0 million women and 2.1 million men had osteoporosis and another 15.4 million women and 3.1 million men had low bone mass.[3] Lifetime probabilities of hip fracture are 14% for white women, 5% to 6% for white men, 6% for African-American women, and 3% for African-American men.[4,5] In 1994, osteoporotic fractures were responsible for 432,447 hospitalizations and 179,222 nursing home stays in the United States.[6]

Many factors contribute to fracture risk. Heredity accounts for approximately 50% of the variability in peak bone mass.[7,8] In the observational Study of Osteoporotic Fractures in 9516 white women more than 65 years of age, a maternal history of a hip fracture doubled the risk of hip fracture, independent of bone mass.[9] In that study, weight was a strong predictor of bone mass, and thinness (being in the lowest quartile for weight) increased hip fracture risk several-fold. Smoking was also a strong determinant of hip fracture. Other risk factors included poor general health, falling in the past year, previous hyperthyroidism, use of anticonvulsants, and a fracture after age 50 years.

Diet is known to influence bone health. Calcium and vitamin D are essential to support bone growth in children and adolescents and to help preserve bone mass in adults. Increasing intake of these nutrients can reduce bone loss in adults, but calcium and vitamin D alone cannot prevent bone loss in every individual. This chapter focuses on the effects of calcium and vitamin D on bone remodeling, bone mass, and fracture risk, and considers the effect of protein and vitamin K intakes on the skeleton.

Calcium and Vitamin D Physiology

An inadequate intake of calcium results in less calcium absorbed, a subtle decline in the ionized calcium concentration in blood, and an increase in parathyroid hormone (PTH) secretion (Figure 1).[10] The same sequence occurs in subjects who have inadequate skin synthesis and intake of vitamin D. The increase in blood PTH concentration stimulates the renal production of 1,25-dihydroxyvitamin D ($1,25[OH]_2D$), the active form of the vitamin that promotes calcium absorption. The increase in PTH concentration also increases bone resorption and bone loss. The level of 25-hydroxyvitamin D (25[OH]D) needed for maximal suppression of PTH differs among individuals and among studies, but has been placed as high as 80 to 100 nmol/L in older men and women.[11,12] It has been estimated that an intake of 800 to 1000 IU/d of vitamin D_3 is needed to bring the group average value to 80 nmol/L.[13]

Aging

Calcium absorption efficiency declines with age in men and women, and the decline is particularly rapid after

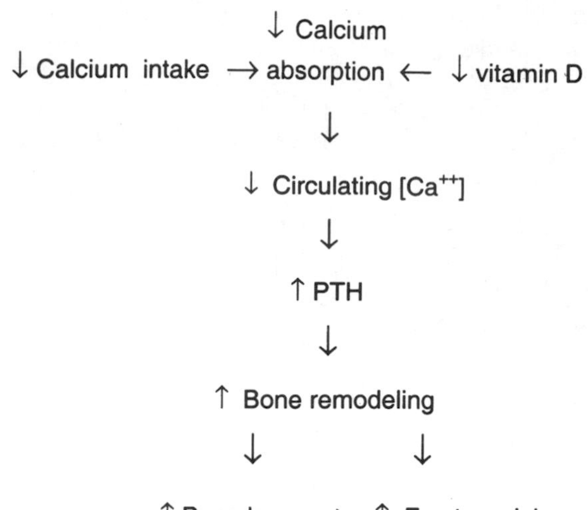

Figure 1. Calcium, vitamin D, and the skeleton. (Used with permission from Dawson-Hughes 1999.[10])

age 60 years.[14] Blood levels of 25(OH)D also decline with age.[15] This decline is in part the result of an age-related decline in skin production of vitamin D.[16] A recent study in 50 subjects found that for daily oral doses of 800 IU of vitamin D_3 given in the winter, older men 62 to 79 years of age had an increase in mean blood 25(OH)D concentration that did not differ significantly from that of younger men 18 to 35 years of age (22.1 vs. 22.5 nmol/L).[17] Initial levels of 25(OH)D in the two groups were similar. This suggests that the intestinal absorption of vitamin D_3 does not change with aging.

Season

Skin production of vitamin D, which is catalyzed by exposure to ultraviolet B radiation, is a major source of the vitamin. In much of the temperate zone, the needed ultraviolet B rays do not reach earth's surface in the winter. Webb et al.[18] demonstrated that in Boston (latitude 42° north), skin exposure to sunlight produced no photoproducts between mid-October and mid-March. A clinical corollary of this finding is evident in a cross-sectional study of 333 healthy postmenopausal women in Boston, mean age 58.0 years, who had serum 25(OH)D and PTH levels measured over 12 months (Figure 2).[11] Mean 25(OH)D levels were higher in summer and fall and lower in winter and spring. The seasonal pattern of PTH levels formed the mirror image.

Because even small, sustained increases in PTH can promote bone resorption and bone loss, we conducted a study to determine whether patterns of bone loss differed in the 6-month intervals when PTH levels were lowest (winter-spring) and highest (summer-fall), and whether supplemental vitamin D would alter the pattern. We recruited 246 postmenopausal women, mean age 61.6 years, and randomly assigned them to treatment for 1 year with placebo or 400 IU/d of vitamin D.[19] All women received 500 mg/d of supplemental calcium throughout the study. Women treated with placebo had a mean spinal BMD gain of 1.5% in summer-fall, a similar loss in winter-spring, and no net change at the end of 1 year. Vitamin D-treated women had a similar summer-fall gain but lost less BMD in the winter-spring (−0.5%), for a net gain of approximately 1% at the end of 1 year ($P = 0.04$). A similar pattern of change was seen in the total body. A subsequent randomized trial with 247 postmenopausal women, mean age 63.0 years, identified seasonal variation in rates of change in femoral neck BMD over 2 years.[20] These studies demonstrate that vitamin D insufficiency contributes to increased bone loss in winter.

Heredity

Calcium absorption seems to have a hereditary component that may be linked to vitamin D receptor alleles. Morrison et al.[21] initially reported that women with alleles designated BB had lower BMD than women with alleles designated bb. Others have sought this association with mixed results. Krall et al.[22] found that the association was present in 229 postmenopausal women and that it was stronger in the subjects who had very low calcium intakes (<400 mg/d) than in women consuming 401 to 650 mg/d of dietary calcium. Calcium absorption at low

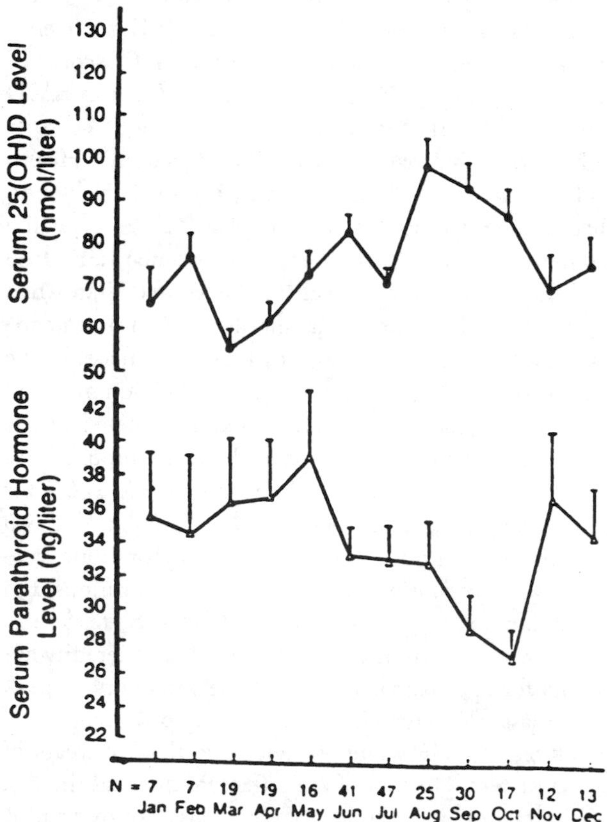

Figure 2. Month to month variations in mean serum 25-hydroxyvitamin D [25(OH)D] and parathyroid hormone concentrations in postmenopausal women. (Used with permission from Krall et al.[11]; copyright 1989 Massachusetts Medical Society. All rights reserved.)

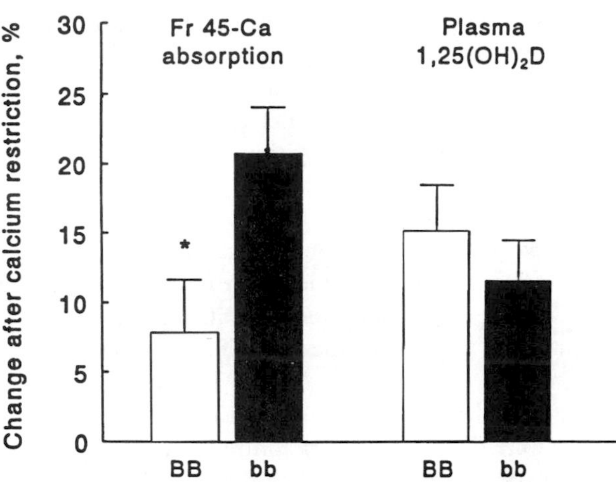

Figure 3. Changes in fractional calcium absorption and circulating 1,25-dihydroxyvitamin D [1,25-$(OH)_2D$] after calcium restriction, adjusted for differences in initial values and expressed as a percentage of the initial values. Genotypes are shown on the abscissa. Asterisk indicates a significant difference between the genotypes ($P = 0.016$). (From Dawson-Hughes et al.[23] copyright 1995 with permission of The Endocrine Society.)

calcium intakes occurs mainly by 1,25$(OH)_2D$-induced active transport, and a 1,25$(OH)_2D$ receptor defect may impair the normal 1,25$(OH)_2D$-mediated increase in fractional calcium absorption that occurs during periods of low calcium intake. This hypothesis was tested in 60 postmenopausal women, mean age 67 years, of whom 26 had BB genotypes and 34 had bb genotypes.[23] Women with BB and bb alleles had similar fractional calcium absorption on 1500 mg calcium diets, but the women with BB alleles had a significantly smaller increase in fractional absorption than did the women with bb alleles when calcium intake was decreased to 300 mg/d (Figure 3).[23] Increases in serum 1,25$(OH)_2D$ levels after the diet change were similar in the two groups. Initial levels of calcium intake, calcium absorption, and 1,25$(OH)_2D$ did not differ significantly between the groups. This study supports the presence of a hereditary-environment interaction in which the ability to adapt to a low calcium intake is genetically determined.

Skeletal Determinants of Fracture

Low BMD has long been recognized as a strong predictor of fracture risk. A site-specific measurement is the strongest predictor of fracture at a given site. For example, Cummings et al.[24] found that among 9516 women over 65 years of age who participated in the observational Study of Osteoporotic Fractures, a 1 SD decline in BMD of the femoral neck was associated with a 2.5-fold increased risk of hip fracture and a 1.6-fold increased risk of spine fracture. A similar decline in spinal BMD is associated with a 2.0-fold increase in risk of spine fracture and a 1.3-fold increase in risk of hip fracture.

Hui et al.[25] observed not only that BMD was inversely related to fracture risk in adults, but also that the magnitude of the risk of fracture at any given BMD increases dramatically with aging. Thus, factors related to aging other than declining BMD contribute to fracture risk. One of these factors seems to be the bone remodeling rate. In women, the bone turnover rate increases at menopause and continues to increase with aging.[26] Garnero et al.[27] performed a nested case-control study in 109 subjects with hip fracture and in 327 control subjects matched for age and time of recruitment and drawn from a prospective cohort study of 7598 healthy French women over 75 years of age (mean 82.5 years). The women with low BMD were at almost a three-fold higher risk of fracture than the women with higher BMD (lowest vs. highest quartile) (Figure 4, left bar). Women with high rates of bone turnover, as measured by urinary deoxypyridinoline and C-telopeptide, were also at significantly higher risk of fracture (highest vs. lowest quartile) (middle bars). Among the women with both low BMD and high bone turnover rates, the risk of hip fracture was additive (right bars: risk ratio 4.8 [95% confidence interval 2.4–9.5]; risk ratio 4.1 [95% confidence interval 2.0–8.2]). The importance of high bone turnover as a risk factor for vertebral fracture has been demonstrated by others.[28]

Bone Turnover

Several randomized trials have assessed the effect of supplemental calcium on serum concentrations of osteocalcin, a biochemical marker of bone formation and turnover in older subjects.[28-30] Two of these studies found that calcium decreased bone turnover by 12% to 14%.[28,29] Elders et al.[30] reported a smaller reduction of 2% in post-

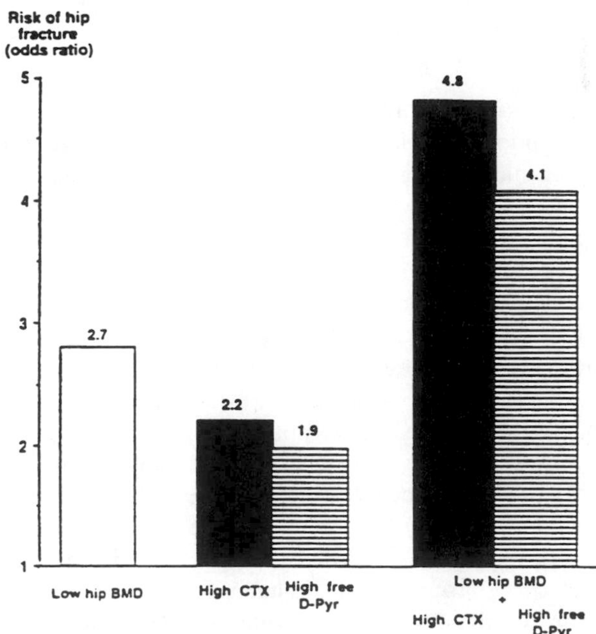

Figure 4. Combination of the assessment of bone mineral density (BMD) and bone resorption rate to predict hip fracture risk in elderly women. CTX, type 1 collagen cross-linked N-telopeptide; D-Pyr, deoxypyridinoline. (Used with permission from Garnero et al., 1996.[27])

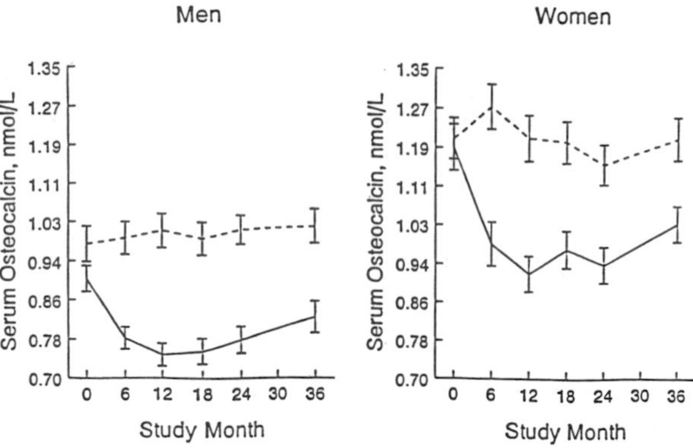

Figure 5. Serum osteocalcin concentrations in men and women treated with placebo (dashed lines) or 500 mg calcium and 700 IU vitamin D (solid lines) daily for 3 years. (Data from Dawson-Hughes et al., 1997.[31]) (Data used with permission from Dawson-Hughes et al.[31]; copyright 1997 Massachusetts Medical Society. All rights reserved.)

menopausal women, probably because these women had a relatively high initial mean dietary calcium intake of more than 1000 mg/d. The effect of combined calcium (500 mg) and vitamin D (700 IU) supplementation on serum osteocalcin concentrations in 176 men and 213 women over 65 years of age (mean 71.5 years) with diets containing an average of 750 mg calcium and 200 IU vitamin D/d is shown in Figure 5.[31] Supplementation decreased serum osteocalcin by 9% in the men and by 14% in the women throughout the 3-year treatment period. The men in this study had lower bone turnover rates than did the women.[32,33] The remodeling rate reductions observed with supplements are small when compared with the 50% reductions induced by estrogen and alendronate. They are sufficient, however, to reverse the increase in bone turnover that occurs with aging.[26]

Bone Mineral Density

Children, Adolescents, and Young Adults. As the major mineral component of bone, calcium is needed to support bone growth and consolidation. During the period of most rapid growth, more than 200 mg of calcium is deposited in the skeleton each day.[34] As indicated in a review by Heaney,[35] 10 randomized, controlled trials examined the effect of added calcium from food or supplements on bone growth in children and adolescents, and each study identified a positive effect of calcium on increase in BMD. For example, in a 3-year study of 45 identical twin pairs 6 to 14 years of age, supplementation with 1000 mg/d of calcium as citrate malate increased distal radius BMD by 1.1% per year and spine BMD by 0.2% per year.[36] Matkovic et al.[37] examined the long-term effect of supplemental calcium on bone accretion in young females. Of the 354 girls enrolled, 226 completed 4 years and 179 completed 7 years in the study. The subjects assigned to placebo had a mean calcium intake of 830 mg/d and those in the supplemented group had a mean intake of 1500 mg/d. There was a significant positive effect of supplementation on distal and proximal radius BMD, total-body BMD, and metacarpal cortical indices during the pubertal growth spurt and a diminishing effect thereafter. By young adulthood, significant effects of calcium remained at the metacarpals and forearm of tall girls only. As indicated by the authors, these findings suggest that standards for calcium intake in adolescents should be based on growth rate and body size.[37]

In several of the shorter-term intervention studies, the investigators continued to measure BMD periodically for up to 2 years after the children discontinued supplemental calcium.[38-41] In most of these studies,[38-40] including the twin study described above,[36] the BMD gains made while taking added calcium were not sustained after supplements were discontinued. In contrast, in a study of 149 prepubertal 11-year-old girls, Bonjour et al.[41] reported a positive residual effect of added calcium on bone mineral content 1 year later in those who had usual calcium intakes below the median intake of 880 mg/d. Residual benefit was not found in the girls who had higher dietary calcium intakes. Although the evidence from these studies is limited by small sample sizes, it is clear that at least some of the supplement-induced gain in BMD reverses when intake is decreased. A calcium-induced increase in mineral acquisition over several years may ultimately affect the peak bone mass achieved at approximately age 20 years, but direct evidence is currently lacking.

BMD tends to be fairly stable in healthy young adults, and as a result very few trials have been performed in this population. One randomized, controlled 3-year trial in 37 healthy women aged 32 to 42 years did find a favorable effect on spinal BMD of increasing calcium intake by an average of 610 mg/d with dairy foods.[42] The women in this study had a usual mean calcium intake of approximately 900 mg/d, and the mean treatment group difference in spinal BMD at the end of 3 years was approximately 2.5%.

Postmenopausal Women. The role of supplemental calcium in the preservation of bone mass in postmenopausal women has been studied extensively. As detailed in the recent review by Heaney,[35] more than 30 randomized, controlled trials have been reported in postmenopausal women, and all but one have demonstrated a positive effect of calcium. In general, women with low usual calcium intakes have benefited most from added calcium, but others have also benefited. In a 4-year trial of 78 women with an initial mean calcium intake of 700 mg/d, supplementation with 1000 mg/d of calcium had a significant beneficial effect on BMD of the spine, femoral neck, and total body.[43]

Most studies have used calcium in supplement form, but Prince et al.[44] compared 1000 mg of added calcium as tablets or milk powder with placebo in a 2-year study of 168 postmenopausal women with an initial mean calcium intake of 750 mg/d. The two calcium forms had similar favorable effects on reducing bone loss from the ultradistal ankle and femoral neck, although changes at the latter site were not statistically significant.

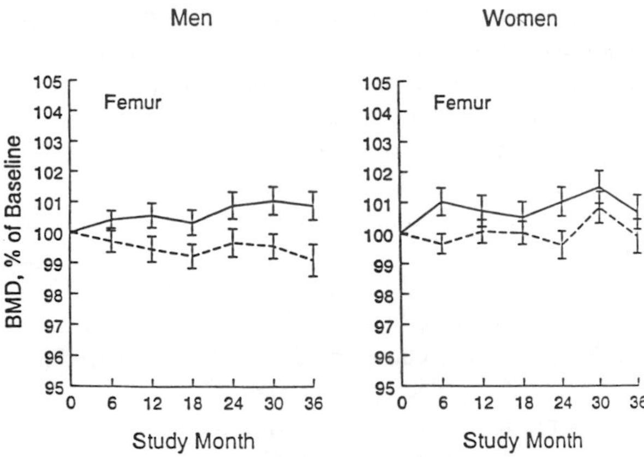

Figure 6. Rates of change in femoral neck BMD in men and women treated with placebo (dashed lines) or 500 mg calcium and 700 IU vitamin D (solid lines). Three-year differences between treatment groups were significant in men ($P = 0.011$). (Data used with permission from Dawson-Hughes et al.[31]; copyright 1997 Massachusetts Medical Society. All rights reserved.)

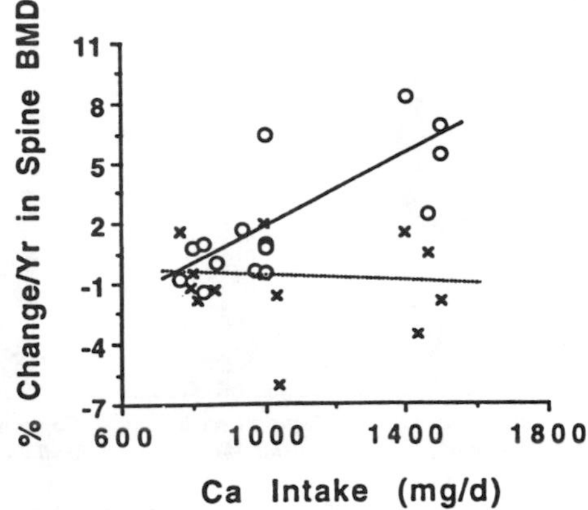

Figure 7. Mean change in spine BMD by mean calcium intake in groups assigned to exercise (o) or to no exercise (x). (Used with permission from Specker 1996.[48])

Several randomized, controlled trials have evaluated supplemental vitamin D in elderly females and found that 400 IU/d reduced bone loss from the spine,[19] femoral neck,[45] and total body,[19] and that 700 IU/d (compared with 100 IU/d) also reduced bone loss from the femoral neck.[20] In two of these studies,[19,20] 500 mg/d of supplemental calcium was given to all study participants.

Men. In the two reported three-year supplement studies in men, vitamin D was given along with calcium.[31,46] In one study, daily supplementation with 500 mg calcium and 700 IU vitamin D (vs. double placebo) reduced bone loss from the spine, femoral neck, and total body in 176 healthy men over 65 years of age (mean 71 years).[31] Figure 6 shows BMD changes at the femoral neck in the men (changes in 213 similar-aged women in the same study are also shown). The men (and women) had usual mean dietary intakes of 750 mg calcium and 200 IU vitamin D. In the other trial conducted in 77 men 30 to 87 years of age (mean age 58 years) with a usual mean calcium intake of 1160 mg/d, supplementation with 1000 mg calcium and 800 IU vitamin D had no effect on the pattern of bone loss from the spine or forearm.[46] The failure of supplementation in the latter study may have been because the men were meeting their requirements for these nutrients through their diets.

One report reveals that when older men and women stop taking supplemental calcium and vitamin D, both the three-year gains in BMD and the suppression of the remodeling rate induced by the supplements are lost over one to two years.[47]

Calcium Interface with Exercise, Estrogen, and Drug Therapy

Exercise is well recognized to be important for the development and preservation of strong bones. A recent meta-analysis of 17 exercise trials (the number for which calcium intake information was available) suggests that the calcium intake may influence the effect of exercise on BMD.[48] The 17 trials lasted from 4 months to 2 years and included young and older populations, mostly women, with mean ages of 30 to 62 years. The types and intensities of the exercise interventions varied widely among the studies. Figure 7 shows the effect of exercise versus no exercise on BMD of the spine in relation to the mean calcium intake. Treatment group differences are greater at higher calcium intakes (slopes of the two regression lines differed significantly at $P < 0.05$). No difference in slopes of regression lines was found for the radius measurements (data not shown). It will be important to test the hypothesis that calcium influences the spinal BMD gains induced by exercise.

Hormone replacement therapy is widely used to prevent bone loss in postmenopausal women. In a different meta-analysis, Nieves et al.[49] looked at the effect of calcium intake on the skeletal effects of exogenous estrogen. Of 31 estrogen intervention trials meeting the study criteria, 20 gave added calcium to both treatment arms (bringing the total mean intake to 1183 mg/d) and 11 did not (total mean intake 563 mg/d). As shown in Figure 8, the mean BMD gain at each skeletal site was significantly greater in the women who took added calcium than in those who did not. This analysis suggests that the importance of maintaining an adequate intake of calcium is not supplanted by use of hormone replacement therapy.

In recent randomized trials evaluating new drug therapies for the prevention and treatment of osteoporotic fractures, supplemental calcium and often vitamin D have been given to the treatment and placebo groups.[50-53] The effectiveness of treatment with alendronate, risedronate, raloxifene, and calcitonin therefore has been assessed in the context of adequate calcium and vitamin D intakes. Similar benefits from these drugs cannot be assumed in patients with low calcium or vitamin D intakes.

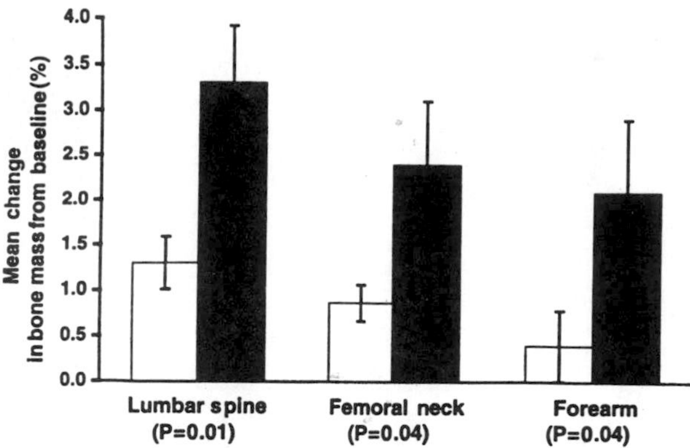

Figure 8. Mean (± SEM) annual percentage change in bone mass in postmenopausal women treated with estrogen alone (open bars) and in women treated with estrogen and calcium (black bars) ($P < 0.05$ for differences at each skeletal site). (Used with permission from Specker 1996.[48])

Falls

In the United States, one in three persons over 65 falls each year.[54] Of those who fall, 20% to 30% sustain moderate or severe injuries,[55] at least half of which are fractures.[54-56] Factors associated with an elevated risk of falling include use of sedatives, gait and balance difficulties, arthritis, poor vision, Parkinson's disease, disabilities of the lower extremities, and diminished muscle strength.[54-57] Vitamin D has been thought to affect fracture risk primarily through its effect on BMD, but several recent studies have suggested a role in muscle strength and risk of falling. In a large, cross-sectional study of men and women age 60 years and older, lower serum 25(OH)D levels were associated with poor lower extremity performance, as defined by prolonged times on sit-to-stand and timed-walk tests.[58] A short-term intervention study reported that 800 IU/d of supplemental vitamin D_3 reduced body sway by 9% in 148 women, mean age 74 years.[59] A recent meta-analysis of five randomized, vitamin D intervention studies involving 1237 subjects revealed that supplemental vitamin D decreased the risk of falling by 22% (corrected odds ratio, 0.78; 95% confidence interval, 0.64–0.92) compared with subjects receiving placebo or calcium.[60] Thus, increasing lower extremity muscle strength and reducing the risk of falling are presumably other ways in which vitamin D influences fracture risk.

Fractures

In the past few years, information on the effect of calcium and vitamin D supplementation on the incidence of fractures has begun to emerge (Table 1). Four calcium intervention studies reported fracture incidence (9 to 61 fractures were reported).[28,29,43,61] In the largest of these studies,[61] supplemental calcium decreased the incidence of new vertebral fractures in postmenopausal women with a prior vertebral fracture but not in women with no prior vertebral fracture. The results of the other studies were also mixed. None of these studies was large enough to establish the antifracture efficacy of supplemental calcium or to determine the size of a potential effect of calcium on fracture rates.

Table 1. Calcium and Vitamin D Intervention Trials and Fracture Incidence

		Calcium Intake (mg/d)		Persons with New Fracture		
Intervention	Study	Diet	Daily Calcium, Vitamin D, or Both	N	Site	Statistically Significant Difference
Calcium	Chevalley et al. 1994[29]	600	800 mg Ca	18	Vertebra	Yes
	Recker et al. 2000[53]	433	1200 mg Ca			
	With prior fracture			36	Vertebra	Yes
	No prior fracture			25	Vertebra	No
	Reid et al. 1990[42]	700	1000 mg Ca	9	All sites	Yes
	Riggs et al. 1998[28]	700	1600 mg Ca	40	All sites	No
Vitamin D	Lips et al. 1988[54]		400 IU Vit D		Hip	No
	Heikinheimo et al. 1992[55]		50,000–300,000 IU Vit D/year IM[a]		All nonvertebral	Yes
Calcium and vitamin D	Dawson-Hughes 1997[31]	700	500 mg Ca, 700 IU Vit D	37	All nonvertebral	Yes
	Chapuy et al. 1989[56]	500	1200 mg Ca, 800 IU Vit D	315	Hip	Yes
				563	All nonvertebral	Yes

[a] IM, intramuscular.

Several large trials have assessed the effect of supplemental vitamin D on fracture rates, with different results.[62-65] The two studies that used 400 IU/d of vitamin D_3[62,63] found no effect on hip[62] or all nonvertebral fracture rates[62,63] in elderly subjects. A subset of the women in the Lips et al.[62] trial had an estimated mean calcium intake of 875 mg/d and a median 25(OH)D level of 27 nmol/L at entry. The intake of the men is unknown. In contrast, studies using higher doses of vitamin D_3 have had positive results. Trivedi et al.[64] found that supplementation with 100,000 IU of vitamin D_3 every 4 months (equivalent to 833 IU/d) significantly decreased all nonvertebral fractures by 33% in 2686 elderly men and women who were living at home. Heikinheimo et al.[65] found that an annual intramuscular injection of vitamin D (150,000 or 300,000 IU) significantly decreased clinical fracture rates in 800 elderly men and women 85 years and older with unspecified calcium intakes.

Three studies have examined the effect of vitamin D in doses of 700 to 800 IU/d in combination with supplemental calcium on fracture incidence.[66,67,31] In more than 3000 women (mean age 84 years) who resided in nursing homes in southern France, daily supplementation with 800 IU vitamin D and 1200 mg calcium as tricalcium phosphate decreased the incidence of hip and other nonvertebral fractures by 25% (Figure 9).[66] No adverse effects were reported. The women had an estimated mean dietary calcium intake of 500 mg/d and low levels of 25(OH)D, indicating vitamin D insufficiency. Similar findings were reported by the same investigators in a second cohort of 583 French women, mean age 85 years.[67] The smaller trial, with a total of 37 verified nonvertebral fractures, identified a similar reduction in fracture incidence after 3 years of daily supplementation with 700 IU vitamin D and 500 mg calcium as citrate malate.[31] As indicated earlier, the participants in this study were 389 healthy men and women over 65 years of age who resided at home in Boston. Their usual diets contained an average of 750 mg/d of calcium and 200 IU/d of vitamin D.

In summary, vitamin D in doses of 700 to 800 IU/d, with and without calcium, has consistently decreased fracture rates in elderly men and women, whereas lower doses have not. Supplementation with 700 to 800 IU/d of vitamin D was effective not only in high-risk institutionalized elderly subjects but also in free-living people whose mean dietary intake of calcium exceeded that of the US national average.[68] The precise contribution of the calcium in the combination studies cannot be determined.

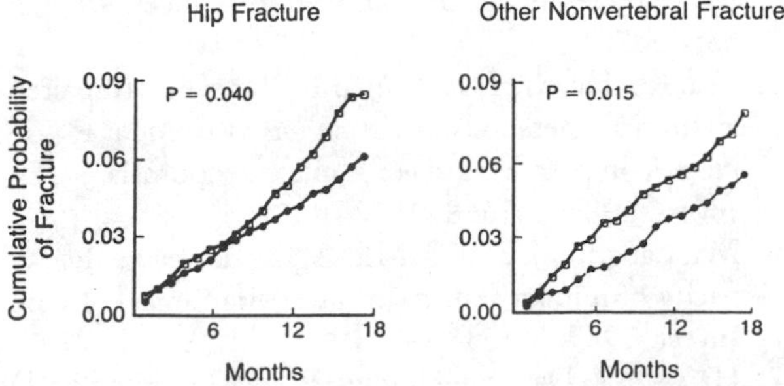

Figure 9. Cumulative probability of hip fracture and other nonvertebral fracture in the placebo group (open squares) and the group treated with calcium and vitamin D (closed circles). (Used with permission from Chapuy et al.[66]; copyright 1992 Massachusetts Medical Society. All rights reserved.)

The National Academy of Sciences increased the recommended intakes of calcium for men and women over 51 years from 800 to 1200 mg/d in 1997.[69] Recommended intakes of vitamin D increased from 200 to 400 IU/d for men and women ages 51 to 70 years and from 200 to 600 IU/d for men and women over 71 years of age.[69] The findings described above suggest that increasing vitamin D intake by 700 to 800 IU/d would decrease fracture rates in the general elderly population. Higher doses could be beneficial, but they have not been tested.

According to the 1994 US Department of Agriculture Continuing Survey of Food Intakes by Individuals, men over 50 years of age consume less than 60% and women over 50 consume less than 50% of the amount of calcium recommended.[68] After age 70, less than 5% of men and less than 1% of women meet the 1200 mg calcium requirement from food.[68] Comparable national data on vitamin D intakes are not available.

Protein and Vitamin K

Historically, dietary protein has been assumed to have a negative effect on the skeleton because of the repeated observation that protein intake and urinary calcium excretion are positively correlated.[70,71] A recent study indicates that the calciuria may be the result, in part, of increased calcium absorption.[72] In the past few years, evidence has been growing that low protein intakes have harmful effects on the skeleton. Kerstetter et al.[73] showed that as protein intake decreased to less than 0.8 g/kg body wt/d in healthy young women, PTH levels increased over the short term. In contrast, Shapses et al.[74] identified no effect of protein restriction from 2.7 to 0.5 g/kg body wt/d on urinary pyridinium cross-links in young subjects, perhaps because the intervention period was only 5 days. Several studies in the elderly have linked lower protein intakes to faster bone loss,[75,76] and one study has associated lower protein intakes with more hip fractures.[77] Protein supplementation of elderly patients with hip fractures has improved clinical outcomes, such as length of hospital stay.[78] In a prospective 6-month study of elderly patients with hip fractures with a mean protein intake of 40 g/d, supplementation with 20 g/d significantly reduced bone loss from the femoral neck.[79] There are probably several mechanisms by which protein is important. A low intake is likely to be a marker for a poor diet in general; it may also be associated with lower levels of the bone growth factor insulin-like growth factor 1.

Vitamin K is required for carboxylation of the bone matrix protein osteocalcin. The established adequate intake of vitamin K, based on clotting parameters, is 0.090 mg/d for women and 0.120 mg/d for men,[80] but more than 0.10 mg/d may be needed to preserve optimal carboxylation of osteocalcin in bone.[81] Among men and women over 65 years of age, mean intakes of phylloquinone, the naturally occurring form of the vitamin, are well below these levels at 0.050 to 0.070 mg/d.[82] Several observation studies have identified associations between low phylloquinone intakes and risk of hip fracture, including the Framingham Osteoporosis Study[83] and the Nurses Health Study.[84] A similar trend was seen in the Study of Osteoporotic Fractures.[85] Long-term prospective intervention studies are needed to determine the effect of supplemental vitamin K on BMD and fracture rates.

Conclusions

A deficiency of calcium or vitamin D results in poor bone mineralization. We now have a new appreciation of the role of vitamin D and the combination of calcium and vitamin D in decreasing the risk of fracture in older men and women. Vitamin D seems to affect fracture risk through effects on muscle strength and risk of falling, and both vitamin D and calcium affect bone mass. Supplementation can decrease bone turnover rates by 10% to 15%, increase BMD by 2% to 5%, and decrease fracture incidence by approximately 25%. Decreasing bone turnover rates by 10% to 15% for extended periods is unlikely to be harmful, because this reduction brings turnover down to levels normally seen in young adults. Finally, meeting the calcium and vitamin D requirements on a continuous basis seems to be important to derive and maintain the maximal skeletal benefit. There is some indication that the recommended intake of vitamin D for older men and women is too low.

Low protein intakes were recently recognized to have adverse effects on bone health in the elderly. It therefore seems advisable to consume protein in recommended amounts.

Strong epidemiologic evidence indicates that subclinical vitamin K insufficiency may contribute to bone loss and fracture risk in the elderly. Direct evidence for this commonly observed association is needed.

Acknowledgment

Any opinions, findings, conclusions, or recommendations expressed in this publication are those of the author and do not necessarily reflect the view of the US Department of Agriculture.

References

1. Kanis JA, Melton LJ III, Christiansen C, et al. The diagnosis of osteoporosis. J Bone Miner Res. 1994; 8:1137–1141.
2. Looker AC, Johnston CC Jr, Wahner HW, et al. Prevalence of low femoral bone density in older US women from NHANES III. J Bone Miner Res. 1995;10:796–802.
3. National Osteoporosis Foundation. *OsteoporosisPrevalence Figures. State-by-State Report.* Washington, DC: National Osteoporosis Foundation; 1997.
4. Melton LJ III, Chrischilles EA, Cooper C, et al. Perspective: how many women have osteoporosis? J Bone Miner Res. 1992;7:1005–1010.
5. Cummings SR, Black DM, Rubin SM. Lifetime risks of hip, Colles, or vertebral fracture and coronary heart disease among white postmenopausal women. Arch Intern Med. 1989;149:2445–2448.
6. Ray NF, Chan JK, Thaemer M, Melton LJ III. Medical expenditures for the treatment of osteoporotic fractures in the United States in 1994. J Bone Miner Res. 1997;12:24–35.
7. Slemenda CW, Hui SL, Longcope C, et al. Predictors of bone mass in perimenopausal women: a prospective study of clinical data using photon absorptiometry. Ann Intern Med. 1990;112:96–101.
8. Pocock NA, Eisman JA, Hopper JL, et al. Genetic determinants of bone mass in adults: a twin study. J Clin Invest. 1987;80:706–710.
9. Cummings SR, Nevitt MC, Browner WS, et al. Risk factors for hip fracture in white women. N Engl J Med. 1995;332:767–773.
10. Dawson-Hughes B. Calcium and vitamin D nutrition. In: Orwoll E, ed. *Osteoporosis in Men, Vol 1.* San Diego: Academic Press; 1999:197–209.
11. Krall EA, Sahyoun N, Tannenbaum S, et al. Effect of vitamin D intake on seasonal variation in intact PTH. N Engl J Med. 1989;321:1777–1783.
12. Dawson-Hughes B, Harris SS, Dallal GE. Plasma calcidiol, season, and serum parathyroid hormone concentrations in healthy elderly men and women. Am J Clin Nutr. 1997;65:67–71.
13. Dawson-Hughes B, Heaney RP, Holick MF, Lips P, Meunier PJ, Vieth R. Estimates of optimal vitamin D status. Osteoporos Int. 2005;16:713–716.
14. Bullamore JR, Wilkinson R, Gallagher JC, et al. Effects of age on calcium absorption. Lancet. 1970;2: 535–537.
15. Tsai KS, Heath H III, Kumar R, Riggs BL. Impaired vitamin D metabolism with aging in women. Possible role in pathogenesis of senile osteoporosis. J Clin Invest. 1984;73:1668–1672.
16. MacLaughlin J, Holick MF. Aging decreases the capacity of human skin to produce vitamin D_3. J Clin Invest. 1985;76:1536–1538.
17. Harris SS, Dawson-Hughes B. Plasma vitamin D and 25OHD responses of young and old men to supplementation with vitamin D_3. J Am Coll Nutr. 2002;21:357–362.
18. Webb AR, Klline L, Holick MF. Influence of season

and latitude on the cutaneous synthesis of vitamin D_3: exposure to winter sunlight in Boston and Edmonton will not promote vitamin D_3 synthesis in human skin. J Clin Endocrinol Metab. 1988;67: 373–378.
19. Dawson-Hughes B, Dallal GE, Krall EA, et al. Effect of vitamin D supplementation on wintertime and overall bone loss in healthy postmenopausal women. Ann Intern Med. 1991;115:505–512.
20. Dawson-Hughes B, Harris SS, Krall EA, et al. Rates of bone loss in postmenopausal women randomized to two dosages of vitamin D. Am J Clin Nutr. 1995; 61:1140–1145.
21. Morrison NA, Qi JC, Tokita A, et al. Prediction of bone density from vitamin D receptor alleles. Nature. 1994;367:284–287.
22. Krall EA, Parry P, Lichter JB, Dawson-Hughes B. Vitamin D receptor alleles and rates of bone loss: influences of years since menopause and calcium intake. J Bone Miner Res. 1995;10:978–984.
23. Dawson-Hughes B, Harris SS, Finneran S. Calcium absorption on high and low calcium intakes in relation to vitamin D receptor genotype. J Clin Endocrinol Metab. 1995;80:3657–3661.
24. Cummings SR, Black DM, Nevitt MC, et al. Bone density at various sites for prediction of hip fractures. Lancet. 1993;341:72–75.
25. Hui SL, Slemenda CW, Johnston CC Jr. Age and bone mass as predictors of fracture in a prospective study. J Clin Invest. 1988;81:1804–1809.
26. Dresner-Pollak R, Parker RA, Poku M, et al. Biochemical markers of bone turnover reflect femoral bone loss in elderly women. Calcif Tissue Int. 1996; 59:328–333.
27. Garnero P, Hausherr E, Chapuy MC, et al. Markers of bone resorption predict hip fracture in elderly women: the EPIDOS prospective study. J Bone Miner Res. 1996;11:1531–1538.
28. Riggs BL, O'Fallon WM, Muhs J, et al. Long-term effects of calcium supplementation on serum parathyroid hormone level, bone turnover, and bone loss in elderly women. J Bone Miner Res. 1998;13: 168–174.
29. Chevalley T, Rizzoli R, Nydegger V, et al. Effects of calcium supplements on femoral bone mineral density and vertebral fracture rate in vitamin-D-replete elderly patients. Osteoporos Int. 1994;4: 245–252.
30. Elders PJM, Netelenbos JC, Lips P, et al. Calcium supplementation reduces vertebral bone loss in perimenopausal women: a controlled trial in 248 women between 46 and 55 years of age. J Clin Endocrinol Metab. 1991;73:533–540.
31. Dawson-Hughes B, Harris SS, Krall EA, Dallal GE. Effect of calcium and vitamin D supplementation on bone density in men and women 65 years of age or older. N Engl J Med. 1997;337:670–676.
32. Delmas PD, Gineyts E, Bertholin A, et al. Immunoassay of pyridinoline crosslink excretion in normal adults and in Paget's disease. J Bone Miner Res. 1993;8:643–648.
33. Epstein S, Poser J, McClintock T, et al. Differences in serum bone GLA protein with age and sex. Lancet. 1984;2:307–310.
34. Martin AD, Bailey DA, McKay HA, Whiting S. Bone mineral and calcium accretion during puberty. Am J Clin Nutr. 1997;66:611–615.
35. Heaney RP. Calcium, dairy products, and osteoporosis. J Am College Nutr. 2000;2:83S–99S.
36. Johnston CC, Miller JZ, Slemenda CW, et al. Calcium supplementation and increases in bone mineral density in children. N Engl J Med. 1992;327:82–87.
37. Matkovic V, Goel PK, Badenhop-Stevens NE, et al. Calcium supplementation and bone mineral density in females from childhood to young adulthood: a randomized controlled trial. Am J Clin Nutr. 2005;81: 175–188.
38. Lloyd TH, Rollings NJ, Chinchilli VM. The effect of enhanced bone gain achieved with calcium supplementation during ages 12 to 16 does not persist in late adolescence. In: Burckhardt P, Dawson-Hughes B, Heaney RP, eds. *Nutritional Aspects of Osteoporosis.* New York: Springer; 1998:11–25.
39. Lee WTK, Leung SSF, Lueng DMY, Cheng JCY. A follow-up study on the effects of calcium-supplement withdrawal and puberty on bone acquisition of children. Am J Clin Nutr. 1996;64:71–77.
40. Slemenda CW, Peacock M, Hui S, et al. Reduced rates of skeletal remodeling are associated with increased bone mineral density during the development of peak skeletal mass. J Bone Miner Res. 1997;12: 676–682.
41. Bonjour JP, Carrie AL, Ferrari S, et al. Calcium-enriched foods and bone mass growth in prepubertal girls: a randomized, double-blind, placebo-controlled trial. J Clin Invest. 1997;99:1287–1294.
42. Baran D, Sorensen A, Grimes J, et al. Dietary modification with dairy products for preventing vertebral bone loss in premenopausal women: a three-year prospective study. J Clin Endocrinol Metab. 1990;70: 264–270.
43. Reid IR, Ames RW, Evans MC, et al. Long-term effects of calcium supplementation on bone loss and fractures in postmenopausal women: a randomized controlled trial. Am J Med. 1995;98:331–335.
44. Prince RL, Devine A, Dick IM, et al. The effects of calcium supplementation (milk powder or tablets) and exercise on bone density in postmenopausal women. J Bone Miner Res. 1995;10:1068–1075.
45. Ooms ME, Roos JC, Bezemer PD, et al. Prevention of bone loss by vitamin D supplementation in elderly women: a randomized double-blind trial. J Clin Endocrinol Metab. 1995;80:1052–1058.
46. Orwoll ES, Oviatt SK, McClung MR, et al. The rate

of bone mineral loss in normal men and the effects of calcium and cholecalciferol supplementation. Ann Intern Med. 1990;112:29–34.
47. Dawson-Hughes B, Harris S, Krall E, Dallal G. Effect of calcium and vitamin D supplement withdrawal on bone mass in elderly men and women. Am J Clin Nutr. 2000;72:745–750.
48. Specker BL. Evidence for an interaction between calcium intake and physical activity on changes in bone mineral density. J Bone Miner Res. 1996;11: 1539–1544.
49. Nieves JW, Komar L, Cosman F, Lindsay R. Calcium potentiates the effect of estrogen and calcitonin on bone mass: review and analysis. Am J Clin Nutr. 1998;67:18–24.
50. Black DM, Cummings SR, Karpf DB, et al. Randomized trial of effect of alendronate on risk of fracture in women with existing vertebral fractures: fracture intervention trial research group. Lancet. 1996; 348:1535–1541.
51. Harris ST, Watts NB, Genant HK, et al. Effects of risedronate treatment on vertebral and nonvertebral fractures in women with postmenopausal osteoporosis. JAMA. 1999;282:1344–1352.
52. Ettinger B, Black DM, Mitlak BH, et al. Reduction of vertebral fracture risk in postmenopausal women with osteoporosis treated with raloxifene. JAMA. 1999;282:637–645.
53. Chestnut HC III, Silverman S, Andriano K, et al. A randomized trial of nasal spray salmon calcitonin in postmenopausal women with established osteoporosis: the Prevent Recurrence of Osteoporotic Fractures study. Am J Med. 2000;109:267–276.
54. Tinetti ME, Speechley M, Ginter SF. Risk factors for falls among elderly persons living in the community. N Engl J Med. 1988;319:1701–1707.
55. Alexander BH, Rivara FP, Wolf ME. The cost and frequency of hospitalization for fall-related injuries in older adults. Am J Public Health. 1992;82: 1020–1023.
56. Nevitt M, Cummings S, Kidd S, Black D. Risk factors for recurrent nonsyncopal falls: a prospective study. J Am Med Assoc. 1989;261:2633–2668.
57. Grisso JA, Kelsey JL, Strom BL, et al. Risk factors for falls as a cause of hip fracture in women. The Northeast hip fracture study group. N Engl J Med. 1991;324:1326–1331.
58. Bischoff-Ferrari HA, Dietrich T, Orav EJ, Zhang Y, Karlson EW, Dawson-Hughes B. Higher 25-hydroxyvitamin D levels are associated with better lower extremity function in both active and inactive adults 60+ years of age. Am J Clin Nutr. 2004;80: 752–758.
59. Pfeifer M, Begerow B, Minne HW, Abrams C, Nachtigall D, Hansen C. Effects of a short-term vitamin D and calcium supplementation on body sway and secondary hyperparathyroidism in elderly women. J Bone Miner Res. 2000;15:1113–1118.
60. Bischoff-Ferrari HA, Dawson-Hughes B, Willett W, et al. Fall prevention by vitamin D treatment: a meta-analysis of randomized controlled trials. J Am Med Assoc. 2004;291:1999–2006.
61. Recker RR Hinders S, Davies KM, et al. Correcting calcium nutritional deficiency prevents spine fractures in elderly women. J Bone Miner Res. 1996;11: 1961–1966.
62. Lips P, Graafmans WC, Ooms ME, et al. Vitamin D supplementation and fracture incidence in elderly persons: a randomized, placebo-controlled clinical trial. Ann Intern Med. 1996;124:400–406.
63. Meyere HE, Smedshaug GB, Kvaavik E, Falch JA, Tverdal A, Pedersen JI. Can vitamin D supplementation reduce the risk of fracture in the elderly? A randomized controlled trial. J Bone Miner Res. 2002; 17:709–715.
64. Trivedi DP, Doll R, Khaw KT. Effect of four monthly oral vitamin D_3 (cholecalciferol) supplementation on fractures and mortality in men and women living in the community: randomized double blind controlled trial. BMJ. 2003;326:469.
65. Heikinheimo RJ, Inkovaara JA, Harju EJ, et al. Annual injection of vitamin D and fractures of aged bones. Calcif Tissue Int. 1992;51:105–10.
66. Chapuy M-C, Arlot ME, Duboeuf F, et al. Vitamin D_3 and calcium to prevent hip fractures in elderly women. N Engl J Med. 1992;327:1637–1642.
67. Chapuy MC, Pamphile R, Paris E, et al. Combined calcium and vitamin D_3 supplementation in elderly women: confirmation of reversal of secondary hyperparathyroidism and hip fracture risk: the Decalyos II study. Osteoporos Int. 2002;13:257–264.
68. Nusser SM, Carriquiry AL, Dodd KW, Fuller WA. A semiparametric transformation approach to estimating usual daily intake distributions. J Am Stat Assoc. 1996;91:1440–1449.
69. Food and Nutrition Board. *Dietary Reference Intakes: Calcium, Phosphorus, Magnesium, Vitamin D, and Fluoride.* Washington, DC: National Academy Press; 1997.
70. Schuette SA, Zemel MB, Linksweiler HM. Studies on the mechanism of protein-induced hypercalciuria in older men and women. J Nutr. 1980;110:305–315.
71. Pannemans DLE, Schaafsma G, Westerterp KR. Calcium excretion, apparent calcium absorption and calcium balance in young and elderly subjects: influence of protein intake. Br J Nutr. 1997;77:721–729.
72. Kerstetter JE, O'Brien KO, Caseria DM, Wall DE, Insogna KL. The impact of dietary protein on calcium absorption and kinetic measures of bone turnover in women. J Clin Endocrinol Metab. 2005;90: 26–31.
73. Kerstetter JE, Svastisalee CM, Caseria DM, et al. A

threshold for low-protein-induced elevations in parathyroid hormone. Am J Clin Nutr. 2000;72: 168–173.
74. Shapses SS, Robins SP, Schwartz EI, Chowdhury H. Short-term changes in calcium but not protein intake alter the rate of bone resorption in healthy subjects as assessed by urinary pyridinium cross-link excretion. J Nutr. 1995;125:2814–2821.
75. Freudenheim JL, Johnson NE, Smith EL. Relationships between usual nutrient intake and bone mineral content in women 35–65 years of age. Am J Clin Nutr. 1986;44:863–876.
76. Hannan M, Tucker K, Dawson-Hughes B, et al. Effect of dietary protein on bone loss in elderly men and women: the Framingham Osteoporosis Study [abstract]. J Bone Miner Res. 1997;12:S151.
77. Munger RG, Chiu BC-H. Prospective study of dietary protein intake and risk of hip fracture in postmenopausal women. Am J Clin Nutr. 1999;69: 147–152.
78. Delmi M, Rapin C-H, Bengoa J-M, et al. Dietary supplementation in elderly patients with fractured neck of the femur. Lancet. 1990;335:1013–1016.
79. Schurch MA, Rizzoli R, Slosman D, et al. Protein supplements increase serum insulin-like growth factor-1 levels and attenuate proximal femur bone loss in patients with recent hip fractures. A randomized, double-blind, placebo-controlled trial. Ann Intern Med. 1998;128:801–809.
80. Food and Nutrition Board: Food and Nutrition Board. *Dietary Reference Intakes for Vitamin A, Vitamin K, Arsenic, Boron, Chromium, Copper, Iodine, Iron Manganese, Molybdenum, Nickel, Silicon, Vanadium, and Zinc.* Washington DC, National Academy Press; 2001.
81. Booth SL, O'Brien-Morse ME, Dallal GE, et al. Response of vitamin K status to different intakes and sources of phylloquinone-rich foods: comparison of younger and older adults. Am J Clin Nutr. 1999;70: 368–377.
82. Booth SL, Webb DR, Peters JC. Assessment of phylloquinone and dihydrophylloquinone dietary intakes among a nationally representative sample of US consumers using 14-day food diaries. J Am Diet Assoc. 1999;99:1072–1076.
83. Booth SL, Tucker KL, Chen H, et al. Dietary vitamin K intakes are associated with hip fracture but not with bone mineral density in elderly men and women. Am J Clin Nutr. 2000;71:1201–1208.
84. Feskanich D, Weber P, Willett WC, et al. Vitamin K intake and hip fractures in women: a prospective study. Am J Clin Nutr. 1999;69:74–79.
85. Stone KL, Duong T, Sellmeyer D, et al. Broccoli may be good for bones: dietary vitamin K1, rates of bone loss and risk of hip fracture in a prospective study of elderly women [abstract]. J Bone Miner Res. 1999:14:S263.

52 Cancer

Young-In Kim

Overview

The development of cancer is thought to be the result of an intimate, and yet poorly understood, interplay between environmental and genetic factors. An impressive body of epidemiologic evidence indicates that dietary and lifestyle factors are among the most important environmental factors implicated in the development of cancer.[1] For instance, in 1981, Doll and Peto[2] estimated that approximately 35% (10%–70%) of all cancers in the United States might be attributable to dietary factors, and that up to 90% of colorectal cancer in the United States may be preventable through dietary modifications. More recently, it was estimated that one-third of the 500,000 cancer deaths that occur in the United States each year are due to dietary factors.[3] Similar estimates were made by the European School of Oncology Task Force on Diet, Nutrition, and Cancer in 1994,[4] and by the World Cancer Research Fund and the American Institute for Cancer Research in 1997.[1] These provocative epidemiologic estimations were supported by a recent study involving 44,788 pairs of twins in Scandinavian countries. In that study, findings suggested that 58%, 65%, and 73% of prostate, colorectal, and breast cancers (3 of the 4 most common cancers in the United States), respectively, are attributable to environmental factors.[5] Much effort has been directed toward defining the relationship between dietary and lifestyle factors and the development of cancer, as well as toward the prevention of cancer through dietary and lifestyle modifications.[1] In this regard, there is evidence that dietary modifications have possibly contributed to a 29% reduction in the colorectal cancer mortality in the US white population from 1950 through 1990, with a more pronounced decrease in women than in men.[6]

However, a cause-and-effect relationship between dietary factors and cancer is difficult to establish. Because of inherent limitations associated with study design, the results from epidemiologic, animal, and interventional studies examining this relationship have often been conflicting. Furthermore, the precise nature of the relationship of cancer with each nutrient and the actual magnitude of the relationship have not been clearly defined. Definitive answers to questions about diet and cancer are probably beyond the reach of both observational epidemiologic studies and randomized, controlled trials.[7] In clinical medicine, the best evidence has been considered to come from well-designed and well-executed double-blind randomized, controlled trials, which minimize a variety of biases. Evidence from randomized, controlled trials is thought to supercede evidence from other sources such as observational studies. The field of nutritional epidemiology has also followed this traditional approach and considered correlation, case-control, and prospective observational epidemiologic studies and intervention trials as a spectrum of increasing weight of evidence for or against a relationship between dietary factors and cancer risk.[1] Thus, general conclusions and recommendations regarding the effect of dietary factors on cancer risk have relied heavily on data from large prospective studies and randomized, controlled intervention human trials.[1] For example, an international panel of experts from the World Cancer Research Fund, in association with the American Institute for Cancer Research, concluded that the dietary constituents and related factors, foods and drinks, and methods of food processing listed in Table 1 modify the risk of colorectal cancer based on the strength of evidence from observational epidemiologic and intervention studies that were available to the panel in 1997.[1]

This traditional approach to grading epidemiologic evidence concerning the relationship between dietary factors and cancer risk has recently been challenged.[7,8] As cancer develops over decades, if not a lifetime, single clinical trials, which normally last up to 5 years, cannot address the whole span of cancer development. In addition, randomized, controlled trials tend to use uncharacteristic levels of exposure. Furthermore, the dietary, nutritional, and physical activity exposures involved are complex and in-

Table 1. Summary of Evidence for the Role of Dietary and Lifestyle Factors in the Development of Colorectal Cancer Presented by the World Cancer Research Fund/American Institute for Cancer Research in 1997

Evidence	Decreased Risk	No Association	Increased Risk
Convincing	Physical activity		
	Vegetables		
Probable			Red meat
			Alcohol
Possible	Nonstarch polysaccharides/fiber	Calcium	High body mass index
	Starch	Selenium	Adult height
	Carotenoids	Fish	Frequent eating
			Sugar
			Total fat
			Saturated/animal fat
			Processed meat
			Eggs
			Heavily cooked meat
Insufficient	Resistant starch		Iron
	Vitamins C, D, E		
	Folate, methionine		
	Cereal		
	Coffee		

Adapted from World Cancer Research Fund/American Institute for Cancer Research, 1997[1] with permission from The American Institute for Cancer Research.

terrelated, making them difficult to manipulate in a controlled fashion. Even if a difference in outcome followed such a clinical intervention, it would not necessarily indicate that reproducing the intervention under other conditions would cause similar outcomes. Thus, it has been argued that drawing a definitive conclusion concerning the effect of dietary factors on cancer risk mainly from randomized, controlled intervention human trials is probably not the right paradigm of nutritional epidemiology.[7,8] Rather, it has been articulated that the totality or "portfolio" of evidence from observational and intervention studies, as well as animal and in vitro experiments, must be analyzed for this purpose.[7,8] The portfolio approach does not set out a hierarchy of evidence. Instead, it recognizes that all types of evidence have advantages and disadvantages. This means that no single kind of study is considered to be definitive. Instead, all of the different types of studies that are used to investigate the link between nutrition and cancer are considered alongside each other, without favoring evidence from one type over another. In support of the portfolio approach, systematic comparisons of the results of randomized intervention studies with observational evidence in several clinical situations have shown that observational data from well-conducted studies do not appear to produce biased results compared with randomized interventions.[9,10]

Furthermore, the importance of experimental studies that contribute to understanding mechanisms that might underlie any observed association between a dietary factor and cancer and might bear on the inference of causation has been increasingly recognized and appreciated in the field of nutrition and cancer. Epidemiologic and experimental evidence indicating a causal association between a dietary factor and cancer is strengthened when a biologic pathway or mechanism by which colorectal carcinogenesis may be modified is identified and when this mechanism is biologically plausible.[7] It can be argued that epidemiologic data, however strong and consistent, are an inadequate basis for any definite judgment of causality unless supported by mechanistic evidence.[7] Although earlier investigations to elucidate potential anticarcinogenic mechanisms associated with dietary factors have focused on physical properties of these factors, more recent work has expanded into physiologic functions and molecular mechanisms. A better mechanistic understanding of how dietary factors can modulate carcinogenesis may lead to a more rational strategy using dietary supplementation to prevent cancer in humans.

Recent advances in molecular epidemiology have added another dimension to the already complex field of nutrition and cancer. Recently identified and characterized single nucleotide polymorphisms and other genetic and epigenetic variants of genes that are involved in absorption, transport, metabolism, and excretion of nutrients have been shown to modify cancer risk and to significantly modulate the effect of nutrients and related compounds on cancer risk.[11] This emerging important topic in the field of nutrition and cancer, termed "gene-nutrient interactions" in carcinogenesis, has a significant implication in designing and interpreting data from observational epidemiologic and intervention studies. Although individuals are subjected to the same level of nutritional exposure, systemic and target tissue bioavailability of nutrients and their metabolites, as well as their functional effects in the target tissue, might be vastly different because of genetic and epigenetic variations. Genetic and epigenetic susceptibility to cancer and the interaction of genetics and epigenetics with diets and other environmental exposures have not been incorporated into the study design of and interpretation of data from previously published epidemiologic and intervention studies. The precise nature and magnitude of gene-nutrient interactions in carcinogenesis are yet to be clearly defined.

Given these considerations, the objective of this chapter is to provide a critical analysis of currently available data from epidemiologic and intervention studies in humans of the effects of nutritional factors on carcinogenesis. A comprehensive review of the entire field of nutrition and cancer including biologic mechanisms of nutritional modulation of cancer risk is beyond the scope of this chapter, and the readers are referred to several recent comprehensive reviews on this topic.[1,12-17] The emphasis here is on colorectal cancer because of its magnitude and impact and because of the large number of studies that have focused on it.

Colorectal Cancer

Colorectal cancer incidence rates vary approximately 10- to 200-fold across different geographic locations around the world, with the highest observed in the developed, Westernized, industrialized, and urbanized parts of the world.[1] The international differences, migrant data, and recent rapid increases in incidence rates in the same geographic location with previously low colorectal cancer incidence rates over time collectively suggest that environmental factors, including diet, play a major role in the development of colorectal cancer.[1]

In the United States, colorectal cancer is the fourth most common cancer and the second most common cause of cancer-specific death for both men and women.[18] In 2005 alone, 145,290 new cases of colorectal cancer were expected to be diagnosed, and approximately 40% of these are expected to die within 5 years.[18] In 2005, an estimated 56,290 deaths will have been caused by colorectal cancer.[18] The lifetime risk of developing colorectal cancer is approximately 6%.[19] Colorectal adenomas, the well-established precursor of colorectal cancer,[19] are found in approximately 25% to 50% of people by 50 years of age in the United States, and the prevalence increases with age.[19] It has been estimated that approximately 25% of adenomas progress to colorectal cancer over 5 to 10 years.[19]

Table 2. Dietary, Lifestyle, and Other Factors that May Modulate Colorectal Cancer Risk

Positive Association	Inverse Association
Energy intake	Fiber
Total, saturated, and animal fat	Vegetables and fruits
Red meat	Calcium
Protein	Vitamin D
Simple sugars	Antioxidant vitamins (A, C, E, and β-carotene)
Alcohol	Selenium
Smoking	Folate
Iron	Fish oil (omega-3 fatty acid)
Body mass index	Physical activity
	Hormonal replacement therapy
	Aspirin, nonsteroidal anti-inflammatory drugs

Colorectal cancer provides an excellent paradigm of gene-nutrient interactions in carcinogenesis because the molecular genetics and epigenetics of this cancer have been well established.[12] As the colorectal epithelium progresses from a normal histology to one that is hyperproliferative, adenomatous, and finally malignant, multiple molecular alterations, including the activation of protooncogenes and inactivation of tumor suppressor and mismatch repair genes, and epigenetic changes accumulate sequentially.[12] Environmental carcinogens and dietary factors can potentially affect each step of colorectal carcinogenesis, thereby modulating these molecular and epigenetic changes. Colorectal cancer is preceded by well-established precursors, including aberrant crypt foci and adenomatous polyps, which are easily accessible, identifiable, and removable.[12] Therefore, colorectal cancer is an ideal cancer for studying the effects of environmental and dietary factors on each stage of carcinogenesis.

Consumption of red meat, animal and saturated fat, refined carbohydrates, and alcohol, as well as total caloric (energy) intake, is generally considered to be positively related to the risk of developing colorectal cancer (Table 1).[1,12,13] On the other hand, the intake of dietary fiber, vegetables, fruits, antioxidant vitamins, calcium, and folate is believed to be negatively associated with the risk of developing colorectal cancer (Table 2).[1,12,13]

Primer of Nutritional Epidemiology

Probably the most challenging problem encountered in nutritional epidemiologic studies examining the relationship between dietary factors and colorectal cancer risk is the difficulty of accurately assessing intake of dietary factors.[20] Dietary intake of nutritional factors is assessed by several different methods, and each method is associated with inherent limitations[20] (see Chapter 58). Qualitative data on food preparation methods, cooking, chewing, and other dietary habits that can alter the physiologic properties of dietary factors are often lacking. In addition, it is often difficult to determine the exact intake of nutritional supplements because of the availability of hundreds of different products, both over the counter and by prescription.[20] Another difficulty in assessing supplement use is that many individuals take supplements inconsistently and in patterns that are hard to characterize.[20]

Four types of human epidemiologic studies and animal studies are used to study the relationship between dietary factors and colorectal cancer risk.[1,13] Broadly, epidemiologic studies are divided into observational (correlation, case-control, and prospective) and intervention studies.[1,13]

Correlation Studies

Correlation studies examine the relationship between the per capita consumption of a dietary factor and the prevalence of, incidence of, or mortality from colorectal cancer in the population. Correlation studies can examine this relationship among populations residing in different countries or among different groups within a country either at a given time or over a certain time (i.e., a time-trend analysis). These studies provide provocative initial evidence that a particular dietary factor plays a role in the development of colorectal cancer and hence is considered worthy only of hypothesis formation. The limitations with the interpretations of data generated from these correlation studies are several, including the inaccuracy with which dietary intake is assessed. Correlation studies often fail to correct for unmeasured confounding factors that may be responsible for the observed association. Correlation studies also do not control for other dietary variables or for any of the other known risk factors associated with colorectal cancer.

Case-Control Studies

Case-control studies compare prior consumption of a dietary factor by subjects with colorectal cancer with that of matched control subjects without colorectal cancer. Many of the weaknesses of correlation studies can be avoided in case-control studies. Known or suspected potential confounding factors can be controlled or eliminated in the study design or controlled in the data analysis. With regard to dietary factors, the most serious limitation in retrospective studies is the accuracy with which intake of dietary factors or supplementation can be established. Case-control studies often fail to incorporated qualitative data on dietary habits and cooking methods into the nutrient estimation. Also, some individual aspects of diet, especially nutrient content, may not vary greatly within a population, so case-control studies may not show wide ranges of colorectal cancer risk within that population. Other common problems are the lack of appropriate controls and selection bias because of the absence of patients who do not survive long enough to be enrolled in the study. Another problem is that it is difficult to adequately control or correct potential confounders in retrospective analyses. Lastly, it is difficult to delineate the effect associated with a dietary factor from other potential anticarcinogens present in the diet in case-control studies. Although inherent problems associated with retrospective analyses often limit the interpretation of results from case-control studies, valuable information can be gathered from well-designed case-control studies in a time- and cost-effective manner.

Prospective Studies

Prospective (or cohort) studies assess the diets of a large group of healthy individuals and follow the participants over time, during which a number of cohort members will develop colorectal cancer. The relationship of colorectal cancer to specific characteristics of individuals' diets is then analyzed. Prospective studies avoid most of the methodologic problems of crude observational and retrospective epidemiologic studies and can control and correct confounding factors more adequately than can correlation and case-control studies. Also, because of the prospective design—with diet being assessed before the occurrence of cancer—there is little likelihood of selection or recording bias in cohort studies.

One of the weaknesses associated with prospective studies is that they correlate dietary consumption of a nutritional factor at baseline to subsequent incidence of colorectal cancer. In other words, the dietary intake at baseline is assumed to reflect past and subsequent consumption. Whether the subjects in these studies change their diet during the follow-up period and how this might affect the study outcome cannot be deduced. However, recent prospective studies obtained repeated assessments of diet at regular intervals, which improves the accuracy of individual dietary assessment. A vast majority of prospective studies are limited by the relatively short follow-up. This issue is important because of the uncertainty regarding the biologically relevant period of exposure before the development of colorectal cancer.

Another potential shortcoming that limits the interpretation of results from prospective studies relates to imprecise estimation of dietary intake (as in other types of epidemiologic studies), as well as the lack of data on food preparation methods, cooking, and chewing, which can alter the physiologic properties of dietary factors. Some prospective studies have selected cohorts with relatively homogeneous lifestyle and dietary habits and therefore may be quite unrepresentative of the general population. Therefore, the applicability of the observations made in these cohorts to the general population is uncertain. Another problem is that the range of dietary intakes of a nutritional factor under investigation may be narrow so that the factor's effects may not be observed.

Intervention Studies

In theory, randomized intervention studies in humans should provide definitive support for the purported cause-and-effect relationship between a dietary factor and colorectal cancer. However, intervention studies are often exceedingly difficult to carry out because of the slowly progressive nature of neoplastic transformation and the large number of subjects necessary to achieve an adequate statistical power. The major weaknesses associated with the majority of published intervention studies are short follow-up periods, small numbers of subjects, poor compliance with dietary interventions, high dropout rates, and use of histologic, molecular, and biochemical surrogate end-point biomarkers of colorectal cancer as the outcome instead of using occurrence or recurrence of colorectal cancer.[21] All surrogate end-point biomarkers have limitations, and most have not been conclusively validated in clinical studies.[21] Furthermore, except for a few biomarkers (e.g., adenomas[19,22]), modulating any of these surrogate end-point biomarkers has not yet clearly led to a reduction in colorectal cancer occurrence and mortality.[21] Even with adenomas, only a very small portion progress to adenocarcinoma, depending on the number, size, and histologic features.[19,22] Therefore, using the recurrence of all adenomas as the end point of intervention trials may not be appropriate; rather, advanced adenomas (defined as those >1 cm in diameter or those with either a villous component or high-grade dysplasia) that have been shown to possess a high degree of neoplastic transformation potential might be a better surrogate end-point biomarker for this purpose.[19,22]

In addition, there are several other limitations associated with intervention trials. Intervention studies attempt to intervene in incompletely understood biologic pathways in special populations of adults at high risk of developing colorectal cancer, who therefore may be at a late, although preclinical, stage of carcinogenesis or have precancerous lesions (Figure 1). Ideally, such interventions should be initiated well before the development of premalignant or precursor lesions in the target organ (Figure 1). Furthermore, interventions to prevent cancer may have to be repositioned to the in utero and early childhood stages of the human life cycle before the target organ is initiated for the subsequent development of cancer (Figure 1).[23] In addition, the time between the change in the level of a dietary factor and any expected change in the incidence of colorectal cancer (i.e., relevant induction time) is usually uncertain and may be decades. Trials should therefore be of a long duration, which is not the case for most of the intervention trials published to date. Another potential problem lies with uncertainty regarding what constitutes biologically relevant doses of dietary intervention that may modulate colorectal carcinogenesis. Also, people who agree to participate in trials tend to be relatively health conscious and highly motivated; people who are at high potential risk on the basis of dietary intake, and thus susceptible to intervention, are liable to be underrepresented. Hence, the validity of generalizing the results is limited. In non-blind studies of foods, individuals in the control group may adopt the dietary behavior of the treatment group if they think the treatment diet is beneficial, which could obscure a real benefit of treatment.

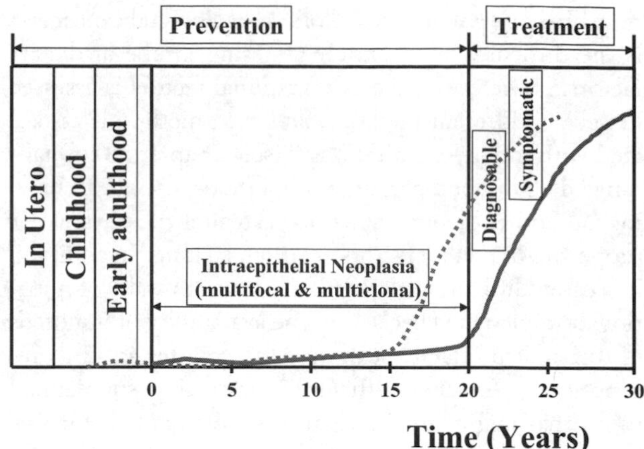

Figure 1. Cancer develops over decades, if not a lifetime, through different stages of premalignant lesions (intraepithelial neoplasia) in the target organ (solid line). Most cancers become diagnosable and symptomatic at advanced ages (solid line). Typically, interventions to prevent cancer are initiated after the establishment of premalignant lesions in the target organ and therefore are actually testing the effect on the regression of or suppression of the progression of these premalignant lesions to cancer. Ideally, strategies to prevent cancer should be initiated well before the development, or at a very early stage, of premalignant lesions in the target organ (i.e., in childhood or early adulthood). In those individuals with genetic predispositions to cancer, the target organ is initiated for subsequent development of cancer at a very young age and may even harbor preneoplastic foci in utero, at birth, or in early infancy (broken line). In these individuals, intervention to prevent cancer may have to be repositioned to the in utero and early childhood stages. (Adapted from Go et al., 2003[23] with permission from the American Society for Nutrition.)

In general, observational epidemiologic studies suggest a stronger association between a dietary factor and cancer risk than do intervention studies.[1,13] Findings from randomized, controlled intervention trials often do not confirm the relationships between nutrients and cancer risk that have been suggested by observational studies (e.g., low fat, high fiber, high vegetables/fruits and colorectal adenoma recurrence;[24] high fiber and colorectal adenoma recurrence;[25] low fat, high fiber and colorectal adenoma recurrence;[26] and antioxidant vitamins and colorectal adenoma recurrence[27]). In some studies, only a modest degree of cancer risk reduction, significantly less than that previously suggested by observation studies, has been demonstrated (e.g., low fat, high fiber and colorectal adenoma recurrence[28] and calcium and colorectal adenoma recurrence[29]). In some cases, trials have even demonstrated that high doses of nutrients previously believed to be beneficial could have unexpected harmful effects (e.g., β-carotene and lung cancer[30,31]). Some intervention studies have uncovered beneficial effects of nutrients on cancer that were not hypothesized a priori as the primary end points (e.g., selenium and colorectal cancer[32]).

It has recently been suggested that intervention studies should not be considered as an epidemiologic "gold standard."[8] According to Byers, controlled trials in which an intervention shows beneficial effects are good evidence that the agents used are protective. Studies in which intervention shows no effect, or even a detrimental effect, however, do not show that the agents used are irrelevant or harmful in the context of whole diets or among normal, healthy populations.[8] Byers argues that the results of intervention studies should not be treated as a refutation of evidence from other types of epidemiologic studies, especially when such other evidence is backed by data from animal studies and identification of plausible biologic pathways.[8]

Animal Studies

Studies utilizing laboratory animals provide for greater control of variables, enable interventions to be used that would not be feasible in humans, and are often less expensive than human trials. Furthermore, potential biologic pathways or mechanisms by which colorectal carcinogenesis may be modified by dietary factors can be investigated in a time- and cost-efficient manner. However, animal studies lack uniform protocols in terms of carcinogen, route of administration, and dose, as well as the species, strain, and age of the animals. Most importantly, they suffer from their inherent differences from human cancer, precluding direct extrapolation of observations from animal studies to humans.

Table 3. Possible Anticarcinogenic Mechanisms of Dietary Fiber

- Increased stool bulk
  - Dilution of potential carcinogens
  - Decrease in transit time (less contact time for carcinogens)
- Binding with potential carcinogens/binding with bile acids
  - Decrease in fecal bile acid concentrations
  - Prevention of the conversion of primary to secondary bile acids
- Lower fecal pH
  - Reduced solubility of free bile acids
  - Inhibition of 7α-dehydroxylase, which converts primary to secondary bile acids
  - Inhibition of bacterial degradation of normal fecal constituents to potential carcinogens
- Alteration of colonic microflora
  - Inhibition of microbial enzymes involved in carcinogen activation
  - Changes in bacterial species
  - Stimulation of bacterial growth, which increases fecal bulk
- Fermentation by fecal flora to short-chain fatty acids
  - Inhibition of cell growth and proliferation
  - Induction of differentiation
  - Induction of apoptosis
  - Modulation of gene expression
- Prevention/reduction of insulin resistance and hyperinsulinemia

Specific Dietary Factors Implicated in Colorectal Carcinogenesis

Evidence for the role of several key dietary factors in colorectal carcinogenesis is discussed using the portfolio approach.

Fiber

The relationship between dietary fiber and colorectal cancer risk provides an excellent case study in nutrition and colorectal cancer and highlights inherent, probably unresolvable, limitations of currently available tools to detect a real effect associated with dietary fiber. The role of dietary fiber in the development of colorectal cancer was first recognized in the early 1970s, when Burkitt[33] noted the rarity of colorectal cancer in most African populations with a high intake of fiber and a low intake of refined carbohydrates. There exist several biologically plausible physiologic, cellular, and molecular mechanisms by which dietary fiber can protect against the development of colorectal cancer, as outlined in Table 3.[34] Most of the published correlation and case-control studies show either a strong or moderate protective effect of dietary fiber or "fiber-rich foods" or show equivocal results that were nevertheless consistent with the fiber hypothesis.[34] Three analyses of case-control studies, conducted in combined analysis or meta-analysis formats, suggest, on average, a 50% reduction in the risk of colorectal cancer in individuals with the highest dietary fiber intake compared with those with the lowest fiber intake.[35-37] Most of the positive case-control studies and one combined analysis of case-control studies show a significant inverse dose-dependent relationship between dietary fiber intake and colorectal cancer risk.[34-37] The strongest argument for the fiber hypothesis that can be made from case-control studies is the remarkable consistency of the protective effect of dietary fiber among studies conducted in populations with different patterns of diet and colorectal cancer.[34,36]

By contrast, published large, prospective studies have produced equivocal findings. The Second Cancer Prevention Study of the American Cancer Society, involving more than 1 million subjects, showed a significant inverse relationship, with a 30% reduction of colorectal cancer mortality in subjects consuming the highest amount of dietary fiber compared with those consuming the lowest amount.[38] Three large prospective studies conducted in the United States—the Nurses' Health Study (N = 88,757; follow-up = 6–16 years),[39,40] the Iowa Women's Health Study (N = 35,216; follow-up = 4 years),[41] and the Health Professionals Follow-up Study (N = 47,949; follow-up = 6 years)[42]—have shown no significant association between dietary fiber intake and colorectal cancer incidence in men and women. These studies, however, have shown a significant protective effect of dietary fiber against distal colon and rectal adenomas in men (35% to 63% reduction in the risk[43,44]) but not in women.[40] The Finnish Alpha-Tocopherol, Beta-Carotene Cancer Prevention Study found no fiber-colorectal cancer association after following more than 27,000 male smokers for 8 years.[45] Two recent prospective studies, however, have demonstrated a significant protective effect of fiber on colorectal cancer.[46,47] The European Prospective Investigation into Cancer and Nutrition, involving 519,978 adults recruited from 10 European countries, showed a significant inverse relationship between fiber intake and colorectal cancer risk after 4.5 years of follow-up.[46] Those in the highest quintile of fiber intake (32 g/d in women and 36 g/d in men) had a significant 40% reduction in colorectal cancer risk compared with the lowest quintile (12.6 g/d in women and 12.8 g/d in men) (relative risk = 0.58, 95% confidence interval (CI), 0.41–0.85).[46] However, no food source of fiber was significantly more protective than others.[46] Another study in 43,611 participants in a multicenter, randomized trial designed to investigate methods for early detection of cancer (the Prostate, Lung, Colorectal, and Ovarian Cancer Screening Trial) in the United States found a significant dose-responsive inverse association between fiber intake and colorectal adenoma risk.[47] Those in the highest quintile of fiber intake were 27% less likely to have adenomas than were those in the lowest quintile (odds ratio = 0.73; 95% CI, 0.62–0.86).[47] The inverse association was significant for fiber from grains, cereals, and fruits but not fiber from legumes and vegetables.[47] The conflicting results from these well-designed and well-conducted large prospective studies naturally beg for possible explanations. The observed differences might be partially explained by different sources, types, and amounts of dietary fiber in different populations studied and by methods used for the analysis of dietary fiber.[48]

Although earlier small pilot trials showed the beneficial effect of fiber supplementation on adenoma recurrence or regression and on other surrogate end-point biomarkers of colorectal cancer,[34] more recent, larger placebo-controlled, randomized trials have generally shown no beneficial effect associated with dietary fiber supplementation, either alone or in combination with other dietary strategies, on adenoma recurrence (Table 4).[24-26,28] Of particular importance is the null effect of dietary fiber from the two largest trials published to date (Table 4).[24,25] The Polyp Prevention Trial, a multiinstitutional intervention study in the United States, was designed to test the effectiveness of a low-fat (20% of total calories), high-fiber (18 g/1000 kcal daily) diet enriched with vegetables and fruits (3.5 servings/1000 kcal daily)

Table 4. Summary of Recent Fiber Colorectal Cancer Chemoprevention Trials

Study (Reference)	Subjects (N)	Intervention	Duration	End Point	Outcome
Toronto Polyp Prevention Group[26]	Adenoma (201)	20% fat calories/d 50 g fiber/d vs. placebo	2 years	Adenoma recurrence	No effect
Australian Polyp Prevention Project[28]	Adenoma (424)	2 × 2 × 2 factorial <25% fat calories/d 25 g wheat bran/d 20 mg β-carotene/d	4 years	Adenoma recurrence	Fiber alone no effect Fiber with low fat protective against >10 mm adenomas
Wheat Bran Fiber Trial[25]	Adenoma (1429)	Wheat bran fiber 13.5 g/d vs. 2.0 g/d	3 years	Adenoma recurrence	No effect
Polyp Prevention Trial[24]	Adenoma (1905)	20% fat calories/d 18 g fiber/100 kcal/d 3.5 servings of fruits & vegetables/1000 kcal/d vs. placebo	4 years	Adenoma recurrence	No effect
European Cancer Prevention Organisation Intervention Study[49]	Adenoma (665)	2 g calcium/d 3.5 g ispaghula husk/d vs. placebo	3 years	Adenoma recurrence	67% increase in adenoma recurrence (P = 0.042)

to decrease the recurrence rate of colorectal adenomas in patients previously treated for them.[24] After 4 years of follow-up, no significant difference in adenoma recurrence was observed between the treatment and placebo groups among the 1905 subjects who completed the trial.[24] The Wheat Bran Fiber trial, a multicenter study conducted in Phoenix, Arizona, randomized 1429 subjects with colorectal adenomas after polypectomy to receive dietary supplementation with either a high (13.5 g/d) or low (2 g/d) amount of wheat bran fiber for 3 years.[25] This study demonstrated no significant protective effect of high-fiber supplementation on adenoma recurrence.[25] One recently published trial, the European Cancer Prevention Organisation Intervention Study (N = 665; follow-up = 3 years),[49] indicated that fiber supplementation (3.5 g/d ispaghula husk) was associated with a significant 67% increase in adenoma recurrence (Table 4). A recent meta-analysis of the randomized, controlled trial data (5 studies, N = 4349) found no evidence that increased dietary fiber reduces either incidence or recurrence of adenomas within a 2- to 4-year period.[50]

As discussed in the previous section, randomized intervention trials utilizing fiber supplementation are limited by several factors: 1) uncertainty concerning optimal timing, duration, and dose of fiber intervention; 2) use of surrogate end-point biomarkers; 3) a small number of subjects; 4) possibility of over- and underreporting of dietary fiber consumption by study participants; and 5) lack of incorporation of genetic variability in metabolism of fiber into the study design. Therefore, randomized intervention trials cannot definitively rule out the beneficial effect of dietary fiber that has been shown to be associated with a lower risk of colorectal cancer in observational studies.

In summary, currently available evidence from observational epidemiologic and intervention studies does not unequivocally support the protective role of fiber against the development of colorectal cancer. However, when the portfolio of evidence from these studies is analyzed critically, the overall conclusion supports an inverse association between dietary fiber intake and colorectal cancer risk. The magnitude of colorectal cancer risk reduction and threshold level above which dietary fiber is associated with a significant degree of colorectal cancer risk reduction are not clearly defined. The duration and timing of fiber supplementation, as well as which specific target groups would benefit most from fiber supplementation, are not well established.

Vegetables and Fruits

Among dietary factors implicated in the development of colorectal cancer, the inverse relationship between vegetable and fruit consumption and colorectal cancer risk has long been considered to represent the strongest epidemiologic evidence. Despite the paucity of supporting data from randomized studies, an international panel of experts from the World Cancer Research Fund concluded that "evidence that diets rich in vegetables protect against cancers of the colon and rectum is convincing. The data on fruit are more limited and inconsistent; no judgment is possible."[1] This strong endorsement for the purported protective role of vegetable consumption in colorectal cancer was based on observational epidemiologic evidence that was available to the panel in 1997. The overwhelming majority of the published correlation and case-control studies suggests the protective effect of high consumption of vegetables and fruits on the risk of colorectal cancer and adenomas; the effect is more pronounced for vegetables than for fruits.[1,12,13,51,52] A meta-analysis of 6 case-control studies of vegetables and colon cancer reported a 52% reduction in the risk of colon cancer associated with the highest consumption of vegetables compared with the lowest consumption.[35]

Large prospective studies published before 1997 also generally support the protective role of high vegetable and fruit consumption in colorectal carcinogenesis. A study of Seventh-Day Adventists (N = 25,943) reported a 30% reduction in the risk of fatal colon cancer in women consuming ≥7 servings of green salad/week compared with those consuming <4 servings/week.[53] In the Second Cancer Prevention Study of the American Cancer Society, a statistically significant inverse association between vegetable consumption and the risk of fatal colon cancer was observed in both men and women, with a 25% to 38% reduction in the risk of fatal colon cancer in subjects consuming the highest amount of vegetables compared with those consuming the lowest.[38]

In a US cohort of elderly persons (the Leisure World Study; N = 11,580), a significantly reduced risk of colon cancer was noted for combined intake of all vegetables and fruits and for fruit intake alone in women but not in men.[54] In the Iowa Women's Health Study involving 98,030 postmenopausal women, the total intake of both vegetables and fruits did not significantly reduce the risk of colorectal cancer.[41] When each vegetable or fruit item was independently analyzed, it was shown that individuals consuming ≥1 garlic clove per week had a 32% reduction in the risk of colorectal cancer compared with those not eating any garlic.[41] The protective effect of garlic on colorectal cancer risk has recently been supported by a meta-analysis of 7 case-control and prospective studies that showed that high garlic consumption (>28.8 g/week) was associated with a significant 30% reduction in colorectal cancer risk compared with low consumption (<3.5 g/week) (relative risk [RR] = 0.69; 95% CI, 0.55–0.89).[55] One study of colorectal adenomas in men (the Health Professionals Follow-up Study) reported an approximate 50% reduction of colorectal adenoma risk associated with high intake of vegetables and fruits.[43]

However, large prospective studies published after 1997 with conflicting results have dampened the enthusiasm for the protective role of vegetable and fruit consumption in colorectal carcinogenesis. The Health Professionals Follow-up Study (N = 47,325, follow-up

= 10 years) and the Nurses' Health Study (N = 88,764, follow-up = 16 years) reported that consumption of vegetables and fruits does not confer protection against colorectal cancer in men and women.[56] There was also no appreciable benefit from any of the specific subgroups of fruits and vegetables considered.[56] The only exception was prune consumption; the RR of colon cancer associated with a 1 serving/d higher prune consumption was 1.46 (95% CI, 0.93–2.31) among women and 1.73 (95% CI, 1.20–2.50) among men.[56] By contrast, a prospective study of a population-based cohort of 61,463 Swedish women (40–74 years; follow-up = 9.6 years) who had been on a mammography-screening program reported a significant dose-dependent inverse relationship between consumption of vegetables and fruits and colorectal cancer risk.[57] Total consumption of >5 servings of vegetables and fruits per day was associated with a 27% reduction in the risk of colorectal cancer (RR = 0.73; 95% CI, 0.56–0.96), compared with those whose total consumption was <2.5 servings per day.[57] Subanalyses showed that this association was due largely to fruit consumption and was stronger for rectal cancer than for colon cancer.[57] This study also showed a significant dose-dependent inverse association between consumption of vegetables and fruits and colorectal cancer risk among individuals consuming less than 2.5 servings per day ($P = 0.001$).[57] Total vegetable and fruit consumption of <1.5 servings per day was associated with a 65% increase in colorectal cancer risk compared with consumption of >2.5 servings per day (RR = 1.65; 95% CI, 1.23–2.20).[57]

In the Netherlands Cohort Study on Diet and Cancer (N = 120,852; follow-up = 6.3 years), no significant association with total vegetable intake or total fruit intake for colon cancer was observed.[58] However, among women, an inverse association was observed with vegetables and fruits combined (for the highest consumption versus the lowest, RR = 0.66 [95% CI, 0.44–1.01]).[58] Brassica vegetables and cooked leafy vegetables showed inverse associations for both men and women.[58] For rectal cancer, no significant associations were found for vegetable consumption or fruit consumption or for specific subgroups of vegetables and fruits.[58] The Breast Cancer Detection Demonstration Project (N = 45,490 women; follow-up = 9 years) reported no significant association between vegetable and fruit intake and the risk of colorectal cancer.[59]

To date, only one randomized intervention human trial that used high consumption of vegetables and fruits as a dietary strategy has been reported.[24] In the Polyp Prevention Trial, a low-fat (20% of total calories), high-fiber (18 g/1000 kcal daily) diet enriched with vegetables and fruits (3.5 servings/1000 kcal daily) did not significantly reduce colorectal adenoma recurrence compared with placebo.[24]

In summary, in contrast to the strong endorsement for the protective role of vegetables in colorectal carcinogenesis by the World Cancer Research Fund,[1] currently available evidence from epidemiologic and intervention studies is conflicting with regard to the association between vegetable and fruit consumption and colorectal cancer risk. Again, this is likely due to limitations of currently available tools to detect a real effect associated with vegetables and fruits, as discussed earlier. Vegetables and fruits contain a large number of substances that possess anticarcinogenic properties (Table 5).[12,60,61] These compounds have both complementary and overlapping mechanisms of action, including the induction of detoxification enzymes; inhibition of nitrosamine formation; provision of substrate for formation of antineoplastic agents, dilution, and binding of carcinogens in the digestive tract; alteration of hormone metabolism; antioxidant activity; stimulation of the immune system; and other mechanisms.[1,60,61] The existence of plausible anticarcinogenic mechanisms and the portfolio of epidemiologic evidence generally support the inverse association between vegetable and fruit consumption and colorectal cancer risk. Collectively, observational epidemiologic studies suggest decreased colorectal cancer risk with raw vegetables, green vegetables, and cruciferous vegetables.[7,12,13,51,52,62] Furthermore, garlic consumption,[41,55] as discussed earlier, and consumption of tomatoes, tomato-based products, and lycopene,[63] as recent evidence indicates, appear to be particularly protective against the development of colorectal cancer.

Table 5. Potential Anticarcinogens in Vegetables and Fruits

Carotenoids	Dithiolthiones
Ascorbate	Glucosinolate/indoles
Tocopherols	Isothiocyanates/thiocyanates
Selenium	Allium compounds
Folate	Plant sterols
Dietary fiber	Isoflavones
	Protease inhibitors
	Coumarins

Fat

The majority of correlation and case-control studies suggest a positive association between dietary fat intake and colorectal cancer incidence and mortality.[1,12,13] However, a number of these studies failed to adjust for total energy intake, another possible risk factor for colorectal cancer.[1,12,13] In this regard, a combined analysis of 13 case-control studies of colorectal cancer involving 5287 cases and 10,478 controls from various populations with differing cancer rates and dietary practices demonstrated no evidence of any increased risk with higher dietary fat after adjustment for total energy intake.[64] There were no statistically significant associations for any type of fat (i.e., total, saturated, monounsaturated, and polyunsaturated fats) in subgroup analyses.[64] Four large, prospective studies—the Iowa Women's Study,[65] the Health Professionals Follow-up Study,[42] and the Netherlands Cohort Study on Diet and Cancer[66,67]—did not find any significant association between total fat intake and colorectal cancer risk. However, in the Nurses' Health Study, the highest intake of total fat was associated with a significant two-fold increase in the risk for colon cancer compared with the lowest intake of total fat.[39] The Nurses' Health Study[39] and the Netherlands Cohort Study[66] demonstrated that a high intake of animal and saturated fat was associated with a significantly increased risk of colorectal cancer in women, whereas the other three prospective studies did not show appreciable association.[42,65,67] Of the four prospective studies that examined the risk of colorectal cancer in association with intake of monounsaturated fatty acids,[39,42,65,66] only the Nurses' Health Study reported a significantly increased risk.[39] Three prospective studies[42,65,66] have demonstrated a weakly decreased risk of colorectal cancer with high intake of polyunsaturated fat. Therefore, there is evidence, albeit not entirely consistent and convincing, that high intake of animal and saturated fat is associated with increased colorectal cancer risk. Evidence for intake of total fat and monounsaturated and polyunsaturated fatty acids is inconsistent.

Three randomized intervention studies have been published concerning the effect of a low-fat diet on colorectal adenoma recurrence. In the trial reported by the Toronto Polyp Prevention Group from Canada,[26] a diet low in fat (<50 g/d or 20% of energy) and high in fiber (50 g/d) did not significantly reduce colorectal adenoma recurrence compared with placebo after 2 years of intervention. In the Australian Polyp Prevention Project,[28] neither the low-fat intervention (<25% of energy) nor high fiber intake (25 g wheat bran supplement/d) significantly reduced the rate of colorectal adenoma recurrence. However, the low-fat diet combined with wheat bran supplementation significantly reduced the recurrence rate of large adenomas (>10 mm) after 4 years of follow-up.[28] The largest randomized study published to date, the Polyp Prevention Trial, demonstrated no protective effect of a low-fat diet (20% of total calories) in conjunction with high fiber (18 g/1000 kcal daily) and high intake of vegetables and fruits (3.5 servings/1000 kcal daily) on the recurrence rate of colorectal adenomas after 4 years of intervention.[24]

Another randomized intervention study utilizing a low-fat component for the nutritional chemoprevention of colorectal cancer in the United States has recently been reported. The Women's Health Initiative is a multicenter clinical trial that included 48,835 postmenopausal women (50–79 years) in a 3 × 2 × 2 factorial intervention involving hormones, calcium, vitamin D, and a low-fat dietary plan.[68] The primary end points of this trial are incident colorectal and breast cancer, coronary heart disease and other cardiovascular disease, and hip and other fractures. After a mean follow-up of 8.1 years, a low-fat dietary pattern intervention (a 10.7% reduction in percentage of energy from fat) did not reduce the risk of colorectal cancer.[69]

Cholesterol

The evidence is conflicting for the effects of cholesterol on colorectal cancer and adenoma incidence and mortality. Earlier case-control and prospective studies, including the Framingham Study, the Multiple Risk Factor Intervention Trial, and the Honolulu Japanese-Hawaiian Study, suggested an inverse association between cholesterol levels and colorectal cancer incidence and mortality.[1] Other prospective studies have not confirmed this purported inverse relationship, and some have found a positive association between serum cholesterol levels and colorectal cancer risk.[1] It was suggested that the inverse association might be caused by the metabolic effects of undiagnosed cancer on serum cholesterol levels.[1] In a combined analysis of 13 case-control studies of colorectal cancer, which involved 5287 cases and 10,478 controls, a weak, albeit significant, increase (of 30%) in risk with higher dietary cholesterol was reported.[64] Two recent, large prospective studies (the Iowa Women's Study[65] and the Health Professionals Follow-up Study[42]), however, found no significant relationship between dietary cholesterol intake and the risk of colorectal cancer.

Meat

The majority of correlation and case-control studies suggest a positive association between meat intake and colorectal cancer risk.[1,12,13] However, the evidence from large prospective studies is conflicting. The Iowa Women's Study,[65] the Second Cancer Prevention Study of the American Cancer Society,[38] the Netherlands Cohort Study on Diet and Cancer,[66] the Finnish study,[70] and the New York University Women's Health Study[71] suggest no association between meat intake and colorectal cancer incidence and mortality. In contrast, the Nurses' Health Study[39] reported that women who consumed red meat frequently had a 2.5-fold increased risk of colon cancer than those who rarely consumed red meat. The Health Professionals Follow-up Study[42] also reported that men who consumed 5 or more servings per week of beef, pork, or lamb had a 1.7-fold increased risk of colon cancer compared with men who consumed these products less than once per month. The Melbourne Collaborative Cohort Study (N = 37,112; follow up = 9 years) recently reported that consumption of fresh red meat and processed meat increases the risk of rectal, but not colon, cancer.[72] The recently reported European Prospective Investigation into Cancer and Nutrition also has demonstrated a significant positive association between colorectal cancer risk and intake of red and processed meat, and a significant inverse association between colorectal cancer risk and fish intake.[73] Furthermore, in the Cancer Prevention Study II Nutrition Cohort (N = 148,610), intake of red and processed meat was positively associated with colorectal cancer risk.[74] A meta-analysis of case-control and prospective studies estimated the mean relative risk of developing colorectal cancer comparing the highest to lowest categories of meat consumption to be

1.35 (95% CI, 1.21–1.51) for red meat and 1.31 (95% CI, 1.13–1.51) for processed meat.[75] Another meta-analysis of 12 prospective studies concluded that a daily increment of 100 g of red or total meat consumption was associated with a 12% to 17% higher risk of colorectal cancer and that an increment of 25 g of processed meat was associated with a 49% higher risk.[76]

It is difficult to accurately assess dietary intake of meat because of variable preparation time (e.g., rare, medium, well done), cooking methods (e.g., charcoal, barbecue, frying), and fat content in meat and uncertainty as to whether fat was removed prior to cooking.[1,13] It is also difficult to rule out the confounding effects of other potential carcinogens present in red meat (e.g., iron). For example, several case-control and large prospective studies using the First National Health and Nutrition Examination Survey in the United States have suggested a positive association between body iron stores and colorectal cancer.[1,77,78] Another potential confounder is protein present in red meat. However, large prospective studies[42,65-67] do not support a positive association between animal protein intake and colorectal cancer risk, as suggested by observations from some case-control studies.[1,12]

Generally, observational studies, including the Iowa Women's Health Study[65] and the Health Professionals Follow-up Study,[42] suggest no appreciable relationship between poultry consumption and colorectal cancer risk.[1,12] In the Nurses' Health Study,[39] however, consumption of chicken without skin at least 5 times per week was associated with a statistically significant decreased risk of colon cancer compared with consumption less than once per month.

For meat and fat, there exist a number of biologically plausible anticarcinogenic mechanisms. Cooked meat, especially when high in fat and cooked at high temperature, produces carcinogens such as heterocyclic amines, polycyclic aromatic hydrocarbons, and nitrosamines, which can potentially induce DNA adduct formation, DNA damage, and mutations.[12] Dietary fat also enhances cholesterol and bile acid synthesis by the liver, increasing the amount of these sterols in the colonic lumen. Colonic bacteria convert these compounds to secondary bile acids, cholesterol metabolites, and other potentially toxic metabolic compounds.[12] These compounds are known to damage the colonic mucosa, increase the proliferative activity of the epithelium, activate secondary cellular transduction signals, alter membrane fluidity, and alter prostaglandin metabolism.[12] More recently, polymorphisms of several genes encoding detoxifying enzymes—including P450, *N*-acetyltransferase, and glutathione-*S*-transferase, which handle toxic compounds resulting from cooking meat and fat—have been observed to modify colorectal cancer risk associated with high dietary fat and meat consumption.[12]

Antioxidant Vitamins

The antioxidant micronutrients—including vitamin A, carotenoids, vitamin C, vitamin E, selenium, zinc, copper, iron, and manganese—are part of the body's defense against free radicals and reactive oxygen species. These antioxidants are thought to convey protection via a host of different mechanisms, including trapping and neutralization of free radicals and reactive oxygen species, protection against lipid peroxidation in cell membranes, potentiation of immune responses, reduction in mutation rates, antiproliferation, and inhibition of nitrosamine and nitrosamide formation.[79]

Relatively few epidemiologic studies have addressed dietary antioxidant intake and the risk of colorectal cancer. Reported studies are plagued by problems of inaccuracy in determining dietary or blood levels of antioxidant vitamins.[79] The Iowa Women's Health Study[80] reported no significant association between intake of vitamins A and C and colorectal cancer risk. However, total vitamin E intake (dietary plus supplemental) and supplemental vitamin E intake, but not dietary vitamin E intake, were inversely associated with colorectal cancer risk in this study.[80] The Nurses' Health study, however, did not show a significant association between vitamin E intake and colon cancer risk.[39] In a US cohort of elderly persons (the Leisure World Study; N = 11,580), a significantly reduced risk of colon cancer was noted for intake of dietary vitamin C and for supplemental use of vitamins A and C in women but not in men.[54] The Second Cancer Prevention Study of the American Cancer Society involving 711,891 men and women followed for 14 years did not find a substantial effect of vitamin C or E supplement use on overall colorectal cancer mortality.[81] In the same cohort, multivitamin use alone or in combination with vitamin A, C, or E had minimal effect on cancer mortality overall, although mortality from all cancers combined was increased among male current smokers but decreased in males who had never or formerly smoked.[82] Other large prospective studies (the Nurses' Health Study, the Health Professionals Follow-up Study, and the Second Cancer Prevention Study of the American Cancer Society) have suggested that long-term use of multivitamins (>10–15 years) containing antioxidants and folic acid reduces colorectal cancer incidence and mortality.[83-86] It is unclear, however, which components of multivitamin preparations have played a major role in colorectal cancer prevention in these studies.

Five small pilot trials suggested that antioxidant vitamins, either alone or in combination, improve proliferation labeling indices,[87] but these studies are severely limited by study design. As shown in Table 6, more recent and larger well-designed and well-conducted randomized human trials (the Toronto Polyp Prevention Study, the Australian Polyp Prevention Project, and the Antioxidant Polyp Prevention Study) do not support the protective role of antioxidant vitamins on colorectal carcinogenesis.[26-28] One exception is an Italian trial that reported a significant protective effect of the combination of vitamins A, C, and E on the rate of colorectal adenoma recur-

Table 6. Summary of Antioxidant Colorectal Cancer Chemoprevention Trials

Study (Reference)	Subjects N	Intervention	Duration	End Point	Outcome
Toronto Polyp Prevention Group[26]	Adenoma 137	Vitamins C (400 mg/d) + E (400 mg/d) vs. placebo	2 years	Adenoma recurrence	No effect
Roncucci L et al.[88]	Adenoma 255	Vitamins A (30,000 IU/d) + C (1000 mg/d) + E (400 mg/d) vs. lactulose vs. placebo	18 months	Adenoma recurrence	Vitamin mixture protective; Lactulose also protective
Australian Polyp Prevention Project[28]	Adenoma 424	2 × 2 × 2 factorial <25% fat calories/d 25 g wheat bran/d 20 mg β-carotene/d	4 years	Adenoma recurrence	β-carotene—no effect
Antioxidant Polyp Prevention Study[27,89]	Adenoma 864	25 mg β-carotene/d vs. 1000 mg ascorbic acid/d vs. 1000 mg ascorbic acid/d + 400 mg α-tocopherol/d vs. placebo	4 years	Adenoma recurrence	No effect; β-carotene reduced risk of recurrence by 44% in nonsmokers and nondrinkers (RR = 0.56; 95% CI, 0.35–0.89) but increased the risk by 2-fold in smokers and drinkers (RR = 2.07; 95% CI, 1.39–3.08)

rence after 18 months of intervention (Table 6).[88] However, this study was not a real randomized trial.

Of particular importance is the Antioxidant Polyp Prevention Study that randomized 864 patients into 4 groups using a factorial design: 1) placebo, 2) β-carotene (25 mg/d), 3) vitamins C (ascorbic acid; 1000 mg/d) and E (α-tocopherol; 400 mg/d), and 4) β-carotene plus vitamin C.[27] After 4 years of follow-up, this study showed no beneficial effect on adenoma recurrence from the antioxidant vitamins. A recent subgroup analysis of this trial demonstrated a very interesting interaction between β-carotene and smoking and alcohol.[89] Among subjects who neither smoked cigarettes nor drank alcohol, β-carotene was associated with a marked decrease in the risk of recurrent adenomas (RR = 0.56; 95% CI, 0.35–0.89), but β-carotene supplementation conferred a modest increase in the risk of recurrence among those who smoked (RR = 1.36; 95% CI, 0.70–2.62) or drank alcohol (RR = 1.13; 95% CI, 0.89–1.43). For those who smoked cigarettes and also drank more than one alcoholic drink per day, β-carotene doubled the risk of adenoma recurrence (RR = 2.07; 95% CI, 1.39–3.08). This analysis therefore suggests that β-carotene may have both proneoplastic and antineoplastic effects depending on smoking and alcohol status. This relationship has recently been confirmed in a French cohort study (N = 700; follow-up = 7.4 years), which clearly showed that β-carotene intake was inversely associated with risk of tobacco-related cancers among nonsmokers with a statistically significant dose-dependent relationship, whereas high β-carotene intake was directly associated with risk among smokers.[90]

Four large trials that adopted β-carotene supplementation as a preventive strategy for cardiovascular disease and cancer have produced either disappointing or alarming results. The Finnish Alpha-Tocopherol, Beta-Carotene Study (male smokers; 50–69 years; N = 29,133; follow-up = 5–8 years) found that β-carotene (20 mg/d) increased the risk of lung cancer (by 18%) and total mortality compared with placebo.[30] The American Beta-Carotene and Retinol Efficacy Trial (smokers 45–74 years of age; N = 18,314; follow-up = 4 years) reported that β-carotene (30 mg/d) administered with retinol (25,000 IU/d) increased the risk of lung cancer by 28% and also increased total mortality.[31] This adverse effect of β-carotene on lung cancer incidence and all-cause mortality in cigarette smokers persisted 6 years after β-carotene was stopped.[91] Even α-tocopherol supplementation (400 IU/d) has recently been shown to increase the occurrence of second primary cancers and decrease cancer-free survival in patients with stage I or II head and neck cancer treated by radiation therapy (N = 540) after 52 months of follow-up.[92]

By contrast, two large trials—the Physicians' Health Study (22,071 male physicians; 40–84 years; follow-up = 12 years[93]) and the Women's Health Study (39,876 healthy female health professionals; 2.1 years of treatment plus another 2.0 years of follow-up[94])—found no benefit or harm from β-carotene supplementation (50 mg/d) on the incidence of cancer. These two latter studies recruited healthy male and female health professionals who had a low prevalence of smoking. These findings collectively suggest that β-carotene likely has no appreciable protective effect on cancer but can increase cancer risk in cigarette smokers. Also, some of these trials suggested that alcohol consumption increases lung cancer risk among β-carotene-supplemented subjects.[95,96] In none of these trials did β-carotene supplementation increase the risk of colorectal cancer, even among subjects who smoked or drank alcohol.[95-98] A recent systemic review and meta-analysis has shown that antioxidant supplements do not prevent gastrointestinal cancers but appear to increase overall mortality from gastrointestinal cancer.[99]

It is evident from the above discussion that antioxidant vitamins should not be routinely used as a chemopreventive agent against colorectal cancer. As a matter of fact, the US Preventive Services Task Force has recently concluded that the evidence is insufficient to recommend for or against the use of supplements of vitamins A, C, or E; multivitamins with folic acid; or antioxidant combinations for the prevention of cancer or cardiovascular disease.[100,101] The US Preventive Services Task Force concluded that β-carotene supplements, either alone or in combination, are unlikely to provide important benefits in the prevention of cancer or cardiovascular disease and might cause harm in some groups.[100,101] β-carotene is an antioxidant at low oxygen pressures, but at ambient or high oxygen pressures, can display prooxidant properties due to the formation of oxidized metabolites that can enhance lipid peroxidation and increase formation of DNA adducts.[102,103] There are several other molecular mechanisms by which β-carotene can promote the development of cancer.[104,105]

Folate

Folate is a water-soluble B vitamin that appears to play an important role in the pathogenesis of several disorders in humans including anemia, cardiovascular disease, neural tube defects, neuropsychiatric disorders, and cancer.[106,107] Folic acid is the fully oxidized monoglutamyl form of this vitamin that is used commercially in supplements and in fortified foods. An accumulating body of evidence over the past decade suggests that folate status (assessed by dietary intake or by the measurement of blood folate levels) is inversely related to the risk of sporadic and ulcerative-colitis-associated colorectal cancer or its precursor, adenomas.[106-109]

Collectively, more than 20 case-control studies suggest an approximately 40% reduction in the risk of colorectal adenomas and cancer in individuals with the highest dietary intake and/or blood concentrations of folate compared with those with the lowest intake and/or blood concentrations.[106-109] Several large prospective studies (the Health Professionals Follow-up Study, the Nurses' Health Study, the First National Health and Nutrition Examination Survey Epidemiologic Follow-up Study, the Iowa Women's Health Study, and the Netherlands Cohort Study on Diet and Cancer) also suggest a 40% reduction in the risk of colorectal adenomas and cancer in those with the highest intake of folate compared with those with the lowest intake.[82,110-115] A recent meta-analysis of 11 prospective studies from the United States, Canada, Netherlands, and Sweden including more than 500,000 male and female subjects demonstrated a significant inverse association between folate intake (dietary and supplemental) and the risk of colorectal cancer.[116] This meta-analysis also showed a 20% reduction in the risk of colorectal cancer in subjects with the highest folate intake compared with those with the lowest intake. Another meta-analysis has also confirmed an inverse relationship between dietary intake of folate and colorectal cancer risk.[117] Some epidemiologic studies have shown a beneficial effect of multivitamin supplements containing ≥400 μg folic acid for ≥15 years on colorectal cancer risk and mortality.[83-85] In some epidemiologic studies, the observed inverse association between folate status and colorectal cancer risk was further modified by the intake of alcohol, a known folate antagonist,[118] and other methyl group donors (e.g., methionine, vitamins B_6 and B_{12}) that are involved in the folate metabolic pathway.[106-109] The role of folate in colorectal carcinogenesis has been further strengthened by the observations that genetic polymorphisms in the folate metabolic pathway (e.g., the methylenetetrahydrofolate reductase C677T polymorphism) modify colorectal cancer risk.[119,120]

Although there is no definitive evidence supporting the protective effect of folate supplementation on colorectal carcinogenesis from human experiments at present, several small intervention studies have demonstrated that folate supplementation can improve or reverse surrogate end point biomarkers of colorectal cancer.[106,107] In contrast, a recent preliminary report of the Aspirin-Folate Polyp Prevention Study (N = 1021) showed that folic acid supplementation (1 mg/d) for 7 years in subjects with previous colorectal adenomas significantly increased the number of adenomas by 44% and nonsignificantly increased the incidence of advanced adenomas with a high malignant potential compared with placebo.[121]

The data from animal studies generally support a causal relationship between folate depletion and colorectal cancer risk and an inhibitory effect of modest levels of folate supplementation on colorectal carcinogenesis.[107] However, animal studies have also shown that folate supplementation may increase colorectal cancer risk and accelerate colorectal cancer progression if too much is given or if it is provided after neoplastic foci are established in the colorectum.[107]

In summary, a growing body of observational epidemiologic studies has suggested that folate deficiency increases whereas folate supplementation decreases the risk of colorectal cancer. Although the results from these stud-

Table 7. Potential Mechanisms of Folate-Deficiency-Mediated Colorectal Carcinogenesis

DNA damage, uracil misincorporation, impaired DNA repair
Increased mutagenesis
Aberrant genomic and site-specific DNA methylation
Hyperproliferation
Abnormal apoptosis
Polymorphisms of genes involved in the folate metabolic pathway and related gene-nutrient interactions

ies are not uniformly consistent, the portfolio of evidence strongly supports the inverse association between folate status and colorectal cancer risk. Several potential mechanisms relating to the disruption of the known biochemical function of folate (mediating the transfer of 1-carbon moieties and consequent DNA synthesis and methylation) exist to support the role of folate in colorectal carcinogenesis (Table 7).[106,118,122,123]

Alcohol

Most correlation and case-control studies that have examined alcohol consumption suggest a positive association between alcohol intake and colorectal neoplasia.[1,12,13,85,124] Some studies have suggested greater risks in the rectum than in the colon and with beer consumption than with other types of liquor.[1,12,13,87,124] Also, these studies have shown a more consistently elevated risk among men than among women, perhaps because of the generally lower consumption of alcohol among women.[1,12,13,87,124] None of six prospective studies that compared the cancer mortality of alcoholics with that of the general population found significant associations with colorectal cancer.[1,87] Interestingly, the Copenhagen Center for Prospective Population Studies, with approximately 25,000 participants, reported that wine drinkers had significantly lower mortality from cancer than did non-wine drinkers ($P = 0.004$).[125] Most of the published large prospective studies in the general population have found significant positive associations between alcohol consumption and the risk of colorectal cancer and adenomas.[1,87,124] A meta-analysis involving a total of 22 studies (six prospective and 16 case-control) showed that alcohol consumption significantly increased the risk of colorectal cancer (pooled RR = 1.08 [95% CI, 1.06–1.10] for alcohol intake of 25 g/d; 1.18 [1.14–1.22] for 50 g/d; and 1.38 [1.29–1.49] for 100 g/d).[126] A recently published pooled analysis of eight cohort studies (the Alpha-Tocopherol Beta-Carotene Cancer Prevention Study, the Canadian National Breast Screening Study, the Health Professionals Follow-up Study, the Iowa Women's Health Study, the Netherlands Cohort Study, the New York State Cohort Study, the Nurses' Health Study, and the Swedish Mammography Cohort Study) demonstrated a significant positive association between alcohol consumption and colorectal cancer risk.[127] Compared with non-drinkers, the pooled multivariate relative risks were 1.16 (95% CI, 0.99–1.36) for those who consumed 30 to <45 g alcohol/d and 1.41 (95% CI, 1.16–1.72) for those who consumed ≥45 g/d.[127] The association was evident for all sites of colorectal cancer, and no clear difference in RR was found among specific alcoholic beverages.[127] The international panel of experts from the World Cancer Research Fund concluded that "high alcohol consumption probably increases the risk of cancers of the colon and rectum. The effect generally seems to be related to total ethanol intake, irrespective of the type of drink."[1]

The mechanisms by which alcohol consumption may contribute to colorectal carcinogenesis appear to relate to the breakdown of alcohol to acetaldehyde, which exerts either a direct or an indirect toxic effect on the colonic epithelium.[128,129] Acetaldehyde is a potent adduct former and is known to inhibit DNA repair.[128,129] Alcohol may exert its carcinogenic effects through associated deficiencies in nutrients, particularly folate.[128,129] Alcohol has also been also shown to induce genomic DNA hypomethylation, which in turn may increase genomic instability, mutations, and expression of protooncogenes.[128,129]

Calcium and Vitamin D

Results from correlation and case-control studies generally suggest an inverse association between calcium intake and colorectal cancer risk.[87] Although earlier prospective studies reported an inverse association between calcium intake and colorectal cancer risk, more recent and larger prospective studies, including the Nurses' Health Study, the Health Professionals Follow-up Study, and the Iowa Women's Study, have failed to demonstrate beneficial effects of calcium on the risk of colorectal cancer and adenomas after multivariate adjustment.[130] A meta-analysis published in 1996 that included 24 case-control and prospective studies did not find a substantial protective effect of calcium on colorectal cancer or adenoma risk.[131] The summary RR of developing colorectal cancer and adenomas in those with the highest intake of calcium compared with those with the lowest intake was 0.89 (95% CI, 0.79–1.01), 0.90 (95% CI, 0.78–1.05), and 0.88 (95% CI, 0.73–1.04) for combined, prospective, and case-control studies, respectively.[131] For adenomas and colorectal cancer, RR was 1.13 (95% CI, 0.91–1.39) and 0.86 (95% CI, 0.74–0.98), respectively.[131] A systematic review published in 1998 of 15 case-control and eight prospective studies that reported results for the association between calcium and colorectal cancer suggests that calcium intake is not associated with a substantially lower risk of colorectal cancer.[130] In particular, findings from large prospective studies were notably consistent in finding weak and nonsignificant inverse associations.[130]

In contrast, a more recent pooled analysis of 10 prospective studies conducted in five countries (N = 534,536) has shown a significant inverse association between colorectal cancer risk and either dietary or total calcium intake, with a risk reduction of 14% to 22% conferred by the highest intake.[132] Furthermore, a fairly consistent modest inverse association (risk reductions of 15% to 40% for the highest versus lowest intake categories) has emerged from several prospective studies (the Nurses' Health Study, the Health Professionals Follow-up Study, the Iowa Women's Study, the Second Cancer Prevention Study Nutrition Cohort, the Breast Cancer Detection Demonstration Project, and the Prostate, Lung, Colorectal and Ovarian Cancer Screening Trial),[133-138] as well as large case-control studies with approximately 2000 colon cancer cases.[139]

Almost all of the uncontrolled intervention trials have demonstrated a protective effect of calcium supplementation on proliferation surrogate end-point biomarkers of colorectal cancer.[87,140] However, less than one-third of the published small, placebo-controlled, randomized human trials have confirmed this protective effect of calcium on proliferation markers.[87,140] One published report on a larger US multicenter study (N = 333) reported no significant protective effect of calcium supplementation (1200 mg elemental calcium daily for 6–9 months) on proliferation biomarkers compared with placebo.[141] Another randomized trial showed that calcium supplementation (1–2 g elemental calcium daily for 6 months) normalized the distribution of proliferating cells without affecting the overall proliferation rate in the colorectal mucosa.[142]

Three placebo-controlled, randomized trials that investigated the effect of calcium supplementation on adenoma recurrence have been published. A small study involved 116 polyp-bearing patients who received a daily mixture of β-carotene (15 mg), vitamin C (150 mg), vitamin E (75 mg), selenium (101 μg), and calcium carbonate (4 g or 1.6 g elemental calcium) or placebo for 3 years.[143] The adenoma recurrence reduction (but not adenoma growth) was statistically significant in this trial, but a separate calcium effect could not be discerned because the intervention combined calcium and antioxidant vitamins.[143] The European Cancer Prevention Organisation Intervention Study (N = 665; follow-up = 3 years) reported a 34% reduction in the recurrence of adenoma associated with 2 g calcium supplementation/d, but this reduction did not attain statistical significance (P = 0.16).[49] The Calcium Polyp Prevention Study (N = 930) showed that calcium supplementation (3 g calcium carbonate [1200 mg of elemental calcium] daily) significantly reduced the recurrence rate of colorectal adenomas by 15% after 4 years of intervention.[29] A further analysis of this trial demonstrated that vitamin D status strongly modified the effect of calcium supplementation on adenoma recurrence.[144] Calcium supplements significantly lowered adenoma risk (by 30%) only among subjects with 25-hydroxyvitamin D levels above the overall median (29.1 ng/mL).[144] Similarly, 25-hydroxyvitamin D was associated with a reduced risk only among subjects randomly assigned to received calcium.[144] The Calcium Polyp Prevention Study has recently reported results from another analysis, which suggests that calcium supplementation has a more profound effect on the risk of recurrence of "histologically advanced neoplasms," which possess a higher potential for progressing to adenocarcinoma (RR = 0.65; 95% CI, 0.46–0.93) compared with tubular adenomas, which are associated with a lower potential to progress to adenocarcinoma (RR = 0.89; 95% CI, 0.77–1.03).[145] The Women's Health Initiative determined the effect of hormones, calcium, vitamin D, and a low-fat dietary plan on colorectal cancer risk in postmenopausal women (50–79 years).[68] Daily supplementation with calcium (1000 mg of elemental calcium as calcium carbonate) with vitamin D (400 IU of vitamin D_3) for 7 years had no effect on the incidence of colorectal cancer among 36,282 postmenopausal women.[146]

The role of vitamin D in colorectal carcinogenesis has not been unequivocally established in epidemiologic studies. Correlation and case-control studies have reported conflicting results.[1,87,130] Although large prospective studies (the Western Electric Workers Study, the Nurses' Health Study, the Health Professionals Follow-up Study, the Iowa Women's Study, and the Second Cancer Prevention Study Nutrition Cohort) have suggested a weak inverse association between vitamin D intake and colorectal cancer and adenoma risk, only a few studies attained statistical significance.[1,87,130]

In summary, the portfolio of observational epidemiologic studies and results from intervention trials generally support the modest protective effect of calcium supplementation on colorectal cancer risk. Also, there is evidence that the chemopreventive effect of calcium supplementation may be enhanced by the concomitant use of vitamin D. The case for calcium as a potential chemopreventive agent against colorectal cancer is further strengthened by the existence of several plausible physiologic and molecular mechanisms, as outlined in Table 8.[147,148] In contrast, given the scarcity of data, additional studies are needed to investigate the relationship between vitamin D and colorectal cancer risk in more detail. Mechanistically, however, the physiologically most active molecular form of vitamin D, 1,25-dihydroxyvitamin D_3, has been shown to restrain cell proliferation and induce differentiation and apoptosis in a large variety of normal and tumor cells, including cells of the colon.[148]

Selenium

Descriptive epidemiologic studies, including many prospective studies, have suggested that dietary intake and/or serum and toenail levels of selenium are inversely related to overall cancer risk.[1,12,13,87] Although most case-control and earlier prospective studies reported a weak inverse association between serum levels of selenium and colorectal cancer risk,[1,12,13,87] a subsequent large prospective study in the Finnish cohort participating in the Social Insurance Institution's Mobile Clinic Health Examination Survey (N = 39,268 men and women; follow-up = 10 years) failed to confirm this relationship.[149] More recent large prospective studies (the Netherlands Cohort

Table 8. Potential Anticarcinogenic Mechanisms of Calcium

Calcium binds free bile acids and fatty acids, forming insoluble calcium soaps, thereby reducing their carcinogenic effects on the colonic epithelium.
Calcium suppresses proliferation and promotes apoptosis of the colonic epithelium.
Calcium reduces or suppresses molecular alterations implicated in colorectal carcinogenesis such as k-*ras* mutations, c-*myc* protooncogene expression, and β-catenin transcriptional activation.
Calcium suppresses the activation of secondary transduction signals such as protein kinase C and alters intracellular calcium regulation.
Calcium activates a calcium-sensing receptor, which results in increased levels of intracellular calcium inducing a wide range of biologic effects, some of which restrain the growth and promote the differentiation of transformed colon cells.
Calcium decreases luminal cytotoxic surfactant concentrations and thus inhibits luminal cytolytic activity.

Study on Diet and Cancer[150] and the Nurses' Health Study[151]) using toenail selenium, an indicator of long-term selenium status, found no significant association between selenium status and colorectal cancer risk. In fact, the Nurses' Health Study found nonsignificant positive associations between selenium status and colorectal cancer, lung cancer, and melanoma.[151] Another large prospective study from Italy reported a 3.9-fold increase in melanoma incidence in 2065 individuals who consumed high levels of inorganic selenium in tap water for 11 years compared with unexposed controls,[152] raising an alarm regarding the role of selenium in cancer chemoprevention. A recent combined analysis of data from three randomized trials—the Wheat Bran Fiber Trial, the Polyp Prevention Trial, and the Polyp Prevention Study—testing the effects of various nutritional interventions on the recurrence of colorectal adenomas has shown that individuals whose blood selenium values were in the highest quartile (median = 150 ng/mL) had significantly lower odds (risk) of developing a new adenoma compared with those in the lowest quartile (OR = 0.66; 95% CI, 0.50–0,87; P trend = 0.006).[153]

The Nutritional Prevention of Cancer Trial in the southeastern United States randomized 1312 patients with a history of basal cell or squamous cell carcinoma of the skin to either selenium (200 μg selenized yeast/d) or placebo to determine the effect of selenium on the incidence of nonmelanoma skin cancers.[32] Although no significant effect of selenium on these primary end points was observed, selenium supplementation significantly reduced total cancer incidence (by 37%) and incidence of lung (by 46%), colorectal (by 58%), and prostate (by 63%) cancers compared with placebo during the 6.4 years of follow-up.[32] A recent report that extends follow-up of the participants of this trial to more than 10 years showed that selenium supplementation significantly increased the risk of squamous cell carcinoma (by 25%) and total nonmelanoma skin cancer (by 17%).[154]

Although potential biologically plausible chemopreventive mechanisms do exist for selenium,[155] the portfolio of evidence from observational and intervention studies does not support the role of selenium in chemoprevention of colorectal cancer at present.

Unifying Hypothesis—Insulin Resistance

There tends to be agreement among epidemiologic studies regarding the risk of colorectal cancer and its relationship with overall diet.[156] However, when many of the findings are examined closely and correlations between colorectal cancer and individual dietary factors are sought, the relationship tends to be less convincing.[156] These observations suggest that overall diet, rather than individual factors, play the more important role, thus underscoring the importance of as-yet-undetermined interactions among dietary components in the development of cancer. This conclusion has lead to several intervention trials in humans that examined combinations of dietary and lifestyle modifications in the prevention of colorectal cancer (e.g., the Polyp Prevention Trial[24] and the Women's Health Initiative[68]).

Furthermore, McKeown-Eyssen[157] and Giovannucci[158] proposed a unifying hypothesis that may explain how obesity, physical inactivity, alcohol consumption, and a typical Western diet (low in fruits, vegetables, and fiber and high in animal and saturated fat, refined carbohydrates, and extensively processed foods) increase colorectal cancer risk. This hypothesis suggests that the putative dietary and lifestyle factors associated with colorectal cancer risk cause insulin resistance and hyperinsulinemia and that hyperinsulinemia in turn may stimulate the growth of colorectal tumors.[157,158] Although it remains unproven whether insulin stimulates the growth of colon tumors in humans, several lines of evidence from animal and in vitro studies support the role of insulin in tumor promotion via the insulin and insulin-like growth factor (IGF) axes.[159] Another indirect line of evidence comes from the observations that subjects with acromegaly, characterized by chronic growth hormone and IGF-1 hypersecretion, have an increased risk of developing colorectal cancer.[160]

Although case-control and earlier prospective epidemiologic studies that examined the relationship between type 2 diabetes mellitus and colorectal cancer risk did not consistently support this hypothesis,[161] more recent large prospective studies generally indicate a significant increase in colorectal cancer risk in subjects with type 2 diabetes compared with nondiabetic controls. A population-based cohort study from Sweden (N = 153,852) has demonstrated that subjects with type 2 diabetes mellitus have, on average, a 40% increased risk of developing colon cancer and a 60% increased risk of dying from colon cancer compared with the general population.[162] The First Cancer Prevention Study of the American Cancer Society, with more than 1 million participants showed that diabetic men had a significant 30% increased risk of developing colorectal cancer compared with nondiabetic men during a 13-year follow-up period.[163] The Nurses' Health Study (N = 118,403; follow-up = 18 years) also reported that type 2 diabetic women had a significant 43% increase in colorectal cancer risk compared with nondiabetic women.[164] The Norwegian National Health Screen Service Study (N = 75,219; follow-up = 12 years) showed that women with a history of type 2 diabetes had a 55% increase in colorectal cancer risk compared with women without diabetes.[165] The European Prospective Investigation into Cancer-Norfolk Study has recently reported a significant 3-fold increase in colorectal cancer risk in diabetic subjects compared with nondiabetic controls.[166] In this study, concentrations of glycated hemoglobin (HbA1c), which is an integrated indicator of average blood glucose concentrations over the preceding 3 months, were continuously related to incident colorectal cancer risk, with the lowest rates observed in those with HbA1c below 5%. The relative risk of incident colorectal cancer per 1% absolute increase in HbA1c was 1.34 (95% CI, 1.12–1.59).[165] Large prospective studies (the Cardiovascular Health Study, the New York University Women's Health Study, the Physicians' Health Study) have also reported a significantly increased colorectal cancer risk in individuals with higher levels of fasting glucose and insulin, with higher levels of glucose and insulin 2 hours after oral glucose challenge, with higher levels of C-peptide (a marker of pancreatic insulin secretion), and with higher circulating levels of IGFs.[167-170]

These epidemiologic observations have been supported by animal studies demonstrating growth-promoting effects of exogenous insulin and dietary-induced hyperinsulinemia on colorectal cancer and aberrant crypt foci, a putative precursor of colon cancer.[171-175] Therefore, the recently proposed hypothesis linking insulin resistance and hyperinsulinemia with colorectal cancer risk provides a very attractive unifying mechanism by which a majority of dietary and lifestyle factors promote the development of colorectal cancer.

Dietary Factors and Colorectal Cancer Risk: Summary

Among the individual dietary factors reviewed here, calcium supplementation may confer a modest protective effect on colorectal cancer risk. It is clear that antioxidant supplementation should not be recommended for this purpose. It appears that high intake of vegetables, fruits, and fiber-rich foods and reduced intake of fat and red meat may provide a protective effect on colorectal cancer risk. Although folic acid and selenium appear to be promising, there are some concerns that these agents may exert procarcinogenic effects depending on the timing and dose of intervention. Overall dietary and lifestyle modifications to reduce insulin resistance appear to be one of the most promising and rational chemopreventive strategies against colorectal cancer.

Conclusions

Although this chapter has focused on the relationship between diet and colorectal cancer risk, the major conclusions can be applied to that between diet and cancer in general. Currently available evidence from epidemiologic, laboratory animal, and intervention studies does not unequivocally support the role of dietary factors in the development of cancer. The precise nature of the relationship to each nutrient and the actual magnitude of the relationship are not clear at present. Disappointingly, recent large, placebo-controlled, randomized intervention trials in humans have not supported the protective role of some of the diets and nutritional supplements thought to lower the risk of cancer. However, when the whole body or portfolio of evidence from these studies is analyzed critically, the overall conclusion supports that dietary factors play a major role in the development of several cancers, particularly of the colorectum. As discussed in this chapter, several inherent limitations are associated with nutritional epidemiologic and intervention studies that are designed to elucidate the relationship between dietary factors and cancer risk. Therefore, definitive answers to questions about diet and cancer are probably beyond the reach of both observational epidemiologic studies and randomized, controlled trials. However, it appears that overall diet, rather than individual factors, plays the more important role in the development of cancer, thus underscoring the importance of as-yet-undetermined interactions among dietary components in the development of cancer. It is likely that dietary factors or components do not act in isolation but as part of a biologic action package.[176] The major difficulty in establishing a relationship between diet and cancer and in translating observations from nutritional epidemiology into progress in cancer prevention has been due to the inability to identify all relevant dietary components that act coordinately to modulate cancer risk and the inability to identify the other relevant nonnutritional factors that interact with dietary components to modify cancer risk.[176]

Recent advances in molecular and cell biology have greatly increased the potential for understanding the mechanistic roles that nutrients play in the development of cancer at the molecular and cellular levels. Also, the topic of nutrient-gene interactions in carcinogenesis, which modifies cancer risk conferred by genetic susceptibility and dietary habits, has just begun to emerge. Identifying and understanding biologically plausible mechanisms by which dietary factors modulate cancer risk further strengthens epidemiologic and experimental evidence.

It is difficult to advise the public with absolute confidence given the insufficient scientific evidence currently available. It is important that the recommendation for prevention of cancer include modifications of overall dietary and lifestyle factors considered to be associated with an increased cancer risk. In other words, a more public health approach that considers the entire biologic action package rather than a reductionist medical approach should be adopted in the matter of diet and cancer. These include decreasing consumption of fat (total, animal, and saturated fat) and red meat, increasing consumption of vegetables, fruits, and all sources and types of fiber-rich foods, avoiding obesity, curtailing alcohol consumption to minimal to moderate amounts, quitting smoking, and engaging in daily physical activity. These dietary recommendations can potentially protect against cancer and provide other health benefits, including decreased cholesterol levels, improved insulin resistance, reduced blood pressure, and prevention of cardiovascular disease. In support of this approach, a recent study analyzed the effect of adherence to the American Institute for Cancer Research recommendations on the incidence and mortality of cancer in the Iowa Women's Health Study Cohort (N = 29,565 women; 55–69 years at baseline; follow-up = 14 years).[177] In this analysis, 14 recommendations related to diet for individuals to reduce cancer incidence and mortality on a global basis[1] and smoking were operationalized into nine recommendations (Table 9).[177] Women who followed no or one recommendation compared with six to nine recommendations were at an increased risk of cancer incidence (RR = 1.35; 95% CI, 1.15–1.58) and cancer mortality (RR = 1.45, 95% CI, 1.11–1.85).[177] The proportion of cancer incidence and cancer mortality that theoretically would have been avoidable if the entire cohort followed six to nine recommendations was 22% for cancer incidence (95% CI, 12–30) and 11% for cancer mortality (95% CI, −5–24).[177] When smoking and the operationalized recommendations were combined these estimates were 31% for cancer incidence (95% CI, 19–37) and for cancer mortality (95% CI, 15–40).[177] Therefore, these data suggest that adherence to the dietary recommendations, independently and in conjunction with not smoking, is likely to have a substantial public health impact on reducing cancer incidence and, to a lesser degree, cancer mortality at the population level.[177]

Table 9. Operationalization of the American Institute for Cancer Research Recommendations Concerning Diet and Cancer

Operationalization	Categories
Body mass index	≤25 vs. >25
Weight gain since age 18	<11 vs. ≥11 pounds
Physical activity	Active vs. not active
Vegetable and fruit consumption	<5 vs. ≥5 servings/d
Complex carbohydrates	<400 vs. ≥400 g/d
Alcohol	<1 vs. 1 drink (14 g)/d
Red meat	<80 vs. ≥80 g/d
Fat as % total calories	≤30% vs. >30%
Sodium consumption	<2400 vs. ≥2400 mg/d
Cigarette smoking	Ever vs. never

Adapted from Cerhan et al., 2004[177] with permission from The American Association for Cancer Research.

References

1. World Cancer Research Fund/American Institute for Cancer Research. *Food, Nutrition, and the Prevention of Cancer: A Global Perspective*. Washington, DC: American Institute for Cancer Research; 1997; 670 pp.
2. Doll R, Peto R. The causes of cancer: quantitative estimates of avoidable risks of cancer in the United States today. J Natl Cancer Inst. 1981;66: 1191–1308.
3. McGinnis JM, Foege WH. Actual causes of death in the United States. JAMA. 1993;270:2207–2212.
4. Miller AB, Berrino F, Hill M, Pietinen P, Riboli E, Wahrendorf J. Diet in the aetiology of cancer: a review. Eur J Cancer. 1994;30A:207–228.
5. Lichtenstein P, Holm NV, Verkasalo PK, et al. Environmental and heritable factors in the causation of cancer—analyses of cohorts of twins from Sweden, Denmark, and Finland. N Engl J Med. 2000;343: 78–85.
6. Chu KC, Tarone RE, Chow WH, Hankey BF, Ries LA. Temporal patterns in colorectal cancer incidence, survival, and mortality from 1950 through 1990. J Natl Cancer Inst. 1994;86:997–1006.
7. Kim YI. Vegetables, fruits, and colorectal cancer risk: what should we believe? Nutr Rev. 2001;59: 394–398.
8. Byers T. What can randomized controlled trials tell us about nutrition and cancer prevention? CA Cancer J Clin. 1999;49:353–361.
9. Benson K, Hartz AJ. A comparison of observational studies and randomized, controlled trials. N Engl J Med. 2000;342:1878–1886.
10. Concato J, Shah N, Horwitz RI. Randomized, controlled trials, observational studies, and the hierarchy of research designs. N Engl J Med. 2000;342: 1887–1892.
11. Rebbeck TR, Ambrosone CB, Bell DA, et al. SNPs, haplotypes, and cancer: applications in molecular epidemiology. Cancer Epidemiol Biomarkers Prev. 2004;13:681–687.

12. Potter JD. Colorectal cancer: molecules and populations. J Natl Cancer Inst. 1999;91:916–932.
13. Kim YI. Nutrition and cancer. In: Bowman BA, Russell RM, eds. *Present Knowledge in Nutrition*. 8th ed. Washington, DC: International Life Science Institute; 2001; 573–689.
14. Courtney ED, Melville DM, Leicester RJ. Review article: chemoprevention of colorectal cancer. Aliment Pharmacol Ther. 2004;19:1–24.
15. Forman MR, Hursting SD, Umar A, Barrett JC. Nutrition and cancer prevention: a multidisciplinary perspective on human trials. Annu Rev Nutr. 2004; 24:223–254.
16. McCullough ML, Giovannucci EL. Diet and cancer prevention. Oncogene. 2004;23:6349–6364.
17. Heavey PM, McKenna D, Rowland IR. Colorectal cancer and the relationship between genes and the environment. Nutr Cancer. 2004;48:124–141.
18. Jemal A, Murray T, Ward E, et al. Cancer statistics, 2005. CA Cancer J Clin. 2005;55:10–30.
19. Winawer SJ, Fletcher RH, Miller L, et al. Colorectal cancer screening: clinical guidelines and rationale. Gastroenterology. 1997;112:594–642.
20. Thompson FE, Byers T. Dietary assessment resource manual. J Nutr. 1994;124:2245S–2317S.
21. Schatzkin A, Gail M. The promise and peril of surrogate end points in cancer research. Nat Rev Cancer. 2002;2:19–27.
22. Winawer S, Fletcher R, Rex D, et al. Colorectal cancer screening and surveillance: clinical guidelines and rationale—Update based on new evidence. Gastroenterology. 2003;124:544–560.
23. Go VL, Butrum RR, Wong DA. Diet, nutrition, and cancer prevention: the postgenomic era. J Nutr. 2003;133:3830S–3836S.
24. Schatzkin A, Lanza E, Corle D, et al, for the Polyp Prevention Trial Study Group. Lack of effect of a low-fat, high-fiber diet on the recurrence of colorectal adenomas. N Engl J Med. 2000;342: 1149–1155.
25. Alberts DS, Martinez ME, Roe DJ, et al, for the Phoenix Colon Cancer Prevention Physicians' Network. Lack of effect of a high-fiber cereal supplement on the recurrence of colorectal adenomas. N Engl J Med. 2000;342:1156–1162.
26. McKeown-Eyssen GE, Bright-See E, Bruce WR, et al, for the Toronto Polyp Prevention Group. A randomized trial of a low fat high fibre diet in the recurrence of colorectal polyps. J Clin Epidemiol. 1994;47:525–536.
27. Greenberg ER, Baron JA, Tosteson TD, et al, for the Polyp Prevention Study Group. A clinical trial of antioxidant vitamins to prevent colorectal adenoma. N Engl J Med. 1994;331:141–147.
28. MacLennan R, Macrae F, Bain C, et al, for the The Australian Polyp Prevention Project. Randomized trial of intake of fat, fiber, and beta carotene to prevent colorectal adenomas. J Natl Cancer Inst. 1995; 87:1760–1766.
29. Baron JA, Beach M, Mandel JS, et al, for the Calcium Polyp Prevention Study Group. Calcium supplements for the prevention of colorectal adenomas. N Engl J Med. 1999;340:101–107.
30. The Alpha-Tocopherol, Beta Carotene Cancer Prevention Study Group. The effect of vitamin E and beta carotene on the incidence of lung cancer and other cancers in male smokers. N Engl J Med. 1994;330:1029–1035.
31. Omenn GS, Goodman GE, Thornquist MD, et al. Effects of a combination of beta carotene and vitamin A on lung cancer and cardiovascular disease. N Engl J Med. 1996;334:1150–1155.
32. Clark LC, Combs GF Jr., Turnbull BW, et al, for the Nutritional Prevention of Cancer Study Group. Effects of selenium supplementation for cancer prevention in patients with carcinoma of the skin. A randomized controlled trial. JAMA. 1996;276: 1957–1963.
33. Burkitt DP. Relationship as a clue to causation. Lancet. 1970;2:1237–1240.
34. Kim YI. AGA technical review: impact of dietary fiber on colon cancer occurrence. Gastroenterology. 2000;118:1235–1257.
35. Trock B, Lanza E, Greenwald P. Dietary fiber, vegetables, and colon cancer: critical review and meta-analyses of the epidemiologic evidence. J Natl Cancer Inst. 1990;82:650–661.
36. Howe GR, Benito E, Castelleto R, et al. Dietary intake of fiber and decreased risk of cancers of the colon and rectum: evidence from the combined analysis of 13 case-control studies. J Natl Cancer Inst. 1992;84:1887–1896.
37. Friedenreich CM, Brant RF, Riboli E. Influence of methodologic factors in a pooled analysis of 13 case-control studies of colorectal cancer and dietary fiber. Epidemiology. 1994;5:66–79.
38. Thun MJ, Calle EE, Namboodiri MM, et al. Risk factors for fatal colon cancer in a large prospective study. J Natl Cancer Inst. 1992;84:1491–1500.
39. Willett WC, Stampfer MJ, Colditz GA, Rosner BA, Speizer FE. Relation of meat, fat, and fiber intake to the risk of colon cancer in a prospective study among women. N Engl J Med. 1990;323: 1664–1672.
40. Fuchs CS, Giovannucci EL, Colditz GA, et al. Dietary fiber and the risk of colorectal cancer and adenoma in women. N Engl J Med. 1999;340: 169–176.
41. Steinmetz KA, Kushi LH, Bostick RM, Folsom AR, Potter JD. Vegetables, fruit, and colon cancer in the Iowa Women's Health Study. Am J Epidemiol. 1994;139:1–15.
42. Giovannucci E, Rimm EB, Stampfer MJ, Colditz GA, Ascherio A, Willett WC. Intake of fat, meat,

and fiber in relation to risk of colon cancer in men. Cancer Res. 1994;54:2390–2397.
43. Giovannucci E, Stampfer MJ, Colditz G, Rimm EB, Willett WC. Relationship of diet to risk of colorectal adenoma in men. J Natl Cancer Inst. 1992;84:91–98.
44. Platz EA, Giovannucci E, Rimm EB, et al. Dietary fiber and distal colorectal adenoma in men. Cancer Epidemiol Biomarkers Prev. 1997;6:661–670.
45. Pietinen P, Malila N, Virtanen M, et al. Diet and risk of colorectal cancer in a cohort of Finnish men. Cancer Causes Control. 1999;10:387–396.
46. Bingham SA, Day NE, Luben R, et al. Dietary fibre in food and protection against colorectal cancer in the European Prospective Investigation into Cancer and Nutrition (EPIC): an observational study. Lancet. 2003;361:1496–1501.
47. Peters U, Sinha R, Chatterjee N, et al. Dietary fibre and colorectal adenoma in a colorectal cancer early detection programme. Lancet. 2003;361:1491–1495.
48. Ferguson LR, Harris PJ. The dietary fibre debate: more food for thought. Lancet. 2003;361:1487–1488.
49. Bonithon-Kopp C, Kronborg O, Giacosa A, Rath U, Faivre J, for the European Cancer Prevention Organisation Study Group. Calcium and fibre supplementation in prevention of colorectal adenoma recurrence: a randomised intervention trial. Lancet. 2000;356:1300–1306.
50. Asano TK, McLeod RS. Dietary fibre for the prevention of colorectal adenomas and carcinomas. Cochrane Database Syst Rev. 2002;(2):CD003430.
51. Steinmetz KA, Potter JD. Vegetables, fruit, and cancer prevention: a review. J Am Diet Assoc. 1996; 96:1027–1039.
52. Steinmetz KA, Potter JD. Vegetables, fruit, and cancer. I. Epidemiology. Cancer Causes Control. 1991;2:325–357.
53. Phillips RL, Snowdon DA. Dietary relationships with fatal colorectal cancer among Seventh-Day Adventists. J Natl Cancer Inst. 1985;74:307–317.
54. Shibata A, Paganini-Hill A, Ross RK, Henderson BE. Intake of vegetables, fruits, beta-carotene, vitamin C and vitamin supplements and cancer incidence among the elderly: a prospective study. Br J Cancer. 1992;66:673–679.
55. Fleischauer AT, Poole C, Arab L. Garlic consumption and cancer prevention: meta-analyses of colorectal and stomach cancers. Am J Clin Nutr. 2000; 72:1047–1052.
56. Michels KB, Edward G, Joshipura KJ, et al. Prospective study of fruit and vegetable consumption and incidence of colon and rectal cancers. J Natl Cancer Inst. 2000;92:1740–1752.
57. Terry P, Giovannucci E, Michels KB, et al. Fruit, vegetables, dietary fiber, and risk of colorectal cancer. J Natl Cancer Inst. 2001;93:525–533.
58. Voorrips LE, Goldbohm RA, van Poppel G, Sturmans F, Hermus RJ, van den Brandt PA. Vegetable and fruit consumption and risks of colon and rectal cancer in a prospective cohort study: The Netherlands Cohort Study on Diet and Cancer. Am J Epidemiol. 2000;152:1081–1092.
59. Flood A, Velie EM, Chaterjee N, et al. Fruit and vegetable intakes and the risk of colorectal cancer in the Breast Cancer Detection Demonstration Project follow-up cohort. Am J Clin Nutr. 2002; 75:936–943.
60. Steinmetz KA, Potter JD. Vegetables, fruit, and cancer. II. Mechanisms. Cancer Causes Control. 1991;2:427–442.
61. Lampe JW. Health effects of vegetables and fruit: assessing mechanisms of action in human experimental studies. Am J Clin Nutr. 1999;70: 475S–490S.
62. Link LB, Potter JD. Raw versus cooked vegetables and cancer risk. Cancer Epidemiol Biomarkers Prev. 2004;13:1422–1435.
63. Giovannucci E. Tomatoes, tomato-based products, lycopene, and cancer: review of the epidemiologic literature. J Natl Cancer Inst. 1999;91:317–331.
64. Howe GR, Aronson KJ, Benito E, et al. The relationship between dietary fat intake and risk of colorectal cancer: evidence from the combined analysis of 13 case-control studies. Cancer Causes Control. 1997;8:215–228.
65. Bostick RM, Potter JD, Kushi LH, et al. Sugar, meat, and fat intake, and non-dietary risk factors for colon cancer incidence in Iowa women (United States). Cancer Causes Control. 1994;5:38–52.
66. Goldbohm RA, van den Brandt PA, van't Veer P, et al. A prospective cohort study on the relation between meat consumption and the risk of colon cancer. Cancer Res. 1994;54:718–723.
67. Kampman E, Verhoeven D, Sloots L, van't Veer P. Vegetable and animal products as determinants of colon cancer risk in Dutch men and women. Cancer Causes Control. 1995;6:225–234.
68. The Women's Health Initiative Study Group. Design of the Women's Health Initiative clinical trial and observational study. Control Clin Trials. 1998; 19:61–109.
69. Beresford SAA, Johnson KC, Ritenbaugh C, et al. Low-fat dietary pattern and risk of colorectal cancer. The Women's Health Initiative Randomized Controlled Dietary Modification Trial. JAMA. 2006;295:643–65.
70. Knekt P, Steineck G, Jarvinen R, Hakulinen T, Aromaa A. Intake of fried meat and risk of cancer: a follow-up study in Finland. Int J Cancer. 1994; 59:756–760.
71. Kato I, Akhmedkhanov A, Koenig K, Toniolo PG,

Shore RE, Riboli E. Prospective study of diet and female colorectal cancer: the New York University Women's Health Study. Nutr Cancer. 1997;28: 276–281.

72. English DR, MacInnis RJ, Hodge AM, Hopper JL, Haydon AM, Giles GG. Red meat, chicken, and fish consumption and risk of colorectal cancer. Cancer Epidemiol Biomarkers Prev. 2004;13: 1509–1514.
73. Norat T, Bingham S, Ferrari P, et al. Meat, fish, and colorectal cancer risk: the European Prospective Investigation into cancer and nutrition. J Natl Cancer Inst. 2005;97:906–916.
74. Chao A, Thun MJ, Connell CJ, et al. Meat consumption and risk of colorectal cancer. JAMA. 2005;293:172–182.
75. Norat T, Lukanova A, Ferrari P, Riboli E. Meat consumption and colorectal cancer risk: dose-response meta-analysis of epidemiological studies. Int J Cancer. 2002;98:241–256.
76. Sandhu MS, White IR, McPherson K. Systematic review of the prospective cohort studies on meat consumption and colorectal cancer risk: a meta-analytical approach. Cancer Epidemiol Biomarkers Prev. 2001;10:439–446.
77. Stevens RG, Jones DY, Micozzi MS, Taylor PR. Body iron stores and the risk of cancer. N Engl J Med. 1988;319:1047–1052.
78. Wurzelmann JI, Silver A, Schreinemachers DM, Sandler RS, Everson RB. Iron intake and the risk of colorectal cancer. Cancer Epidemiol Biomarkers Prev. 1996;5:503–507.
79. Dorgan JF, Schatzkin A. Antioxidant micronutrients in cancer prevention. Hematol Oncol Clin North Am. 1991;5:43–68.
80. Bostick RM, Potter JD, McKenzie DR, et al. Reduced risk of colon cancer with high intake of vitamin E: the Iowa Women's Health Study. Cancer Res. 1993;53:4230–4237.
81. Jacobs EJ, Connell CJ, Patel AV, et al. Vitamin C and vitamin E supplement use and colorectal cancer mortality in a large American Cancer Society cohort. Cancer Epidemiol Biomarkers Prev. 2001;10: 17–23.
82. Watkins ML, Erickson JD, Thun MJ, Mulinare J, Heath CW Jr. Multivitamin use and mortality in a large prospective study. Am J Epidemiol. 2000;152: 149–162.
83. Giovannucci E, Rimm EB, Ascherio A, Stampfer MJ, Colditz GA, Willett WC. Alcohol, low-methionine—low-folate diets, and risk of colon cancer in men. J Natl Cancer Inst. 1995;87:265–273.
84. Giovannucci E, Stampfer MJ, Colditz GA, et al. Multivitamin use, folate, and colon cancer in women in the Nurses' Health Study. Ann Intern Med. 1998;129:517–524.
85. Jacobs EJ, Connell CJ, Patel AV, et al. Multivitamin use and colon cancer mortality in the Cancer Prevention Study II cohort (United States). Cancer Causes Control. 2001;12:927–934.
86. Jacobs EJ, Connell CJ, Chao A, et al. Multivitamin use and colorectal cancer incidence in a US cohort: does timing matter? Am J Epidemiol. 2003;158: 621–628.
87. Kim YI, Mason JB. Nutrition chemoprevention of gastrointestinal cancers: a critical review. Nutr Rev. 1996;54:259–279.
88. Roncucci L, Di Donato P, Carati L, et al, for the Colorectal Cancer Study Group of the University of Modena and the Health Care District 16. Antioxidant vitamins or lactulose for the prevention of the recurrence of colorectal adenomas. Dis Colon Rectum. 1993;36:227–234.
89. Baron JA, Cole BF, Mott L, et al. Neoplastic and antineoplastic effects of beta-carotene on colorectal adenoma recurrence: results of a randomized trial. J Natl Cancer Inst. 2003;95:717–722.
90. Touvier M, Kesse E, Clavel-Chapelon F, Boutron-Ruault MC. Dual association of beta-carotene with risk of tobacco-related cancers in a cohort of French women. J Natl Cancer Inst. 2005;97:1338–1344.
91. Goodman GE, Thornquist MD, Balmes J, et al. The Beta-Carotene and Retinol Efficacy Trial: incidence of lung cancer and cardiovascular disease mortality during 6-year follow-up after stopping beta-carotene and retinol supplements. J Natl Cancer Inst. 2004;96:1743–1750.
92. Bairati I, Meyer F, Gelinas M, et al. A randomized trial of antioxidant vitamins to prevent second primary cancers in head and neck cancer patients. J Natl Cancer Inst. 2005;97:481–488.
93. Hennekens CH, Buring JE, Manson JE, et al. Lack of effect of long-term supplementation with beta carotene on the incidence of malignant neoplasms and cardiovascular disease. N Engl J Med. 1996; 334:1145–1149.
94. Lee IM, Cook NR, Manson JE, Buring JE, Hennekens CH. Beta-carotene supplementation and incidence of cancer and cardiovascular disease: the Women's Health Study. J Natl Cancer Inst. 1999; 91:2102–2106.
95. Albanes D, Heinonen OP, Taylor PR, et al. Alpha-tocopherol and beta-carotene supplements and lung cancer incidence in the Alpha-Tocopherol, Beta-Carotene Cancer Prevention Study: effects of base-line characteristics and study compliance. J Natl Cancer Inst. 1996;88:1560–1570.
96. Omenn GS, Goodman GE, Thornquist MD, et al. Risk factors for lung cancer and for intervention effects in CARET, the Beta-Carotene and Retinol Efficacy Trial. J Natl Cancer Inst. 1996;88: 1550–1559.
97. Albanes D, Malila N, Taylor PR, et al. Effects of supplemental alpha-tocopherol and beta-carotene

on colorectal cancer: results from a controlled trial (Finland). Cancer Causes Control. 2000;11: 197–205.

98. Cook NR, Le IM, Manson JE, Buring JE, Hennekens CH. Effects of beta-carotene supplementation on cancer incidence by baseline characteristics in the Physicians' Health Study (United States). Cancer Causes Control. 2000;11:617–626.
99. Bjelakovic G, Nikolova D, Simonetti RG, Gluud C. Antioxidant supplements for prevention of gastrointestinal cancers: a systematic review and meta-analysis. Lancet. 2004;364:1219–1228.
100. U.S. Preventive Services Task Force. Routine vitamin supplementation to prevent cancer and cardiovascular disease: recommendations and rationale. Ann Intern Med. 2003;139:51–55.
101. Morris CD, Carson S. Routine vitamin supplementation to prevent cardiovascular disease: a summary of the evidence for the U.S. Preventive Services Task Force. Ann Intern Med. 2003;139:56–70.
102. Burton GW, Ingold KU. Beta-carotene: an unusual type of lipid antioxidant. Science. 1984;224: 569–573.
103. Wang XD, Russell RM. Procarcinogenic and anticarcinogenic effects of beta-carotene. Nutr Rev. 1999;57:263–272.
104. Liu C, Wang XD, Bronson RT, Smith DE, Krinsky NI, Russell RM. Effects of physiological versus pharmacological beta-carotene supplementation on cell proliferation and histopathological changes in the lungs of cigarette smoke-exposed ferrets. Carcinogenesis. 2000;21:2245–2253.
105. Lotan R. Lung cancer promotion by beta-carotene and tobacco smoke: relationship to suppression of retinoic acid receptor-beta and increased activator protein-1? J Natl Cancer Inst. 1999;91:7–9.
106. Kim YI. Folate and carcinogenesis: evidence, mechanisms, and implications. J Nutr Biochem. 1999; 10:66–88.
107. Kim YI. Role of folate in colon cancer development and progression. J Nutr. 2003;133:3731S–3739S.
108. Bailey LB, Rampersaud GC, Kauwell GP. Folic acid supplements and fortification affect the risk for neural tube defects, vascular disease and cancer: evolving science. J Nutr. 2003;133:1961S–1968S.
109. Giovannucci E. Epidemiologic studies of folate and colorectal neoplasia: a review. J Nutr. 2002;132: 2350S–2355S.
110. Giovannucci E, Stampfer MJ, Colditz GA, et al. Folate, methionine, and alcohol intake and risk of colorectal adenoma. J Natl Cancer Inst. 1993;85: 875–884.
111. Fuchs CS, Willett WC, Colditz GA, et al. The influence of folate and multivitamin use on the familial risk of colon cancer in women. Cancer Epidemiol Biomarkers Prev. 2002;11:227–234.
112. Wei EK, Giovannucci E, Wu K, et al. Comparison of risk factors for colon and rectal cancer. Int J Cancer. 2004;108:433–442.
113. Su LJ, Arab L. Nutritional status of folate and colon cancer risk: evidence from NHANES I epidemiologic follow-up study. Ann Epidemiol. 2001;11: 65–72.
114. Harnack L, Jacobs DR Jr., Nicodemus K, Lazovich D, Anderson K, Folsom AR. Relationship of folate, vitamin B-6, vitamin B-12, and methionine intake to incidence of colorectal cancers. Nutr Cancer. 2002;43:152–158.
115. Konings EJ, Goldbohm RA, Brants HA, Saris WH, van den Brandt PA. Intake of dietary folate vitamers and risk of colorectal carcinoma: results from The Netherlands Cohort Study. Cancer. 2002; 95:1421–1433.
116. Hunter D. Folate and folate-metabolism gene variants and colorectal cancer. Paper presented at: Environmental Mutagen Society: Impact of the Environment on Colon Cancer; May 14–16, 2003; Miami Beach, Fl.
117. Sanjoaquin MA, Allen N, Couto E, Roddam AW, Key TJ. Folate intake and colorectal cancer risk: a meta-analytical approach. Int J Cancer. 2005;113: 825–828.
118. Hillman RS, Steinberg SE. The effects of alcohol on folate metabolism. Annu Rev Med. 1982;33: 345–354.
119. Potter JD. Methyl supply, methyl metabolizing enzymes and colorectal neoplasia. J Nutr. 2002;132: 2410S–2412S.
120. Sharp L, Little J. Polymorphisms in genes involved in folate metabolism and colorectal neoplasia: A HuGE review. Am J Epidemiol. 2004;159: 423–443.
121. Cole BF, Baron JA, Sandler RS. A randomized trial of folic acid to prevent colorectal adenomas. Proc Am Assoc Cancer Res. 2005;46:4399.
122. Kim YI. Folate, colorectal carcinogenesis, and DNA methylation: lessons from animal studies. Environ Mol Mutagen. 2004;44:10–25.
123. Kim YI. Folate and DNA methylation: a mechanistic link between folate deficiency and colorectal cancer? Cancer Epidemiol Biomarkers Prev. 2004;13: 511–519.
124. Kune GA, Vitetta L. Alcohol consumption and the etiology of colorectal cancer: a review of the scientific evidence from 1957 to 1991. Nutr Cancer. 1992;18:97–111.
125. Gronbaek M, Becker U, Johansen D, et al. Type of alcohol consumed and mortality from all causes, coronary heart disease, and cancer. Ann Intern Med. 2000;133:411–419.
126. Bagnardi V, Blangiardo M, La Vecchia C, Corrao G. A meta-analysis of alcohol drinking and cancer risk. Br J Cancer. 2001;85:1700–1705.
127. Cho E, Smith-Warner SA, Ritz J, et al. Alcohol

intake and colorectal cancer: a pooled analysis of 8 cohort studies. Ann Intern Med. 2004;140: 603–613.
128. Garro AJ, Lieber CS. Alcohol and cancer. Annu Rev Pharmacol Toxicol. 1990;30:219–249.
129. Seitz HK, Matsuzaki S, Yokoyama A, Homann N, Vakevainen S, Wang XD. Alcohol and cancer. Alcohol Clin Exp Res. 2001;25:137S–143S.
130. Martinez ME, Willett WC. Calcium, vitamin D, and colorectal cancer: a review of the epidemiologic evidence. Cancer Epidemiol Biomarkers Prev. 1998;7:163–168.
131. Bergsma-Kadijk JA, van't Veer P, Kampman E, Burema J. Calcium does not protect against colorectal neoplasia. Epidemiology. 1996;7:590–597.
132. Cho E, Smith-Warner SA, Spiegelman D, et al. Dairy foods, calcium, and colorectal cancer: a pooled analysis of 10 cohort studies. J Natl Cancer Inst. 2004;96:1015–1022.
133. Zheng W, Anderson KE, Kushi LH, et al. A prospective cohort study of intake of calcium, vitamin D, and other micronutrients in relation to incidence of rectal cancer among postmenopausal women. Cancer Epidemiol Biomarkers Prev. 1998;7: 221–225.
134. Wu K, Willett WC, Fuchs CS, Colditz GA, Giovannucci EL. Calcium intake and risk of colon cancer in women and men. J Natl Cancer Inst. 2002; 94:437–446.
135. McCullough ML, Robertson AS, Rodriguez C, et al. Calcium, vitamin D, dairy products, and risk of colorectal cancer in the Cancer Prevention Study II Nutrition Cohort (United States). Cancer Causes Control. 2003;14:1–12.
136. Sellers TA, Bazyk AE, Bostick RM, et al. Diet and risk of colon cancer in a large prospective study of older women: an analysis stratified on family history (Iowa, United States). Cancer Causes Control. 1998;9:357–367.
137. Flood A, Peters U, Chatterjee N, Lacey JV Jr., Schairer C, Schatzkin A. Calcium from diet and supplements is associated with reduced risk of colorectal cancer in a prospective cohort of women. Cancer Epidemiol Biomarkers Prev. 2005;14: 126–132.
138. Peters U, Chatterjee N, McGlynn KA, et al. Calcium intake and colorectal adenoma in a US colorectal cancer early detection program. Am J Clin Nutr. 2004;80:1358–1365.
139. Kampman E, Slattery ML, Caan B, Potter JD. Calcium, vitamin D, sunshine exposure, dairy products and colon cancer risk (United States). Cancer Causes Control. 2000;11:459–466.
140. Bostick RM. Human studies of calcium supplementation and colorectal epithelial cell proliferation. Cancer Epidemiol Biomarkers Prev. 1997;6: 971–980.
141. Baron JA, Tosteson TD, Wargovich MJ, et al. Calcium supplementation and rectal mucosal proliferation: a randomized controlled trial. J Natl Cancer Inst. 1995;87:1303–1307.
142. Bostick RM, Fosdick L, Wood JR, et al. Calcium and colorectal epithelial cell proliferation in sporadic adenoma patients: a randomized, double-blinded, placebo-controlled clinical trial. J Natl Cancer Inst. 1995;87:1307–1315.
143. Hofstad B, Almendingen K, Vatn M, et al. Growth and recurrence of colorectal polyps: a double-blind 3-year intervention with calcium and antioxidants. Digestion. 1998;59:148–56.
144. Grau MV, Baron JA, Sandler RS, et al. Vitamin D, calcium supplementation, and colorectal adenomas: results of a randomized trial. J Natl Cancer Inst. 2003;95:1765–1771.
145. Wallace K, Baron JA, Cole BF, et al. Effect of calcium supplementation on the risk of large bowel polyps. J Natl Cancer Inst. 2004;96:921–925.
146. Wactawski-Wende J, Kotchen JM, Anderson GL, et al. Calcium plus vitamin D supplementation and the risk of colorectal cancer. N Engl J Med. 2006; 354:684–696.
147. Pence BC. Role of calcium in colon cancer prevention: experimental and clinical studies. Mutat Res. 1993;290:87–95.
148. Lamprecht SA, Lipkin M. Chemoprevention of colon cancer by calcium, vitamin D and folate: molecular mechanisms. Nat Rev Cancer. 2003;3: 601–614.
149. Knekt P, Aromaa A, Maatela J, et al. Serum selenium and subsequent risk of cancer among Finnish men and women. J Natl Cancer Inst. 1990;82: 864–868.
150. van den Brandt PA, Goldbohm RA, van't Veer P, et al. A prospective cohort study on toenail selenium levels and risk of gastrointestinal cancer. J Natl Cancer Inst. 1993;85:224–229.
151. Garland M, Morris JS, Stampfer MJ, et al. Prospective study of toenail selenium levels and cancer among women. J Natl Cancer Inst. 1995;87: 497–505.
152. Vinceti M, Rothman KJ, Bergomi M, Borciani N, Serra L, Vivoli G. Excess melanoma incidence in a cohort exposed to high levels of environmental selenium. Cancer Epidemiol Biomarkers Prev. 1998;7:853–856.
153. Jacobs ET, Jiang R, Alberts DS, et al. Selenium and colorectal adenoma: results of a pooled analysis. J Natl Cancer Inst. 2004;96:1669–1675.
154. Duffield-Lillico AJ, Slate EH, Reid ME, et al. Selenium supplementation and secondary prevention of nonmelanoma skin cancer in a randomized trial. J Natl Cancer Inst. 2003;95:1477–1481.
155. Ip C. Lessons from basic research in selenium and cancer prevention. J Nutr. 1998;128:1845–1854.

156. Helzlsouer KJ, Block G, Blumberg J, et al. Summary of the round table discussion on strategies for cancer prevention: diet, food, additives, supplements, and drugs. Cancer Res. 1994;54: 2044s–2051s.
157. McKeown-Eyssen G. Epidemiology of colorectal cancer revisited: are serum triglycerides and/or plasma glucose associated with risk? Cancer Epidemiol Biomarkers Prev. 1994;3:687–695.
158. Giovannucci E. Insulin and colon cancer. Cancer Causes Control. 1995;6:164–179.
159. Sandhu MS, Dunger DB, Giovannucci EL. Insulin, insulin-like growth factor-I (IGF-I), IGF binding proteins, their biologic interactions, and colorectal cancer. J Natl Cancer Inst. 2002;94:972–980.
160. Ritter MM, Richter WO, Schwandt P. Acromegaly and colon cancer. Ann Intern Med. 1987;106: 636–637.
161. Kim YI. Diet, lifestyle, and colorectal cancer: is hyperinsulinemia the missing link? Nutr Rev. 1998;56: 275–279.
162. Weiderpass E, Gridley G, Nyren O, Ekbom A, Persson I, Adami HO. Diabetes mellitus and risk of large bowel cancer. J Natl Cancer Inst. 1997;89: 660–661.
163. Will JC, Galuska DA, Vinicor F, Calle EE. Colorectal cancer: another complication of diabetes mellitus? Am J Epidemiol. 1998;147:816–825.
164. Hu FB, Manson JE, Liu S, et al. Prospective study of adult onset diabetes mellitus (type 2) and risk of colorectal cancer in women. J Natl Cancer Inst. 1999;91:542–547.
165. Nilsen TI, Vatten LJ. Prospective study of colorectal cancer risk and physical activity, diabetes, blood glucose and BMI: exploring the hyperinsulinaemia hypothesis. Br J Cancer. 2001;84:417–422.
166. Khaw KT, Wareham N, Bingham S, Luben R, Welch A, Day N. Preliminary communication: glycated hemoglobin, diabetes, and incident colorectal cancer in men and women: a prospective analysis from the European prospective investigation into cancer—Norfolk study. Cancer Epidemiol Biomarkers Prev. 2004;13:915–919.
167. Schoen RE, Tangen CM, Kuller LH, et al. Increased blood glucose and insulin, body size, and incident colorectal cancer. J Natl Cancer Inst. 1999; 91:1147–1154.
168. Kaaks R, Toniolo P, Akhmedkhanov A, et al. Serum C-peptide, insulin-like growth factor (IGF)-I, IGF-binding proteins, and colorectal cancer risk in women. J Natl Cancer Inst. 2000;92:1592–1600.
169. Ma J, Pollak MN, Giovannucci E, et al. Prospective study of colorectal cancer risk in men and plasma levels of insulin-like growth factor (IGF)-I and IGF-binding protein-3. J Natl Cancer Inst. 1999; 91:620–625.
170. Ma J, Giovannucci E, Pollak M, et al. A prospective study of plasma C-peptide and colorectal cancer risk in men. J Natl Cancer Inst. 2004;96:546–553.
171. Tran TT, Medline A, Bruce WR. Insulin promotion of colon tumors in rats. Cancer Epidemiol Biomarkers Prev. 1996;5:1013–1015.
172. Corpet DE, Jacquinet C, Peiffer G, Tache S. Insulin injections promote the growth of aberrant crypt foci in the colon of rats. Nutr Cancer. 1997;27: 316–320.
173. Koohestani N, Tran TT, Lee W, Wolever TM, Bruce WR. Insulin resistance and promotion of aberrant crypt foci in the colons of rats on a high-fat diet. Nutr Cancer. 1997;29:69–76.
174. Koohestani N, Chia MC, Pham NA, et al. Aberrant crypt focus promotion and glucose intolerance: correlation in the rat across diets differing in fat, n-3 fatty acids and energy. Carcinogenesis. 1998; 19:1679–1684.
175. Tran TT, Gupta N, Goh T, et al. Direct measure of insulin sensitivity with the hyperinsulinemic-euglycemic clamp and surrogate measures of insulin sensitivity with the oral glucose tolerance test: correlations with aberrant crypt foci promotion in rats. Cancer Epidemiol Biomarkers Prev. 2003;12: 47–56.
176. Meyskens FL Jr., Szabo E. Diet and cancer: the disconnect between epidemiology and randomized clinical trials. Cancer Epidemiol Biomarkers Prev. 2005;14:1366–1369.
177. Cerhan JR, Potter JD, Gilmore JM, et al. Adherence to the AICR cancer prevention recommendations and subsequent morbidity and mortality in the Iowa Women's Health Study cohort. Cancer Epidemiol Biomarkers Prev. 2004;13:1114–1120.

53 Gastrointestinal Disease

Charles L. Baum and Catherine McIsaac

Introduction

The digestion of food and the absorption of nutrients require the synchronized action of a number of digestive organs (Table 1). The process is initiated before eating when the sight and smell of food trigger a neurohormonal response that stimulates gastric motility and secretion. Nutrient digestion begins in the mouth with the chewing action of the jaws and teeth and the secretion of salivary amylase, which initiates the breakdown of ingested starch. Mastication allows the tongue and other structures of the mouth to shape food into a bolus, which is propelled into the oropharynx and esophagus by a complex set of highly coordinated neuromuscular actions. Waves of esophageal peristalsis carry the food bolus into the stomach, where acid and the proteolytic enzyme pepsin begin the process of protein digestion. The stomach is also the site of production of intrinsic factor, a specific vitamin B_{12}-binding protein that transports vitamin to receptors located on enterocytes in the ileum. Gastric chyme, composed of partly digested food, hydrochloric acid, and a range of enzymes, is slowly released into the duodenum, where acid and partially digested fats and proteins stimulate the secretion of cholecystokinin and secretin, which in turn stimulate pancreatic digestive enzyme secretion and gallbladder contraction. Bile, produced in the liver and released from the gallbladder in coordination with gastric emptying, contains bile acids that facilitate dietary lipid emulsification and absorption. Digestive end products, peptides, amino acids, oligosaccharides, di- and monosaccharides, lipids, and other micronutrients, are taken up and transported across the microvillus membrane by a number of different processes ranging from diffusion to receptor-mediated endocytosis. During the process of luminal digestion, the intrinsic gut neuromuscular system maintains a synchronized peristalsis that shuttles intestinal contents down the length of the bowel.

The small and large intestines have evolved specialized barrier and immunologic functions that play a critical role in host defense and compensate for the complex spatially organized digestive and absorptive functions that demand a large surface area and a thin epithelium. In Westernized countries, critical research efforts are focusing on the link between alterations in gut mucosal function and the growing burden of food allergy, idiopathic inflammatory bowel diseases, and colon cancer. A number of recent reports suggest that the dysregulation of the amount, location, or composition of intestinal commensal microorganisms (collectively referred to as the microbiota) may play a role in the growing incidence of these bowel diseases. Intestinal microbiota exist throughout the gastrointestinal (GI) tract but are largely confined to the distal bowel (Table 2).[1] Through an assortment of metabolic attributes, different microbiota co-exist and serve as a "microbial organ" within the host GI tract, providing a critical interface between ingested food, chemicals, antigens, and the host immune system.[2,3] Recent data indicate that the complex consortium of gut microorganisms are determined by multiple factors, including host genotype, GI physiology, immunologic function, and external factors such as diet, lifestyle, and antibiotic use.[1,4,5] The extent of microbial functional diversity is illustrated by the wide range of physiologic processes associated with intestinal microflora: 1) bacterial fermentation and generation of products such as short-chain fatty acids that serve as nutrients and growth modulators for colonocytes; 2) transformation of xenobiotics, bile acids, and dietary phytoestrogens; 3) binding and inactivation of toxins and pathogenic microorganisms; 4) regulation of gut immune reactions through direct and indirect interactions with Peyer's patches and lymphoid cells; and 5) maintenance of mucosal structure.[5]

Intestinal Microflora: Prebiotics and Probiotics

Recent molecular studies have confirmed the regulatory impact of dietary patterns and macronutrient compo-

Table 1. Function of Digestive Organs

Organ/Location	Physical Function	Secretory Function (Substrate)
Oral cavity	Mastication	
Salivary glands		Fluid/salivary amylase (starch)
Oropharynx/esophagus	Swallowing	
Stomach	Grinding Emulsification	Hydrochloric acid Pepsin (proteolytic enzyme–protein) Gastric lipase (triglyceride) Intrinsic factor (vitamin B_{12} absorption)
Small intestine (duodenum/jejunum)	Peptide, oligosaccharide digestion Nutrient absorption Fluid/electrolyte absorption Muscular propulsion of food	Fluid/bicarbonate
Ileum	Bile acids, vitamin B_{12} absorption	
Pancreas		Fluid and bicarbonate Proteolytic enzymes (protein) Amylase (starch) Lipolytic enzymes (triglyceride, cholesteryl ester, phospholipid) Nucleases (DNA, RNA)
Liver	Bile acid synthesis	Bile
Gallbladder	Bile storage	Meal-induced bile secretion

sition (e.g., cereal fiber, pectin, fat, or protein) on gut microbiota. For example, a high fat intake is associated with higher numbers of anaerobes, whereas a high protein intake enriches colonic aerobic bacteria. This observation stimulated an extensive evaluation of global differences in colonic microflora, dietary correlates, and colon cancer risk, which found that indigenous rural diets were associated with higher levels of *Lactobacillus* species and a lower risk of colon cancer than Western-style high-fat diets.[6] Further use of molecular genotyping will revolutionize the characterization of microfloral effects on intestinal and extra-intestinal diseases.[7] Orally administered bacterial cultures, particularly yogurt, have led to extensive research on the health benefits of specific bacterial species, primarily lactic acid-fermenting bacteria, used in the production of fermented dairy products.[8] Metchnikoff,[9] the first to propose the use of lactic acid-producing bacteria therapeutically, spawned the now large body of evidence indicating that a healthy population of commensal microbiota can regulate and suppress colonization by enteropathogens.

The therapeutic administration of a live active culture that improves the balance of gut microflora and functional potential is known as probiotic therapy. Probiotics have been used for a variety of conditions associated with unbalanced or altered concentrations of indigenous microflora: food allergy, atopic dermatitis, infectious and antibiotic-associated diarrhea, irritable bowel syndrome (IBS), inflammatory bowel diseases, and arthritis.[1] The common thread in all of these conditions relates to either an inadequate or hyperreactive immune response, perhaps mediated by alterations in the gut immune system. Probiotics have been shown to modulate immune function and inflammation through inhibition of the transcription factor NF-κB pathway.[10] The precise requirements for probiotic-induced immunomodulatory activity, such as adherence and colonization, remain poorly understood. Nevertheless, a number of studies have demonstrated direct immunomodulatory effects of probiotic treatment, principally lactobacilli and bifidobacteria (Table 3)[11-18]; others suggest an indirect effect on gut function through changes in substrate availability. For example, lactose intolerance, which is due to a single nucleotide polymorphism (C-13910T) that disrupts mucosal lactase gene expression and causes lactose malabsorption, is often associated with a wide range of clinical responses to dietary lactose. Some individuals have minimal symptoms; others suffer gas production, bloating, and abdominal discomfort. The variability in symptoms can be explained by higher rates of microbial lactose metabolism to lactate and short-chain fatty acids in intolerant individuals.[19] Administration of yogurt and probiotic bacteria improves symptoms of lactose intolerance through microbial beta-galactosidase action and suppression of the adverse population of lactose-fermenting organisms.[20] Gut microbiota may also affect the salvage of dietary energy, and it has recently been proposed that variations in "bioreactor" effi-

Table 2. The Gut Microbiota Ecosystem

Gastrointestinal Tract	Resident Microbiota	Microbiota Concentration (CFU/g)
Mouth	Streptococci	Variable
	Bacteroides	
	Lactobacilli	
	Yeasts	
Esophagus	None	
Stomach	*Candida albicans*	10^4*
	Helicobacter pylori	
	Lactobacillus	
	Streptococcus	
Duodenum	*Bacteroides*	10^3–10^4
	C. albicans	
	Lactobacillus	
	Streptococcus	
Jejunum	*Bacteroides*	10^5–10^7
	Candida albicans	
	Lactobacillus	
	Streptococcus	
Ileum	*Bacteroides*	10^7–10^8
	Clostridium	
	Enterobacteriaceae	
	Enterococcus	
	Lactobacillus	
	Veillonella	
Colon	*Bacteroides*	10^{10}–10^{11}
	Bacillus	
	Bifidobacterium	
	Clostridium	
	Enterococcus	
	Eubacterium	
	Fusobacterium	
	Peptostreptococcus	
	Ruminococcus	
	Streptococcus	
	Veillonella	

*CFU/g, colony forming units per gram.
Adapted from Isolauri et al.[1] Copyright 2004 with permission from Elsevier.

ciencies may affect energy balance.[21] These authors argue that genetically determined variations in the composition of microbiota may determine whether an individual has a high- or low-efficiency bioreactor, in the former case promoting energy storage (obesity) and in the latter leanness.

A wide range of clinical research evidence supports the utility of probiotics. Probiotic treatment of acute childhood diarrhea, most of which can be accounted for by rotavirus infection, has been demonstrated to shorten the duration of diarrhea and reduce stool frequency.[11-13] Similarly, preliminary reports indicate the benefit of probiotics in the modulation of the immunologic disturbances characteristic of Crohn's disease. A growing number of randomized, double-blind clinical trials indicate that selected probiotic species have efficacy equivalent to and in some cases superior to traditional medications in maintaining remission and preventing recurrent disease in Crohn's disease, ulcerative colitis, and pouchitis.[16] Early studies demonstrated alterations in intestinal microflora in patients with IBS, with a shift from the dominant anaerobic species to *Clostridium* species.[22] Subsequent studies have extended this observation and shown that differences in microflora are associated with abnormal colonic fermentation and the development of symptoms in patients with IBS.[23] Further evidence linking alterations in colonic microflora to IBS symptoms comes from studies demonstrating a 10-fold relative risk of IBS after bacterial gastroenteritis.[24] Clinical evidence of the effectiveness of probiotics in IBS comes from a number of randomized, controlled trials demonstrating short- and long-term improvement in pain scores, bloating symptoms, and stool consistency.[17,18]

The aging process is associated with several impaired GI functions. Reserve capacity of the intestine and pancreas limits functional impairment in most elderly persons; however, aging-associated changes in gut motility and gastric acid production and loss of intestinal immunity increase the likelihood of adverse changes in intestinal microflora.[25] An increased susceptibility to *Clostridium difficile* and small bowel bacterial overgrowth have profound effects on morbidity and mortality in the elderly. Tube-feeding formulas increase the risk of *C. difficile* infection and diarrhea by increasing the ratio of aerobic to anaerobic colonic bacteria.[25] Probiotics supplied either in capsules or as a yogurt-based product with antibiotics significantly reduce the risk of antibiotic-associated diarrhea.[26] The progressive loss of gastric acid production with aging has been attributed in part to *Helicobacter pylori* colonization. *H. pylori* has resided in the stomach of humans for millions of years, generally as a commensal organism, but under certain conditions *H. pylori* becomes pathogenic and results in atrophic gastritis and ulceration. Recent epidemiologic studies have shown a relation between *H. pylori* colonization, hypertension, and dietary salt intake, suggesting a pathophysiologic link to a common lifestyle factor.[27] *H. pylori*-induced atrophic gastritis allows colonization with other bacteria, including species that increase nitrosamine production, which has been associated with an increased risk of gastric cancer.[28]

Prebiotics are nondigestible food ingredients that beneficially affect host's health by selectively stimulating the growth of resident microbiota. The health implications of dietary fiber are well known; however, the prebiotic

Table 3. Immunomodulatory Effects of Probiotic Treatment

Treatment Target	Potential Mechanism	Reference
Acute diarrhea	Reduction in duration of viral shedding. Increase in IgA-secreting cells. Normalization of gut microflora. Increase in mucin production.	Huang et al., 2002[11]; van Niel et al., 2002[12]; de Roos and Katan, 2000[13]
Allergic disease	Degradation and/or structural modification of enteral antigens. Normalization of gut permeability and microflora.	Kalliomaki et al., 2001[14]; Kalliomaki et al., 2003[15]
Inflammatory bowel disease	Normalization of gut permeability and microflora. Reduction in local and systemic inflammatory response. Increase in mucin production.	Sartor, 2004[16]
Irritable bowel disease	Normalization of gut microflora and improved intestinal motility	Verdu and Collins, 2004[17]; Saggioro, 2004[18]

properties appear to be limited to a small group of constituent complex carbohydrate ingredients or synthetic analogues: lactulose, fructo-oligosaccharides, inulin, and transgalactosides.[29] Prebiotics require activation by bacterial fermentation to the short-chain fatty acids acetate, propionate, and butyrate, which in turn have physiologic effects on gut mucosal function.[30] Perhaps the best known prebiotic action is on bowel laxation, which is due to both increased stool bulk and short-chain fatty acid effects on colonic motility.[29] Prebiotics have also been shown to improve tolerance to enteral tube feeding, particularly in the elderly; to increase colonic calcium and magnesium absorption; to reduce colonic DNA synthesis in high-risk colon polyp patients; to reduce absenteeism and the incidence of fever and diarrhea in kindergarten children; to lower cholesterol and glucose levels; and to heal ileal pouchitis in patients with an ileal-anal anastomosis.[31-34] Prebiotics are generally well tolerated but may cause undesirable effects, including excessive flatus, abdominal pain, and diarrhea.[35] Recent studies have called into question the health benefits of dietary fructo-oligosaccharides, which are nondigestible carbohydrates found in varying concentrations in foods such as wheat, bananas, asparagus, and garlic and which are also added to infant formulas. Early studies with fructo-oligosaccharides supported a powerful role as probiotics; however, more recently studies in healthy men have revealed increased bloating, gas, and mucin production, suggesting mucosal irritation.[36] Thus, while short-term treatment with prebiotics may have positive benefits on fecal microflora, clearly there is a need for longer-term studies.

Diet, Nutrition, and GI Diseases

Most GI diseases alter digestion, nutrient assimilation, or luminal nutrient processing. In some cases, specific nutrients increase GI symptoms and/or lead to GI disease (e.g., lactose intolerance and celiac sprue disease). Disruption of any number of steps in the digestive and absorptive process can lead to GI symptoms and clinically significant malabsorption with varying degrees of protein, energy, and micronutrient deficiency. In general, malabsorption presents with overt signs of macronutrient deficiency and symptoms of intestinal nutrient loss such as steatorrhea; however, certain conditions such as pernicious anemia and celiac sprue disease are often diagnosed before overt symptoms based on an incidental discovery of subclinical micronutrient deficiency. Proper diagnosis of malabsorption syndromes requires detailed functional and morphologic studies of the GI tract that are beyond the scope of this discussion. Careful attention must be given to the impact of disease status and behavioral- and cytokine-mediated effects on appetite and nutrient assimilation.

The management of digestive/nutrient disorders requires strategies that often include multiple routes of nutrient repletion and repeated longitudinal assessment of nutritional status. GI dysfunction is managed with a variety of pharmacologic agents, including motility and antimotility agents, digestive enzyme supplements, and judicious use of antibiotics, prebiotics, and probiotics in situations where there is overgrowth or alteration in the composition of intestinal microflora (Table 4). The following discussion elaborates on specific disease states and indications for these different treatment options.

Gastroesophageal Reflux Disease

Gastroesophageal reflux disease (GERD) is an example of a condition in which food, both in terms of the amount and composition, affects gastroesophageal function. GERD is a complex disorder resulting from the reflux of gastric contents, gastric acid, pepsin, and/or bile into the esophagus, with resultant stimulation of pain receptors and subsequent damage to the mucosa. Common etiologies include lower esophageal sphincter dysfunction, delayed gastric emptying, or increased intragastric pressure. Both the length of exposure and the amount of gastric acid eventually determine the degree of mucosal injury, which manifests as GERD symptoms: substernal burning pain (heartburn), chest pressure, and/or acid regurgitation. GERD is common in industrialized nations, with an estimated 15% to 20% of US and European

Table 4. Stepwise Approach to the Management of Malabsorption

1. Provide additional micro- and macronutrients to compensate for anorexia, catabolism, and stool losses.
2. Modify meal frequency, diet composition, and portion size (e.g., small frequent meals for postgastrectomy patients or frequent low-osmolality meals for short bowel patients).
3. Pharmacotherapy
   a. Short course of appetite stimulants (megestrol acetate, dronabinol, oxandralone)
   b. Pancreatic enzyme supplements
   c. Antimotility agents (opiates, loperamide)
   d. Antisecretory agents (H_2 antagonists, proton pump inhibitors, octreotide)
   e. Antibiotics in cases of suspected bacterial overgrowth
4. Prebiotics and probiotics
5. Nutrition supplements (oral and enteral)
6. Parenteral nutrition support (vitamins, minerals, total parenteral nutrition)

adults experiencing GERD symptoms at least once per week.[37] Over the past several decades, the increasing incidence of GERD has resulted in an increase in complications: esophagitis, stricture formation, metaplastic Barrett's lesions, and esophageal adenocarcinoma.[38]

The relationship between nutrition and GERD is particularly evident in obese patients. Several studies have shown the adverse impact of obesity on GERD symptoms, hospitalizations, and progression to esophagitis.[39–41] Obesity produces an increased gastroesophageal pressure gradient resulting from the weight of abdominal fat and overeating-induced gastric distention. In addition, obesity is associated with a higher incidence of hiatal hernia, which can act to lower esophageal sphincter pressure.[42] Further proof of the pathophysiologic link between obesity and GERD comes from studies demonstrating the beneficial effects of weight loss on GERD symptoms.[43] In view of these findings and based on the current understanding of the pathophysiology of GERD, it is not surprising to find that obesity also increases the risk of premalignant Barrett's mucosa and esophageal adenocarcinoma.[44,45] The association between body weight and esophageal adenocarcinoma may be more complex than a simple physical effect of obesity on lower esophageal sphincter function and GERD frequency. The association between obesity and esophageal cancer risk is well recognized and raises the possibility that there may be tumor-promoting effects of excess adipose tissue. Insulin and leptin, both of which are elevated in parallel with body fat, have been implicated as possible mediators of the increased cancer risk through their growth-promoting effects.[46] Trends in the incidence of obesity and esophageal adenocarcinoma support the need for large randomized, controlled trials to critically evaluate the independent effects of body weight on intermediate markers of carcinogenesis and cancer risk. Recent studies indicate that the incidence of GERD is as high as 50% in morbidly obese patients and that bariatric surgical approaches improve GERD through both direct anatomic changes and indirectly through weight loss.[47,48]

Celiac Disease

Gluten-sensitive enteropathy, celiac sprue, and nontropical sprue are different names for celiac disease. Celiac disease is an autoimmune disease characterized by an immune reaction to tissue transglutaminase (TTG) and a strong association with class II haplotypes of human leukocyte antigen (HLA) DR17-DQ2 and, to a lesser extent, DR4-DQ8. Anti-TTG and endomysial antibodies are the serologic hallmarks of celiac disease.[49] TTG is a ubiquitously distributed cytosolic enzyme that deamidates dietary gliadin to a peptide that binds to TTG, and together this complex is recognized as foreign, resulting in autoantibody production and gut-derived T-cell activation.[50] This series of events can be triggered by other dietary prolamins; gliadin in wheat gluten is the most common, but others include secalins in rye and hordeins in barley.

An abnormality in intestinal permeability appears to allow the entry of gliadin peptides not entirely degraded by the intraluminal and brush border-bound peptidases and not normally allowed to cross the intestinal barrier. The epithelial barrier may also be disrupted in the course of a viral infection, allowing disease activation in otherwise susceptible individuals. The subsequent immune activation results in a dramatic mucosal inflammatory reaction that manifests histologically as total or subtotal villous flattening, hyperplastic elongated crypts, and chronic inflammatory infiltration of the lamina propria. The absorptive cells that remain are functionally compromised, with reduced levels of digestive enzymes and absorptive capacity. The extent of small bowel involvement varies and is correlated with the severity of clinical symptoms. Patients with severe villous atrophy are typically malnourished at presentation, in contrast to patients with predominantly patchy or proximal small bowel involvement, who may be asymptomatic.

The advent of reliable serologic screening tests for anti-endomysial and TTG antibodies has facilitated a more accurate estimation of the population-based incidence of celiac disease, and recent studies suggest that celiac sprue is as common as 1 in 122 people in Northern Ireland[51] and 1 in 250 to 300 people in the United States.[52] As these findings suggest, diagnosis of celiac disease before the typical presentation of malabsorption, steatorrhea, abdominal pain, fatigue, weight loss, and growth failure in children has been made possible by the use of serologic screening tests. A diagnostic workup for celiac disease is often prompted by unexplained folate or iron deficiency,[53] accelerated bone disease with severe osteopenia (and in some cases multiple fractures due to alterations in calcium and vitamin D metabolism)[54], and vitamin K deficiency with resultant bleeding diathesis.[55]

In most cases, strict adherence to a gluten-free diet will normalize small bowel histology, lead to a prompt resolution of symptoms, and improve or prevent further nutrient deficiencies. During the initial phase of treatment, it may be necessary to administer pancreatic supplements because intestinal mucosal damage may prevent the normal dietary-induced release of cholecystokinin and secretin, which mediate the release of pancreatic enzymes.[56] The benefit of gluten exclusion is usually rapid, and most patients show improvement within days, with complete resolution occurring by 4 to 6 weeks. Patients whose GI symptoms persist after gluten withdrawal need to be examined by hydrogen breath testing for small intestinal bacterial overgrowth.[57] If positive, a short course of antibiotics can have a dramatic effect on symptoms.[58]

A gluten-free diet requires not only elimination of the primary sources of prolamins, such as bread and related grain products, but also meticulous label reading to avoid the sources of gluten commonly used in processed foods. Recent legislation will facilitate patients' efforts; after Jan. 1, 2006, US manufacturers are required to identify in plain English any ingredient that is or contains protein from wheat. Unfortunately, relapses are common because of the difficulty associated with recognizing and avoiding sources of toxic gluten. Wheat flour is ubiquitous in the normal American diet, being frequently used as an extender in processed foods. Organizations such as the Celiac Sprue Association and websites such as Celiac.com have produced extensive lists of ingredients, handbooks, recipes, and gluten-free products.[59]

Although it is clear that wheat, rye, and barley have harmful effects on the small intestinal mucosa of patients with celiac disease, the toxic effects of oats have been debated. Oats belong to the same subfamily of grasses as wheat, rye, and barley (Pooideae), but differ in the makeup of their prolamin fraction. Oats do not contain gliadin, the toxic component of wheat; instead they contain avenin. Whereas prolamins represent half of the protein content in wheat, rye, and barley, avenin constitutes only 5% to 15% of the total protein content in oats, suggesting that a much higher intake of oats would be needed to produce the same toxic effect as wheat. Therefore, some have advocated that strict oat restriction may not be necessary. Data support this contention: in a randomized, controlled trial of a gluten-free diet supplemented with 70 g of oats in adults with newly diagnosed celiac disease and celiac disease in remission, dietary supplementation with 70 g of oats (the equivalent of approximately 1.5 cups of cooked oatmeal) had no effect on small bowel morphology or serologic tests.[60] In this study, a comparison of the gluten-free diet containing oats with a conventional gluten-free diet revealed that the rate of disappearance of serologic markers and the decrease in the number of intraepithelial lymphocytes were the same on the two diets. A small amount of oats in the diet provides a needed source of micronutrients, fiber, and dietary variety and may help patients with celiac disease better comply with the other diet restrictions.

Unfortunately, recent data highlight the potential for contamination of oat products with gluten during harvesting, processing, and packaging. Analysis of three commercially available brands of oatmeal by ELISA revealed a gluten level of more than 20 ppm in samples of all three brands, with some samples containing as much as 1800 ppm.[61] For this reason, celiac disease organizations continue to advise against the consumption of oats.

Pancreatic Insufficiency

There are a number of causes of pancreatitis, but alcoholic pancreatitis is by far the most common etiology. Over time, repeated acute attacks of pancreatitis lead to progressive loss of exocrine pancreatic function, with resultant maldigestion, malabsorption, and vitamin and mineral deficiency. Patients with pancreatic insufficiency require digestive enzyme replacement therapy. Early in the course of chronic pancreatitis, patients may have chronic abdominal pain that produces sitophobia and contributes to altered nutritional status. Typically, steatorrhea and azotorrhea occur only after lipase and trypsin secretion is reduced by 90%, at which point fecal fat losses may exceed 100 g/d. Administration of commercially available enzyme supplements may require large numbers of pills to replace the normal lipase production of approximately 28,000 IU per meal. Loss of pancreatic bicarbonate production also affects digestive capacity by allowing gastric acid inactivation of pancreatic enzymes. Therefore, patients with persistent steatorrhea may benefit from the use of an H_2 histamine antagonist or proton-pump inhibitor. Alternatively, enteric-coated enzyme replacements, which typically have a higher concentration of lipase per pill, may be tried, but there does not seem to be an advantage in terms of a reduction in steatorrhea compared with preparations that are not enteric coated.[62] Preparations with higher amounts of lipase have been withdrawn from the market because of colonic strictures in children with pancreatic insufficiency secondary to cystic fibrosis. Finally, pancreatic enzymes that are not enteric coated have been shown to improve pancreatic pain, presumably by digesting a cholecystokinin-releasing peptide, providing negative feedback inhibition of pancreatic secretion.[63]

Approximately 5% of patients with pancreatic insufficiency have severe malnutrition and maldigestion that fails to respond to oral diet modifications or enzyme supplements. Recent data suggest that the use of gastric acid suppression therapy in combination with the loss of pancreatic antibacterial activity may lead to alterations in intestinal microflora that exacerbate malabsorption.[64] Anecdotal experience suggests selected benefit from the use of antibiotic therapy or probiotics. If additional nutrition support is necessary, studies suggests that patients tolerate lower-cost standard polypeptide formulas.[65]

Short Bowel Syndrome

The loss of nutrient-, fluid-, and electrolyte-absorptive capacity associated with partial or near-complete loss of the small intestine often results in the need for nutrition support. Nutritional complications of short bowel syndrome include macronutrient and micronutrient deficiencies, fluid and electrolyte abnormalities, weight loss, complications of parenteral nutrition, and metabolic bone disease. The most important determinant of residual bowel function after loss of the small intestine is mucosal surface area, which determines absorptive capacity and is functionally related to the number and height of villi and microvilli. For example, loss of the proximal small bowel (duodenum and jejunum) is less well tolerated than loss of the distal small bowel because of the greater villous density. Certain areas of the small intestine provide specialized functions that affect the outcome in patients with short bowel syndrome. The distal small bowel (ileum) is the site of vitamin B_{12} and bile acid absorption, and the ileocecal valve plays a critical role in determining intestinal transit time and preventing the reflux of colonic bacteria into the small bowel, causing secondary bacterial overgrowth.

Estimating residual bowel in terms of length and functional status is at best qualitative. In adults with short bowel syndrome, there is a poor correlation between the absolute length of remnant small bowel and the incidence of complications, but in general the length has prognostic importance. Less than 100 cm of remnant jejunum in the absence of a colon (end-jejunostomy patients) usually necessitates parenteral nutrition support. A similar prognosis has been observed with less than 50 to 60 cm of small intestine and a jejuno-colonic anastomosis.[66]

In adults, the leading cause of short bowel syndrome is Crohn's disease, accounting for 77% of reported cases.[67] Other common causes include arterial/venous mesenteric infarction, radiation enteritis, and volvulus. Mesenteric infarction is the major cause of near-total small bowel loss and severe short bowel syndrome, defined as remnant postduodenal small bowel length of 150 cm or less.[67] In the pediatric population, congenital abnormalities (e.g., intestinal atresia and gastroschisis) account for two-thirds of all cases and necrotizing enterocolitis accounts for about one-third of cases.[68]

The true incidence of short bowel syndrome in the United States is difficult to ascertain. Data from The Oley Foundation indicated that in 1992 there were 40,000 patients with intestinal failure receiving total parenteral nutrition; more recent data indicate that the number of patients dependent on total parenteral nutrition with short bowel syndrome may have decreased to less than 50%.[69]

Most patients with short bowel syndrome begin the postsurgical period on parenteral nutrition support. The first 1 to 2 years after intestinal resection represent a critical recovery phase marked by a series of adaptive changes in the remaining small bowel. These changes are most pronounced when the remaining distal small bowel is ileum, but to some extent there is an increase in absorptive capacity along the entire length of the remaining small intestine. The anatomy of the residual bowel has prognostic significance (Table 5).[69] In many patients, nutrient absorption increases because of both molecular and structural changes that result in an increase in the expression of brush-border membrane enzymes, villous height, crypt depth, bowel diameter, blood flow, increased pancreatico-biliary secretions, and length.[69] The adaptive hyperplasia that occurs along the crypt-villous axis is mediated by a number of growth factors released in response to the presence of food and pancreatic secretions.[70] Therefore, early enteral feeding helps to facilitate the process of adaptation. This may not be possible in the first 1 to 2 weeks after resection because of massive diarrhea resulting from remnant intestinal fluid secretion and electrolyte losses. In addition, in the first year after resection, malabsorption may be worsened by transient gastric hypersecretion due to hypergastrinemia and rapid liquid gastric emptying caused by the loss of the colonic or ileal brake mediated by neuropeptide YY.[71] Parenteral H_2 antagonists are recommended to reduce secretion and to prevent peptic ulceration. In the transition from parenteral to enteral nutrition, patients are prone to dehydration and ongoing electrolyte and divalent cation losses, specifically calcium, magnesium, and zinc. Loss of the terminal ileum results in vitamin B_{12} and bile salt malabsorption. Depletion of the bile salt pool impedes fat absorption, which in turn allows for the formation of complexes between free fatty acids and divalent cations, with a further reduction in divalent cation absorption.

Table 5. Prognostic Determinants in Patients with SBS

1. Jejunal resection $<$ 50%–60% is usually well tolerated.
2. Ileal resection $>$ 30% is poorly tolerated.
3. Total small bowel $<$ 60 cm is associated with severe malabsorption, dependence on total parenteral nutrition, and a high risk of liver and kidney failure.
4. End-jejunostomy is associated with severe fluid and electrolyte loss.
5. Colon and ileocecal valve in continuity increase tolerance to small bowel resection.

Adapted from O'Keefe et al.,[69] copyright 2006, with permission from the American Gastroenterological Association.

In general, short bowel syndrome patients with an end-jejunostomy absorb nutrients, fluids, and electrolytes in proportion to bowel length. Below a critical bowel length, consumption of hypotonic fluids should be avoided because these commonly result in a rapid flux of sodium into the bowel lumen and an increase in sodium loss. In patients with a high jejunostomy, liquids consumed should contain a sodium concentration of at least 90 mmol/L; unfortunately, at this concentration of sodium these solutions are not very palatable. When ostomy output is more than 2 to 3 L/d, it is often difficult to maintain sodium balance with an oral supplement. It has been proposed that the addition of glucose polymers may augment fluid and sodium absorption in jejunostomy patients, but supporting data are limited.[72]

In summary, the dietary management of jejunostomy patients requires a large total energy intake of an iso-osmolar diet with added salt. In patients with a strong secretory component to their ostomy output, nutrient absorption may be enhanced by the use of H_2 antagonists or high doses of antimotility agents such as loperamide, Lomotil, or narcotics.

Patients with a short bowel and a retained colon present different nutritional management issues. A diet high in complex carbohydrate (but lactose-free) is beneficial because of colonic fermentation to short-chain fatty acids. Short-chain fatty acids are readily absorbed in the colon and may provide a mechanism for the salvage of up to 4.2 MJ/d.[73] On the other hand, persistent bloating symptoms in patients with short bowel syndrome and colonic continuity have recently been shown to correlate with small intestinal bacterial overgrowth (despite shortened intestinal transit times) and to improve with antibiotic therapy.[74] Moreover, improvement in symptoms is correlated with improvement in breath hydrogen levels, suggesting that breath hydrogen testing is a useful tool for monitoring symptoms in patients with short bowel syndrome. Anecdotal reports have suggested that probiotics may have limited value in patients with short bowel syndrome; however, larger-scale trials are needed before this approach can be recommended.[75]

Patients with intractable short bowel syndrome ultimately depend on home parenteral nutrition. This is a life-saving measure that allows a period of nutrition support for maximal gut adaptation. Attention must be paid to the provision of adequate protein and calories to prevent weight loss and provide fluid, electrolytes, and base-equivalents to compensate for GI losses. Gut adaptation is maximal within the first 3 years after resection and is dependent in part on appropriate luminal nutrition, highlighting the need for enteral intake during the adaptive phase. In this regard, pharmacologic and nutritional treatments aimed at facilitating gut adaptation have become an area of active research interest. Early data from uncontrolled trials using glutamine, growth hormone, and a modified fiber-containing diet were encouraging, but subsequent controlled trials showed little effect on nutrient absorption or morphometric changes in gut mucosa.[76-78] A recent preliminary report suggests that glucagon-like peptide-2 analog may have benefit in inducing functional and morphologic small bowel adaptation; a controlled trial is in progress.[79]

Several surgical treatments have been proposed for the treatment of short bowel syndrome. Prior work has focused on attempts to either slow intestinal transit or increase intestinal surface area, but with very little success.[80] Small intestinal transplantation has evolved from an experimental procedure to a potential therapeutic alternative to long-term parenteral nutrition for selected patients with short bowel syndrome.[81] With improvements in immunosuppressive medications, there has been a proportional increase in graft and patient survival, but the outcome is still poor compared with other organ transplantation outcomes (55% graft survival after 1 year). The lack of adequate HLA matching and prolonged cold ischemia times have resulted in an unacceptably high rate of rejection and have prompted the use of segmental bowel transplant from living related donors.[82] To date, the results have been very promising and suggest that a well-matched segmental ileal graft from a living donor can provide complete rehabilitation for patients with short bowel syndrome.[83]

Inflammatory Bowel Disease

Ulcerative colitis and Crohn's disease, chronic inflammatory GI disorders of unknown cause, are collectively termed inflammatory bowel disease (IBD). Adults with Crohn's disease and ulcerative colitis are at high risk for micronutrient deficiency and protein-calorie malnutrition, and children commonly suffer from growth failure. The mechanisms of malnutrition are complex and relate in part to cytokine-induced anorexia as well as sitophobia. IBD patients may develop significant malabsorption from extensive small bowel inflammation or as a result of stricture formation with bacterial overgrowth. Inflammation of the terminal ileum is common in patients with Crohn's disease and can lead to vitamin B_{12} deficiency as well as fat malabsorption. Protein depletion may be compounded by intestinal protein losses from inflamed and ulcerated mucosa.

Medications used in the treatment of IBD often contribute to the development of nutrient deficiencies. Sulfasalazine is a competitive inhibitor of the brush-border folate transporter and conjugase enzyme,[84] metronidazole treatment may leave a metallic taste and reduce appetite, and corticosteroids result in negative calcium balance through effects on both intestinal calcium absorption and urinary calcium loss.[85]

Nutrition support is necessary in many IBD patients to reverse nutrient depletion. Enteral nutrition is preferred over total parenteral nutrition because of cost and a reduced incidence of serious complications. Recent data indicate that enteral nutrition support has the added advantage of reducing a range of inflammatory parameters, often within the first 3 to 7 days after initiation.[86] Nevertheless, although enteral feedings clearly improve nutritional status, data indicate that corticosteroids are more effective as a single therapy than enteral nutrition in the treatment of active Crohn's disease.[87] Furthermore, analysis of elemental versus non-elemental formulas revealed similar remission rates and maintenance of remission in Crohn's disease, suggesting that there is no advantage to the use of more expensive and less palatable defined-formula diets.[88]

For patients who cannot tolerate enteral nutrition support, total parenteral nutrition therapy improves nutritional status for severely malnourished IBD patients. Total parenteral nutrition has the added advantage of reducing complication rates in those requiring surgical treatment.[89] Similar to enteral feeding, total parenteral nutrition has benefit as a form of bowel rest. The response, however, varies depending on whether the underlying disease is Crohn's disease or ulcerative colitis, with a poor long-term response noted in ulcerative colitis patients.[90]

Several small-scale trials of butyrate enemas as primary therapy for left-sided ulcerative colitis have demonstrated remission rates comparable to those seen in patients treated with corticosteroids and mesalamine. Recently, topical butyrate treatment combined with 5-ASA in patients with refractory distal ulcerative colitis showed significant improvement in endoscopic, histologic, and clinical end points, supporting the value of combining two or more active drugs.[91] Similarly, an open controlled trial of the prebiotic germinated barley foodstuff in patients with ulcerative colitis demonstrated increased fecal butyrate levels and decreased fecal concentrations of bifidobacterium and *Eubacterium limosum*, and clinical activity and mucosal inflammation.[92] A growing number of randomized, double-blind, controlled studies have shown superior or equal effects of probiotics compared with placebo or mesalamine in the treatment or maintenance of remission of Crohn's disease, ulcerative colitis, or pouchitis.[93] Finally, a recent randomized, controlled trial examined the combined effect of probiotic and prebiotic treatment on sigmoidoscopy scores, histologic features, and markers of inflammation in patients with active ulcerative colitis. After 1 month of treatment, transcript levels for beta-defensins 2, 3, and 4, which are upregulated in patients with active ulcerative colitis, were significantly reduced, as were TNF-alpha and interleukin-1 levels and colonic inflammation.[94] Overall, the data to date support efficacy in ulcerative colitis more so than in Chrohn's disease, but it is clear that prebiotics and probiotics have emerged as modalities for the monotherapy and combined therapy of IBD.

Future Directions

Several new treatments are under development for GI diseases with nutritional complications. A growing understanding of intestinal neuromuscular function has allowed for the development of new approaches for motility disorders. For example, disorders of gastric motility result from disruption of autonomic innervation and commonly result in nausea, vomiting, abdominal pain, and distention, with associated limitations to dietary intake. The use of high-frequency gastric electrical stimulators appears to have utility in the treatment of diabetic gastroparesis, with improvement in upper GI symptoms, nutritional status, glucose tolerance, and quality of life.[95]

The dramatic growth in bariatric surgical procedures has resulted in a number of reports of vitamin and nutrient deficiencies[96,97]; for example, protein, iron, vitamin B_{12}, folate, calcium, and the fat-soluble vitamins (A, D, E, K). Nutrient deficiencies occur more commonly after malabsorptive procedures such as biliopancreatic diversion, but may also occur with restrictive procedures such as gastric bypass. As many as 25% of bariatric surgery patients develop nutrient deficiencies, in some cases with severe complications such as Wernicke's encephalopathy, blindness secondary to unrecognized vitamin A deficiency, and severe protein malnutrition.[98-100] In addition, long-term follow-up data suggest a significant recidivism rate, with as many as 20% of patients developing significant postoperative weight regain, re-emergence of psychosocial and behavioral problems, and obesity comorbidities.[101,102] An understanding of the individual behavioral and physiologic factors that differentiate those with long-term success from those who develop nutritional complications is remedial at best. Clearly, blanket micronutrient supplementation is appropriate, but whether this is sufficient to prevent micronutrient deficiency in all cases is unclear. Prevention of postoperative weight gain requires routine follow-up and monitoring of body weight and eating behavior. Preliminary data suggest that preoperative eating behavior may predict postoperative response, but much more research is needed.[101] Better systems for maintaining long-term follow-up that incorporate postoperative weight gain prevention and multidisciplinary weight management options are needed.

On another front, work is needed to more clearly define the important role played by the gut microbiota in health and disease. The use of unique nutrient-based pharmacotherapies for patients with alterations in gut structure (e.g., patients with IBD and short bowel syndrome) is emerging as a useful way to modulate gut function. Studies are needed on the utility of probiotics in the prevention of childhood diarrhea, the relative efficacy of different probiotic agents, the synergy between prebiotics and probiotics, optimal dosage, and application to specific patient groups. In addition, studies are needed to clarify concerns regarding the safety and tolerability of prebiotics and probiotics.

References

1. Isolauri E, Salminen S, Ouwehand AC. Microbial-gut interactions in health and disease. Probiotics.

Best Pract Res Clin Gastroenterol. 2004;18: 299–313.
2. Backhead F, Ley RE, Sonnenburg JL, et al. Host-bacterial mutualism in the human intestine. Science. 2005;307:1915–1920.
3. MacDonald TT, Monteleone G. Immunity, inflammation and allergy in the gut. Science. 2005; 307:1920–1925.
4. Zoetendal EG, Akkermans ADL, Akkermans-van Vliet WM, et al. The host genotype affects the bacterial community in the human GI tract. Microbial Ecol Health Dis. 2001;13:129–134.
5. Mai V. Dietary modification of the intestinal microbiota. Nutr Rev. 2004;62:235–242.
6. Moore WE, Moore LH. Intestinal floras of populations that have a high risk of colon cancer. Appl Environ Microbiol. 1995;61:3202–3207.
7. Peltonen R, Nenonen M, Helve T, et al. Faecal microbial flora and disease activity in rheumatoid arthritis during vegan diet. Br J Rheumatol. 1997; 36:64–68.
8. Adolfsson O, Meydani SN, Russell RM. Yogurt and gut function. Am J Clin Nutr. 2004;80: 245–256.
9. Farthing MJG. Bugs and the gut: an unstable marriage. Best Prac Res Clin Gastro. 2004;18:233–239.
10. Neish AS, Gewirtz AT, Zeng H, et al. Prokaryotic regulation of epithelial responses by inhibition of ikappaB-alpha ubiquitination. Science. 2000;289: 1560–1563.
11. Huang JS, Bousvaros A, Lee JW, et al. Efficacy of probiotic use in acute diarrhea in children: a meta-analysis. Dig Dis Sci. 2002;47:2625–2634
12. van Niel CW, Fewudtner C, Garrison MM, et al. *Lactobacillus* therapy for acute infectious diarrhea in children: a meta-analysis. Pediatrics. 2002;109: 678–684.
13. de Roos N, Katan M. Effects of probiotic bacteria on diarrhea, lipid metabolism, and carcinogenesis: a review of papers published between 1988 and 1998. Am J Clin Nutr. 2000;71:405–411.
14. Kalliomaki M, Salminen S, Kero P, et al. Probiotics in the primary prevention of atopic disease: a randomized, placebo-controlled trial. Lancet. 2001; 357:1076–1079.
15. Kalliomaki M, Salminen S, Kero P, et al. Probiotics and prevention of atopic disease—a 4-year follow-up of a randomized placebo-controlled trial. Lancet. 2003;361:1869–1870.
16. Sartor B. Therapeutic manipulation of the enteric microflora in inflammatory bowel diseases: antibiotics, probiotics, and prebiotics. Gastroenterology. 2004;126:1620–1633.
17. Verdu EF, Collins SM. Irritable bowel syndrome. Best Prac Res Clin Gastro. 2004;18:315–321.
18. Saggioro A. Probiotics in the treatment of irritable bowel syndrome. J Clin Gastroenterol. 2004;38: S104–S106.
19. He T, Priebe MG, Harmsen HJM, et al. Colonic fermentation may play a role in lactose intolerance in humans. J Nutr. 2006;136:58–63.
20. de Vrese M, Stegelmann A, Richter B, et al. Probiotics—compensation for lactase insuffiency. Am J Clin Nutr. 2001;73(2 Suppl):421S–429S.
21. Backhed F, Ley RE, Sonnenburg JL, et al. Host-bacterial mutualism in the human intestine. Science. 2005;307:1915–1920.
22. Balsari A, Ceccarelli A, Dubini F, et al. The fecal microbial population in the irritable bowel syndrome. Microbiologica. 1982;5:185–194.
23. King TS, Elia M, Hunter JO. Abnormal colonic fermentation in irritable bowel syndrome. Lancet. 1998;352:1187–1189.
24. Rodriguez LA, Ruigomez A. Increased risk of irritable bowel syndrome after bacterial gastroenteritis: cohort study. Br Med J. 1999;318:565–566.
25. Hebuterne X. Gut changes attributed to ageing: effects on intestinal microflora. Curr Opin Clin Nutr Metab Care. 2003;6:49–54.
26. D'Souza A, Rajkumar C, Cooke J, et al. Probiotics in prevention of antibiotic associated diarrhoea: meta-analysis. Br Med J. 2002;324:1361–1366.
27. Beevers DG, Lip G, Blann AD. Salt intake and *Helicobacter pylori* infection. J Hypertens. 2004;22: 1475–1477.
28. Husbebye E. The pathogenesis of GI bacterial overgrowth. Chemotherapy. 2005;51(suppl 1):1–22.
29. Van Loo JAE. Prebiotics promote good health: the basis, the potential, and the emerging evidence. J Clin Gastroenterol. 2004;38:S70–S75.
30. Manning TS, Gibson GR. Prebiotics. Best Prac Res Clin Gastroenterol. 2004;18:287–298.
31. Nakao M, Ogura Y, Satake S. Usefulness of soluble dietary fiber for the treatment of diarrhea during enteral nutrition in elderly patients. Nutrition. 2002;18:35–39.
32. Van Loo J, Clune Y, Bennett M, et al. The SYN-CAN project: goals, set-up, first results and settings of the human intervention study. Br J Nutr. 2005; 93(Suppl 1):S91–98.
33. Saavedra JM, Tschernia A. Human studies with probiotics and prebiotics: clinical implications. Br J Nutr. 2002;87(suppl 2):S241–S246.
34. Welters CFM, Heineman E, Thunnissen FBJM. Effect of dietary inulin supplementation on inflammation of pouch mucosa in patients with an ileal pouch-anal anastomosis. Dis Colon Rectum. 2002; 45:621–627.
35. Marteau P, Seksik P. Tolerance of probiotics and prebiotics. J Clin Gastroenterol. 2004;38:S67–S69.
36. Ten Bruggencate SJM, Bovee-Oudenhoven IMJ, Lettink-Wissink MLG, et al. Dietary fructooligosaccharides affect intestinal barrier function in healthy men. J Nutr. 2006;136:70–74.
37. Locke GR III, Talley NJ, Gett SL, et al. Prevalence and clinical spectrum of gastroesophageal reflux: a

population-based study in Olmsted county, Minnesota. Gastroenterology. 1997;112:1448–1456.
38. Blot WJ, McLaughlin JK. The changing epidemiology of esophageal cancer. Semin Oncol. 1999; 26(Suppl 15):2–8.
39. Locke GR III, Talley NJ, Gett SL, et al. Risk factors associated with symptoms of gastroesophageal reflux. Am J Med. 1999;106:642–649.
40. Ruhl CE, Everhart JE. Overweight, but not high dietary fat intake, increases risk of gastroesophageal reflux disease hospitalization: the NHANES I Epidemiologic Followup Study. Ann Epidemiol. 1999; 9:424–435.
41. Stene-Larsen G, Weberg R, Larsen F. Relationship of overweight to hiatus hernia and reflux esophagitis. Scand J Gastroenterol. 1988;23:427–432.
42. Wilson LJ, Ma W, Jirschowitz BI. Association of obesity with hiatal hernia and esophagitis. Am J Gastroenterol. 1999;94:2840–2844.
43. Fraser-Moodie CA, Norton B, Gornall C, et al. Weight loss has an independent beneficial effect on symptoms of gastro-oesophageal reflux in patients who are overweight. Scand J Gastroenterol. 1999; 34:337–40
44. Chow WH, Blot WJ, Vaughan TL, et al. Body mass index and risk of adenocarcinomas of the esophagus and gastric cardia. J Natl Cancer Inst. 1998;90:150–155.
45. Ford ES. Body mass index and colon cancer in a national sample of adult U.S. men and women. Am J Epidemiol. 1999;150:390–398.
46. Tessitore L, Vizio B, Jenkins O, et al. Leptin expression in colorectal and breast cancer patients. Int J Mol Med. 2000;5:421–426.
47. Ortega J, Escudero MD, Mora F, et al. Outcome of esophageal function and 24-hour esophageal pH monitoring after vertical banded gastroplasty and Roux-en-Y gastric bypass Obesity Surg. 2004;14: 1086–1094.
48. Iovino P, Angrisani L, Tremolaterra F, et al. Abnormal esophageal acid exposure is common in morbidly obese patients and improves after a successful Lap-band system implantation. Surg Endosc. 2002;16:1631–1635.
49. Dieterich W, Ehnis T, Bauer M, et al. Identification of tissue transglutaminase as the autoantigen of celiac disease. Nat Med. 1997;3:797–801.
50. Molberg O, McAdam SN, Korner R, et al. Tissue transflutaminase selectively modifies gliadin peptides that are recognized by gut-derived T cells in celiac disease. Nat Med. 1998;4:713–717.
51. Johnston SD, Watson RG, McMillan SA, et al. Prevalence of coeliac disease in Northern Ireland. Lancet. 1997;350:1370.
52. Not T, Horvath K, Hill ID, et al. Celiac disease risk in the USA: high prevalence of antiendomysium antibodies in healthy blood donors. Scand J Gastroenterol. 1998;33:494–498.
53. Kemppainen TA, Kosma VM, Janatuinen EK, et al. Nutritional status of newly diagnosed celiac disease patients before and after the institution of a celiac disease diet: association with the grade of mucosal villous atrophy. Am J Clin Nutr. 1998;67:482–487.
54. Vazquez H, Mazure R, Gonzalez D, et al. Risk of fractures in celiac disease patients: a cross-sectional, case-control study. Am J Gastroenterol. 2000;95: 183–189.
55. Bhattacharyya A, Patel MK, Tymms DJ. Coeliac disease in adults: variations on a theme. J R Soc Med. 1999;92:286–289.
56. Nousia-Arvanitakis S, Karagiozoglou-Lamboudes T, Aggouridaki C, et al. Influence of jejunal morphology changes on exocrine pancreatic function in celiac disease. J Pediatr Gastroenterol Nutr. 1999; 29:81–85.
57. Tursi A, Brandimarte G, Giorgetti G. High prevalence of small intestinal bacterial overgrowth in celiac patients with persistence of GI symptoms after gluten withdrawal. Am J Gastroenterol. 2003;98: 839–843.
58. Ghoshal UC, Ghoshal U, Misra A, etal. Partially responsive celiac disease resulting from small intestinal overgrowth and lactose intolerance. BMC Gastroenterol. 2004:4:10.
59. Celiac Sprue Association Website Directory. Available at http://www.csaceliacs.org/index.php. Accessed Jan. 16, 2006. Gluten Disease and Gluten-free Diet Support Page. Available at http://www.celiac.com. Accessed Jan. 16, 2006.
60. Janatuinen EK, Pikkarainen PH, Kemppainen TA, et al. A comparison of diets with and without oats in adults with celiac disease. N Engl J Med 1 995; 333:1033–1077.
61. See J, Murray JA. Gluten-free diet: the medical and nutrition management of celiac disease. Nutr Clin Pract. 2006;21:1–15.
62. Regan PT Malagelada JR, DiMagno EP, et al. Comparative effects of antacids, cimetidine and enteric coating on the therapeutic response to oral enzymes in severe pancreatic insufficiency. N Engl J Med. 1977;297:854–858.
63. Halgreen H, Pedersen NT, Wroning H. Symptomatic effect of pancreatic enzyme therapy in patients with chronic pancreatitis. Scand J Gastroenterol. 1986;21:104–108.
64. Kruszewska D, Ljungh A, Hunes SO, et al. Effect of the antibacterial activity of pig pancreatic juice on human multiresistant bacteria. Pancreas. 2004; 28:191–199.
65. Stanga Z, Giger U, Marx A, et al. Effect of jejunal long-term feeding in chronic pancreatitis. JPEN. 2005; 29:12–20.
66. Messing B, Crenn P, Beau P, et al. Long-term sur-

vival and parenteral nutrition dependence in adult patients with the short bowel syndrome. Gastroenterology. 1999;117:1043–1050.
67. Scolapio JS, Fleming CR. Short bowel syndrome. Gastroenterol Clin North Am. 1998;27:467–479.
68. Goulet O. Short bowel syndrome in pediatric patients. Nutrition. 1998:14:784–787.
69. O'Keefe SJ, Buchman AL, Fishbein TM, et al. Short bowel syndrome and intestinal failure: consensus definitions and overview. Clin Gastroenterol Hepatol. 2006;4:6–10.
70. Buchman AL. Short-bowel syndrome. Clin Gastroenterol Hepatol. 2005;3:1066–1070.
71. Wen J, Phillips SF, Sarr MG, et al. PYY and GLP-1 contribute to feedback inhibition from the canine ileum and colon. Am J Physiol, 1995;269:G945–952.
72. Nightingale JM, Lennard-Jones JE, Walker ER, et al. Oral salt supplements to compensate for jejunostomy losses: comparison of sodium chloride capsules, glucose electrolyte solution, and glucose polymer electrolyte solution. Gut. 1992;33:759–761.
73. Nordgaard I, Hansen BS, Mortensen PB. Importance of colonic support for energy absorption as small-bowel failure proceeds. Am J Clin Nutr. 1996;64:222–231.
74. Justino SR, Dias MCG, Maculevicius J, et al. Fasting breath hydrogen concentration in short bowel syndrome patients with colon incontinuity before and after antibiotic therapy. Nutrition. 2004;20: 187–191.
75. Dibaise JK, Young RJ, Vanderhood JA. Enteric microbial flora, bacterial overgrowth, and short-bowel syndrome. Clin Gastroenterol Hepatol. 2006;4: 11–20.
76. Byrne TA, Morrissey TB, Nattakom TV, et al. Growth hormone, glutamine, and a modified diet enhance nutrient absorption in patients with severe short bowel syndrome. JPEN. 1995;19:296–302.
77. Scolapio JS, Camilleri M, Fleming CR, et al. Effect of growth hormone, glutamine, and diet on adaptation in short-bowel syndrome: a randomized, controlled study. Gastroenterology. 1997;113:1074–1081.
78. Ellegard L, Bosaeus I, Nordgren S, et al. Low-dose recombinant human growth hormone increases body weight and lean body mass in patients with short bowel syndrome. Ann Surg. 1997;225:88–96.
79. Jeppesen PB, Sanguinetti EL, Buchman A, et al. Teduglutide (ALX-0600), a dipeptidyl peptidase IV resistant glucagon-like peptide 2 analogue, improves intestinal function in short bowel syndrome patients. Gut. 2005;54:1224–1231.
80. Thompson JS, Quigley EM, Adrian TE. Effect of intestinal tapering and lengthening on intestinal structure and function. Am J Surg. 1995;169: 111–119.
81. Abu-Elmagd K, Reyes J, Todo S, et al. Clinical intestinal transplantation: new perspectives and immunologic considerations. J Am Coll Surg. 1998; 186:512–525.
82. Benedetti E, Baum C, Raofi V, et al. Living related small bowel transplantation: progressive functional adaptation of the graft. Transplant Proc. 2000;32: 1209.
83. Fryer JP. Intestinal transplantation: an update. Curr Opin Gastroenterol. 2005;21:162–168.
84. Darcy-Vrillon B, Selhub J, Rosenberg IH. Analysis of sequential events in intestinal aborption of folypolyglutamate. Am J Physiol. 1988;255:C361–366.
85. Ziegler R, Kasperk, C. Glucocorticoid-induced osteoporosis: prevention and treatment. Steroids. 1998;63:344–348.
86. Bannerjee K, Camacho-Hubner C, Babinska K et al. Anti-inflammatory and growth-stimulating effects precede nutritional restitution during enteral feeding in Crohn disease. J Pediatr Gastroenterol Nutr. 2004;38:270–275.
87. Fernandez-Banares F, Cabre E, Esteve-Comas M, et al. How effective is enteral nutrition in inducing clinical remission in active Crohn's disease? A meta-analysis of the randomized clinical trials. JPEN. 1995;19:356–364.
88. Beattie RM, Bentsen BS, MacDonald TT. Childhood Crohn's disease and the efficacy of enteral diets. Nutrition. 1998;14:345–350.
89. Gouma DJ, von Meyenfeldt MF, Fourlart M, et al. Preoperative total parenteral nutrition in severe Crohn's disease surgery. Surgery. 1988;103:648–662.
90. Han PD, Burke A, Baldassano RN, et al. Nutrition and inflammatory bowel disease. Gastroenterol Clin North Am. 1999;28:423–443.
91. Vernia P, Annese V, Bresci G, et al. Topical butyrate improves efficacy of 5-ASA in refractory distal ulcerative colitis: results of a multicentre trial. Eur J Clin Invest. 2003;33:244–248.
92. Kanauchi O, Suga T, Tochihara M, et al. Treatment of ulcerative colitis by feeding with germinated barley foodstuff: first report of a multicenter open control trial. J Gastroenterol. 2002;37(suppl 14):67–72.
93. Dolan I, Rachmilewitz D. Probiotics in inflammatory bowel disease: possible mechanisms of action. Curr Opin Gastroenterol. 2005;21:426–430.
94. Bousvaros A, Guandalini S, Baldassano RN, et al. A randomized, double-blind trial of lactobacillus GG versus placebo in addition to standard maintenance therapy for children with Crohn's disease. Inflamm Bowel Dis. 2005;11:833–839.
95. Lin Z, Forster J, Sarosiek I, et al. Treatment of diabetic gastroparesis by high-frequency gastric electrical stimulation. Diabetes Care. 2004;27: 1071–1076.

96. Encinosa WE, Bernard DM, Steiner CA, et al. Use and costs of bariatric surgery and prescription weight-loss medications. Health Affairs. 2005;24: 1039–1046.
97. Bloomberg RD, Fleishman A, Nalle JE, et al. Nutritional deficiencies following bariatric surgery: what have we learned? Obes Surg. 2005;15:145–154.
98. Escalona A, Perez G, Leon F, et al. Wernicke's encephalopathy after Roux-en-Y gastric bypass. Obes Surg. 2004;14:1135–1137.
99. Lee WB, Hamilton SM, Harris JP, et al. Ocular complications of hypovitaminosis A after bariatric surgery. Ophthalmology. 2005;112:1031–1034.
100. Faintuch J, Matsuda M, Cruz ME, et al. Severe protein-calorie malnutrition alter bariatric surgery. Obes Surg. 2004;14:175–181.
101. Sarwer DB, Wadden TA, Fabricatore AN. Psychosocial and behavioral aspects of bariatric surgery. Obes Res. 2005;13:639–648.
102. Sjostrom L, Lindroos A, Peltonen M, et al. Lifestyle, diabetes and cardiovascular risk factors 10 years after bariatric surgery. N Engl J Med. 2004; 351:2683–2693.

54 Kidney Disease

Tahsin Masud and William E. Mitch

Background and Definitions

Each kidney is made up of about 1 million tiny functional units called nephrons. Each nephron consists of the glomerulus, which is composed of a tight knot of fine blood vessels from which water and waste products filter into a tubule (Figure 1). The tubule selectively reabsorbs water, electrolytes, and different metabolic products to maintain homeostasis. Important synthetic and degradative functions are also performed by glomerular and tubular epithelial cells (Table 1).

Each nephron appears to act independently. Consequently, a change in the sum of their filtering capabilities (i.e., the glomerular filtration rate, or GFR) reflects a change in the number of functioning nephron units. Thus, the degree of damage or the loss of nephrons is assessed by a fall in GFR and/or a rise in waste products present in plasma. The two waste products used most frequently to estimate the severity of chronic kidney disease (CKD) are urea and creatinine. If the loss of renal function is rapid, but potentially reversible, the condition is called acute renal failure, but if the function is lost gradually and irreversibly, the process is CKD. Nephrotic syndrome is a type of renal disease characterized by excessive urinary loss of albumin and other plasma proteins plus hypoalbuminemia (low plasma albumin levels), hyperlipidemia (elevated plasma lipids levels), and edema formation (salt and water retention leading to swelling of limbs and, in severe cases, the whole body). When kidney function deteriorates to a level that metabolic homeostasis can no longer be maintained, a patient is defined as having approached end-stage renal disease (ESRD). At this stage, renal replacement therapy is provided by dialysis or renal transplantation. Basically, two types of dialysis exist: 1) hemodialysis, a process that removes waste products by circulation of the patient's blood through an artificial filter, and 2) peritoneal dialysis, in which waste products diffuse into dialysis fluid placed in the peritoneal cavity and then removed and discarded.

The topics to be discussed in this chapter are the effects of protein-calorie malnutrition (PCM) on kidney function; the effects of renal insufficiency on nutrient metabolism; mechanisms causing loss of protein stores in renal disease; the assessment of nutritional status in patients with CKD; the effects of low protein diets on the progression of renal disease; and the requirements for protein, calories, fat, and other nutrients in patients with CKD,

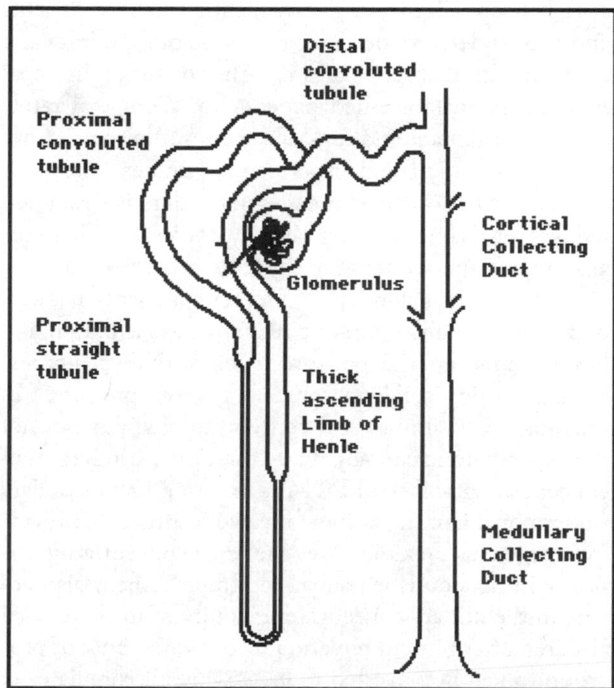

Figure 1. A diagram of a nephron and its various components.

Table 1. Principal Functions of the Kidney

1. Excretion of metabolic waste products (urea, uric acid, creatinine, peptides, etc.) derived from metabolism of protein-rich foods
2. Elimination and detoxification of drugs and toxins
3. Maintenance of the volume and ionic composition of body fluids
4. Regulation of systemic blood pressure
5. Production of erythropoietin
6. Control of mineral metabolism through synthesis of vitamins (1,25-dihydroxycholecalciferol and 24,25-dihydroxycholecalciferol)
7. Degradation and catabolism of hormones (insulin, glucagon, parathyroid hormone) and low-molecular-weight peptides (β_2-macroglobulin and light chains)
8. Regulation of metabolic processes (gluconeogenesis, lipid metabolism)

Adapted with permission from Klahr S. Effects of renal insufficiency on nutrient metabolism and endocrine function. In: Mitch WE, Klahr S, eds. *Handbook of Nutrition and the Kidney.* Boston: Lippincott, Williams & Wilkins; 1998; 25–44.

nephrotic syndrome, or patients treated by either peritoneal dialysis or hemodialysis.

Effects of Malnutrition on Renal Function

Malnutrition, as detected by weight for age, is highly prevalent in children in underdeveloped countries.[1] In developed countries, PCM is found in 20% to 50% of acutely hospitalized and elderly institutionalized patients and is considered to be the major cause of morbidity and mortality in that population.[2] Abnormalities in renal function in malnourished patients are silent and rarely cause clinical manifestations of renal insufficiency. However, both clinical and experimental studies have confirmed that PCM causes changes in renal hemodynamics, reduces renal concentrating capacity, increases sodium reabsorption, and reduces the capacity to excrete acid.[3]

Reduced renal blood flow in severe malnutrition is secondary to a combination of a reduced cardiac output and low systemic arterial pressure along with hypoalbuminemia, causing a fall in capillary oncotic pressure.[4] In humans, PCM limits renal concentrating ability but not the capacity to maximally dilute the urine. Limitation of concentrating ability in PCM is due to a low medullary (inner portion of the kidney) urea concentration; providing exogenous urea improves the renal concentrating capacity in malnourished subjects.[5] Improvement also occurs in the urinary concentrating ability of malnourished children after protein repletion, because the bulk of protein nitrogen is converted to urea, which accumulates in the kidney medulla to improve concentrating ability.[6] Patients with PCM usually maintain normal blood pH and serum bicarbonate concentrations unless given an acid load that induces a greater degree of metabolic acidosis than in normal individuals.[7] An inability to maximally acidify urine also occurs in malnourished children who were hypokalemic (low serum potassium), a condition that usually increases acid excretion. The decreased capacity to excrete acid may result from the combined contributions of a reduced proximal tubule Na^+/H^+ exchange, reduced ammonia production, and decreased titratable acid excretion (measured by the amount of sodium hydroxide that must be added to titrate the urine pH back to the same pH as that in plasma, approximately 7.40 in normal subjects). Phosphates and sulfates represent the major fraction of titratable anions in the urine.

Renal Insufficiency and Changes in Nutrient Metabolism

Carbohydrate Metabolism

The abnormal glucose metabolism of patients with renal insufficiency is characterized by an abnormal glucose tolerance test, but fasting blood sugar is generally normal. A delayed fall in blood glucose in response to insulin and elevated plasma insulin and glucagon levels is also present. Although the majority of nondiabetic uremic patients are insulin resistant, and about half of them have glucose intolerance, they rarely develop clinical diabetes. Inadequate insulin secretion, increased hepatic gluconeogenesis, and reduced insulin clearance by renal and extrarenal mechanisms all play a role in abnormal glucose tolerance in CKD.[8] However, the most prominent metabolic disturbance in uremic patients is insulin resistance caused by a post-receptor defect. The cellular basis for insulin resistance in CKD remains unclear. Possible causes include a circulating factor, an increase in growth hormone because of impaired removal of peptide hormones by the damaged kidney, and metabolic acidosis. A deficiency of 1,25-dihydroxycalciferol, the active metabolite of vitamin D, also known as calcitriol, may contribute to insulin resistance because intravenous administration of calcitriol during dialysis significantly improves insulin resistance.[9] Impaired release of insulin in response to hyperglycemia (the sign of reduced sensitivity of pancreatic β cells) can be related to the high level of parathyroid hormone (PTH). Excess PTH stimulates movement of calcium into the β cells, thereby impairing insulin secretion. In contrast, the insulin requirement of a diabetic patient often decreases as renal failure develops due to decreased degradation of insulin by the diseased kidney. This sequence of events leads to hypoglycemic episodes, and the insulin dose must be closely monitored as CKD progresses toward ESRD.

Lipid Metabolism

In patients diagnosed with nephrotic syndrome, lipid abnormalities are characterized by high levels of serum total cholesterol and triglycerides, particularly the low-density lipoprotein, very-low-density lipoprotein, and intermediate-density lipoprotein fractions.[10] A lower level of high-density lipoprotein cholesterol is also present. This pattern of lipid abnormalities contributes to accelerated atherosclerosis. In non-nephrotic CKD patients, or in patients treated with hemodialysis, the most common abnormalities are an increase in plasma triglyceride levels that is linked to accumulation of triglyceride-enriched apolipoprotein-B particles and a decrease in plasma concentration of high-density lipoprotein; plasma cholesterol levels are modestly high or within the normal range. Chronic peritoneal dialysis patients also have increased total cholesterol and low-density lipoprotein-cholesterol levels.[11] The primary cause of hypertriglyceridemia is reduced removal of triacylglycerol-rich lipoproteins due to suppression of both lipoprotein lipase and hepatic triglyceride lipase activities. Insulin resistance and hyperparathyroidism have been implicated as agents causing these changes, because both insulin and PTH can directly or indirectly regulate the synthesis of lipoprotein lipase.[12] Inflammation, genetics, and dialysis-related factors such as heparin, dialysis membranes, and dialysate composition contribute to the pathogenesis of lipid abnormalities in chronic peritoneal dialysis patients.

Protein and Amino Acid Metabolism

Metabolism of protein and amino acids is distinctly abnormal in patients with renal insufficiency, and contributes to uremia by causing an excessive accumulation of nitrogenous waste products generated during protein metabolism. In patients with advanced CKD, serum albumin and serum transferrin may be decreased but not simply as a reflection of PCM (see following discussion of assessment of nutritional status in renal failure).

Abnormal plasma amino acid concentrations are generally present in patients with CKD. These include a decrease in ratio of essential to nonessential amino acids, a pattern that mimics subjects with PCM. However, other abnormalities in the plasma amino acids pattern present in patients with CKD cannot be explained on the basis of malnutrition, because the same pattern occurs when protein intake is sufficient. This suggests that abnormal plasma amino acid levels may be the result of defects in amino acid metabolism brought about by the development of renal insufficiency. For example, metabolic acidosis reduces the plasma levels of the branched-chain amino acids valine, leucine, and isoleucine (and their respective ketoacids); valine is reduced to the greatest extent. The mechanism for this finding is that metabolic acidosis activates branched-chain ketoacid dehydrogenase, resulting in accelerated, irreversible oxidation of branched-chain amino acids.[13] Decreased plasma concentrations of threonine, lysine, serine, as well as tyrosine are also present.[14] Tyrosine levels are low because uremia limits the activity of the enzyme phenylalanine hydrolase, which converts phenylalanine to tyrosine. Consequently, the plasma levels of phenylalanine are usually normal. Total tryptophan is decreased; however, the level of free tryptophan is normal due to reduced threonine binding by plasma proteins. Certain amino acids are increased in the plasma of patients with CKD, including homocysteine, methionine, glycine, citrulline, cystine, aspartate, and both 1- and 3-methylhistidines.[15] Clinical studies of the general population and CKD patients have demonstrated a significant correlation between cardiovascular and peripheral vascular morbidity and mortality and the level of circulating homocysteine.[16]

Phosphate and Calcium

The regulation of calcium and phosphate homeostasis depends on two major regulatory hormone systems, PTH and vitamin D. As renal function is lost (i.e., as the GFR decreases), there is a reduction in the amount of filtered phosphate and its excretion. The result is a mild increase in plasma phosphate concentration, which leads to stimulation of parathyroid glands (secondary hyperparathyroidism). However, when the GFR decreases below about 30 mL/min, even the inhibition of tubular phosphate reabsorption is insufficient to prevent the development of hyperphosphatemia. The increase in serum phosphate reduces ionized calcium, which stimulates secretion of PTH. This general scheme, known as the "trade-off hypothesis," explains how secondary hyperthyroidism develops.[17] Other mechanisms that increase PTH secretion in CKD patients include vitamin D deficiency and decreased renal production of the active vitamin D sterol (calcitriol).[18] Serum levels of 25-dihydroxyvitamin D (not 1,25-dihydroxyvitamin D) are the measure of body stores of vitamin D. The prevention and treatment of vitamin D insufficiency (defined as serum 25-hydroxyvitamin D level <30 ng/mL) in moderate to advanced CKD patients reduce the frequency and severity of secondary hyperparathyroidism.[19] Calcitriol inhibits PTH production by inhibiting synthesis of pre- and pro-PTH and, indirectly, by raising serum calcium levels following an increase in intestinal calcium absorption. The key event is a decrease in serum ionized calcium concentration that is attributable to three factors: 1) an increase in serum phosphate that binds ionized calcium and decreases its level; 2) suppression of calcitriol production, which decreases absorption of calcium from the gastrointestinal tract; and 3) skeletal resistance to the action of PTH, resulting in decreased release of calcium from bone despite abnormally high levels of PTH. Nutritional therapy is critical, because these abnormalities can be largely, if not entirely, eliminated by dietary phosphorus restriction. Because high-protein foods are rich in phosphates, achieving this goal requires compliance with a low-protein diet and avoiding foods that are especially rich in phosphates (e.g., milk products).

Magnesium

Magnesium, like calcium, is partially bound to proteins and anions in plasma. Approximately 70% of plasma magnesium is filtered by kidneys, but only 3% to 5% is excreted because most of it is reabsorbed by the tubules. As the GFR decreases, magnesium reabsorption by the tubule is inhibited, preventing a significant increase in plasma magnesium. Clinically important hypermagnesemia (elevated serum magnesium level) is rarely seen in CKD, unless certain preparations of antacids, enemas, or laxatives with a high magnesium content are consumed.

Vitamins

Vitamin deficiencies can be present in all stages of renal failure and may be related to a poor dietary intake, interference with vitamin absorption by other drugs, altered metabolism of vitamins, and, in dialysis patients, a loss of vitamins during dialysis. Reduced serum, erythrocyte, and leukocyte concentrations of several water-soluble vitamins have been reported in uremic patients, but clinical syndromes that are caused by a deficiency of water-soluble vitamins are rare because elimination of vitamins by the diseased kidney is also reduced. In contrast to water-soluble vitamins, the concentrations of lipid-soluble vitamins can be elevated. For example, the levels of retinol (vitamin A) and retinol-binding proteins are increased in patients with CKD.

No persuasive evidence documents that supplements of cobalamin, biotin, niacin, pantothenic acid, or vitamin A and E are required to correct deficiencies in CKD patients. But in some reports, a combination of vitamin B_6, folic acid, and vitamin B_{12} has produced partial reduction in homocysteine levels in patients with advanced CKD.[20] Whether vitamin supplements should be prescribed for patients with renal disease depends on the degree of renal insufficiency, the mode of replacement therapy, the dietary prescription, concurrent medication, and the patient's nutritional status. Supplements of thiamine, riboflavin, pyridoxine, and vitamin C are required in patients with advanced CKD or patients on dialysis.[20] Nephrologists routinely use a commercially available renal formulation of vitamins providing an appropriate amount of vitamins B_1, B_2, B_6, B_{12}, folic acid, niacin, pantothenic acid, biotin, and vitamin C. For patients with hyperhomocysteinemia, folic acid supplementation of at least 2.5 mg/d is recommended.

Loss of Protein Store in Kidney Disease

Distinguishing the loss of protein store abnormalities present in CKD patients from that in patients with PCM is important because PCM indicates that the diet is inadequate in protein and that correction of the dietary deficiency will correct the abnormality. In contrast, loss of kidney function results in several conditions that cause loss of protein stores; for example, metabolic acidosis, decreased insulin responses and inflammation. A change in the diet may not correct these causes of protein wasting. The diagnosis of "malnutrition" in patients with CKD is confounded by the lack of uniform criteria for its diagnosis and, as discussed above, there are serious difficulties in separating abnormal nutritional parameters due to a poor diet from those caused by complications of uremia.[21] In cross-sectional and longitudinal surveys, the reported prevalence of lost protein stores in dialysis patients varies from 25% to 75%.[22,23] Although some ESRD patients may have true PCM, there are several other reasons for the loss of protein mass being mistakenly assigned to malnutrition (Figure 2). Another problem is the lack of precision in determining actual protein and calorie intake.

Kidney failure disturbs one or more steps in the complex process of protein synthesis and degradation. In Western societies, a typical protein intake by healthy individuals is 1 to 2 g/kg body wt/d, well above the World Health Organization's recommended daily protein allowance of 0.8 g/kg body wt/d (the minimum daily requirement is 0.6 g/kg body wt/d). In response to variations in the amount of protein eaten, healthy subjects will activate the following adaptive mechanisms to promote neutral nitrogen balance: As dietary protein is reduced, amino acid oxidation is suppressed, allowing more efficient use of dietary, essential amino acids. Then, as dietary protein intake approaches 0.6 g/kg body wt/d, another adaptive response is activated; there is suppression of protein degradation along with increasing protein synthesis, but the magnitude of the latter response is less than the limitation of protein degradation.[24] Patients with uncomplicated CKD will activate the same metabolic responses to dietary protein restriction, even if the patient is eating only approximately 0.3 g protein/kg body wt/d plus a supplement with nitrogen-free analogs of essential amino acids (ketoacids).[25] However, if the diet contains less than 0.6 g protein/kg body wt/d (without a supplement of essential amino acids), such as the Giordano-Giovannetti diet, nitrogen balance generally becomes negative and causes a loss of lean body mass.[26] Similar responses are activated in CKD patients with nephrotic syndrome. In these patients, however, the degree of suppression of amino acid oxidation is proportional to the net protein intake (the amount of dietary protein minus the urinary loss of protein).[27] The mechanism explaining this fascinating obser-

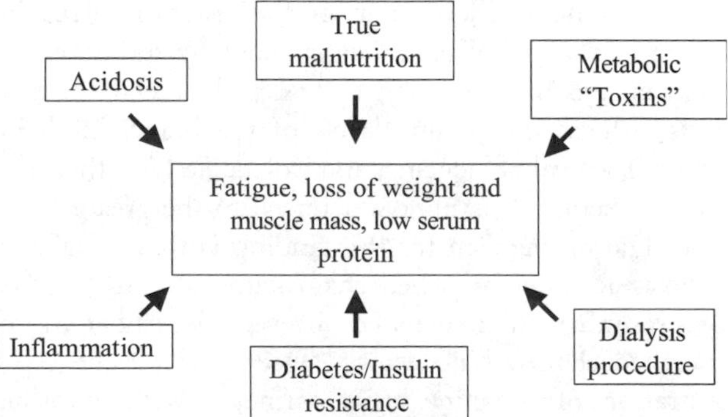

Figure 2. Factors leading to the fatigue, loss of lean body mass, and low serum proteins associated with loss of kidney function. (Used with permission from Mitch 2002.[21])

vation is unknown. These critical adaptive responses that act to maintain protein balance can be impaired by factors that are commonly present in CKD patients, such as metabolic acidosis, inflammation, infection, sepsis, and the prescription of certain medications. Metabolic acidosis is common in CKD and will stimulate the irreversible destruction of essential branched-chain amino acids. Acidosis also accelerates the degradation of protein, especially muscle protein.[28] Evidence also suggests that acidosis contributes to the low level of serum albumin in dialysis patients.[29] Therefore, acidosis in CKD could contribute substantially to the abnormalities that are incorrectly assigned to a diagnosis of malnutrition.

Assessment of Nutritional Status in Renal Diseases

As already stated, loss of lean body mass is common in patients with renal failure. Therefore, it is important to repeatedly assess nutritional status to recognize substrate deficiencies early. No single assessment method has been identified to evaluate all of the variables that affect nutritional status. Consequently, a complete nutritional evaluation that includes all of the categories in Table 2 should be conducted by a physician and/or a renal dietitian every 3 months. A nutritional evaluation will be needed more frequently in patients at higher risk for malnutrition, for example, the elderly and those with preexisting illnesses or other chronic diseases.

Table 2. Categories of Nutritional Assessment in Renal Patient

Clinical
Medical and psychosocial history
Physical examination
Dietary History
Diet history
Appetite assessment
Food habits and patterns
Fluid intake
Dietary Nutrient Intake
Food intake records and dietary recall
Normalized protein equivalent of total nitrogen appearance
Biochemical Measurements
Serum albumin, serum prealbumin,* serum transferrin*
Serum bicarbonate, serum potassium, serum glucose
Serum creatinine, urea nitrogen, cholesterol, calcium, and phosphorus
Kinetic clearance or urea reduction ratio
Body Composition Measurements
Anthropometric measurements
Creatinine kinetics*
Subjective Global Assessment

*Not routinely recommended.

The most common methods for estimating dietary intake in patients with renal disease are dietary recalls, dietary diaries, and determination of the protein equivalent of nitrogen appearance. The dietary recall (dietary intake of previous 24 hours) is a simple, rapid method of obtaining a crude assessment of dietary intake.[30] Dietary diaries are written reports of foods consumed during a specified length of time (3–7 days). Unfortunately, dietary diaries do not provide a reliable estimate of an individual's intake, but do provide the pattern of foods ingested and some insights into energy intake.[31] The validity and reliability of dietary interviews and diaries depend on the patient's ability to provide accurate data and the ability of the dietitian to conduct detailed and probing interviews. A dietary history includes portions and patterns of nutrient intake, current energy level, appetite, physical activity, medications and use of dietary and herbal supplements, alcohol, and illicit drugs. A concomitant medical history and physical examination should identify the type of renal disease, comorbid conditions, and current socioeconomic circumstances that might interfere with a necessary diet.

Protein Equivalent of Total Nitrogen Appearance

This method for estimating protein intake is based on the concept that ingested protein plus the products arising from endogenous protein are metabolized to several nitrogenous products (e.g., urea, amino acids, peptides, urate, or creatinine). If nitrogen balance is neutral (neither catabolism nor anabolism), the nitrogenous products that are removed from the body through urine, stool, and skin, plus any change in the body urea nitrogen pool, are equal to the dietary nitrogen intake.[32] Based on this principle, protein intake in CKD patients can be estimated from the urea appearance rate using a simple method described by Maroni et al.[32] To understand this technique (and its limitations), one must recognize that waste nitrogen arising from degraded protein is excreted as urea and non-urea nitrogen. The urea nitrogen appearance rate (i.e., urea excretion plus accumulation) parallels protein intake, but non-urea nitrogen excretion (i.e., the nitrogen in feces and urinary creatinine, uric acid, ammonia, peptides, etc.) does not vary substantially with dietary protein and averages 0.031 g of nitrogen/kg daily. In the steady state (when blood urea nitrogen and weight are constant), the urea nitrogen appearance equals urinary urea nitrogen excretion. Consequently, nitrogen intake equals urinary urea nitrogen plus 0.031 g nitrogen/kg (Table 3). To convert nitrogen grams into a protein equivalent, multiply it by 6.25, assuming all proteins consist of 16% nitrogen.

In ESRD patients, depending on the residual urine production, the urea nitrogen accumulates in the body and can be removed only through diffusion into the dialysate. Therefore, the calculation of protein nitrogen ap-

Table 3. Estimating Protein Intake from Urea Nitrogen Appearance Rate

Formulas

1. $B_N = I_N - U -$ NUN, where U = urea nitrogen appearance rate (urea nitrogen excretion plus accumulation) and NUN = 0.031 g N/kg body wt
2. If $B_N = 0$, then $I_N = U + 0.031$ g N/kg body wt
3. When BUN is not changing, then U = UUN, so I_N = UUN + 0.031 g N/kg body weight

Example

A 40-year-old woman weighing 60 kg is seen 1 month after instruction in a diet providing 0.6 protein/kg body wt/d (i.e., 60 kg × 0.6 protein/kg body wt = 36 g protein). The 24-hour urine is collected and UUN = 4.1 g/d; NUN = 0.031 g N × 60 kg = 1.86 g N/d

If $B_N = 0$, then I_N = UUN + NUN
= 4.1 + 1.86 = 5.96 g N
= 5.96 g N × 6.25 g protein/g N
= 37.3 g protein/d, so the patient is compliant with the diet.

N, nitrogen; B_N, nitrogen balance (g N/d); I_N, nitrogen intake (g N/d); BUN, blood urea nitrogen; U, urea nitrogen appearance (g N/d); UUN, urinary urea nitrogen (24-hour) (g N/d); NUN, non-urea nitrogen (g N/d).

pearance in an hemodialysis patient requires complex equations, taking into account the pre- and post-dialysis blood urea nitrogen, properties of the dialyzer, duration of dialysis treatment, and amount of ultrafiltration performed.[34] The calculation of protein intake for a chronic peritoneal dialysis patient is simpler; it requires only the urea nitrogen excretion in the urine and that present in the dialysate. Numerous equations proposed for calculating dietary protein have been developed for chronic ambulatory peritoneal dialysis patients, but they also apply to patients treated by automated peritoneal dialysis.[30] Protein nitrogen appearance is usually normalized to some function of body weight (e.g., edema-free body weight or body weight derived from the urea distribution space [V_{urea}/0.58]).[30]

Important limitations occur in interpreting estimates of dietary protein intake in ESRD patients from a urea kinetic analysis. First, in catabolic states (acidosis, infection, etc.), a breakdown of endogenous protein will increase the urea appearance, suggesting that dietary protein exceeds the prescribed protein intake. Conversely, when a patient becomes anabolic, the protein nitrogen appearance will underestimate actual protein intake. Second, day-to-day variations in protein intake are reflected rapidly by the protein nitrogen appearance. Consequently, a single measurement may not represent the average protein intake over a month. Third, the protein nitrogen appearance method does not accurately estimate the extremes in protein intake. Increased nitrogen losses occur through unmeasured pathways of excretion when the protein intake is high, and excessive endogenous protein catabolism occurs when protein intake is low. Finally, normalizing protein nitrogen appearance to body weight can be misleading in obese, malnourished, or edematous patients. Therefore, individuals who are less than 90% or greater than 115% of the standard body weight should have their values adjusted to reflect edema-free body weight, as recommended by the Kidney Disease Outcome Quality Initiative guidelines.[30]

Biochemical Values and Nutritional Assessment

Serum albumin, prealbumin, transferrin, and retinol-binding protein are the biochemical markers that are often used to assess visceral protein stores, to monitor the adequacy of responses to a nutritional intervention, and to identify which patients are at risk for developing complications or responding poorly to medical/surgical treatment. Hypoalbuminemia is a major risk factor for morbidity and mortality in both hemodialyis and chronic peritoneal dialysis patients.[35,36] The serum albumin concentration, however, is influenced by age, fluid overload, capillary leakage, evidence of inflammation, and dietary protein stores.[37] Regarding its clinical relevance, there is a strong association among presence of atherosclerosis, a low serum albumin and a high C-reactive protein level in predialysis patients.[38] In dialysis patients, albumin generation and serum albumin levels are negatively correlated with markers of inflammation, including C-reactive protein, fibrinogen, and interleukin-6.[39] These findings suggest that inflammation, mediated by proinflammatory cytokines, results in decreased serum albumin levels, loss of lean body mass, and the development of cardiovascular disease in kidney disease patients. The decline in protein stores, in this case, is linked to increased protein breakdown initiated by responses to inflammation rather than to an abnormal diet (as would be the case in malnutrition). The reason for emphasizing this distinction is the persuasive evidence indicating that serum albumin increases when dietary protein is restricted in patients with renal insufficiency.[40] The complexity of these responses indicate that the serum albumin concentration may not accurately reflect total albumin mass and should not be used as the sole indicator of protein stores. Prealbumin is a carrier protein for retinol-binding protein, with a short half-life (2–3 days vs. 20 days for serum albumin), theoretically making it more sensitive to acute changes in protein status. However, prealbumin, like albumin, decreases when there is inflammation. The serum prealbumin level, like serum albumin, is a powerful predictor of survival in dialysis patients and correlates directly with markers of visceral (albumin and cholesterol), somatic protein stores (creatinine), and recent protein intake.[41] But, as noted, serum prealbumin is affected by many of the same factors as serum albumin, and there is insufficient evidence to recommend that prealbumin should be used as an indicator of nutritional status that is more sensitive or accurate than changes in serum albumin.

Serum transferrin also has a short half-life (8 days) compared with serum albumin's half-life (20 days); however, the plasma transferrin concentration is frequently reduced in renal failure, independent of malnutrition.[41] Serum transferrin increases with iron deficiency, pregnancy, and in the early phases of acute hepatitis; it decreases with certain chronic infections, liver disease, cancer, or iron loading. Finally, its concentration, like that of albumin, varies with hydration. In summary, no single serum protein measurement is ideal for detecting early malnutrition; however, repeatedly low values generally indicate some degree of protein depletion but do not provide insight into the mechanism causing the low value.

Assessment of Body Composition

Methods to assess adipose stores and lean body mass range from simple techniques such as anthropometric and creatinine kinetics to more complex measurements such as bioelectrical impedance, dual-energy x-ray absorptiometry, neutron activation, magnetic resonance imaging, and computed tomography.

Anthropometry consists of a series of noninvasive, inexpensive, and easy-to-perform indices, including body weight, skeletal frame size, BMI, body fat, and fat-free mass.[30] The reliability of anthropometric measurements depends heavily on the skill of the observer, the sites examined (e.g., the circumference of the dominant or nondominant arm to assess muscle mass), and the degree of hydration. In hemodialysis patients, it is recommended that measurements be made after a treatment using the arm that does not bear the dialysis access. Loss of fat from subcutaneous tissues occurs proportionately, so repeated measures from a selected group of sites in an individual patient will provide reasonably reliable information on trends in gain or loss of adipose stores. Only with careful, repeated evaluations will the investigator be confident that there has been a decline in lean body mass or fat mass.

The creatinine index is used to assess creatinine production and therefore provides some estimate of skeletal muscle protein intake and muscle mass or fat-free body mass in an ESRD patient.[30] This method has several limitations. First, the rate of creatinine appearance is affected by dietary meat as well as residual renal function. Second, mathematical coupling is involved between weekly creatinine clearance and lean body mass in chronic peritoneal dialysis patients because both are calculated from the same 24-hour urine and dialysate collection. Third, the creatinine-based calculation of lean body mass in chronic peritoneal dialysis patients is highly variable compared with lean body mass that is measured from total body potassium.

Management of Nutritional Issues in CKD and ESRD

The goals of dietary therapy for CKD patients are: 1) to diminish the accumulation of nitrogenous wastes and limit the metabolic disturbances caused by uremia; 2) prevent loss of protein stores; and 3) to slow the progression of renal failure. It has been known for more than 150 years that protein-restricted diets improve uremic symptoms as they reduce the levels of uremic toxins, most of which result from the metabolism of protein.[42] A low-protein diet also ameliorates specific complications of CKD, including metabolic acidosis, renal osteodystrophy, hyperkalemia, and hypertension, because such a diet is invariably restricted in the quantities of sulfates, phosphates, potassium, and sodium eaten each day. These considerations explain why dietary protein restriction has been used for decades to treat chronically uremic patients.

Protein Restriction and the Progression of Renal Disease

An unexplained complication of CKD is that the remaining renal function continues to decline at a constant rate even when the disease that initially damaged the kidney is no longer active. This means that once established, CKD progresses toward ESRD. Interestingly, each patient progresses at a different rate even when the same type of underlying renal disease is present.[43] Despite intensive investigation, the mechanism(s) causing the progressive loss of renal function has not been identified. Risk factors for progression of kidney disease include hypertension, proteinuria, male gender, obesity, diabetes mellitus, hyperlipidemia, smoking, high-protein diets, phosphate retention, and metabolic acidosis.[44] The randomized, controlled trials that have enrolled only insulin-dependent diabetes patients have shown improved preservation of kidney function in patients assigned to a low-protein diet compared with patients eating unrestricted amounts of dietary protein. The number of diabetic patients studied in these trials were generally small, and the duration of follow-up was short. To examine this question in a larger number of patients, meta-analyses were performed combining results from several studies. The results published by Fouque et al[45] and Pedrini et al[46] indicate a significant benefit from low-protein diets in preserving the renal function of diabetic patients.

Trials enrolling nondiabetic and noninsulin-dependent, diabetic CKD patients in a randomized fashion have not consistently demonstrated that dietary protein restriction slows progression, at least when analyzed according to the diet prescribed.[47] In the largest trial to address this question, the Modification of Diet in Renal Disease (MDRD), patients were randomized to protein intakes of 1.3 and 0.6 g/kg body wt/d, with or without aggressive blood pressure control or when renal failure was more advanced, to 0.6 g of protein/kg body wt/d or a lower protein intake (0.28 g/kg body wt/d) supplemented with ketoacids.[48] The intention-to-treat analysis of the results (i.e., the outcome regardless of whether patients did or did not ingest the prescribed diet) did not demonstrate a statistically significant benefit of the low-protein diet on the rate of GFR loss. However, when the results were analyzed according to the degree of compliance with the low-protein diet, GFR loss showed a significant slowing and a substantial delay until patients reached the stage of disease when dialysis was required.[49] The MDRD study produced other shortcomings that explain why the study did not find a slowing of renal function loss in CKD patients eating low-protein diets.[47] First, the criteria for entering the MDRD study did not include a requirement that patients were, in fact, losing renal function; approximately 15% of the Study A control group had no evidence of progressive GFR loss. This factor would increase the number of patients required to demonstrate a benefit from dietary manipulations. Second, the overall rate of renal function loss in this study was slower than predicted. Third, a disproportionate number of patients (approximately 20%) had polycystic kidney disease, because these patients had been known to benefit least from the dietary restriction and might have obscured a benefit of the dietary manipulation. Fourth, patients in the MDRD study were not controlled for taking angiotensin-converting enzyme inhibitor therapy. Because these drugs can slow the loss of kidney function, it would make it more difficult to detect any benefit of eating a low-protein diet on preserving residual kidney function. Finally, the MDRD study lasted an average of only 2.2 years. This factor is important because the patients with modest CKD (Study A) had an initial rapid loss of GFR just after initiation of the low-protein diet followed by a slower loss of GFR. If the study had lasted longer, a significant slowing of GFR loss may have occurred. The concern about the poor prognosis of ESRD patients (approximately 20% deaths per year) and the frequent occurrence of low levels of serum proteins and evidence of lost muscle mass in ESRD patients has led some to suggest that low-protein diets should be used cautiously or avoided in predialysis patients.[50] Early initiation of dialysis has also been recommended. Indeed, if CKD patients are not properly instructed and supervised, there may be a spontaneous decrease in protein intake and deterioration of nutritional status. Another worrisome report is the association between hypoalbuminemia and increased mortality in hemodialysis patients, but hypoalbuminemia in these patients can be linked more to inflammation than to any dietary inadequacy.[51] In fact, CKD patients treated with low-protein diets were found to have an increase in serum protein concentrations at the initiation of dietary therapy.[40] Further, a low-protein diet is also associated with improved survival of CKD patients who subsequently began dialysis.[52] Finally, clear evidence shows that with proper implementation, a low-protein diet yields neutral nitrogen balance and maintenance of normal serum proteins and anthropometric indices during long-term therapy.[53] Once dialysis therapy begins, patients who were treated with amino acid/ketoacid and supplemented with low-protein diets can increase their protein intake and gain lean body mass.[54] In summary, when low-protein diets are properly applied, they do not lead to malnutrition. No substantial evidence shows that early initiation of dialysis in ESRD improves survival or that it is associated with a better health-related quality of life.[47] For these reasons, we recommend instituting a low-protein diet in all patients who have symptoms attributable to uremia (and patients who exhibit progressive renal insufficiency, despite the proper management of risk factors for progression, such as hypertension and hyperglycemia) and are already receiving drugs that block the angiotensin II responses so that proteinuria is minimized. This requires patient education by the medical team plus interaction with a skilled dietitian who will monitor the intake of protein and calories while documenting periodic assessments of the patient's nutritional status.

Dietary Recommendations

Dietary Protein Prescription for CKD Patients

Patients with advanced renal disease (GFR <25 mL/min with or without symptoms attributable to uremia or with uncontrolled progressive renal insufficiency should be treated with a well-planned, low-protein diet providing 0.6 g of protein/kg body wt/d following Kidney Disease Outcome Quality Initiative committee recommendations (Table 4).

For individuals who do not comply with this diet or who are unable to maintain adequate protein-energy intake, dietary protein intake can be increased up to 0.8 g of protein/kg body wt/d. Further increment in protein intake will not only generate more urea, but will also contribute to metabolic acidosis and renal osteodystrophy because of hyperphosphatemia. At least 50% of the protein intake for these patients should be of high biological value. The diet should be designed by a dietitian with experience in implementing diets for CKD patients. The dietitian should take advantage of the patient's food preferences and tailor a diet plan to his or her preferences while ensuring an adequate intake of calories, vitamins, etc.

Dietary Protein Prescription for Nephrotic Patients

Until recently, nephrotic patients were advised to consume high-protein diets to compensate for urinary albumin losses and to promote anabolism. However, low-protein diets suppress proteinuria and reduce hypercholesterolemia in nephrotic patients. Proteinuria is an established risk factor for progressive renal insufficiency; therefore, dietary protein restriction should be used as adjunctive therapy in nephrotic syndrome patients. A recommended protein intake of 0.8 g/kg body wt/d (plus 1 g of protein/1 g of proteinuria) will promote neutral nitrogen balance and is considered safe for nephrotic patients.[47]

Table 4. Recommended Nutrient Intake in Chronic Renal Failure and Dialysis Patients

	Chronic Renal Failure and Renal Transplant	End-Stage Renal Disease
Protein* (g/kg of ideal body weight)	GFR (mL/min/1.73m^2) > 50 No restriction recommended 25–50 0.6 to 0.75 controlled <25 0.6 For early transplant recipient† For nephrotic patient‡	MHD 1.2 CPD 1.2 to 1.3 Revise goals to 1.0 to 1.1 if serum phosphorus difficult to control
Energy (kcal/kg of ideal body weight)	< age 60 ≥35 > age 60 30 to 35	< age 60 ≥35 > age 60 30 to 35
Carbohydrates	35% of nonprotein calories	35% of nonprotein calories
Fat	Polyunsaturated to saturated ratio of 2:1	Polyunsaturated to saturated ratio of 2:1
Phosphorus (mg)	800–1000 No restriction in transplant recipient if serum phosphorus is normal	800–1000
Potassium	Individualized	Individualized
Sodium and Water	As tolerated, to maintain body weight and blood pressure	As tolerated, to maintain body weight and blood pressure

*At least 50% of proteins should be of high biological value.
†Protein intake of 1.3 to 1.5 g/kg/d while on high doses of steroids.
‡For nephrotic patients, 0.8 g of protein/kg, and add 1 g of protein/g of proteinuria.
CPD, chronic peritoneal dialysis; GFR, glomerular filtration rate; MHD, maintenance hemodialysis.

Dietary Protein Prescription for Dialysis Patients

Hemodialysis patients have increased protein and amino acid losses into dialysate and increased catabolism from the chronic inflammatory state of uremia, acidemia, or the dialysis procedure itself (e.g., exposure to hemodialyzer membranes, tubing, and catheters). Protein losses into and glucose absorption from the dialysate can have important nutritional consequences for patients treated by peritoneal dialysis. Protein losses into dialysate average between 5 and 15 g/d and consist primarily of albumin; however, during an episode of peritonitis, protein losses may increase by as much as 50% to 100% and often remain elevated for several weeks following successful treatment of the infection.[55] Measurement of nitrogen balance is the "gold standard" for determining dietary protein requirements, but only a small number of these measurements have been performed in hemodialysis patients. Some of the weaknesses of nitrogen balance studies in hemodialysis patients include: small numbers of patients, short periods of observation, patients that were not always in a steady-state, inclusion of acidotic patients, and reliance on dietary histories for measuring nitrogen intake instead of duplicate diet analysis.[30] Measurements reported in chronic peritoneal dialysis patients have the same limitations. Notwithstanding these limitations, the available nitrogen balance studies suggest that the average protein intake necessary to maintain nitrogen balance in hemodialysis patients is about 1.0 to 1.10 g of protein/kg body wt/d and 1.05 to 1.20 g of protein/kg body wt/d in chronic peritoneal dialysis patients. The Kidney Disease Outcome Quality Initiative Work Group recommended adding 25% to the average protein intake to obtain safe protein intake (Table 4). Some experts believe that this is too much protein, especially in anuric chronic peritoneal dialysis, because it will increase the likelihood of developing hyperphosphatemia.[56] Virtually all patients will require restriction of sodium, potassium, and phosphorus in their diet. Fluid intake should also be restricted to 100 mL/d in hemodialysis patients unless there is residual kidney function.

Energy Requirements

Few studies have examined the calorie requirements of CKD patients. In predialysis patients, nitrogen balance with a low-protein diet improves when calorie intake rises. The recommended caloric intake is 30 to 35 kcal/kg body wt/d.[30] The same amount is recommended for dialysis patients. Monitoring calorie intake is important because a diet containing too few calories could compromise the patient's ability to achieve nitrogen balance and thus cause loss of muscle mass. Unfortunately, no simple method exists for estimating calorie intake, so the clinician and dieticians must rely on repeated measurements of weight and muscle mass with knowledge of shortcomings of the technique.[31]

Renal failure is a major public health problem, and the number of patients with ESRD in the United States is expected to increase by 48% from 1998 to 2010.[57] In 1998, this represented $12 billion in Medicare expenditures, or approximately 5% of the annual Medicare budget. By 2010, expenditures for the ESRD population are expected to increase to $28.3 billion. The economic benefit associated with delaying CKD progression to ESRD by dietary protein restriction could provide substantial cost savings. For example, with successful control of the diet, results from the MDRD study showed that the rate of decline in GFR was 28% lower in the low-protein group and 19% slower in the very-low-protein group compared with the expected loss of kidney function. For a 10%, 20%, and 30% decrease in GFR in all patients with a GFR of 30 mL/min or less, an estimated cumulative savings through 2010 could rise to $9.1, $20, and $33.4 billion, respectively, for the same groups of patients.[58] Based on these estimates, even if only 10% of CKD patients successfully followed low-protein regimens, there would be tremendous cost savings. To lower the increasing burden of ESRD, other strategies for slowing the progression of CKD must be included with the dietary interventions, including control of hypertension and diabetes, use of renin-angiotensin system blockade, and prevention of cardiovascular disease. Research in renal nutrition should be directed at identifying more sensitive indices of early malnutrition, better understanding the interrelationship between inflammation and nutrition, and understanding how nutritional intervention can affect the clinical outcomes in CKD and dialysis patients.

Acknowledgment

The authors wish to thank Peggy Bush, MS, RD, for assistance and valuable suggestions in the preparation of the manuscript.

References

1. World Development Indicators. Malnutrition prevalence, weight for age (% of children under 5). Washington, DC: The World Bank; 2002.
2. Bistrian BR, Blackburn GL, Vitale J, et al. Prevalence of malnutrition in general medical patients. JAMA. 1976;235:1567–1570.
3. Benabe JE, Martinez-Maldonado M. The impact of malnutrition on kidney function. Miner Electrolyte Metab. 1998;24:20–26.
4. Abel RM, Grimes JB, Alonso D, et al. Adverse hemodynamic and ultrastructural changes in dogs hearts subjected to protein-calorie malnutrition. Am Heart J. 1979;97:733–744.
5. Klahr S, Alleyne GA. Effects of chronic protein-calorie malnutrition on the kidney. Kidney Int. 1973; 3:129–141.
6. Alleyne GA. The effects of severe protein-calorie malnutrition on the renal function in Jamaican children. Pediatrics. 1967;39:400–410.
7. Klahr S, Tripathy K, Lotero H. Renal regulation of acid-base balance in malnourished man. Am J Med. 1970;48:325–331.
8. Sechi LA, Catena C, Zingaro L, et al. Abnormalities of glucose metabolism in patients with early renal failure. Diabetes. 2000;51:1226–1232.
9. Kautzky-Willer A, Pacini G, Barnas U, et al. Intravenous calcitriol normalizes insulin sensitivity in uremic patients. Kidney Int. 1995;47:200–206.
10. Vega GL, Toto RD, Grundy SM. Metabolism of low density lipoproteins in nephrotic dyslipidemia: comparison of hypercholesterolemia alone and combined hyperlipidemia. Kidney Int. 1995;47:579–586.
11. Massy ZA, Keane WF. Management of lipid abnormalities in the patients with renal disease. In: Mitch WE, Klahr S, eds. *Handbook of the Nutrition and the Kidney,* 3rd ed. Philadelphia: Lippincott-Raven; 1998; 126–134.
12. Massary SG, Akmal M. Lipid abnormalities, renal failure, and parathyroid hormone. Am J Med. 1989; 87:42N–44N.
13. Lofberg E, Wernerman J, Anderstam B, et al. Correction of acidosis in dialysis patients increases branched-chain and total essential amino acid levels in muscle. Clin Nephrol. 1997;48:230–237.
14. Betts PR, Green A. Plasma and urine amino acid concentrations in children with chronic renal insufficiency. Nephron. 1977;18:132–139.
15. Furst P. Amino acid metabolism in uremia. J Am Coll Nutr. 1989;8:310–323.
16. Moustapha A, Naso A, Nahalawi M, et al. Prospective study of hyperhomocysteinemia as an adverse cardiovascular risk factor in end-stage renal disease. Circulation. 1998;97:138–141.
17. Slatopolsky E, Bricker NS. The role of phosphorus restriction in the prevention of secondary hyperparathyroidism in chronic renal failure. Kidney Int. 1973; 4:141–145.
18. Coburn J. An update on vitamin D as related to nephrology practice: 2003. Kidney Int. 2003;87(Suppl): S125–S130.
19. Thomas MK, Lloyd-Jones DM, Thandani RI, et al. Hypovitaminosis D in medical inpatients. N Engl J Med. 1998;338:777–783.
20. Masud T. Trace elements and vitamins in renal disease. In: Mitch WE, Klahr S, eds. *Handbook of Nutrition and Kidney*, 4th ed. Philadelphia: Lippincott Williams & Wilkins; 2002; 233–252.
21. Mitch WE. Malnutrition: a frequent misdiagnosis for hemodialysis patients. J Clin Invest. 2002;110: 437.
22. Marckmann P. Nutritional status of patients on hemodialysis and peritoneal dialysis. Clin Nephrol. 1998;29:75–78.
23. Cianciaruso B, Brunori G, Kopple JD, et al. Cross-sectional comparison of malnutrition in continuous

ambulatory peritoneal dialysis and hemodialysis patients. Am J Kidney Dis. 1995;26:475–486.
24. Mitch WE. Mechanisms causing loss of lean body mass in kidney disease. Am J Clin Nutr. 1998;67: 359–366.
25. Masud T, Young VR, Chapman T, et al. Adaptive responses to a very low protein diets: the first comparison of ketoacids to essential amino acids. Kidney Int. 1994;45:1182–1192.
26. Maroni BJ. Requirements for protein, calories, and fat in the predialysis patient. In: Mitch WE, Klahr S, eds. *Handbook of Nutrition and the Kidney.* Philadelphia: Lippincott-Raven; 1998; 144–165.
27. Maroni BJ, Staffeld C, Young VR, et al. Mechanisms permitting nephrotic patients to achieve nitrogen equilibrium with a protein restricted diet. J Clin Invest. 1997;99:2479–2487.
28. Hara Y, May RC, Kelly RA, et al. Acidosis, not azotemia, stimulates branched-chain amino acid catabolism in uremic rats. Kidney Int. 1987;32: 808–814.
29. Movilli E, Zani R, Carli O, et al. Correction of metabolic acidosis increases serum albumin concentration and decreases kinetically evaluated protein intake in hemodialysis patients: a prospective study. Nephrol Dial Transplant. 1998;13:1719–1722.
30. National Kidney Foundation: K/DOQI clinical practice guidelines for nutrition in chronic renal failure. Am J Kidney Dis. 2000;6(Suppl 2):S1–S140.
31. Avesani CM, Kamimura MA, Draibe SA, et al. Is energy intake underestimated in nondialyzed chronic kidney disease patients? J Renal Nutr. 2005;15: 159–165.
32. Maroni BJ, Stienman TI, Mitch WE. A method for estimating nitrogen intake in patients with chronic renal failure. Kidney Int. 1985;27:58–65.
33. Masud T, Mitch WE. The precision of estimating protein intake of patients with chronic renal failure. Kidney Int. 2002;62:1750–1756.
34. Depner TA. Quantification of dialysis. Urea modeling: the basics. Semin Dial. 1991;4:179–184.
35. Lowrie EG, Lew NL. Death risk in hemodialysis patients: the predicative value of commonly measured variables and evaluation of death rate differences between facilities. Am J Kidney Dis. 1990;5:458–482.
36. Spiegel DM, Breyer JA. Serum albumin: a predictor of long-term outcome in peritoneal dialysis patients. Am J Kidney Dis. 1994;23:283–285.
37. Kaysen GA. Biological basis of hypo-albuminemia in ESRD. J Am Soc Nephrol. 1998;9:2368–2376.
38. Stenvinkle P, Heimburger O, Paultre F, et al. Strong association between malnutrition, inflammation, and atherosclerosis in chronic renal failure. Kidney Int. 1999;55:1899.
39. Caglar K, Peng Y, Pupim L, et al. Inflammatory signals associated with hemodialysis. Kidney Int. 2002;62:1408–1416.
40. Aparicio M, Chauveau P, De Precigout V, et al. Nutrition and outcome on renal replacement therapy of patients with chronic renal failure treated by a supplemented very low protein diet. J Am Soc Nephrol. 2000;11:708.
41. Neyra NR, Hakim RM, Shyr Y, et al. Serum transferrin and serum prealbumin are early predictors of serum albumin in chronic hemodialysis patients. J Renal Nutr. 2000;10:184–190.
42. Beale LS. *Kidney Diseases, Urinary Deposits and Calculous Disorders: their Nature and Treatment.* Philadelphia: Lindsay & Blakiston; 1869.
43. Maroni BJ, Mitch WE. Role of nutrition in prevention of the progression of renal disease. Ann Rev Nutr. 1997;17:435–455.
44. Mitch WE. Nutrition therapy and the progression of renal disease. In: Mitch WE, Klahr S, eds. *Handbook of Nutrition and the Kidney.* Philadelphia: Lippincott-Raven; 1998; 237–252.
45. Fouque D, Laville M, Boissel JP, et al. Controlled low protein diets in chronic renal insufficiency: meta-analysis. Br Med J. 1992;304:216–220.
46. Pedrini MT, Levey AS, Lau J, et al. The effect of dietary protein restriction on the progression of diabetic and nondiabetic renal diseases: a meta-analysis. Ann Intern Med. 1996;124:627–632.
47. Masud T, Mitch WE. Nutrition in end-stage renal disease. In: Pereira BJ, Sayegh MH, eds. *Chronic Kidney Disease, Dialysis, & Transplantation.* Philadelphia: Elsevier Saunders; 2005; 214–231.
48. Klahr S, Levey AS, Beck GJ, et al. The effects of dietary protein restriction and blood pressure control on the progression of chronic renal disease. N Engl J Med. 1994;330:878–884.
49. Levey AS, Adler S, Caggiula AW, et al. Effects of dietary protein restriction on the progression of advanced renal disease in the Modification of Diet in Renal Disease study. Am J Kidney Dis. 1996;27: 652–663.
50. Ikizler TA, Greene JH, Wingard RL, et al. Spontaneous dietary protein intake during progression of chronic renal failure. J Am Soc Nephrol. 1995;6: 1386–1391.
51. Kaysen GA, Dubin JA, Muller HG, et al. Inflammation and reduced albumin synthesis associated with stable decline in serum albumin in hemodialysis patients. Kidney Int. 2004;65:1408–1415.
52. Coresh J, Walser M, Hill S. Survival on dialysis among chronic renal failure patients treated with a supplemented low-protein diet before dialysis. J Am Soc Nephrol. 1995;6:1379–1385.
53. Tom K, Young VR, Chapman T, et al. Long-term adaptive responses to dietary protein restriction in chronic renal failure. Am J Physiol. 1995;268: E668–E677.
54. Vendrely B, Chauveau P, Barthe N, et al. Nutrition in hemodialysis patients previously on a supple-

mented very low protein diet. Kidney Int. 2003;63: 1491–1498.

55. Blumenkrantz MJ, Gahl GM, Kopple JD, et al. Protein losses during peritoneal dialysis. Kidney Int. 1981;19:593–602.
56. Uribarri J. DOQI guidelines for nutrition in long-term peritoneal dialysis patient: a dissenting view. Am J Kidney Dis. 2001;37:1313–1318.
57. Xue JL, Ma JZ, Louis TA, et al. Forecast of the number of patients with end-stage renal disease in the United States to the year 2010. J Am Soc Nephrol. 2001;12:2753–2758.
58. Trivedi HS, Pang MM, Campbell A, et al. Slowing the progression of chronic renal failure: economic benefited and the patients' perspectives. Am J Kidney Dis. 2002;39:721–729.

55
Liver Disease

Craig J. McClain, Daniell B. Hill, and Luis Marsano

The liver is the largest organ in the body, weighing approximately 1.5 kg in adults, and it is possibly the most complex organ in terms of metabolism. It has a unique dual blood supply, being perfused by both the portal vein and hepatic artery, and comprises multiple cell types having differing functions. Hepatocytes make up over 80% of total liver mass and play a critical role in the metabolism of amino acids and ammonia; biochemical oxidation reactions; and detoxification of a variety of drugs, vitamins, and hormones. Kupffer cells represent the largest reservoir of fixed macrophages in the body. They play a protective role against gut-derived toxins that have escaped into the portal circulation, and are a major producer of cytokines, which can markedly influence nutrition. Hepatic stellate cells are the major storehouse for vitamin A in the body and play an important role in collagen formation during liver injury. Other specific cell types also have unique functions (e.g., bile duct epithelium in bile flow, sinusoidal endothelial cells in adhesion molecule expression and endocytosis). The liver plays a vital role in protein, carbohydrate, and fat metabolism as well as micronutrient metabolism. It synthesizes plasma proteins, nonessential amino acids, urea (for ammonia excretion), glycogen, and critical hormones such as the anabolic molecule insulin-like growth factor-1. The liver is a major site for fatty acid metabolism, and bile from the liver is needed for fat absorption from the intestine. Thus, it seems obvious that the liver is important for proper nutrition.

A strong association exists between advanced liver disease and malnutrition. However, malnutrition is not always recognized in patients with liver disease, at least in part because weight loss in these patients can be masked by fluid retention. The loss of glycogen stores predisposes patients with advanced liver disease to enter a starvation state within a few hours of fasting that can lead to further protein catabolism and loss of function. Therefore, it is important to recognize malnutrition and initiate nutrition support early in these patients. Moreover, obesity and the metabolic syndrome are increasingly recognized as a major cause of abnormal liver enzymes and a spectrum of nonalcoholic fatty liver disease (NAFLD). Thus, both undernutrition and obesity play important roles in liver disease.

This chapter begins with a discussion of the prevalence of malnutrition and nutritional assessment in patients with liver disease. Causes of malnutrition and cytokine nutrient interactions are then discussed, followed by a review of nutritional support, including obesity, in liver disease, as well as nutrition and liver transplantation.

Assessment and Prevalence of Malnutrition

Malnutrition is widely present in liver disease, especially in more severe, chronic forms. When evaluating information concerning the prevalence of malnutrition in cirrhosis, it is important to use tests that accurately define nutritional status. Unfortunately, assessment of nutritional status in patients with liver disease is often quite difficult. Tests that are most frequently used include serum visceral protein concentrations, some assessment of immunity (total lymphocyte count or delayed hypersensitivity), anthropometry, percentage of ideal body weight, creatinine-height index, dietary history, subjective global assessment, and—in more sophisticated clinical settings—bioelectric impedance and body composition determinations. Unfortunately, almost all of these tests can be influenced either by underlying liver disease or factors that may be causing the liver disease, such as chronic alcohol consumption or viral infection. Visceral protein concentrations are probably the tests most frequently used by nutritionists in evaluating nutritional status, especially protein malnutrition. The visceral proteins such as albumin, prealbumin, and retinol-binding protein are all produced in the liver and correlate better with severity of underlying liver disease than with malnutrition.[1] Alcohol and viral infection can influence immune function, and edema and ascites can influence anthropometry and bioelectric impedance.[2-6] Impaired renal function frequently occurs in more severe liver disease and influences indicators such as creatinine-height index.[7] Thus, no ideal single indicator of malnutrition in liver disease exists, and often subjective global assessment in conjunction with a combination of tests most appropriate for the particular patient will provide the best possible evaluation.[8,9]

Probably the most extensive studies of nutritional status in patients with liver disease are in patients with alcoholic liver disease, and we will focus on abnormalities in alcoholic liver disease which can be extrapolated to other forms of liver disease. The best recent studies are two large studies in the Veterans Health Administration (VA) Cooperative Studies Program dealing with patients having alcoholic hepatitis.[10-14] The first of these studies (#119) demonstrated that virtually every patient with alcoholic hepatitis had some degree of malnutrition.[12] Patients (284 with complete nutritional assessments) were divided into groups with mild, moderate, or severe alcoholic hepatitis based on clinical and biochemical parameters. Patients had a mean alcohol consumption of 228 g/d (with almost 50% of energy intake coming from alcohol). The severity of liver disease was generally correlated with the severity of malnutrition (Table 1). Similar data were generated in a follow-up VA study on alcoholic hepatitis (#275).[13] In both of these studies, patients were given a balanced, 2500 kcal (10.5 MJ) hospital diet, monitored carefully by a dietitian, and encouraged to consume the diet. In the second study, patients in the therapy arm of the protocol also received an enteral nutritional support product high in branched-chain amino acids, as well as the anabolic steroid oxandrolone (80 mg/d). In neither of these studies were patients fed by tube if voluntary oral intake was inadequate (probably a study design flaw in retrospect). Voluntary oral food intake correlated in a stepwise fashion with 6-month mortality data. Thus, patients who voluntarily consumed over 3000 kcal/d (12.6 MJ/d) had virtually no mortality, whereas those consuming under 1000 kcal/d (4.2 MJ/d) had more than an 80% 6-month mortality (Figure 1).[10] Moreover, the degree of malnutrition correlated with the development of serious complications such as encephalopathy, ascites, and hepatorenal syndrome.[10] In the VA Cooperative Studies, the chronic alcohol-consuming control population without liver disease also frequently had some degree of protein-energy malnutrition. This is in contrast to many other studies in which only alcoholics with liver disease demonstrated significant protein-energy malnutrition.[15]

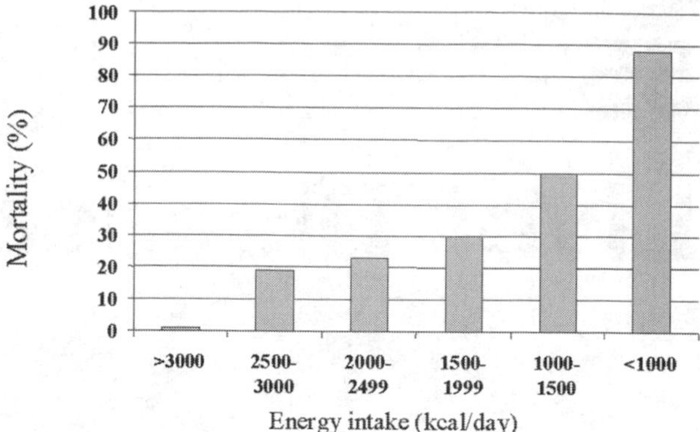

Figure 1. A direct relationship was noted between voluntary caloric intake in Veterans Health Administration studies in patients with moderate and severe alcoholic hepatitis. It is not known whether providing enteral feeding to patients with inadequate caloric intake would have improved mortality. (From Lolli et al., 1992[18]; copyright 1992, with permission from Editrice Gastroentrologica Italiana S.r.L.)

Because both of these VA studies evaluated patients with acute inflammatory response (hepatitis), it was important to determine nutritional status in patients with stable alcoholic liver disease without alcoholic hepatitis. We evaluated patients with stable cirrhosis followed in an ascites clinic who were not actively drinking, were free of alcoholic hepatitis, and had bilirubin levels under 51 mmol/L (3 mg/dL). They had indicators of malnutrition almost as severe as patients with alcoholic hepatitis (e.g., a creatinine-height index of 71%).[15]

It could be argued that alcohol, rather than the underlying liver pathology, is the critical variable in malnutrition in liver disease. There have been several major studies evaluating patients having both alcoholic liver disease and nonalcoholic- (especially viral) induced liver disease.[16-20]

Table 1. Nutritional Status in Alcoholic Hepatitis

	Severity of Liver Disease		
Initial Laboratory Test	**Mild**	**Moderate**	**Severe**
Lymphocytes (1000–4000/mm³)	2067 ± 148	1598 ± 90	1366 ± 83
Albumin (35–51 g/L)	37 ± 1	27 ± 1	23 ± 1
Creatinine-height index (% of standard)	75.7 ± 2.84	62.9 ± 3.3	64.0 ± 4.65

From Mendenhall et al., 1984.[12] Copyright 1984, used with permission from Excerpta Medica, Inc.

Table 2. Major Causes of Malnutrition

Anorexia
Diarrhea and malabsorption
Nausea and vomiting
Poor food availability and quality
Metabolic disturbances (e.g., hypermetabolism and catabolism)
Cytokines
Liver complications (portal-systemic encephalopathy, ascites, gastrointestinal bleed)
Unpalatable diets (low sodium, protein)
No feeding (nothing by mouth) for procedures

Although the prevalence of malnutrition in liver disease varied somewhat in the different studies, there was a compelling consistent observation that no difference in malnutrition occurred between alcoholic and nonalcohol-related causes of cirrhosis in the individual studies. In one of the most carefully designed studies, Sarin et al.[16] demonstrated that protein-energy malnutrition was equally severe in alcoholic and nonalcoholic liver disease and that dietary intake decreased equally in both diseases. Caregaro et al.[17] from Italy found that the prevalence, characteristics, and severity of protein-energy malnutrition were comparable in alcoholic and viral-induced cirrhosis. Malnutrition was correlated with the severity of the liver disease. Thus, multiple studies now document that the degree of liver injury, rather than the etiology, is critical in the development of nutritional disorders.

Causes of Malnutrition in Liver Disease

Multiple factors combine to cause malnutrition in patients with liver disease (Table 2). Poor nutritional intake can result from gastrointestinal disturbances, prolonged periods eating nothing during hospitalizations for complications of cirrhosis, and iatrogenic causes. Maldigestion and malabsorption may occur in liver disease and play an important role in causing malnutrition. Typical gastrointestinal disturbances in liver disease include dysgeusia, anorexia, nausea, and early satiety.[21] Although the exact pathophysiology of how liver dysfunction causes these manifestations is still debated, local and systemic neurohormonal mechanisms are likely involved in causing delayed gastric emptying, small-bowel dysmotility and bacterial overgrowth, and constipation.[22-26] Liver transplantation improves or reverses many of these gastrointestinal manifestations.[27] Concomitant complications typical of liver disease, such as upper gastrointestinal bleeding, portal systemic encephalopathy, and sepsis, also cause prolonged periods of poor oral intake. Dietary management of fluid retention with salt and water restriction; dietary management of encephalopathy with protein restriction; and carbohydrate and lipid restrictions used in patients with diabetes mellitus, chronic pancreatic insufficiency, and cholestatic liver disease can all affect diet palatability and can severely restrict patients' food choices.

Impaired lipid metabolism is also multifactorial in liver disease. Decreased intraluminal bile salts, small-bowel bacterial overgrowth, coexistent pancreatic insufficiency or intestinal disease (e.g., inflammatory bowel disease, sprue), and mucosal vascular hypertension and edema can worsen maldigestion and malabsorption. Cholestatic liver disorders are associated with decreased intraluminal concentration of bile salts, resulting in lipid and lipid-soluble vitamin malabsorption.[28] Impaired intestinal capacity for absorption of long-chain fatty acids, interference of lipid absorption by neomycin, binding of bile salts by cholestyramine, and exocrine pancreatic insufficiency may also contribute to lipid malabsorption[29-31]; as a result, patients with liver disease may have decreased plasma levels of essential fatty acids and their polyunsaturated derivatives.[31]

Low-grade endotoxemia facilitated by portal hypertension and gut bacterial translocation leads to a low-grade increase in proinflammatory cytokines that further affects nutrient management and overall metabolism[32] (Figure 2). Glycogen storage is impaired in cirrhotic livers partly because of hyperglucagonemia. This results in peripheral muscle proteolysis to provide amino acids for gluconeogenesis, thus contributing to protein malnutrition. Liver disease patients with portal hypertension and ascites are at increased risk of developing a hypermetabolic state

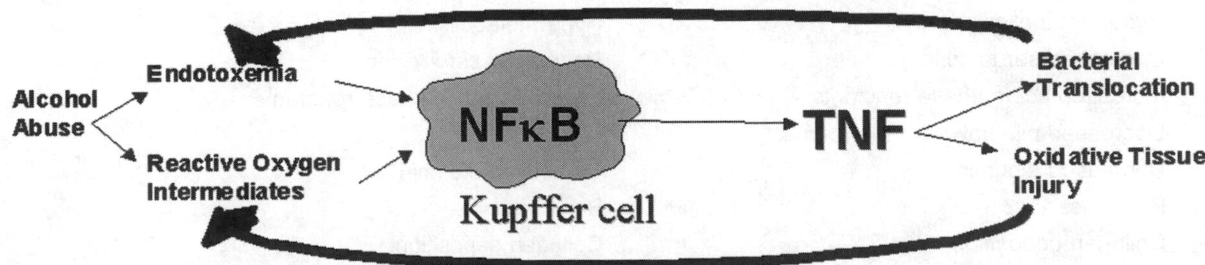

Figure 2. Endotoxemis and oxidative stress occur in virtually all forms of liver disease, especially in alcoholic liver disease. Both endotoxin and reactive intermediates activate the critical redox sensitive transcription factor NFκB in hepatic Kupffer cells, with subsequent cytokine production. This activation will lead to further bacterial translocation with endotoxemia and further oxidative tissue injury. Antioxidants may have a role in blocking this cycle of tissue destruction.

(resting energy expenditure >110% of its expected value), which contributes to overall malnutrition.[33-36]

Health care providers have to exert great care to improve nutritional status instead of inadvertently compounding the problem (e.g., long periods of fasting for procedures, unpalatable low-sodium diets). This concern is highlighted by the fact that 67% of patients in a VA cooperative study on alcoholic hepatitis did not consume the recommended 2500 kcal/d (10.5 MJ/d), even though these patients received expert care by nutritionists and hepatologists who knew that nutrition was a major outcome variable of the study.[14]

Cytokine-Nutrient Interactions

Dysregulated cytokine metabolism (with elevated proinflammatory cytokines such as tumor necrosis factor [TNF] and interleukin 8 [IL-8]) is well documented in many forms of liver disease, with alcoholic liver disease having been studied in the greatest detail[32,37] (Figure 2). The cytokine interferon-α is used to treat both hepatitis B and C. Increased levels of cytokines have been postulated to cause many of the metabolic and nutritional abnormalities observed in liver disease, especially in more decompensated liver disease.[32,37] Thus, abnormalities such as fever, anorexia, muscle breakdown and wasting, and altered mineral metabolism are likely to be at least partially cytokine mediated (Table 3). We will briefly review alterations in mineral metabolism, visceral proteins, hypermetabolism, and anorexia in relationship to cytokines and liver disease.

Mineral Metabolism

Cytokines such as TNF and IL-1 generally cause a decrease in the serum zinc concentration and an internal redistribution of zinc, with zinc being sequestered in the liver and being lost from other tissues such as bone marrow and thymus.[38-40] This internal redistribution of zinc is thought to facilitate priority protein synthesis in the liver, and it also makes the plasma a less favorable environment for bacterial growth (zinc withholding).[38-40] There frequently is an increase in urinary zinc loss that can contribute to overall zinc deficits in patients with increased cytokine activity. Patients with liver disease regularly have decreased serum zinc concentrations and increased urinary zinc losses.[41] This zinc deficiency may play a role in the anorexia, sexual dysfunction, and immune impairment in liver disease. Although the serum and zinc concentrations are decreased with increased cytokine levels, the serum copper level generally increases, as does the binding protein for copper (ceruloplasmin).[42] Increased copper can enhance hepatic oxidative stress and worsen liver injury.

Visceral Proteins

With increased cytokines, there is generally a depression in plasma proteins that are used as indicators of nutritional status, including albumin, transferrin, prealbumin, and retinol-binding protein. This reduction in protein occurs initially because cytokines generally cause an increase in endothelial permeability, which then causes a decrease in these visceral proteins.[43] Cytokines also generally decrease production (mRNA) of these visceral proteins, which partially accounts for long-term depression of the proteins.[44] At the same time that these visceral protein decrease, hepatic acute-phase proteins increase. Certain of these acute-phase reactants play a role in attenuating the ongoing toxic effects of cytokines (e.g., α-1 acid glycoprotein attenuates toxic effects of TNF).[45]

Table 3. Biological Activities of Cytokines

Cytokine Effects	Metabolic Complications of Alcoholic Hepatitis
Fever	Fever
Anorexia	Anorexia
Neutrophilia	Neutrophilia
Altered amino acids, decreased glutathione, catabolism with muscle wasting	Altered amino acids, decreased glutathione, catabolism with muscle wasting
Hypermetabolism	Hypermetabolism
Decreased serum zinc	Decreased serum zinc
Increased acute phase reactants	Increased acute phase reactants
Decreased bile flow	Cholestasis
Decreased albumin	Decreased albumin
Bone loss	Bone loss
Collagen deposition	Collagen deposition
Increased triacylglycerols	Increased triacyglycerols (Zieve's syndrome)
Increased endothelial permeability	Ascites and peripheral edema
Slow wave sleep	Encephalopathy

Hypermetabolism and Hypercatabolism

Increased cytokine production can induce a hypermetabolic or hypercatabolic state. For example, TNF infusion into experimental animals causes a decrease in protein synthesis with an overall increase in net protein breakdown.[46] This may relate to the hypermetabolism and wasting seen in liver disease.[36]

Anorexia and Decreased Gastric Emptying

Cytokines frequently induce anorexia; indeed, TNF was initially termed cachectin.[37] Interferon is used as a therapeutic agent in certain forms of viral hepatitis, and it has anorexia and flu-like symptoms as major side effects that generally improve as therapy progresses. Several cytokines such as IL-1 and TNF also impair gastric emptying, which occurs as a complication of liver disease.[47] Some patients will respond to prokinetic agents such as metoclopramide.

Nutrition Support

Interest was first stimulated regarding nutritional therapy in cirrhosis when Patek et al.[48] demonstrated that a nutritious diet improved the 5-year outcome of patients with cirrhosis compared with control subjects consuming an inadequate diet. These low-income patients had alcoholic cirrhosis. Several recent studies further support the concept of improved outcome with nutritional support in patients with cirrhosis. Hirsch et al.[49] demonstrated that outpatients taking an enteral nutritional support product (1000 kcal [4.2 MJ], 34 g protein) had significantly improved protein intake and significantly fewer hospitalizations. These same investigators subsequently gave an enteral supplement to outpatients with alcoholic cirrhosis and observed an improvement in nutritional status and immune function.[50] In the VA Cooperative Study on nutritional support in alcoholic liver disease using both an anabolic steroid and an enteral nutritional supplement, improved mortality was seen with the combination of oxandrolone plus nutrition supplementation in patients who had moderate protein-energy malnutrition.[10] Those with severe malnutrition did not significantly benefit from therapy, possibly because their malnutrition was so advanced that no intervention, including nutrition, could help. Studies by Kearns et al.[51] showed that patients with alcoholic liver disease hospitalized for treatment and given an enteral nutritional supplement via feeding tube had significantly improved serum bilirubin levels and liver function as assessed by antipyrine clearance. A multicenter randomized study of enteral nutrition versus steroids in patients with alcoholic hepatitis showed similar overall short-term results.[52] Moreover, those receiving enteral nutrition (rich in BCAAs) had a better long-term outcome with less infectious deaths. Thus, traditional nutritional supplementation clearly improves nutritional status and, in some instances, hepatic function and other indicators of outcome in cirrhosis.

Table 4. Nutritional Recommendations for Patients with Liver Disease

- Early nutrition assessment and regular follow-ups
- Total energy: 1.2–1.4 × resting energy expenditure
- Protein: 1.0–1.5 g/kg/d
- Fat: 30–40% of non-protein energy
- Formulate water and electrolyte intake to individual needs, renal function, diuretic sensitivity
- Replace vitamins and minerals (avoid excessive iron and copper intake)
- Complement daily requirements with enteral feedings (parenteral if enteral route otherwise contraindicated)

A defined approach is necessary to achieve appropriate nutritional support in patients with liver disease[53-57] (Table 4). For the patient who has been actively drinking alcohol, it is useful first to correct electrolyte imbalances and to treat and control withdrawal symptoms when present. (This will facilitate control of electrolyte disorders and decrease the risk of having a feeding tube or parenteral nutrition line pulled out.) During this period (2–3 days), if the mental status of the patient is adequate, the patient can be offered a nutritious diet and energy intake can be measured. If the patient is able to ingest adequate amounts of energy and protein, this diet should be continued. If the patient develops portal-systemic encephalopathy (PSE) and there is no evidence of other precipitating disorders (gastrointestinal bleeding, sedative use, hypoxia, electrolyte or acid-base disturbances, volume depletion, infection, etc.), then protein can be restricted to as low as 20 g/d for only 1 to 2 days. Protein restriction is utilized too often and too long in most clinical situations. If employed, it should be only short term to prevent further muscle catabolism. Indeed, recent research casts doubt on the use of protein restriction even during clinical encephalopathy.[58,59] Most PSE episodes have a precipitating factor, and long-term protein intolerance is not a frequent problem. As soon as mental status improves, protein intake must be increased to at least 60 g/d and perhaps to 1 to 1.5 g/kg/d while lactulose and neomycin are given as needed. If, despite maximal medical therapy with lactulose and neomycin, an adequate protein intake cannot be obtained, the protein intake should be kept at the highest tolerated amount, and a BCAA-enriched formula can be administered to supplement nitrogen intake.

Another option is to use only vegetable protein.[60] Vegan diets have a high carbohydrate-to-protein ratio that favors insulin secretion, with a corresponding anabolic effect. In addition, the high-fiber content of vegan diets has a laxative action that can ameliorate hepatic encephalopathy. These diets also have fewer sulfur amino acids and aromatic amino acids than do animal protein diets. Unfortunately, vegan diets are not palatable and are rarely accepted. Their use is almost exclusively limited to research settings. Late-evening meals and snacks are another approach that may improve nitrogen balance.[61] BCAA-enriched diets were developed in an attempt to correct the abnormal ratios of BCAAs to aromatic amino acids observed in liver disease (<2.5 vs. 3.5–4 in normal subjects), with even greater disturbances in hepatic coma (0.8–1.2). Theoretical advantages of BCAA-enriched formulas include increased protein synthesis and decreased protein breakdown as a result of high leucine; use of BCAAs as an energy source for brain, muscle, and heart; better regulation of amino acid efflux from muscle during catabolism and hypoinsulinemia; improved ammonia metabolism by skeletal muscle; increased protein synthesis and decreased proteolysis; increased norepinephrine synthesis in brain; and decreased penetration of aromatic amino acids into the brain (BCAAs compete for the blood-brain amino acid transport system).

Because of the high cost of BCAA-enriched formulas and their limited role in hepatic encephalopathy, these formulas unfortunately are not considered cost effective in the United States. The major exception may be for the few patients who have chronic stable PSE who require multiple admissions to the hospital. In these patients, the enteral formula cost is more than offset by the savings of fewer hospitalizations. A recent randomized trial of BCAA in advanced cirrhosis from Italy reported that BCAA supplementation attenuated progression of liver disease and improved markers of nutrition. However, compliance was poor and use of this product remains limited in the United States, as noted above.[62,63]

If the patient cannot take in adequate kilocalories and has a functioning gastrointestinal tract, then a feeding tube should be used and a standard enteral formula should be given following the guidelines already mentioned above. If the patient develops PSE without other precipitating factors, the amount of protein may be decreased until lactulose and neomycin control the PSE, and then protein must be increased to satisfy nitrogen requirements.[64,65] If, despite medical therapy, the standard enteral formula leads to the development of PSE, then the amount of standard enteral formula can be decreased until well tolerated, and a BCAA-enriched formula can be supplemented to meet nitrogen needs.[62,64]

One infrequent problem in enterally fed patients with alcoholic liver disease is the development of steatorrhea secondary to pancreatic insufficiency. In this situation, supplementation with medium-chain fatty acids while restricting long-chain fatty acids may be helpful. On the other hand, the use of pancreatic enzyme supplements, with or without control of gastric acidity (e.g., proton pump inhibitors) may correct most of the steatorrhea.

Enteral nutrition is desired over parenteral nutrition because of cost, risk of sepsis of the parenteral nutrition line, preservation of the integrity of the gut mucosa, and prevention of bacterial translocation and multiple organ failure. Moreover, total parenteral nutrition can, in some instances, cause liver disease as one of its complications.

If enteral nutrition is not possible, then total parenteral nutrition can be used with the knowledge that it is important to return to the enteral route as soon as the small bowel shows evidence of recovered function. Total parenteral nutrition can be started with a standard amino acid formula in amounts that are increased until nitrogen needs are met. If the patient develops PSE, then standard therapy with lactulose and neomycin must be given. If the patient is still unable to tolerate the amount of amino acids needed to satisfy nitrogen requirements, then the standard amino acids can be replaced by a BCAA-enriched solution specifically designed for liver disease.[64]

Individual Nutrients and Complementary and Alternative Medicine

A recent major thrust in therapy for liver disease has been supplementation with individual nutrients, or the use of complementary and alternative medicine (CAM).[66,67] A detailed discussion of CAM is necessary because it is estimated that >40% of the US population uses CAM; patients with chronic disease processes such as cirrhosis are frequent users of CAM. Moreover, CAM use is frequently not reported to traditional physicians.[67] A variety of forms of CAM have been used effectively to treat or prevent liver injury in animal models, and preliminary data with some agents suggest efficacy in human liver disease. It is the responsibility of health care workers to be aware of the potential benefits and toxicities of these agents and to demand well-designed randomized human trials on such products.

The specific CAM agents that will be reviewed in relation to liver disease include vitamin E, glutathione (GSH) pro-drugs, *S*-adenosylmethionine (SAM), polyenylphosphatidylcholine (lecithin), silymarin (milk thistle), herbals, and glycyrrhizin.

Vitamin E

Vitamin E is a potent antioxidant that is widely used as a nutritional supplement. In patients with alcoholic liver disease and in experimental models of liver disease, depressed serum and hepatic levels of vitamin E have been documented. Vitamin E has been used extensively to protect against experimental models of liver injury, such as that induced by carbon tetrachloride. Zern's laboratory[68] demonstrated that vitamin E inhibited hepatic activation of the oxidative-stress-sensitive transcription factor NFκB in the carbon tetrachloride model, and postulated that inhibition of this critical transcription factor for proinflammatory cytokine production (e.g., TNF) resulted in attenuation of liver injury. Hill et al.[69] treated human peripheral blood monocytes and rat Kupffer cells in vitro with vitamin E, inhibiting both NFκB activation and TNF production. Vitamin E also inhibits activation of hepatic stellate cells and collagen production in vitro.[70]

Vitamin E was reported to have beneficial effects in some but not all studies of patients with fatty liver (nonalcoholic steatohepatitis [NASH]).[71-73] A study in children[71] showed improvement in liver enzymes, and a study from Japan[72] showed that vitamin E not only improved liver enzymes but also decreased serum levels of the profibritin cytokine transforming growth factor β. A recent study in alcoholic hepatitis patients showed improvement in hyaluronic acid (a marker of fibrosis) but no improvement in mortality. However, this possibly was the wrong study population and study duration. Lastly, preliminary studies in hepatitis C patients showed positive results, but longer duration studies with liver histology are required.[74] Thus, vitamin E has been shown to attenuate liver injury in a variety of experimental animal models, and may positively influence liver injury in humans by attenuating proinflammatory cytokine production, inhibiting activation of stellate cells and fibrosis, and blocking oxidant injury in hepatocytes.

Glutathione Pro-Drugs

GSH is a tripeptide synthesized from glutamate, cysteine, and glycine. Glutathione, in its reduced form, is the main non-protein thiol in cells and has an important role in detoxification of electrophiles and in protection against reactive oxygen toxicity. This includes protection against intracellular free radicals, reactive oxygen intermediates, and several endogenous and exogenous toxins.[75] GSH also protects against toxicity from certain drugs (e.g., acetaminophen). GSH cannot be taken up by hepatocytes, but a number of pharmacologic agents have been devised to enhance intracellular pools (e.g., *N*-acetylcysteine, 2-oxothiazolidine-4-carboxylic acid). There are two distinct intercellular GSH pools: cytosolic (approximately 80%) and mitochondrial (approximately 20%). Mitochondrial GSH detoxifies hydrogen peroxide and other organic peroxides produced in mitochondria. Chronic alcohol consumption has been reported to deplete GSH levels.[75] Moreover, alcohol causes a marked depletion of GSH in the mitochondrial pool, with at least part of that depletion attributed to its impaired transport from the cytosolic pool.[76] This depletion renders hepatocytes more vulnerable to oxidative stress. The molecular basis for the impaired GSH transport into mitochondria is unclear, but it has been reported that exogenous SAM—but not *N*-acetylcysteine or other pro-GSH molecules—restores mitochondrial functions, enhances mitochondrial transport, and corrects mitochondrial GSH deficiency.

GSH precursors also can regulate production of proinflammatory cytokines such as TNF and IL-8 by Kupffer cells and monocytes, with increased GSH levels decreasing cytokine production.[77] This occurs at least in part through inhibition of the oxidative-stress-sensitive transcription factor NFκB, which plays a central role in lipopolysaccharide-stimulated TNF production.

S-Adenosylmethionine

Abnormal methionine metabolism is well documented in liver disease (especially alcoholic liver disease), with

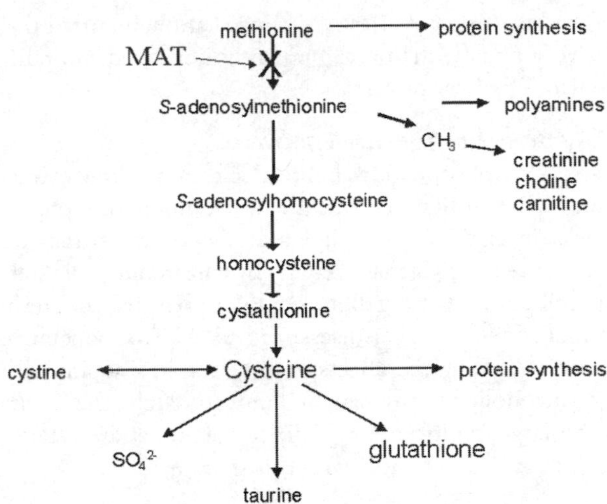

Figure 3. In most forms of liver injury, there is a defect in the enzyme methionine adenosyltransferase (MAT) and an impaired conversion of methionine to adenosylmethionine. These can lead to inadequate levels of critical downstream products such as cysteine, that are needed for glutathione production, which provides one of the rationales for providing S-adenosylmethionine therapy in liver disease.

patients regularly having elevated plasma methionine concentrations and decreased clearance of intravenously or orally administered methionine (Figure 3). The enzyme methionine adenosyltransferase is responsible for the initial conversion of methionine to SAM. SAM is important for its role as a methyl donor, and the process of methylation is critical in a host of cellular processes. Oxidative stress and depletion of GSH play a role in methionine adenosyltransferase inactivation,[78] and hepatic hypoxia can cause a decrease in activity.[79] Both oxidative stress and hepatic hypoxia are prominent features of many forms of liver injury, including alcoholic liver disease.

Thus, for multiple reasons, depletion of downstream products of methionine metabolism such as SAM and GSH may occur in liver disease.[80] Depletion of mitochondrial GSH in the liver is thought to be an important early event in the development of alcoholic liver disease as assessed in rodent models. Recent studies have suggested that SAM therapy attenuates mitochondrial GSH depletion in alcohol-fed rats, presumably by preventing changes in mitochondrial membrane fluidity and maintaining the mitochondrial transport of GSH. Moreover, rats fed a diet to induce SAM deficiency developed increased serum TNF levels and marked sensitivity to endotoxin (lipopolysaccharide) hepatotoxicity that could be blocked by SAM injection.[81] This supports the concept that SAM may have hepatoprotective functions and that it attenuates lipopolysaccharide-stimulated TNF production. SAM decreases production of the proinflammatory cytokine TNF and increases lipopolysaccharide-stimulated production of the anti-inflammatory cytokine IL-10.[82] SAM has also been used to protect against a variety of forms of experimental liver injury, including that caused by acetaminophen, carbon tetrachloride, galactosamine, and others.[83] Lastly, a clinical study reported that SAM supplementation significantly improved mortality in alcoholic liver disease.

Polyenylphosphatidylcholine

Polyenylphosphatidylcholine (lecithin) is a lipid extract from soybeans that prevents the development of septal fibrosis and cirrhosis in alcohol-fed baboons and stimulates the release of collagenase activity by cultured hepatic stellate cells. Studies using dilinoleoylphosphatidyl-choline in animal models of liver disease led to a VA Cooperative Study evaluating the effects of this drug in humans with early alcoholic liver disease, and unfortunately, the results of this large, multicenter trial did not demonstrate a statistically significant benefit with this therapy.[85]

Silymarin

Silymarin, the active ingredient extracted from *Silybum marianum* (also known as milk thistle), was shown in experimental animals to protect against multiple types of liver injury, including that induced by carbon tetrachloride, acetaminophen, and iron overload and, very importantly, mushroom poisoning.[86] Silymarin is probably the most widely used form of CAM in the treatment of liver disease. Clinically, it has been suggested to have hepatoprotective effects in various forms of toxic hepatitis, fatty liver, cirrhosis, ischemic injury, and viral-induced liver disease.[86] It has antioxidant activities, protects against lipid peroxidation, has anti-inflammatory effects, and has antifibrotic effects. Large controlled trials of silymarin performed in Europe have had variable results.[87,88] Silymarin may become one of the most popular forms of CAM therapy for liver disease because it has a good safety profile, it has been extensively investigated in multiple forms of experimental liver injury in animals, and some positive results have been reported in humans. Clearly, further clinical studies are required on this form of therapy, especially in chronic hepatitis C as an antifibrotic agent.

Herbals

Herbals are widely used for a variety of chronic inflammatory processes, such as rheumatoid arthritis, and the use of herbal products for liver disease was recently reviewed.[67,89] Green tea, green tea polyphenols, and grape seed polyphenols were reported to have anti-inflammatory properties and to protect against certain forms of experimental liver injury.[90] TJ9 is commonly used in China and Japan and comes from an aqueous extract of the roots from a variety of plants. This agent has been shown to be hepatoprotective in certain animal models of liver injury and to down-regulate proinflammatory cytokine production. It is frequently used to treat hepatitis B and hepatitis C in Asia. Compound 861 is an aqueous extract of 10 defined herbs reported to have very potent antifibrotic activity. It has been used extensively in China as an antifibrotic agent and has been reported to actually decrease fibrosis in hepatitis B in repeat liver biopsies. It is also effective in carbon-tetrachloride-induced liver injury and has antiproliferative effects on stellate cells in vitro.

A major problem with herbals is that they are actually a combination of agents that have been poorly characterized and are not highly reproducible from one lot to the next. Moreover, some herbal compounds cause severe hepatotoxicity.[67,89,90]

Glycyrrhizin

Glycyrrhizin is an aqueous extract of the licorice root. It inhibits collagen deposition in animal models of hepatic fibrosis and decreases pro-collagen mRNA in hepatic stellate cells in vitro. It has antioxidant effects and decreases NFκB activation. However, it has aldosterone-like effects and can produce electrolyte abnormalities.[67]

Potential Nutritional Toxicities in Liver Disease: Vitamin, Electrolyte, and Mineral Supplementation

Vitamins

In liver disease, vitamin deficiencies can occur not only because of decreased dietary intake, but also because of problems with malabsorption, especially of the fat-soluble vitamins. The use of antioxidant vitamins such as vitamin E has been proposed as therapy in some types of liver disease. However, supplementation, especially if large doses of specific vitamins such as vitamin A or niacin are used, also can cause liver toxicity or exacerbate the underlying liver disease.

Malabsorption of the fat-soluble vitamins A, D, E, and K is well described in patients with advanced cholestatic liver disease.[91] The malabsorption and deficiencies have been classically described in patients with primary biliary cirrhosis and primary sclerosing cholangitis. However, cholestasis can occur with advanced liver disease from other etiologies such as alcoholic or viral liver disease. Overt night blindness is unusual; however, subclinical vitamin A deficiency can be detected by testing a subject's dark adaptation.[92] Because zinc deficiency can also affect dark adaptation, it must be corrected before the test is valid to test for vitamin A deficiency.

Fortunately, vitamin A deficiency in patients with cholestatic liver disease usually responds to dietary vitamin A supplements. However, parenteral vitamin A may be required for patients with night blindness. Caution must be used in giving vitamin A supplements to alcoholics and patients with alcoholic liver disease.[93] Vitamin A toxicity can occur even at the dosages of vitamin A present in some multivitamin preparations with the concomitant use of alcohol. Liver toxicity has also been described in patients with type 1 hyperlipidemia and in the elderly, despite only modest ingestion of vitamin A supplements. Long-term use of multivitamin preparations containing higher amounts of vitamin A (500–1000 IU) should be avoided by patients with advanced liver disease, especially if there is ongoing alcohol consumption. The stellate cell in the liver is the major storage site for vitamin A in the body.

Vitamin D deficiency can occur because of malabsorption of vitamin D and because the liver produces a metabolite of vitamin D, calcidiol, or 25-hydroxy vitamin D.[91] Metabolic bone disease is well documented in advanced liver disease, especially in primary biliary cirrhosis and primary sclerosing cholangitis.[94] Vitamin D and calcium supplements (discussed below) are frequently given to these patients, especially if there is evidence of osteoporosis. Patients with low plasma calcidiol levels should receive vitamin D supplementation (400–800 IU/d). If plasma calcidiol levels do not normalize on vitamin D, then calcidiol, which is more water soluble, can be given.[91] However, the effectiveness of this practice is not well documented.

Deficiencies in the antioxidant vitamin E may lead to lipid peroxidation and cell membrane instability. Decreased serum levels of vitamin E have been reported in advanced liver disease. However, the value of vitamin E supplements has not been well documented in adults. If vitamin E is given to children with cholestatic liver disease before age 3 years, neurologic symptoms such as areflexia, ataxia, and sensory neuropathy can be improved.[91] A new water-soluble form, tocopherol polyethylene glycol succinate, has theoretic advantages over standard lipid-soluble forms of vitamin E. Vitamin E supplementation in the range of 800 to 1200 IU/d has generally been thought to be safe in liver disease, even long term; however, dosages in the higher part of this range may potentiate the effect of oral anticoagulants and interfere with platelet function. A recent meta-analysis of vitamin E therapy reported an increased mortality in patients (not liver disease patients) receiving high-dose vitamin E supplementation, and this has tempered enthusiasm for high-dose vitamin E therapy in liver disease.[95]

Vitamin K malabsorption can occur in cholestatic liver disease and lead to prolongation of the prothrombin time because of deficiencies of vitamin K-dependent coagulation factors.[91] In patients with liver disease and a prolonged prothrombin time, vitamin K is often given parenterally to help determine whether the prolonged prothrombin time is due to vitamin K deficiency or malabsorption or to the severity of parenchymal liver disease itself.

Deficiencies of water-soluble vitamins can occur in liver disease. The best dietary sources for most water-soluble vitamins are fruits and vegetables. Patients with liver disease, especially advanced liver disease, can have problems with anorexia and develop dietary deficiencies of these vitamins. In addition, chronic alcohol usage has played a role in many patients with advanced liver disease. Thus, deficiencies of vitamins related to alcohol usage per se can also occur in patients with liver disease. As for most other adults, the intake of a daily multivitamin preparation is recommended. In addition, we usually give folic acid (1 mg/d) for several months to replete dietary inadequacies. The amount of niacin contained in multivitamins (20 mg niacinamide) is unlikely to cause liver problems. When controlled-release niacin is used as a blood-lipid-lowering agent in dosages of 1 to 3 g/d, a dose-related increase in liver enzymes occurs.[96] Although hepatotoxicity is infrequent, it can occur with doses above 3 g/d and result in fulminant hepatic failure. Thus, the use of niacin as an antihyperlipidemic agent is contraindicated in patients with liver dysfunction.

The use of antioxidants, including antioxidant vitamins A, C, and E, has become popular because of the hypothesis that antioxidants can prevent cancer and slow the aging process by detoxifying toxic free radicals. The use of large doses of some of these agents should be avoided in patients known to have liver disease. As mentioned above, vitamin A toxicity can occur in patients with liver disease and other predisposed individuals. Excessive vitamin C supplementation should be avoided in patients with iron overload states, because vitamin C enhances iron uptake and potentiates free radical generation by transition metals.[97]

Electrolytes and Minerals

Sodium is the primary electrolyte present in body fluids outside cells, with only 5% of the sodium concentration of the body occurring intracellularly. This electrolyte, together with potassium, assists in the maintenance of the body's electrolyte and water balance. In addition, sodium and potassium play important roles in nerve conduction, muscle contraction, and transport of substances across membranes. Hyponatremia (low serum sodium) is a frequent complication of liver disease.[98] This usually occurs with normal or increased amounts of sodium being offset by greater increases in total water volume. The increased volume of water and sodium is expressed as edema or ascites. Many factors contribute to decreased sodium concentrations, with two of the most important being impaired free water clearance and the use of diuretics. In patients with decompensated liver disease, the main way of treating hyponatremia is fluid restriction. Hypernatremia occurs much less frequently in liver disease, and it is usually due to medical interventions with agents such as diuretics or lactulose therapy.

Hypokalemia is frequently observed in liver disease.[98] Unlike sodium, potassium is predominantly an intracellular electrolyte. Hypokalemia may occur as a result of poor nutrition; losses because of nausea, vomiting, or diarrhea; or use of diuretics to control edema or ascites. Various metabolic factors (e.g., increased insulin levels and respiratory alkalosis) may shift potassium from the extracellular fluid into cells, thus decreasing the serum potassium concentration. Hypokalemia can produce a spectrum of consequences ranging from muscular weakness to cardiac arrhythmias and even cardiac arrest. Hyperkalemia is much less commonly observed in liver disease and usually accompanies renal failure and use of potassium-sparing diuretics. It is vital that patients not be placed on potassium-containing salt substitutes while on potassium-sparing diuretics because severe hyperkalemia can occur.

In liver disease, hypocalcemia can occur because of hypoalbuminemia. If hypocalcemia is due to hypoalbuminemia, there is a reduction in total serum calcium, but the ionized calcium remains normal and no treatment is necessary. However, hypocalcemic crisis due to transient hypoparathyroidism associated with magnesium deficiency has been reported in acute alcoholic fatty liver.[99] This hypocalcemia improves with magnesium replacement and improvement in the acute liver disease.

Chronic calcium deficiencies also can occur with liver disease because of dietary insufficiencies and malabsorption. Reduced total and ionized plasma calcium levels can occur with vitamin D deficiency, such as that occurring with cholestatic liver disease, because calcium absorption is reduced with vitamin D deficiency. However, additional factors are thought to be involved in the low-turnover osteoporosis that can occur with cholestatic liver disease, because this osteoporosis can occur despite normal plasma vitamin D and calcium levels.[100] Calcium supplementation in a dose of 1500 mg/d is usually given in cholestatic liver disease, although the effectiveness of such therapy is not well documented. This calcium supplementation is often given along with vitamin D supplementation, especially if plasma calcidiol levels are low.

Hypomagnesemia is frequently observed in liver disease, especially alcoholic liver disease.[101] Major causes of the deficiency in liver disease include poor intake, impaired absorption, renal-related losses, and effects of drugs such as diuretics. Moreover, anti-rejection drugs such as cyclosporine and tacrolimus can cause a variety of metabolic and nutritional effects, including hypomagnesemia and hypophosphatemia, alterations in potassium, glucose intolerance, and hyperlipidemia. Hypophosphatemia may occur in very malnourished patients with liver disease and can be exacerbated by refeeding. Thus, serum levels need to be monitored, especially in aggressive refeeding of malnourished patients.

The role of trace elements in liver disease has been reviewed.[41,42] Trace elements are present in the body in amounts equal to or less than iron, the most abundant trace metal. Iron overload is a well-documented cause of liver disease. Chronic iron overload can result in fibrosis, cirrhosis, and ultimately even hepatocellular carcinoma. Mechanisms for injury are thought to be multifactorial and most likely relate to oxidative stress and lipid peroxidation. The genetic defect for hereditary hemochromatosis has been identified, and genetic analysis for hemochromatosis is now clinically available.[102,103] Iron deficiency can also occur in liver disease, usually caused by gastrointestinal bleeding, especially from esophageal varices or portal hypertensive gastropathy. Care must be taken with iron supplementation in patients with liver disease to avoid iron overload.

Zinc deficiency, as discussed previously, is well documented in liver disease. This is usually due to poor dietary zinc intake as well as increased losses, especially in the urine.[41,42] Zinc deficiency in liver disease may present as neurosensory defects (with alterations in cognitive function, night vision, or appetite), skin lesions, hypogonadism, immune dysfunction, or altered protein metabolism. A major and frequently unrecognized complication of mineral deficiency in cirrhosis is severe muscle cramps. This is often associated with deficiencies of zinc and magnesium, and replacement with these two minerals often improves or corrects these disturbing symptoms.

Increased copper levels may cause hepatotoxicity, the classic example of which is Wilson disease (an autosomal recessive genetic disorder of copper overload).[104-106] Copper is excreted in the bile, and cholestatic liver diseases such as primary biliary cirrhosis and sclerosing cholangitis frequently have prominent copper overload. Interestingly, zinc has been used as a therapy for Wilson's disease. Zinc blocks copper absorption by inducing intestinal metallothionein, thus preferentially reducing copper absorption at the intestinal level.[105]

Other trace metals of particular relevance to liver disease include selenium (potential antioxidant function), chromium (role in glucose tolerance), and manganese, which is excreted via the biliary route.[42]

Obesity and Nonalcoholic Steatohepatitis

In 1980, the term "NASH" (nonalcoholic steatohepatitis) was coined to describe a new syndrome occurring in patients who usually were obese (often with type 2 diabetes) females who had liver consistent with alcoholic hepatitis but who denied alcohol use.[107] The causes of this syndrome were unknown, and there was no defined therapy. More than two decades later, this clinical syndrome is only somewhat better understood, and still there is no Food and Drug Administration-approved or even generally accepted drug therapy. Men are now proving to be equally affected, and terminology has been expanded to include NAFLD, which encompasses just fatty liver as well as fat plus inflammation/fibrosis.[108] Patients with "primary" NASH typically have insulin resistance syndrome (synonymous with metabolic syndrome, syndrome X, etc.), which is characterized by obesity, type 2 diabetes, hyperlipidemia, hypertension, and, in some instances, other metabolic abnormalities such as polycystic ovary disease. "Secondary" NASH may be caused by drugs such as tamoxifen, certain industrial toxins, rapid weight loss, etc. The etiology of NASH remains elusive, but most investigators agree that a baseline of steatosis requires a second "hit" capable of inducing inflammation, fibrosis, or necrosis to develop NASH. Second hits or insults that are thought to be etiologic in the development of NASH include oxidative stress, mitochondrial dysfunction, increased proinflammatory cytokines such as TNF and low levels of the anti-inflammatory adipokine adiponectin, and insulin resistance.[109]

The clinical features of NASH are generally nonspecific. Patients are typically diagnosed in the fifth or sixth decade of life, although there is an increasing recognition of NASH in children. Most patients are asymptomatic, although some complain of fatigue and/or right upper quadrant discomfort. Many patients are diagnosed on routine physical examination (mild hepatomegaly) and laboratory evaluation (mild increase in aspartate aminotransferase and alanine aminotransferase <5 times normal). The aspartate aminotransferase/alanine aminotransferase ratio is usually less than 1 in NASH, thus helping to distinguish it from alcoholic steatohepatitis. The natural history of steatosis relates to histologic severity.[110] Fatty liver without inflammation has a relatively more benign course, while the presence of fibrosis and inflammation indicate a more ominous prognosis. Fat may decrease as NASH patients develop cirrhosis. NASH is a major cause of cryptogenic cirrhosis, an increasingly recognized cause of hepatomas, and an indicator for liver transplantation. Lastly, obesity can accelerate the course of other liver diseases such as alcoholic liver disease and hepatitis C.[111,112]

The cornerstone of therapy for NAFLD/NASH is lifestyle modification and appropriate nutritional support. As noted above, oxidative stress is a major feature and potential second hit in NAFLD. Obesity and metabolic syndrome are states of increased oxidative stress, and weight loss can reduce indicators of oxidative stress.[113] The most important thing that patients with NAFLD can do is institute gradual weight reduction through diet and exercise. Several studies have shown that this will improve liver enzymes and liver histology. Moreover, obese patients who undergo gastric bypass surgery also have improvement in liver enzymes and liver histology. Obese patients have increased cytochrome P4502E1 activity as one etiologic factor for their increased oxidative stress, and this activity decreases following gastric bypass surgery and weight loss.[114]

As mentioned previously, antioxidant therapy has been utilized in NASH patients. While initial pilot studies universally showed positive results, small randomized trials demonstrated somewhat more variable results. A recent study by Sanyal et al.[115] evaluated the effects of vitamin E versus vitamin E plus pioglitazone in the treatment of NASH patients. Vitamin E caused a significant decrease in steatosis, but the combination therapy was significantly more effective and improved pericellular fibrosis, Mallory hyaline, clearance of glucose, and decreased free fatty acid and insulin.[115] Thus, treatment with vitamin E in conjunction with weight loss or another therapeutic agent such as pioglitazone is promising. However, concerns about risks with high-dose vitamin E therapy have likely reduced its overall usage except in the context of therapeutic trials.

Insulin-sensitizing agents, such as metformin and pioglitazone, have been effective in experimental animals, and small studies in humans also have reported benefit.[116] The downside to agents such as pioglitazone is that they may induce weight gain, an obvious undesired effect.

Another group of therapeutic agents are drugs that improve alterations in the hepatic transmethylation and transsulfuration pathways.[109] A decrease in SAM and an increase in *S*-adenosyl-homocysteine and homocysteine occur in many forms of liver disease, including NASH. Betaine therapy has been shown in a pilot study to improve liver enzymes in patients with NASH. This agent also helped remove fat from the liver in a variety of animal models of fatty liver. SAM therapy modulates cytokine profiles, provides an important substrate for glutathione production, and is vital for methylation reactions. Both of these drugs are currently under investigation for the treatment of human NASH.

Nutrition and Liver Transplantation

Malnutrition in Liver Transplantation

Malnutrition is a risk factor for general postoperative morbidity (e.g., poor wound healing, infections, mortality), and this holds true for liver transplantation. In one study, malnutrition was the only variable of six studied that significantly affected outcome that was potentially alterable and not completely dependent on underlying hepatic function[117]. In that study, a risk stratification scoring system, including encephalopathy, ascites, nutritional status, serum bilirubin, prothrombin time, age, and intraoperative blood loss, was used to assign patients a low, intermediate, or high risk for liver transplantation. The actuarial 1-year survival after liver transplantation was significantly poorer for high-risk patients than for intermediate- or low-risk patients (44.5%, 85.2%, and 90.5%, respectively).[117] Moderately to severely malnourished patients had prolonged ventilator times, ICU lengths of stay, total hospital lengths of stay, and total hospitalization costs. Others validated these data.[118,119] Mortality increased 3.2-fold when significant loss in body cell mass was present preoperatively.[120] Using a modified subjective global assessment of malnutrition, Pikul et al.[119] found a 79% incidence of malnutrition in 68 adult liver transplant recipients; in those with moderate and severe malnutrition, they found a significant increase in the number of days requiring ventilatory support, number of days in the ICU and in the hospital, and a higher incidence of tracheostomy. In this study, patients with moderate and severe malnutrition had a significantly higher mortality than did those with an adequate status or mild malnutrition. The pediatric literature presents similar information. In a study of 119 pediatric liver transplants, malnutrition (assessed as failure to grow in height) was also shown to predict postoperative complications.[118]

Moreover, infants appear to be more susceptible to malnutrition associated with chronic liver disease than do older children; infants show both acute and chronic malnutrition with more severe reductions in weight and fat body mass because their accelerated growth phase is affected.[121]

Nutritional Intervention Before Liver Transplantation

Dietary restrictions are necessary but often detrimental in maintaining adequate nutritional intake in patients with liver disease. Restricting fat intake is seldom necessary and only justified in the minority of patients with fat malabsorption. Sodium restriction is probably the single most important restriction in the diet of patients with decompensated portal hypertension, but 1 to 2 g sodium diets are usually well tolerated and easily followed by well-coached patients. Fluid restriction is sometimes necessary to correct hyponatremia.[122] Simple interventions can be tried before restricting protein intake for the management of hepatic encephalopathy in liver disease patients. These simple interventions include ensuring an adequate intestinal transit time; preventing small- and large-bowel bacterial overgrowth (by decreasing portal hypertension and using broad-spectrum antibiotics and lactulose); replacing electrolytes, vitamins, and minerals; and maybe adding casein or vegetable protein to the diet. Maintaining an adequate nutritional status might prevent proteolysis from providing substrate for gluconeogenesis. This would theoretically prevent excessive use of BCAAs for gluconeogenesis and may prevent worsening hepatic encephalopathy. A large body of evidence has been accumulated on the use and safety of BCAA preparations in the management of overt hepatic encephalopathy. Many physicians and nutritionists have also extended the use of BCAA preparations to malnourished patients with cirrhosis in an attempt to improve nutritional states. One reviewer summarizes current data regarding that practice: "The cost to benefit ratio makes it impossible to justify the use of BCAA in every malnourished patient with cirrhosis."[123]

Although a strong body of work suggests that malnutrition is a risk factor for morbidity and mortality after liver transplantation, limited data actually document the benefit of nutritional intervention before this surgery. One of the reasons for this lack of data is that as the survival after liver transplantation improves, the number of patients needed for such studies grows, making it more difficult to perform them. Another reason is that, as we have discussed above, the reasons for malnutrition are multiple and vary from patient to patient. Nevertheless, nutritional intervention improves nutritional status in the pediatric population, and postoperative nutritional intervention decreases ICU and ventilatory-support days in adult liver transplant recipients.[124,125]

When adequate oral intake cannot be maintained, nutritional goals should be supplemented by using nighttime enteral feedings via small-bore nasoenteric tubes. Only in rare instances when the enteral route fails or is contraindicated should total parenteral nutrition be used.

Nutrition Support After Liver Transplantation

Nutrition support after liver transplantation is generally simple because a patient's health improves remarkably fast after the surgery. Although increased protein catabolism and a negative nitrogen balance have been documented up to 4 weeks after transplantation, these have not been associated with a poor outcome.[126] Immediate enteral feeding was well tolerated by 25 patients who were fed via a nasojejunal tube within 12 hours after liver transplantation. When compared with 24 control patients with a sham nasogastric tube, the only significant benefit seen was a decrease in viral infections.[127] Nevertheless, nutrition support guidelines have been published for the post-transplant patient.[128] For patients who have a longer ICU stay after transplantation, the experience of Reilly et al.[125] suggests that parenteral nutrition may reduce ICU length of stay (although a shortcoming of this study was that there were no patients fed enterally). Nutrition support will be needed in the minority of patients with complicated postoperative courses and prolonged hospital stays. The rule of using the gut whenever possible stands true in this setting as well.

Starting weeks to months after transplantation, patients are prone to developing hyperglycemia, hypertension, and hypercholesterolemia as drug-related side effects. Necessary traditional nutrition intervention is warranted in these circumstances. Certain foodstuffs may alter immunosuppressive medications (e.g., grapefruit juice increases tacrolimus blood levels), whereas others can cause disease (e.g., raw seafood can transmit bacteria and promote life-threatening infections in immunosuppressed individuals).

In addition, after liver transplantation, there is a period of accelerated loss of bone due to corticosteroid therapy and decreased patient mobility. After this period of accelerated bone loss, there is a progressive increase in bone mineral density that can continue for several years post-transplant.[129] Calcium supplementation is important during the period of increased bone formation.

Conclusions

The liver is a unique metabolic organ that metabolizes and detoxifies nutrients, toxins, and drugs from the portal circulation and the arterial blood supply. It is responsible for the production of visceral proteins such as albumin and anabolic hormones such as insulin-like growth factor-1, and it is the reservoir for the largest source (Kupffer cells) of fixed macrophages, which are responsible for clinical scavenging functions and cytokine production. When liver disease occurs, there are derangements in metabolic functions, with malnutrition being one critical consequence. The prevalence of malnutrition is high and correlates with the severity of liver disease, and the causes of malnutrition are multiple. It is important to initiate early assessment of nutritional status in patients with liver disease and to begin early nutritional support. Patients may have generalized protein calorie malnutrition or more selected depletion of individual nutrients (e.g., zinc, magnesium, or folate deficiency). Nutritional supplementation has been shown to improve nutritional status, and in some situations improve liver function or clinical outcome in patients with chronic liver disease.

References

1. Merli M, Romiti A, Riggio O, Capocaccia L. Optimal nutritional indexes in chronic liver disease. JPEN J Parenter Enteral Nutr. 1987;11(suppl): 130S–134S.
2. O'Keefe SJ, El-Zayadi AR, Carraher TE, Davis M, Williams R. Malnutrition and immuno-incompetence in patients with liver disease. Lancet. 1980;2: 615–617.
3. Shronts EP, Teasley KM, Thoele SL, Cerra FB. Nutritional support of the adult liver transplant candidate. J Am Diet Assoc. 1987;87:441–451.
4. Shronts EP. Nutritional assessment of adults with end stage hepatic failure. Nutr Clin Pract. 1988;3: 113–119
5. McCullough AJ, Mullen KD, Kalhan SC. Measurements of total body and extracellular water in patients with and without ascites. Hepatology. 1991;14:1102–1111.
6. Guglielmi FW, Contento F, Laddaga L, Panella C, Francavilla A. Bioelectric impedance analysis: experience with male patients with cirrhosis. Hepatology. 1991;13:892–895.
7. Pirlich M, Selberg O, Boker K, Schwarze M, Muller MJ. The creatinine approach to estimate skeletal muscle mass in patients with cirrhosis. Hepatology. 1996;24:1422–1427.
8. Baker JP, Detsky AS, Wesson DE, et al. Nutritional assessment: A comparison of clinical judgment and objective measurements. N Engl J Med. 1982;306:969–972
9. Detsky AS, McLaughlin JR, Baker JP, et al. What is subjective global assessment of nutritional status? JPEN J Parenter Enteral Nutr. 1987;11:8–13.
10. Mendenhall C, Roselle GA, Gartside P, Moritz T. Relationship of protein calorie malnutrition to alcoholic liver disease: a reexamination of data from two Veterans Administration cooperative studies. Alcohol Clin Exp Res 1995;19:635–641.
11. Mendenhall CL, Tosch T, Weesner RE, et al. VA cooperative study on alcoholic hepatitis II: prognostic significance of protein-calorie malnutrition. Am J Clin Nutr. 1986;43:213–218.
12. Mendenhall CL, Anderson S, Weesner RE, Goldberg SJ, Crolic KA, for the Veterans Administration Cooperative Study Group on Alcoholic Hepatitis. Protein-calorie malnutrition associated with alcoholic hepatitis. Am J Med. 1984;76:211–222.
13. Mendenhall CL, Moritz TE, Roselle GA, et al. A study of oral nutritional support with oxandrolone in malnourished patients with alcoholic hepatitis: results of a Department of Veterans Affairs cooperative study. Hepatology. 1993;17:564–576.
14. Mendenhall CL, Moritz TE, Roselle GA, et al, for the VA Cooperative Study Group #275. Protein energy malnutrition in severe alcoholic hepatitis: diagnosis and response to treatment. JPEN J Parenter Enteral Nutr. 1995;19:258–265.
15. Antonow DR, McClain CJ. Nutrition and alcoholism. In: Tarter RE, Van Thiel DH, eds. *Alcohol and the Brain: Chronic Effects.* New York: Plenum; 1985; 81–120.
16. Sarin SK, Dhingra N, Bansal A, Malhotra S, Guptan RC. Dietary and nutritional abnormalities in alcoholic liver disease: a comparison with chronic alcoholics without liver disease. Am J Gastroenterol. 1997;92:777–783.
17. Caregaro L, Alberino F, Amodio P, et al. Malnutrition in alcoholic and virus-related cirrhosis. Am J Clin Nutr. 1996;63:602–609.
18. Lolli R, Marchesini G, Bianchi G, et al. Anthropometric assessment of the nutritional status of patients with liver cirrhosis in the Italian population. Ital J Gastroenterol. 1992;24:429–435.
19. Thuluvath PJ, Triger DR. Evaluation of nutritional status by using anthropometry in adults with alcoholic and nonalcoholic liver disease. Am J Clin Nutr. 1994;60:269–273.
20. DiCecco SR, Wieners EJ, Wiesner RH, Southorn PA, Plevak DJ, Krom RA. Assessment of nutritional status of patients with end-stage liver disease undergoing liver transplantation. Mayo Clin Proc. 1989;64:95–102.
21. Madden AM, Bradbury W, Morgan MY. Taste perception in cirrhosis: its relationship to circulating micronutrients and food preferences. Hepatology. 1997;26:40–48.
22. Galati JS, Holdeman KP, Bottjen PL, Quigley EM. Gastric emptying and orocecal transit in portal hypertension and end-stage chronic liver disease. Liver Transpl Surg. 1997;3:34–38.
23. Galati JS, Holdeman KP, Dalrymple GV, Harrison KA, Quigley EM. Delayed gastric emptying of both the liquid and solid components of a meal in chronic liver disease. Am J Gastroenterol. 1994;89: 708–711.
24. Isobe H, Sakai H, Satoh M, Sakamoto S, Nawata H. Delayed gastric emptying in patients with liver cirrhosis. Dig Dis Sci. 1994;39:983–987.
25. Thuluvath PJ, Triger DR. Autonomic neuropathy

and chronic liver disease. QJ Med. 1989;72: 737–747.
26. Quigley EMM. Gastrointestinal dysfunction in liver disease and portal hypertension. Gut-liver interaction revisited. Dig Dis Sci. 1996;41:557–561.
27. Madrid AM, Brahm J, Buckel E, Silva G, Defilippi C. Orthotopic liver transplantation improves small bowel motility disorders in cirrhotic patients. Am J Gastroenterol. 1997;92:1044–1045.
28. Vlahcevic ZR, Buhac I, Farrar JT, Bell CC Jr, Swell L. Bile acid metabolism in patients with cirrhosis. I. Kinetic aspects of cholic acid metabolism. Gastroenterology. 1971;60:491–498
29. Malagelada JR, Pihl O, Linscheer WG. Impaired absorption of molecular long-chain fatty acid in patients with alcoholic cirrhosis. Am J Dig Dis. 1974; 19:1016–1020.
30. Thompson GR, Barrowman J, Gutierrez L, Dowling RH. Actions of neomycin on the intraluminal phase of lipid absorption. J Clin Invest. 1971;50: 321–323.
31. Cabre E, Peraigo JL, Abad-Lucruz A, et al. Plasma fatty acid profile in advanced cirrhosis: unsaturation deficit of lipid fractions. Am J Gastroenterol. 1990; 85:1597–1604.
32. McClain CJ, Barve S, Deaciuc I, Kugelmas M, Hill D. Cytokines in alcoholic liver disease. Semin Liver Dis. 1999;19:205–219.
33. Ksiazyk J, Lyszkowska M, Kierkus J. Energy metabolism in portal hypertension in children. Nutrition. 1996;12:469–474.
34. Dolz C, Raurich JM, Ibanez J, Obrador A, Marse P, Gaya J. Ascites increases the resting energy expenditure in liver cirrhosis. Gastroenterology. 1991; 100:738–744.
35. Muller MJ, Lautz HU, Plogmann B, Burger M, Korber J, Schmidt FW. Energy expenditure and substrate oxidation in patients with cirrhosis: the impact of cause, clinical staging and nutritional state. Hepatology. 1992;15:782–794.
36. John WJ, Phillips R, Ott L, Adams LJ, McClain CJ. Resting energy expenditure in patients with alcoholic hepatitis. JPEN J Parenter Enteral Nutr. 1989;13:124–127.
37. McClain CJ, Song Z, Barve SS, Hill DB, Deaciuc I. Recent advances in alcoholic liver disease. IV. Dysregulated cytokine metabolism in alcoholic liver disease. Am J Physiol Gastrointest Liver Physiol. 2004; 287:G497–G502.
38. Gaetke L, McClain CJ, Talwalkar RT, Shedlofsky SI. Effects of endotoxin on zinc metabolism in human volunteers. Am J Physiol. 1997;272: E952–E956.
39. McClain CJ, McClain ML, Boosalis MG, Hennig B. Zinc and the stress response. Scand J Work Environ Health. 1993;19(Supp 1):132–133.
40. Goldblum SE, Cohen DA, Jay M, McClain CJ. Interleukin-1-induced depression of iron and zinc: role of granulocytes and lactoferrin. Am J Physiol. 1987;252:E27–E32.
41. McClain CJ, Kasarskis EJ, Marsano L. Zinc and alcohol. In: Watson RR, Watzl B, eds. *Nutrition and Alcohol.* Boca Raton: CRC Press; 1992; 281–307.
42. McClain CJ, Marsano L, Burk RF, Bacon B. Trace metals in liver disease. Semin Liver Dis. 1991;11: 321–339.
43. Hennig B, Honchel R, Goldblum SE, McClain CJ. Tumor necrosis factor-mediated hypoalbuminemia in rabbits. J Nutr. 1988;118:1586–1590.
44. Boosalis MG, Ott L, Levine AS, et al. Relationship of visceral proteins to nutritional status in chronic and acute stress. Crit Care Med. 1989;17:741–747.
45. Libert C, Brouckaert P, Fiers W. Protection by α1-acid glycoprotein against tumor necrosis factor-induced lethality. J Exp Med. 1994;180:1571–1575.
46. Sakurai Y, Zhang X-J, Wolfe RR. Effect of tumor necrosis factor on substrate and amino acid kinetics in conscious dogs. Am J Physiol. 1994;266: E936–E945.
47. Suto G, Kiraly A, Tache Y. Interleukin-1β inhibits gastric emptying in rats: mediation through prostaglandin and corticotropin-releasing factor. Gastroenterology. 1994;106:1568–1575.
48. Patek AJ Jr., Post J, Ralnoff OD, et al. Dietary treatment of cirrhosis of the liver. JAMA. 1948; 139:543–549
49. Hirsch S, Bunout D, de la Maza P, et al. Controlled trial on nutrition supplementation in outpatients with symptomatic alcoholic cirrhosis. JPEN J Parenter Enteral Nutr. 1993;17:119–124.
50. Hirsch S, de la Maza MP, Gattas V, et al. Nutritional support in alcoholic cirrhotic patients improves host defenses. J Am Coll Nutr. 1999;18: 434–441.
51. Kearns PJ, Young H, Garcia G, et al. Accelerated improvement of alcoholic liver disease with enteral nutrition. Gastroenterology. 1992;102:200–205.
52. Cabré E, Rodríguez-Iglesias P, Caballería J, et al. Short- and long-term outcome of severe alcohol-induced hepatitis treated with steroids or enteral nutrition: a multicenter randomized trial. Hepatology. 2000;32:36–42.
53. Marsano L, McClain CJ. Nutrition and alcoholic liver disease. JPEN J Parenter Enteral Nutr. 1991; 15:337–344.
54. Marsano L, McClain CJ. Nutritional support in alcoholic liver disease. In: Watson RR, Watzl B, eds. *Nutrition and Alcohol.* Boca Raton: CRC Press; 1992; 385–402.
55. McCullough AJ. Malnutrition in liver disease. Liver Transpl. 2000;6(4 Suppl 1):S85–S96.
56. Campillo B, Richardet JP, Scherman E, Bories PN.

Evaluation of nutritional practice in hospitalized cirrhotic patients: results of a prospective study. Nutrition. 2003;19:515–521.

57. Stickel F, Hoehn B, Schuppan D, Seitz HK. Review article: Nutritional therapy in alcoholic liver disease. Aliment Pharmacol Ther. 2003;18: 357–373.
58. Cordoba J, Lopez-Hellin J, Planas M, et al. Normal protein diet for episodic hepatic encephalopathy: results of a randomized study. J Hepatol. 2004;41: 38–43.
59. Mullen KD, Dasarathy S. Protein restriction in hepatic encephalopathy: necessary evil or illogical dogma? J Hepatol. 2004;41:147–148.
60. Greenberger NJ, Carley J, Schenker S, Bettinger I, Stamnes C, Beyer P. Effect of vegetable and animal protein diets in chronic hepatic encephalopathy. Am J Dig Dis. 1977;22:845–855.
61. Swart GR, Zillikens MC, van Vuure JK, van den Berg JW. Effect of a late evening meal on nitrogen balance in patients with cirrhosis of the liver. BMJ. 1989;299:1202–1203.
62. Charlton M. Branched-chain amino acid-enriched supplements as therapy for liver disease: Rasputin lives. Gastroenterology. 2003;124:1980–1982.
63. Marchesini G, Bianchi G, Merli M, et al, for the Italian BCAA Study Group. Nutritional supplementation with branched-chain amino acids in advanced cirrhosis: a double-blind, randomized trial. Gastroenterology. 2003;124:1792–1801.
64. Marsano L, McClain CJ. How to manage both acute and chronic hepatic encephalopathy. J Crit Illness. 1993;8:579–600.
65. Mizock BA. Nutritional support in hepatic encephalopathy. Nutrition. 1999;15:220–228.
66. Haas L, McClain CJ, Varilek G. Complementary and alternative medicine and gastrointestinal diseases. Curr Opin Gastroenterol. 2000;16:188–196.
67. McClain CJ, Dryden G, Krueger K. Complementary and alternative medicine in gastroenterology. In: Yamada T, Kaplowitz N, Laine L, Owyang C, Powell DW, eds. *Textbook of Gastroenterology*. 4th ed. Philadelphia: Lippincott Williams & Wilkins; 2003; 1135–1146.
68. Liu S-L, Degli Esposti S, Yao T, Diehl AM, Zern MA. Vitamin E therapy of acute CC14-induced hepatic injury in mice is associated with inhibition of nuclear factor kappa B binding. Hepatology. 1995;22:1474–1481.
69. Hill DB, Devalarja R, Joshi-Barve S, Barve S, McClain CJ. Antioxidants attenuate nuclear factor-kappa B activation and tumor necrosis factor-alpha production in alcoholic hepatitis patient monocytes and rat Kupffer cells, in vitro. Clin Biochem. 1999; 32:563–570.
70. Lee KS, Buck M, Houglum K, Chojkier M. Activation of hepatic stellate cells by TGFα and collagen type I is mediated by oxidative stress through c-myb expression. J Clin Invest. 1995;96:2461–2468.
71. Lavine JE. Vitamin E treatment of nonalcoholic steatohepatitis in children: a pilot study. J Pediatr. 2000;136:734–738.
72. Hasegawa T, Yoneda M, Nakamura K, Makino I, Terano A. Plasma transforming growth factor-beta1 level and efficacy of alpha-tocopherol in patients with non-alcoholic steatohepatitis: a pilot study. Aliment Pharmacol Ther. 2001;15:1667–1672.
73. Adams LA, Angulo P. Vitamins E and C for the treatment of NASH: duplication of results but lack of demonstration of efficacy. Am J Gastroenterol. 2003;98:2348–2350.
74. Mezey E, Potter JJ, Rennie-Tankersley L, Caballeria J, Pares A. A randomized placebo controlled trial of vitamin E for alcoholic hepatitis. J Hepatol. 2004; 40:40–46.
75. Lauterburg BH, Velez ME. Glutathione deficiency in alcoholics: risk factor for paracetamol hepatotoxicity. Gut. 1988;29:1153–1157.
76. Fernandez-Checa JC, Hirano T, Tsukamoto H, Kaplowitz N. Mitochondrial glutathione depletion in alcoholic liver disease. Alcohol. 1993;10: 469–475.
77. Pena LR, Hill DB, McClain CJ. Treatment with glutathione precursor decreases cytokine activity. JPEN J Parenter Enteral Nutr. 1999;23:1–6.
78. Sanchez-Gongora E, Ruiz F, Mingorance J, An W, Corrales FJ, Mato JM. Interaction of liver methionine adenosyltransferase with hydroxyl radical. FASEB J. 1997;11:1013–1019.
79. Chawla RK, Watson WH, Jones DP. Effect of hypoxia on hepatic DNA methylation and tRNA methyltransferase in rat: similarities to effects of methyl-deficient diets. J Cell Biochem. 1996;61: 72–80.
80. McClain CJ, Hill DB, Song Z, et al. S-adenosylmethionine, cytokines, and alcoholic liver disease. Alcohol. 2002;27:185–192.
81. Chawla RK, Watson WH, Eastin CE, Lee EY, Schmidt J, McClain CJ. S-adenosylmethionine deficiency and TNF-alpha in lipopolysaccharide-induced hepatic injury. Am J Physiol. 1998;275: G125–G129.
82. Song Z, Barve S, Chen T, et al. S-adenosylmethionine (AdoMet) modulates endotoxin stimulated interleukin-10 production in monocytes. Am J Physiol Gastrointest Liver Physiol. 2003;284: G949–G955.
83. Song Z, McClain CJ, Chen T. S-adenosylmethionine protects against acetaminophen-induced hepatotoxicity in mice. Pharmacology. 2004;71: 199–208.
84. Mato JM, Camara J, Fernandez de Paz J, et al. S-adenosylmethionine in alcoholic liver cirrho-

sis: a randomized, placebo-controlled, double-blind, multicenter clinical trial. J Hepatol. 1999;30: 1081–1089.
85. Lieber CS, Weiss DG, Groszmann R, Paronetto F, Schenker S, for the Veterans Affairs Cooperative Study 391 Group. II. Veterans Affairs Cooperative Study of polyenylphosphatidylcholine in alcoholic liver disease. Alcohol Clin Exp Res. 2003;27: 1765–1772.
86. Luper S. A review of plants used in the treatment of liver disease: part 1. Altern Med Rev. 1998;3: 410–421.
87. Ferenci P, Dragosics B, Dittrich H, et al. Randomized controlled trial of silymarin treatment in patients with cirrhosis of the liver. J Hepatol. 1989;9: 105–113.
88. Pares A, Planas R, Torres M. Effects of silymarin in alcoholic patients with cirrhosis of the liver: results of a controlled, double-blind, randomized and multicenter trial. J Hepatol. 1998;28:615–621.
89. Schuppan D, Jia J-D, Brinkhaus B, Hahn EG. Herbal products for liver diseases: a therapeutic challenge for the new millennium. Hepatology. 1999; 30:1099–1104.
90. Yang F, de Villiers WJS, McClain CJ, Varilek GW. Green tea polyphenols block endotoxin-induced tumor necrosis factor-x production and lethality in a murine model. J Nutr. 1998;128:2334–2340.
91. Sokol RJ. Fat-soluble vitamins and their importance in patients with cholestatic liver diseases. Gastroenterol Clin North Am. 1994;23:673–705.
92. Russell RM. The vitamin A spectrum: from deficiency to toxicity. Am J Clin Nutr. 2000;71: 878–884.
93. Leo MA, Lieber CS. Alcohol, vitamin A, and β-carotene: adverse interactions, including hepatotoxicity and carcinogenicity. Am J Clin Nutr. 1999; 69:1071–1085.
94. Bonkovsky HL, Hawkins M, Steinberg K, et al. Prevalence and prediction of osteopenia in chronic liver disease. Hepatology. 1990;12:273–280.
95. Miller ER 3rd, Pastor-Barriuso R, Dalal D, Riemersma RA, Appel LJ, Guallar E. Meta-analysis: high-dosage vitamin E supplementation may increase all-cause mortality. Ann Intern Med. 2005; 142:37–46.
96. Gray DR, Morgan T, Chretien SD, Kashyap ML. Efficacy and safety of controlled-release niacin in dyslipoproteinemic veterans. Ann Intern Med. 1994;121:252–258.
97. Sokol RJ. Antioxidant defenses in metal-induced liver damage. Semin Liver Dis. 1996;16:39–46.
98. Marsano L, McClain CJ. Effects of alcohol on electrolytes and minerals. Alcohol Health Res World. 1989;13:255–260.
99. Chiba T, Okimura Y, Inatome T, Inoh T, Watanabe M, Fujita T. Hypocalcemic crisis in alcoholic fatty liver: transient hypoparathyroidism due to magnesium deficiency. Am J Gastroenterol. 1987; 82:1084–1087.
100. Hay JE. Bone disease in cholestatic liver disease. Gastroenterology. 1995;108:276–283.
101. Flink EB. Magnesium deficiency: causes and effects. Hosp Prac. 1987;116A–116P.
102. Bacon BR, Schilsky ML. New knowledge of genetic pathogenesis of hemochromatosis and Wilson's disease. Adv Intern Med. 1999;44:91–116.
103. Fleming RE, Britton RS, Waheed A, Sly WS, Bacon BR. Pathogenesis of hereditary hemochromatosis. Clin Liver Dis. 2004;8:755–773.
104. Harris ZL, Gitlin JD. Genetic molecular basis for copper toxicity. Am J Clin Nutr. 1996;63: 836S–841S.
105. Brewer GJ. Zinc therapy induction of intestinal metallothionein in Wilson's disease. Am J Gastroenterol. 1999;94:301–302.
106. Brewer GJ. The treatment of Wilson's disease. Adv Exp Med Biol. 1999;448:115–126.
107. Ludwig J, Viggiano, TR, McGill, DB, Oh, BJ. Nonalcoholic steatohepatitis: Mayo Clinic experiences with a hitherto unnamed disease. Mayo Clin Proc. 1980;55:434–438.
108. Neuschwander-Tetri BA, Caldwell SH. Nonalcoholic steatohepatitis: summary of an AASLD Single Topic Conference. Hepatology. 2003;37:1202–1219.
109. McClain CJ, Mokshagundam SPL, Barve SS, et al. Mechanisms of non-alcoholic steatohepatitis. Alcohol. 2004;34:1–13.
110. Brunt EM. Nonalcoholic steatohepatitis: definition and pathology. Semin Liver Dis. 2001;21:3–16.
111. Naveau S, Giraud V, Borotto E, Aubert A, Capron F, Chaput JC. Excess weight risk factor for alcoholic liver disease. Hepatology. 1997;25:108–11.
112. Patton HM, Patel K, Behling C, et al. The impact of steatosis on disease progression and early and sustained treatment response in chronic hepatitis C patients. J Hepatol. 2004;40:484–490.
113. Furukawa S, Fujita T, Shimabukuro M, et al. Increased oxidative stress in obesity and its impact on metabolic syndrome. J Clin Invest. 2004;114: 1752–1761.
114. Emery MG, Fisher JM, Chien JY, et al. CYP2E1 activity before and after weight loss in morbidly obese subjects with nonalcoholic fatty liver disease. Hepatology. 2003;38:428–435.
115. Sanyal AJ, Mofrad PS, Contos MJ, et al. A pilot study of vitamin E versus vitamin E and pioglitazone for the treatment of nonalcoholic steatohepatitis. Clin Gastroenterol Hepatol. 2004;2:1107–1115.
116. Marchesini G, Brizi M, Bianchi G, Tomassetti S, Zoli M, Melchionda N. Metformin in non-alcoholic steatohepatitis. Lancet. 2001;358:893–894.

117. Shaw BW Jr, Wood RP, Gordon RD, Iwatsuki S, Gillquist WP, Starzl TE. Influence of selected patient variables and operative blood loss on six-month survival following liver transplantation. Semin Liver Dis. 1985;5:385–393.
118. Moukarzel AA, Najm I, Vargas J, McDiarmid SV, Busuttil RW, Ament ME. Effect of nutritional status on outcome of orthotopic liver transplantation in pediatric patients. Transplant Proc. 1990;22: 1560–1563.
119. Pikul J, Sharpe MD, Lowndes R, Ghent CN. Degree of preoperative malnutrition is predictive of postoperative morbidity and mortality in liver transplant recipients. Transplantation. 1994;57:469–472.
120. Muller MJ, Lautz HU, Plogmann B, Burger M, Korber J, Schmidt FW. Energy expenditure and substrate oxidation in patients with cirrhosis: the impact of cause, clinical staging and nutritional state. Hepatology. 1992;15:782–794.
121. Roggero P, Cataliotti E, Ulla L, et al. Factors influencing malnutrition in children waiting for liver transplants. Am J Clin Nutr. 1997;65:1852–1857.
122. Lowell JA. Nutritional assessment and therapy in patients requiring liver transplantation. Liver Transpl Surg. 1996;2(5 Suppl 1):79–88.
123. Munoz SJ. Nutritional therapies in liver disease. Semin Liver Dis. 1991;11:278–291.
124. Charlton CPJ, Buchanan E, Holden CE, et al. Intensive enteral feeding in advanced cirrhosis: reversal of malnutrition without precipitation of hepatic encephalopathy. Arch Dis Child. 1992;67:603–607.
125. Reilly J, Mehta R, Teperman L, et al. Nutritional support after liver transplantation: a randomized prospective study. JPEN J Parenter Enteral Nutr. 1990;14:386–391.
126. Plevak DJ, DiCecco SR, Wiesner RH, et al. Nutritional support for liver transplantation: identifying caloric and protein requirements. Mayo Clin Proc. 1994;69:225–230.
127. Hasse JM, Blue LS, Liepa GU, et al. Early enteral nutrition support in patients undergoing liver transplantation. JPEN J Parenter Enteral Nutr. 1995;19: 437–443.
128. Hasse JM. Nutritional implications of liver transplantation. Henry Ford Hops Med J. 1990;38: 235–240.
129. Porayko MK, Wiesner RH, Hay JE, et al. Bone disease in liver transplant recipients: incidence, timing, and risk factors. Transplant Proc. 1991;23: 1462–1465.

56 Hypertension

Heather McGuire and Jamy D. Ard

Introduction

Etiologic causes of hypertension include nutritional, hygienic, environmental, and genetic interactions. Strictly speaking, it is defined as elevated systolic and/or diastolic blood pressure. The absolute level of blood pressure considered to denote hypertension has changed over time,[1] and, recently, more emphasis has been placed on the importance of elevated systolic blood pressure. The most recent Joint National Committee on the Prevention, Detection, Evaluation, and Treatment of High Blood Pressure (JNC-7)[2] defines hypertension as a systolic blood pressure greater than or equal to 140 mmHg and/or a diastolic blood pressure greater than or equal to 90 mmHg, on the average of two or more properly measured, seated blood pressure readings on each of two or more office visits. A strong linear correlation exists between risk of death from stroke and ischemic heart disease beginning at systolic blood pressure levels as low as 115 mmHg and diastolic blood pressure levels of 75 mmHg.[3] Thus, the cutoff points used to define hypertension are somewhat arbitrary but serve as a guide to help evaluate, classify, and treat patients.

Hypertension is an international problem. Suboptimal blood pressure control (systolic blood pressure > 115 mmHg) is responsible for 62% of cerebrovascular disease and 49% of ischemic heart disease.[4] Hypertension is estimated to account for 6% of deaths worldwide.[5] In 2000, 26.4% of the worldwide adult population had hypertension.[6] Based on national and regional surveys, hypertension prevalence is greater in Europe than in Canada and the United States.[7] In the United States, 23.4% of the population, approximately 50 million people, have hypertension,[8,9] whereas 44% of the European population has blood pressure levels greater than 140/90 mmHg.[7] The reason for this striking difference in hypertension prevalence is not clear, but may be related to differences in nutrient intake, physical activity, obesity, alcohol intake, environmental toxins, psychosocial stressors, and genetic susceptibility.[10] The continued aging of the population contributes to the increasing incidence of hypertension. Analysis of Framingham data suggests that the residual lifetime risk of hypertension is 90%.[11] In the United States, more than one of every two adults older than 60 years has hypertension.[8] By 2025, the prevalence of hypertension is projected to increase to 29.2%[6]; economically developing countries will have a majority of the burden of hypertension, with a projected 1.15 billion cases of hypertension.[6]

A large percentage of hypertension is related to nutrition. Observational and experimental studies in numerous populations have shown that dietary intake influences blood pressure. Specific dietary components associated with blood pressure range from sodium to soy protein. In addition, recent trials suggest that combinations of nutrients in a comprehensive dietary pattern are effective in reducing blood pressure. This chapter will review the pathophysiology and treatment of hypertension, with special emphasis on the role of nutrition in the development and management of hypertension.

Pathogenesis of Hypertension

Patients with hypertension can be divided into those with monogenic hypertension, secondary hypertension, or essential hypertension. Monogenic hypertension is caused when a single genetic defect leads to hypertension, usually via abnormal sodium handling in the kidney. Several forms of monogenic hypertension have been discovered, such as Liddle's disease and glucocorticoid remedial hypertension. Hypertension is considered secondary when it is caused by an identifiable disease. Examples of this include primary hyperaldosteronism, Cushing's disease, pheochromocytoma, renal vascular disease, renal parenchymal disease, and medication-induced hypertension. Secondary hypertension is usually suspected in people who develop hypertension either early (age <30) or later (age >60) in life.

The vast majority of people with hypertension (≥95%), however, have primary (or essential) hypertension. The pathogenesis of essential hypertension is complex and multifactorial. Several factors are known to be associated with the development of elevated blood pressure. These include obesity, insulin resistance, high or low dietary intake of certain nutrients, excessive alcohol intake, and aging. Genetic susceptibility may also be important in the development of hypertension. In any given person, one or multiple factors may contribute to the development of elevated blood pressure.

Prospective studies have reported that persons with hypertension are insulin resistant/hyperinsulinemic compared with those with normotension. For example, a large European study found that blood pressure was directly related to both insulin resistance and insulin concentration among normotensive individuals.[12] A study of 2130 men examined risk factors for the development of hypertension over 10 years.[13] When baseline blood pressure was controlled for, independent predictors of the progression to hypertension were obesity (as estimated by the body-mass index), fasting and post-glucose challenge plasma insulin concentrations, and family history of hypertension; similar results have been reported in women.[14] In a prospective study involving African Americans and European Americans, plasma insulin levels and insulin-to-glucose ratios were found to be positively associated with the development of hypertension regardless of race.[15] Despite the evidence supporting an association between insulin and elevated blood pressure, this is not always the case, and cross-sectional studies suggest that less than half of those with essential hypertension have insulin resistance/hyperinsulinemia.[16,17] The exact mechanism by which insulin resistance/hyperinsulinemia may lead to elevated blood pressure is not clear. Insulin resistance may lead to elevated blood pressure through the action of the compensatory hyperinsulinemia. For example, insulin infusion into normal individuals and hypertensives increase sodium retention in the kidney.[18,19] Complex interactions with nitric oxide may also contribute to elevated blood pressure mediated by hyperinsulinemia.[20] The sympathetic nervous system is activated by insulin, leading to increased heart rate, thereby predisposing to hypertension.[21,22] Other possible mechanisms likely exist as well, including volume expansion due to increased renal sodium reabsorption,[23-25] endothelial dysfunction,[26] and up-regulation of angiotensin II receptors.[26]

The prevalence of obesity is greater in patients with hypertension compared with normotensive individuals.[27,28] Based on long-term follow-up of participants in the Framingham Heart Study, an elevated body mass index accounted for approximately 26% of the cases of hypertension in men and 28% in women.[29] Weight gain is also an important determinant of the blood pressure rise associated with aging.[30] How obesity causes elevated blood pressure is not entirely clear, and several possible mechanisms have been proposed. Obesity is associated with insulin resistance, often as part of the metabolic syndrome, and may affect blood pressure in ways primarily related to hyperinsulinemia, as discussed earlier. Obstructive sleep apnea is also more common among patients with obesity. The repetitive hypoxia caused by obstructive sleep apnea leads to activation of the sympathetic nervous system, enhanced aldosterone levels, and increased levels of endothelin.[31,32] Treatment of obstructive sleep apnea with continuous positive airway pressure improves blood pressure control.[33] Another potential mechanism by which obesity increases blood pressure is suggested in recent studies showing that the hormone leptin may play a role in hypertension.[34,35] Leptin is a protein that acts as a negative feedback signal to the brain when adequate energy stores are present. The clearest indication that obesity is related to blood pressure is provided by therapy studies of weight reduction. When overweight or obese individuals lose weight, their blood pressure decreases.

Potassium intake has been linked to blood pressure levels in epidemiological and experimental studies. Among societies with naturally high potassium intake, blood pressure levels tend to be lower than those with low intake.[36] Although the association has been related to sodium intake in some studies,[37,38] other reports suggest that there may be an independent association between potassium intake and blood pressure. In the United States, African Americans have a higher prevalence of hypertension than European Americans, whereas their diets tend to be lower in both potassium and sodium.[39] In Japan, sodium intake is generally high, but among farmers who have a high potassium intake, blood pressure is lower than among fisherman who have a low potassium intake.[40,41] An inverse relationship between potassium intake and blood pressure was also found in an international study involving 32 countries, the INTERSALT study.[42] Using urinary excretion of potassium as a measure of potassium intake, a significant negative correlation between blood pressure and potassium intake was found in a large, diverse population.[43] In experimental animal models of hypertension[44,45] and in genetically predisposed and "salt-sensitive" human studies,[46-48] supplemental potassium either reduced the rise in blood pressure or prevented the development of hypertension. Several mechanisms have been proposed for how potassium affects blood pressure. In animal[49,50] and human studies,[51,52] potassium loading leads to a natriuretic effect, and potassium may also suppress the renin-angiotensin system.[49] Other possible mechanisms include vasodilation, effects on eicosanoid metabolism, and the kallikrein-kinin system.

The role of sodium in hypertension has been the subject of controversy, but the majority of evidence suggests that elevated sodium intake is related to increased blood pressure levels. In unindustrialized populations with little or no salt intake, blood pressure does not increase with age and there is little hypertension.[53] Additionally, when normotensive people from unindustrialized countries adopt modern lifestyles, they experience elevations in blood pressure and the development of hypertension.[54] Observational studies have also demonstrated a relationship between sodium intake and blood pressure. In the INTERSALT study described previously, a 24-hour urinary sodium excretion was positively correlated with both systolic and diastolic blood pressures.[43] In experimental studies in which sodium intake is manipulated, increasing sodium intake increases blood pressure. When chimpanzees were fed a diet with up to 15 g of sodium added for over 20 months, their blood pressure increased by 33/10 mmHg above baseline.[55] Although long-term feeding trials of dietary salt modifications are not feasible, low-sodium diets were fed to approximately 250 newborn infants for 6 months, whereas another 250 received diets with 50% more sodium. At follow-up 15 years later, the infants who were assigned the low-sodium diet had 3.6/2.2 mmHg lower blood pressure.[56]

The elderly and African Americans appear to be the most sensitive to sodium and are thought to have "salt-sensitive" blood pressure.[57] Several mechanisms for salt-sensitive hypertension have been studied. Abnormal kidney function from subtle renal injury leading to an inability to excrete sodium likely plays an important role.[58] Other possible mechanisms include increased activity of the sodium-hydrogen exchanger in the proximal tubule of the kidney[59]; increased calcium entry into vascular smooth muscles cells from elevated sodium intake, which causes vasoconstriction[60]; and a defect in the adducin gene that encodes a cytoskeletal protein.[61]

Essential hypertension is a complex disease with roots in genetics and environmental factors.[62] Identification of the exact variant genes that cause hypertension is complicated by the numerous factors that regulate blood pressure. However, family studies support a genetic predisposition to hypertension, with greater similarity of blood pressures within families than between families. Twin studies document greater concordance of blood pressure in monozygotic than dizygotic twins. Greater concordance of blood pressure is also found among biological siblings than adoptive siblings, suggesting that more than shared environment accounts for these findings. The "hypertensinogenic factors" (obesity, diet, etc.) discussed previously interact with a person's inherited blood pressure, leading to elevations in blood pressure and a shift in the population distribution of blood pressures.[63] Genetics and environment likely interact to influence a series of intermediate phenotypes, such as sympathetic nervous system activity and the renin-angiotensin-aldosterone system that, in turn, effect downstream phenotypes and lead to elevated blood pressures. These interactions are important because they may have therapeutic implications.[64]

Hypertension and Cardiovascular Risk

Elevated blood pressure is a leading risk factor for stroke, heart disease, and renal failure. Observational studies have found a linear relationship between increasing levels of both systolic and diastolic blood pressures and mortality from strokes and ischemic heart disease.[3] Mortality from stroke and ischemic heart disease doubles for every 20 mmHg systolic or 10 mmHg diastolic increase in blood pressure. This relationship begins at levels of systolic and diastolic blood pressures considered normal. Indeed, people with high-normal blood pressure (130–139/85–89 mmHg) have more than a two-fold increased risk of having an adverse cardiovascular event than those who are normotensive (<120/80 mmHg).[65] Therefore, small reductions in systolic blood pressure can lead to clinically important reductions in cardiovascular disease. It has been estimated that a population-wide decrease in systolic blood pressure of 3 mmHg will decrease total mortality by 4%, stroke mortality by 8%, and coronary heart disease mortality by 5%.[28] Development of hypertensive renal disease is also linearly related to blood pressure.[66,67] Hypertension is the second leading cause of end-stage renal disease, second only to diabetes; lowering systolic blood pressure by 20 mmHg decreases the risk of end-stage renal disease by two-thirds.[68]

Elevated blood pressure tends to co-segregate with other cardiovascular risk factors; hypertension is twice as common in persons with diabetes mellitus.[69] Hypercholesterolemia occurs in approximately 40% of patients with hypertension. Hypertension also occurs in combination with other metabolic abnormalities, including insulin resistance, dyslipidemia, and obesity.[70] This has been termed the metabolic syndrome[71] and is associated with increased cardiovascular risk. Although elevated blood pressure is independently associated with cardiovascular events, each additional risk factor compounds the risk from hypertension.[72]

Hypertension Classification

JNC-7 has classified elevated blood pressure into several categories based on blood pressure level (Table 1). Blood pressure <120/80 mmHg is considered normal, whereas a systolic blood pressure of 140 to 159 mmHg or diastolic blood pressure of 90 to 99 mmHg is stage 1 hypertension, and systolic blood pressure ≥160 mmHg or diastolic blood pressure ≥100 mmHg is stage 2 hypertension.[73] People whose blood pressure is 120 to 139 mmHg systolic or 80 to 89 mmHg diastolic, previously categorized as high-normal blood pressure, are now considered to have prehypertension.

Guidelines for the treatment of hypertension have been published by several countries (JNC-7, WHO-ISH, Canadian guidelines, European guidelines). In the United States, JNC-7 guidelines recommend a combination of lifestyle modifications and medications based on level of blood pressure.

Table 1. Joint National Committee on the Prevention, Detection, Evaluation, and Treatment of High Blood Pressure (JNC-7) Classification of Hypertension Based on Blood Pressure Measurement

Blood Pressure Classification	Systolic Blood Pressure (mmHg)*		Diastolic Blood Pressure (mmHg)†
Normal	<120	and	<80
Prehypertension	120–139	or	80–89
Stage 1 hypertension	140–159	or	90–99
Stage 2 hypertension	≥160	or	≥100

*†Classification determined by highest blood pressure category.
Adapted with permission from Chobanian et al., 2003.[2]

Treatment Based on Hypertension Stage

As stated earlier, recommendations for treatment of hypertension are based on the patient's blood pressure level. Prehypertension is not considered a disease category and antihypertensive drug therapy is not recommended. However, given the risks associated with this level of blood pressure, patients should be counseled on lifestyle modifications. Lifestyle modifications proven to reduce blood pressure and recommended for all patients include weight reduction, adopting the Dietary Approaches to Stop Hypertension (DASH) dietary pattern, dietary sodium reduction, physical activity, and moderation of alcohol intake (Table 2). Thirty minutes of aerobic activity per day on most days a week are also recommended to help with blood pressure control.[74] These interventions appear to independently reduce blood pressure levels as well as positively influence other cardiovascular risk factors. Smoking cessation will also have a positive influence on cardiovascular risk factors, but has no long-term effect on blood pressure.

In patients with stage 1 or 2 hypertension, medication therapy is necessary. Lifestyle modifications remain a key component of hypertension management. Indeed, as described previously, patients with stage 1 hypertension and no evidence of target organ damage are candidates for a trial of the lifestyle modifications for at least 6 months.[75] If not at goal blood pressure after a trial of lifestyle modification, antihypertensive medications should be initiated. In addition, lifestyle modifications may enhance the efficacy of antihypertensive medications. In patients with stage 2 hypertension, antihypertensive medication should be initiated concomitantly with lifestyle modifications.

Table 2. Lifestyle Modifications Recommended to Improve Blood Pressure Control

Modification	Recommendation	Approximate Systolic Blood Pressure Reduction Range
Weight reduction	Maintain a normal body weight (BMI 18.5–24.9)	5–20 mmHg/10 kg weight loss
Adopt DASH dietary pattern	Consume a diet rich in fruits, vegetables, and low-fat dairy products, with a reduced content of saturated and total fat.	8–14 mmHg
Dietary sodium reduction	Reduce dietary sodium intake to no more than 100 mEq/L (2.4 g sodium or 6 g sodium chloride).	2–8 mmHg
Physical activity	Engage in regular aerobic physical activity, such as brisk walking (at least 30 minutes per day, most days of the week).	4–9 mmHg
Moderation of alcohol consumption	Limit consumption to no more than two drinks per day (1 oz or 30 mL ethanol [e.g., 24 oz beer, 10 oz wine, or 3 oz 80-proof whiskey]) in most men, and no more than one drink per day in women and lighter-weight persons.	2–4 mmHg

BMI, body mass index; BP, blood pressure; DASH, Dietary Approaches to Stop Hypertension.
Adapted with permission from Chobanian et al., 2003.[2]

A large selection of medications is available for treating hypertension. Trials have shown the efficacy of these drugs for lowering blood pressure; however, for most patients, therapy should be initiated with a diuretic (e.g., hydrochlorothiazide).[76] The majority of patients will require two or more medications from different classes to control blood pressure. In patients with stage 2 hypertension, some experts recommend starting with two antihypertensive medications. Specific drugs/drug classes are indicated for patients with certain comorbid conditions.

When treating patients, the target blood pressure to reduce cardiovascular disease outcomes should be <140/90 mmHg for most patients.[77] Based on trial data, those with diabetes or chronic kidney disease have a lower blood pressure goal of <130/80 mmHg.[78]

Nutritional Considerations when Treating with Antihypertensives

Many antihypertensive therapies have untoward side effects, ranging from constipation to elevations of fasting glucose and increased risk of diabetes. These side effects, in many instances, are treatable and often preventable with consideration of nutritional adjuncts to antihypertensive therapy. A wide variety of prospective, randomized trials have shown that thiazide diuretics and beta-blockers increase the risk of type 2 diabetes relative to angiotensin-converting enzyme inhibitors and calcium channel blockers in treated hypertensives.[76,79-81] Caution should be used when initiating antihypertensive therapy with beta-blockers or diuretics in patients who have a body mass index ≥ 30 kg/m^2 or fasting glucose > 100 mg/dL. Prescriptions for energy restriction and physical activity are prudent, in addition to promoting a healthful dietary pattern, such as DASH. The DASH diet has been shown to lower blood pressure, independently of any other intervention, emphasizing fruits, vegetables, and low-fat dairy products, and contains reduced amounts of saturated fat, total fat, cholesterol, and sweets. All of these interventions can improve insulin sensitivity[82] and may be helpful in preventing progression to diabetes.

Thiazide diuretics also result in potassium wasting by increasing delivery of sodium and water to renal collecting tubules, where aldosterone-sensitive potassium secretion occurs, and by increasing secretion of aldosterone as a result of diuretic-induced volume depletion. Patients on thiazide diuretics should receive potassium supplementation for hypokalemia.[83] Because potassium will reach a new steady state approximately 2 to 3 weeks following initiation of the diuretic, those patients who do not experience hypokalemia in that initial time period have a lower risk of hypokalemia later if there are no significant changes in potassium intake. Dietary consumption of potassium-rich food, while taking a thiazide diuretic, may be the key to preventing hypokalemia. Using the lowest effective dose (12.5–25 mg) is also recommended as a way to reduce the risk of hypokalemia.

Tenets of Nutritional Therapy for Hypertension

Low Sodium Intake

Because of the recognized impact of sodium intake on blood pressure, this micronutrient is generally the first target of therapy in the nonpharmacological management of hypertension. Sodium reduction can be difficult because of its ubiquitous nature in the food supply. In the United States, the majority of sodium intake is from the processing of foods, accounting for approximately 75% of sodium intake.[84] Discretionary sodium, or salt added at the table or during cooking, accounts for only 10% of sodium intake. Naturally occurring sodium in foods accounts for the remaining sodium intake. Therefore, guidelines such as the US Department of Agriculture's Dietary Guidelines for Americans focus on choosing foods that have a low sodium content, whereas previous guidelines focused on using less salt and sodium.[85] To be successful at achieving sodium reduction in the current food environment, patients need to be aware of high-sodium foods and potential alternatives.

Although highly industrialized countries such as the United States and Britain have high levels of sodium in their food supply, primarily as a result of food processing, rural populations and residents of less industrialized countries have lower sodium intake. Lower population dietary sodium intake is associated with lower blood pressure; the INTERSALT study provides the best evidence of this. Four populations (Yanomamo and Xingu Indians of Brazil and rural populations in Kenya and Papua, New Guinea) with the lowest salt intake had the lowest blood pressure of the 52 populations included in the study.[53] A lower population salt intake was not associated with a significant increase in blood pressure with age, as is typically seen in the United States and Britain. However, even within industrialized populations, there are significant differences in sodium intake. The INTERMAP study of nutrient and blood pressure associations in the United States, Britain, China, and Japan revealed that the eastern Asian populations had higher sodium intake than those of the Western countries.[86] Combined with a lower potassium intake, the higher sodium intake is hypothesized to be responsible for the high prevalence of stroke seen in China and Japan.

The 2004 Institute of Medicine Report on fluids and electrolytes reviews the evidence for recommended dietary sodium intake levels.[87] The median intake of sodium in the United States is 4300 mg/d for men and 2900 mg/d for women, with a large majority being provided by processed foods.[88] A level of 1.5 g/d is recommended as the minimum adequate intake (AI). This level of intake allows for adequate intake of other nutrients in the dietary pattern. Although some concerns have been raised regarding low levels of sodium intake and adverse effects on lipids, insulin sensitivity, and cardiovascular disease risk, these effects are transient and have generally been reported in association with extremely low levels of sodium intake (<500 mg/d). Moderate sodium intake has not been associated with any adverse effects on total cholesterol or plasma glucose.[2,89]

Because blood pressure increases progressively with increased sodium intake, the Institute of Medicine and the US Department of Agriculture recommend an upper limit of sodium intake of 2300 mg/d. The changes in blood pressure in response to sodium are nonlinear, with the greatest change occurring at levels below the recommended upper limit. The limit of 2300 mg/d was chosen because it is the level above the minimum intake that has been routinely studied in clinical trials of sodium intake and blood pressure response. Approximately 95% of adult men and 75% of adult women consume more than the recommended upper limit of sodium.[88] No benefit can be expected for consuming higher amounts of sodium, and the upper limit should not be considered the recommended intake of sodium. Indeed, for some groups, such as those with hypertension, diabetes, chronic kidney disease, African Americans, and the elderly, the upper limit may need to be considerably lower.[88] These groups of individuals are more prone to experience larger increases in blood pressure with increases in dietary sodium intake or a greater salt sensitivity. Sensitivity to sodium can be modified by increasing dietary potassium intake, thereby blunting the increase in blood pressure seen with higher sodium intake.

Sodium reduction has been shown to lead to clinically significant decreases in blood pressure in several clinical trials. One of the clearest demonstrations of this efficacy was in the DASH-Sodium trial.[90] In this study of 412 middle-aged, prehypertensive and stage 1 hypertensive adults on no medications, there was a clear dose-response to feeding lower levels of sodium intake. While consuming a typical American dietary pattern, reductions in sodium intake from 3300 to 2500 mg resulted in a mean change in systolic blood pressure of 2.1 mmHg, and further reductions to 1500 mg/d resulted in additional decreases in systolic blood pressure of 4.6 mmHg. The same levels of sodium reduction were tested in individuals consuming the DASH dietary pattern; this resulted in blunting of the sodium effect (reductions in systolic blood pressure of 1.3 and 1.7 mmHg, respectively), primarily because of the high potassium content of DASH. Subgroup analyses revealed that those who were hypertensive and older (age >45) had the greatest blood pressure reduction in response to sodium reduction.[91]

Additional randomized, controlled clinical trials using behavior modification and dietary advice have established the effectiveness of sodium reduction in lowering blood pressure or preventing incident hypertension. The Trials of Hypertension Prevention Phase II included a sodium-reduction-only intervention group that achieved a sodium intake of approximately 2300 mg/d. This intake was 1150 mg/d lower than the control group and resulted in an 18% risk reduction for developing hypertension over the 48-month study follow-up.[92] The Trial of the Nonpharmacologic Interventions in the Elderly demonstrated that sodium reduction can be useful therapy in the elderly population. A targeted 1150 mg/d reduction in sodium intake decreased blood pressure to an average of 4.6/2.3 mmHg compared with 0.4/0.2 in the usual-lifestyle group. During the follow-up period of over 2 years, the blood pressure reduction achieved with sodium reduction decreased the risk of requiring antihypertensive medication or suffering a clinical cardiovascular event by 32%.[93]

Before the publication of DASH-Sodium, The Trials of Hypertension Prevention Phase II, and The Trial of the Nonpharmacologic Interventions in the Elderly, Cutler et al[94] conducted a meta-analysis of 32 randomized clinical trials, including over 2600 patients. Even though this meta-analysis predated these major clinical trials, the findings were consistent. Cutler reported a dose response relationship between sodium reduction and blood pressure, such that for every 2300 mg/d decrease in sodium, blood pressure decreased 5.8/2.5 mmHg in patients with hypertension and 2.3/1.4 mmHg in those without hypertension. The wealth of evidence supports moderate sodium reduction as a safe and effective therapy for lowering blood pressure in hypertensives and the elderly, and for preventing increases in blood pressure in normotensives. In another meta-analysis by Hooper et al.[95] 11 trials of dietary advice to reduce sodium intake were pooled. Their results showed that the advice to reduce sodium intake resulted in 1.1 mmHg systolic and 0.6 mmHg diastolic reductions in blood pressure for the 3491 patients included in the studies. They also considered the relationship between urinary sodium excretion and blood pressure; no relationship was present between blood pressure at follow-up and follow-up urinary sodium excretion. This meta-analysis highlights the behavioral challenge associated with achieving long-term sodium reduction in a typical clinical care setting complicated by a food environment that promotes high sodium intake. It can be expected that adherence to sodium reduction will wane over time. The lack of a relationship between maintenance of some long-term blood pressure reduction and urinary sodium excretion, however, suggests that other behavioral factors, such as increases in potassium intake or reductions in alcohol or total energy intake, may be responsible for some of the long-term changes.

Moderate Alcohol Intake

Early epidemiological studies have identified a relationship between increasing alcohol intake and higher blood pressure starting at an intake of more than two drinks per day (a standard drink is defined as 14 g of ethanol—12 ounces beer, 5 ounces table wine, or 1.5 ounces distilled spirits).[96] Recent studies, such as the Atherosclerosis Risk in Communities study, have shown that intake of >210 g of alcohol per week is an independent risk factor for incident hypertension.[97] Intervention studies have also confirmed the impact of alcohol on blood pressure. Puddey et al.[98] demonstrated, in a crossover study, the pressor effect of alcohol in normotensive men. When alcohol consumption was decreased from 350 to 70 mL per week, a decrease in systolic blood pressure of 3.1 mmHg resulted, after adjusting for weight loss resulting from decreased caloric intake. Blood pressure increased when alcohol consumption at previous levels resumed. Estimates from experts suggest that 5% to 7% of hypertension is attributable to alcohol intake, comprising a larger cause of hypertension than all secondary causes.[99]

Although increased alcohol intake has a pressor effect, the mechanistic link between alcohol and blood pressure is unclear. In addition to the absolute volume of alcohol intake, it is becoming clearer that drinking pattern has a significant influence on blood pressure. A study of men and women in the United States showed that those drinking mostly outside of meals or snacks had a higher risk of hypertension compared with those who drank primarily with meals or abstainers.[100] This has also been seen in an Italian population.[101] The pattern of weekend-only drinking can also influence the effect of alcohol on blood pressure; a higher blood pressure on the Monday following weekend drinking was noted in an Irish population compared with a French population who drank daily during the week.[102] No evidence supports the idea that beverage choice plays an important role in the risk of hypertension or blood pressure elevation.[99] For example, in a group of Australian men, 40 g of daily alcohol consumption as either red wine or beer increased blood pressure equally.[103]

The largest study designed specifically to test the effect of alcohol reduction on blood pressure was the Prevention and Treatment of Hypertension Study.[104] A total of 641 outpatient, US military veterans with an average intake of more than three drinks per day and diastolic blood pressure of 80 to 99 mmHg, were randomized into a 6-month cognitive-behavioral program designed to reduce alcohol intake or to an observational control group. At 6 months, there was a significant decrease in alcohol intake for the intervention group (432–230 g/wk). The target separation between the groups was two drinks per day, but the actual difference was only 1.3 drinks per day, resulting in a nonstatistically significant decrease in blood pressure of 1.2/0.7 mmHg compared with the controls.

However, when the results of this single trial were combined with 14 other trials focused on alcohol reduction in a meta-analysis, the results were more impressive for alcohol reduction. A 3.31 mmHg systolic and a 2.04 mmHg diastolic reduction in blood pressure was seen for a median 76% decrease in self-reported alcohol intake.[105] Based on this strength of evidence, expert panel such as the JNC-7 recommend limiting alcohol intake to less than two drinks a day for men and less than one drink a day for women.[2] Also, abstinence is an option for everyone and may be the best choice for some, such as pregnant women or those with a history of alcoholism.

Weight Control

Overweight and obesity are increasing problems for populations worldwide. Globally, over 1 billion adults are overweight and nearly 300 million are obese.[106] The typical pattern of obesity in developing countries is usually a higher prevalence in higher-income and urban populations. In industrialized nations, women of lower socioeconomic status are more commonly obese, and those in rural settings are more likely to be obese compared with those in urban environments. Since the 1980s, the rates of obesity have increased three-fold in some areas of North America, the United Kingdom, Eastern Europe, the Middle East, the Pacific Islands, Australasia, and China. Rates range from as low as 5% in China, Japan, and some African countries to 75% in urban Samoa.[106] The increase in obesity is directly associated with increased mechanization and transportation efficiency, higher availability of low-cost, energy-dense food, and decreased energy expenditure through decreased leisure time physical activity.

As the prevalence of obesity increases, weight loss as a therapeutic strategy for blood pressure control will be more relevant for a growing number of patients. Weight loss of relatively small amounts can significantly reduce blood pressure levels, so the weight loss targets needed to show benefits are realistic goals for most patients. Weight loss of as little as 5% of initial body weight can have a significant impact on blood pressure. Several studies have demonstrated that hypertension can be successfully treated and prevented using weight-reducing diets.[92,107-110] In a review of studies of weight reduction and its maximum effect on blood pressure, at an average of 35.3 weeks, blood pressure had decreased by 1.05 mmHg systolic and 0.92 mmHg diastolic for each kilogram of weight lost.[111] Weight loss also reduces the incidence of hypertension. In the Trial of Hypertension Prevention Phase I study, follow-up at 18 months found that a 3.9-kg weight loss using energy restriction and physical activity was associated with a 34% reduction in risk for hypertension.[112]

Theoretically, changes in blood pressure following weight loss of 5% to 10% of initial body weight could be related to acute changes in energy intake, fluid status, or other dietary factors. However, maintenance of a lower body weight following initial weight loss has been associated with long-term blood pressure reduction. In a meta-analysis of 14 trials, after 2 years of follow-up, studies estimated that a sustained weight reduction of 10 kg was associated with 6 mmHg systolic and a 4.6 mmHg diastolic blood pressure reductions.[113] Interestingly, in this meta-analysis, there was little long-term impact on blood pressure for those who had a weight reduction through surgical procedures. This does not mean that weight loss following surgery has no benefit on blood pressure, but various confounders, such as medication usage and baseline blood pressure, combined with a follow-up time that was well beyond 2 years for the surgical studies, may have been responsible for a weaker relationship between blood pressure and weight loss. The results of the meta-analysis are supported by other observational data. Results from the Framingham, Massachusetts, cohort showed that older persons with a sustained weight loss over 4 years decreased risk of hypertension by 36%.[114] Even though a large proportion of people who lose weight will regain a portion of the weight, it appears that efforts to maintain weight loss can result in long-term benefits to blood pressure.

DASH Diet

Lowering blood pressure within the context of a dietary pattern may offer several advantages. Because foods are not consumed in isolation, a comprehensive dietary pattern is obviously more natural to the patient than attempting to manipulate individual nutrients. Synergy between various dietary components thought to impact blood pressure may also occur when consumed together in a dietary pattern. In addition, this framework for nutritional therapy might lead to additional beneficial effects on other cardiovascular risk factors.

Some of the key nutrients observed to be related to lower blood pressure in population studies included potassium, magnesium, calcium, protein, and fiber. However, when these nutrients are delivered as supplements, the effect on blood pressure has been variable. Potassium, found in fruits and vegetables, has been associated with lower blood pressure in epidemiological studies and in some supplementation interventions. The hypotensive effects of potassium are primarily greatest at higher sodium intakes. The reductions in blood pressure with a net urinary potassium increase of 50 mmol/d are approximately 4.4/2.5 mmHg in hypertensives and 1.8/1.0 mmHg in normotensives.[115] Intervention studies and meta-analyses of randomized, controlled trials have been less impressive for the effects on blood pressure of magnesium or calcium supplementation. For example, two meta-analyses of calcium supplementation showed only modest reductions in systolic blood pressure and no significant effect on diastolic blood pressure.[116,117] A randomized trial of multiple supplements, including a combination of calcium and magnesium, did not result in any significant blood pressure reduction.[118] The Trials of Hypertension Prevention also failed to show a reduction in blood pressure for potassium, calcium, or magnesium supplements in normotensives patients.[109]

Some nutrients are in higher concentrations in plant-based dietary patterns. For example, vegetarians have been shown to have lower blood pressures than omnivores in similar environments.[119] A vegetarian dietary pattern provides various minerals and nutrients that are associated with lower blood pressure, including potassium, magnesium, and fiber. However, attempts to isolate the key factor in the vegetarian dietary pattern that might be responsible for lowering blood pressure have been less than definitive. Vegetarian diets also have other characteristics that are associated with lower blood pressure, including lower amounts of total and saturated fats.

Table 3. Dietary Approaches to Stop Hypertension (DASH) Diet Components Based on 2000-Calorie Intake

Food Group	Servings	Nutrient Contribution
Whole grains and grain products	7–8/d	Energy, fiber
Vegetables	4–5/d	Potassium, magnesium, fiber
Fruit	4–5/d	Potassium, magnesium, fiber
Low-fat or fat-free dairy products	2–3/d	Calcium, protein
Meat, fish, poultry	2 or less/d	Protein
Nuts, seeds, dry beans	4–5/wk	Energy, protein, fiber, magnesium, potassium
Fat	2–3/d	27% of calories from fat
Sweets	5/wk	

The DASH dietary pattern attempts to include all of these dietary factors, taking into account the micronutrients, minerals, and macronutrient proportions observed to have an association with lower blood pressure in various populations.[120]

The DASH diet emphasizes fruits, vegetables, and low-fat dairy products, and contains reduced amounts of saturated fat, total fat, cholesterol, and sweets. The DASH food group servings per day are shown in Table 3. The DASH dietary pattern is high in potassium, magnesium, and calcium, all near the 75th percentile of US consumption.[121] Fiber intake is approximately three times the average US intake, and, because the total fat content is low at 27%, nutrient goals can be met without excess calories. In the original feeding study that established the efficacy of DASH, sodium intake was not reduced (3000 mg/d in each treatment group), and caloric intake was adjusted to maintain a stable weight throughout the 8-week study period. This dietary pattern resulted in an average blood pressure reduction of 5.5/3.0 mmHg for the entire study population and 11.4/5.5 mmHg for those with stage 1 hypertension.[122] The dietary pattern was effective for all subgroups studied, especially in hypertensive African Americans.[123] When combined with sodium reduction, the effect on blood pressure is greater than either intervention in isolation[90] (Figure 1); however, the combination is subadditive, possibly as a result of the blunted

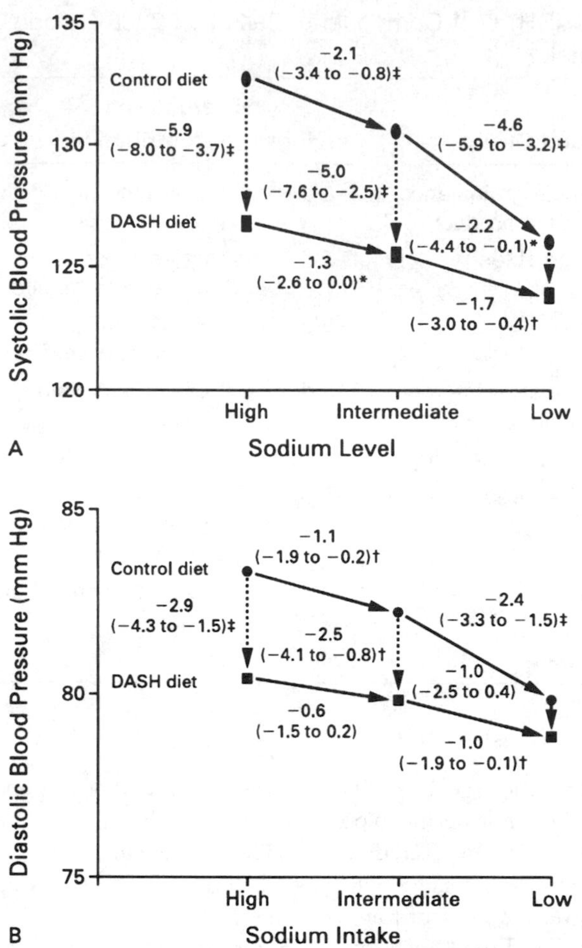

Figure 1. The effect on systolic (A) and diastolic (B) blood pressure of reduced sodium intake with and without the DASH dietary pattern. The mean changes in blood pressure for various levels of sodium intake are represented by the solid arrows. Differences in blood pressure between the control diet and the DASH diet at each level of sodium are represented by the dotted arrows. Mean differences in blood pressure are shown with 95% confidence intervals in parentheses. Asterisks ($P < 0.05$), daggers ($P < 0.01$), and double daggers ($P < 0.001$) indicate significant differences in blood pressure between groups or between dietary sodium categories.

sodium effect associated with the higher potassium intake of the DASH dietary pattern.

The dietary components of the DASH dietary pattern also have health benefits in addition to lowering blood pressure. The high fiber and magnesium content have a significant impact on blood glucose and insulin sensitivity.[82] DASH has been shown to also improve lipid profiles and serum homocysteine,[124,125] likely as a result of its low saturated and total fat and high folate content, respectively. Self-reported quality of life also improved with the DASH intervention.[126]

Behavior Modification

Although a dietary change is efficacious for lowering blood pressure, it is only as effective as the implementation and maintenance of a behavioral change. The health care provider must be consistent in providing brief counseling and support for healthful lifestyle modifications. Even in the span of a brief visit, it may be possible to use some efficient strategies for promoting a behavioral change.[127] The first task is to assess current dietary behavior. A simple 24-hour dietary recall, making sure to include snacks, desserts, and alcoholic and nonalcoholic beverages, can accomplish this step. From this quick survey, one can determine the area of the diet that might be most easily modified to lower blood pressure. The next step is to assess the patient's willingness to change by simply asking the patient whether he or she has considered using or has tried some method other than medication for lowering blood pressure. If the patient answers affirmatively, then potential plans should be explored. This plan should be endorsed and follow-ups scheduled to assess the results of the behavioral change. If the patient does not have a plan but is willing to institute behavioral changes, a strategy should be chosen that the patient considers feasible. Patients who are not ready to make changes should be reminded of the importance of these recommendations at each visit until they are ready. Specific goals and clear timelines should be outlined, and self-monitoring should be encouraged. Expectations should be reasonable, and caregivers should express confidence that the goals can be achieved. Last, a prescription should be written outlining the goals, a strategy to achieve the goals, and a timeline. Giving this "lifestyle prescription" to the patient sends the message that this behavioral intervention is as important as drug therapy.

Impact of Instituting More than One Dietary Intervention

Often it will be necessary to institute more than one dietary intervention because of multiple risk factors, such as in a patient with the metabolic syndrome. Combining interventions has definite advantages, particularly in the highly motivated patient. Synergy between interventions may likely result in greater effects on blood pressure than if using only one intervention alone. A clear example of this is using the DASH dietary pattern as the basis of a weight reduction plan. Because of the high fiber content and low-fat nature of the dietary pattern, the DASH diet is low in energy density, making it an ideal means for facilitating weight reduction. When the DASH diet has been used in a weight loss intervention for men, greater reductions in blood pressure were seen than with a standard low-fat weight loss diet.[128] The PREMIER study, a test of multiple lifestyle interventions for the control of blood pressure, demonstrated that combining all of the nonpharmacological dietary and physical activity interventions can be an effective method for lowering blood pressure in prehypertensive and hypertensive patients.[129] Therefore, despite some of the apparent complexities, lifestyle behavioral change can be successfully implemented and lead to meaningful clinical changes in blood pressure.

Conclusion and Future Directions

Beyond the impact on individual patients, widespread implementation of lifestyle modifications could result in a small decrease in mean blood pressure levels across the population, which could have a highly significant impact on cardiovascular disease outcomes. For example, it is estimated that a population-wide decrease in systolic blood pressure of 5 mmHg would result in a 14% reduction in mortality due to stroke, a 9% reduction in mortality due to coronary heart disease, and a 7% decline in all-cause mortality.[28] The following are at least three facts that underscore the importance of population-wide lifestyle changes to minimize the risk for developing hypertension:

1. Hypertension is permanent in most cases.
2. Many adults are unaware that they have prehypertension.
3. The increase in blood pressure that occurs as people age appears to be lifestyle related.

Further research is needed to determine the most effective methods of implementation on a large-scale population basis. As societies become more industrialized, innovative targets that include the environment and food manufacturing and delivery systems will need to be altered to encourage, achieve, and sustain any beneficial impact on blood pressure and cardiovascular health through lifestyle modification.

References

1. The 1980 Report of the Joint National Committee on Detection, Evaluation, and Treatment of High Blood Pressure. Arch Intern Med. 1980;140(10): 1280–1285.
2. Chobanian AV, Bakris GL, Black HR, et al. The Seventh Report of the Joint National Committee on Prevention, Detection, Evaluation, and Treatment of High Blood Pressure: The JNC 7 report. JAMA. 2003;289(19):2560–2572.
3. Lewington S, Clarke R, Qizilbash N, et al. Age-specific relevance of usual blood pressure to vascular mortality: a meta-analysis of individual data for one million adults in 61 prospective studies. Lancet. 2002;360(9349):1903–1913.
4. Brundtland GH. From the World Health Organization. Reducing risks to health, promoting healthy life. JAMA. 2002;288(16):1974.
5. Murray CJ, Lopez AD. Mortality by cause for eight regions of the world: Global Burden of Disease Study. Lancet. 1997;349(9061):1269–1276.
6. Kearney PM, Whelton M, Reynolds K, et al. Global burden of hypertension: analysis of worldwide data. Lancet. 2005;365(9455):217–223.
7. Wolf-Maier K, Cooper RS, Banegas JR, et al. Hypertension prevalence and blood pressure levels in 6 European countries, Canada, and the United States. JAMA. 2003;289(18):2363–2369.
8. Burt VL, Whelton P, Roccella EJ, et al. Prevalence of hypertension in the U.S. adult population. Results from the Third National Health and Nutrition Examination Survey, 1988–1991. Hypertension. 1995;25(3):305–313.
9. Hajjar I, Kotchen TA. Trends in prevalence, awareness, treatment, and control of hypertension in the United States, 1988–2000. JAMA. 2003;290(2): 199–206.
10. Kotchen TA, Kotchen JM. Regional variations of blood pressure: environment or genes? Circulation. 1997;96(4):1071–1073.
11. Vasan RS, Beiser A, Seshadri S, et al. Residual lifetime risk for developing hypertension in middle-aged women and men: the Framingham Heart Study. JAMA. 2002;287(8):1003–1010.
12. Ferrannini E, Natali A, Capaldo B, et al. Insulin resistance, hyperinsulinemia, and blood pressure: role of age and obesity. European Group for the Study of Insulin Resistance (EGIR). Hypertension. 1997;30(5):1144–1149.
13. Skarfors ET, Lithell HO, Selinus I. Risk factors for the development of hypertension: a 10-year longitudinal study in middle-aged men. J Hypertens. 1991; 9(3):217–223.
14. Lissner L, Bengtsson C, Lapidus L, et al. Fasting insulin in relation to subsequent blood pressure changes and hypertension in women. Hypertension. 1992;20(6):797–801.
15. He J, Klag MJ, Caballero B, et al. Plasma insulin levels and incidence of hypertension in African Americans and whites. Arch Intern Med. 1999; 159(5):498–503.
16. Marigliano A, Tedde R, Sechi LA, et al. Insulinemia and blood pressure. Relationships in patients with primary and secondary hypertension, and with or without glucose metabolism impairment. Am J Hypertens. 1990;3(7):521–526.
17. Zavaroni I, Mazza S, Dall'Aglio E, et al. Prevalence of hyperinsulinaemia in patients with high blood pressure. J Intern Med. 1992;231(3):235–240.
18. Muscelli E, Natali A, Bianchi S, et al. Effect of insulin on renal sodium and uric acid handling in essential hypertension. Am J Hypertens. 1996;9(8): 746–752.
19. DeFronzo RA, Cooke CR, Andres R, et al. The effect of insulin on renal handling of sodium, potassium, calcium, and phosphate in man. J Clin Invest. 1975;55(4):845–855.
20. Facchini FS, DoNascimento C, Reaven GM, et al. Blood pressure, sodium intake, insulin resistance, and urinary nitrate excretion. Hypertension. 1999; 33(4):1008–1012.

21. Paffenbarger RS Jr, Thorne MC, Wing AL. Chronic disease in former college students. VIII. Characteristics in youth predisposing to hypertension in later years. Am J Epidemiol. 1968;88(1): 25–32.
22. Selby JV, Friedman GD, Quesenberry CP Jr. Precursors of essential hypertension: pulmonary function, heart rate, uric acid, serum cholesterol, and other serum chemistries. Am J Epidemiol. 1990; 131(6):1017–1027.
23. Williams B. Insulin resistance: the shape of things to come. Lancet. 1994;344(8921):521–524.
24. Hall JE, Louis K. Dahl Memorial Lecture. Renal and cardiovascular mechanisms of hypertension in obesity. Hypertension. 1994;23(3):381–394.
25. Rocchini AP, Katch V, Kveselis D, et al. Insulin and renal sodium retention in obese adolescents. Hypertension. 1989;14(4):367–374.
26. Steinberg HO, Chaker H, Leaming R, et al. Obesity/insulin resistance is associated with endothelial dysfunction. Implications for the syndrome of insulin resistance. J Clin Invest. 1996;97(11): 2601–2610.
27. Thompson D, Edelsberg J, Colditz GA, et al. Lifetime health and economic consequences of obesity. Arch Intern Med. 1999;159(18):2177–2183.
28. Whelton PK, He J, Appel LJ, et al. Primary prevention of hypertension: clinical and public health advisory from the National High Blood Pressure Education Program. JAMA. 2002;288(15):1882–1888.
29. Wilson PW, D'Agostino RB, Sullivan L, et al. Overweight and obesity as determinants of cardiovascular risk: the Framingham experience. Arch Intern Med. 2002;162(16):1867–1872.
30. Sonne-Holm S, Sorensen TI, Jensen G, et al. Independent effects of weight change and attained body weight on prevalence of arterial hypertension in obese and non-obese men. Br Med J. 1989; 299(6702):767–770.
31. Phillips BG, Narkiewicz K, Pesek CA, et al. Effects of obstructive sleep apnea on endothelin-1 and blood pressure. J Hypertens. 1999;17(1):61–66.
32. Goodfriend TL, Calhoun DA. Resistant hypertension, obesity, sleep apnea, and aldosterone: theory and therapy. Hypertension. 2004;43(3):518–524.
33. Becker HF, Jerrentrup A, Ploch T, et al. Effect of nasal continuous positive airway pressure treatment on blood pressure in patients with obstructive sleep apnea. Circulation. 2003;107(1):68–73.
34. Aizawa-Abe M, Ogawa Y, Masuzaki H, et al. Pathophysiological role of leptin in obesity-related hypertension. J Clin Invest. 2000;105(9):1243–1252.
35. Agata J, Masuda A, Takada M, et al. High plasma immunoreactive leptin level in essential hypertension. Am J Hypertens. 1997;10(10 Pt 1): 1171–1174.
36. Oliver WJ, Cohen EL, Neel JV. Blood pressure, sodium intake, and sodium related hormones in the Yanomamo Indians, a "no-salt" culture. Circulation. 1975;52(1):146–151.
37. Beevers DG, Hawthorne VM, Padfield PL. Salt and blood pressure in Scotland. Br Med J. 1980; 281(6241):641–642.
38. Harlan WR, Harlan LC. An epidemiological perspective on dietary electrolytes and hypertension. J Hypertens Suppl. 1986;4(5):S334–S339.
39. Frisancho AR, Leonard WR, Bollettino LA. Blood pressure in blacks and whites and its relationship to dietary sodium and potassium intake. J Chronic Dis. 1984;37(7):515–519.
40. Yamori Y, Kihara M, Fujikawa J, et al. Dietary risk factors of stroke and hypertension in Japan—part 3: comparative study on risk factors between farming and fishing villages in Japan. Jpn Circ J. 1982; 46(9):944–947.
41. Sasaki N. High blood pressure and the salt intake of the Japanese. Jpn Heart J. 1962;3:313–324.
42. INTERSALT Study: an international co-operative study on the relation of blood pressure to electrolyte excretion in populations. I. Design and methods. The INTERSALT Co-operative Research Group. J Hypertens. 1986;4(6):781–787.
43. INTERSALT: an international study of electrolyte excretion and blood pressure. Results for 24 hour urinary sodium and potassium excretion. INTERSALT Cooperative Research Group. Br Med J. 1988;297(6644):319–328.
44. Sugden AL, Straw JA, Bean BL. Effects of a high K+/low Na+ diet on blood pressure in young spontaneously hypertensive rats. Clin Sci (Lond). 1987;72(3):313–319.
45. Louis WJ, Tabei R, Spector S. Effects of sodium intake on inherited hypertension in the rat. Lancet. 1971;2(7737):1283–1286.
46. Parfrey PS, Vandenburg MJ, Wright P, et al. Blood pressure and hormonal changes following alteration in dietary sodium and potassium in mild essential hypertension. Lancet. 1981;1(8211):59–63.
47. Skrabal F, Aubock J, Hortnagl H. Low sodium/high potassium diet for prevention of hypertension: probable mechanisms of action. Lancet. 1981; 2(8252):895–900.
48. Tannen RL. Effects of potassium on blood pressure control. Ann Intern Med. 1983;98(5 Pt 2): 773–780.
49. Vander AJ. Direct effects of potassium on renin secretion and renal function. Am J Physiol. 1970; 219(2):455–459.
50. Kahn M, Bohrer NK. Effect of potassium-induced diuresis on renal concentration and dilution. Am J Physiol. 1967;212(6):1365–1375.
51. Tabuchi Y, Ogihara T, Gotoh S, et al. Hypotensive mechanism of potassium supplementation in salt-

loaded patients with essential hypertension. J Clin Hypertens. 1985;1(2):145–152.
52. MacGregor GA, Smith SJ, Markandu ND, et al. Moderate potassium supplementation in essential hypertension. Lancet. 1982;2(8298):567–570.
53. Carvalho J, Baruzzi R, Howard P, et al. Blood pressure in four remote populations in the INTERSALT Study. Hypertension. 1989;14(3): 238–246.
54. Poulter NR, Khaw KT, Hopwood BE, et al. The Kenyan Luo migration study: observations on the initiation of a rise in blood pressure. Br Med J. 1990; 300(6730):967–972.
55. Denton D, Weisinger R, Mundy NI, et al. The effect of increased salt intake on blood pressure of chimpanzees. Nat Med. 1995;1(10):1009–1016.
56. Geleijnse JM, Hofman A, Witteman JC, et al. Long-term effects of neonatal sodium restriction on blood pressure. Hypertension. 1997;29(4):913–917.
57. Weinberger MH. Salt sensitivity of blood pressure in humans. Hypertension. 1996;27(3 Pt 2): 481–490.
58. Johnson RJ, Herrera-Acosta J, Schreiner GF, et al. Subtle acquired renal injury as a mechanism of salt-sensitive hypertension. N Engl J Med. 2002; 346(12):913–923.
59. Siffert W, Dusing R. Sodium-proton exchange and primary hypertension. An update. Hypertension. 1995;26(4):649–655.
60. Iwamoto T, Kita S, Zhang J, et al. Salt-sensitive hypertension is triggered by Ca2+ entry via Na+/Ca2+ exchanger type-1 in vascular smooth muscle. Nat Med. 2004;10(11):1193–1199.
61. Cusi D, Barlassina C, Azzani T, et al. Polymorphisms of alpha-adducin and salt sensitivity in patients with essential hypertension. Lancet. 1997; 349(9062):1353–1357.
62. Oparil S, Zaman MA, Calhoun DA. Pathogenesis of hypertension. Ann Intern Med. 2003;139(9): 761–776.
63. Carretero OA, Oparil S. Essential hypertension. Part I: definition and etiology. Circulation. 2000; 101(3):329–335.
64. Hunt SC, Cook NR, Oberman A, et al. Angiotensinogen genotype, sodium reduction, weight loss, and prevention of hypertension: trials of hypertension prevention, phase II. Hypertension. 1998; 32(3):393–401.
65. Vasan RS, Larson MG, Leip EP, et al. Impact of high-normal blood pressure on the risk of cardiovascular disease. N Engl J Med. 2001;345(18): 1291–1297.
66. Whelton PK. Challenges and evolving contributions of epidemiology in nephrology and hypertension. Curr Opin Nephrol Hypertens. 1996;5(3): 203–204.
67. Klag MJ, Whelton PK, Randall BL, et al. Blood pressure and end-stage renal disease in men. N Engl J Med. 1996;334(1):13–18.
68. Perry HM Jr, Miller JP, Fornoff JR, et al. Early predictors of 15-year end-stage renal disease in hypertensive patients. Hypertension. 1995;25(4 Pt 1): 587–594.
69. Haffner SM, Lehto S, Ronnemaa T, et al. Mortality from coronary heart disease in subjects with type 2 diabetes and in nondiabetic subjects with and without prior myocardial infarction. N Engl J Med. 1998;339(4):229–234.
70. Reaven GM, Lithell H, Landsberg L. Hypertension and associated metabolic abnormalities—the role of insulin resistance and the sympathoadrenal system. N Engl J Med. 1996;334(6):374–381.
71. Executive Summary of The Third Report of The National Cholesterol Education Program (NCEP) Expert Panel on Detection, Evaluation, And Treatment of High Blood Cholesterol In Adults (Adult Treatment Panel III). JAMA. 2001;285(19): 2486–2497.
72. Anderson KM, Wilson PW, Odell PM, et al. An updated coronary risk profile. A statement for health professionals. Circulation. 1991;83(1):356–362.
73. Chobanian AV, Bakris GL, Black HR, et al. The Seventh Report of the Joint National Committee on Prevention, Detection, Evaluation, and Treatment of High Blood Pressure: the JNC 7 report [see comment][erratum appears in JAMA. 2003;9; 290(2):197]. JAMA. 2003;289(19):2560–2572.
74. Whelton SP, Chin A, Xin X, et al. Effect of aerobic exercise on blood pressure: a meta-analysis of randomized, controlled trials. Ann Intern Med. 2002; 136(7):493–503.
75. Anonymous. The Sixth Report of the Joint National Committee on Prevention, Detection, Evaluation, and Treatment of High Blood Pressure. Arch Intern Med. 1997;157(21):2413–2446.
76. The ALLHAT Officers and Coordinators for the ALLHAT Collaborative Research Group. Major Outcomes in High-Risk Hypertensive Patients Randomized to Angiotensin-Converting Enzyme Inhibitor or Calcium Channel Blocker vs Diuretic: The Antihypertensive and Lipid-Lowering Treatment to Prevent Heart Attack Trial (ALLHAT). JAMA. 2002;288(23):2981–2997.
77. Hansson L, Zanchetti A, Carruthers SG, et al. Effects of intensive blood-pressure lowering and low-dose aspirin in patients with hypertension: principal results of the Hypertension Optimal Treatment (HOT) randomised trial. HOT Study Group. Lancet. 1998;351(9118):1755–1762.
78. The Expert Committee on the Diagnosis and Classification of Diabetes Mellitus. Follow-up report on

the diagnosis of diabetes mellitus. Diabetes Care. 2003;26(11):3160–3167.

79. Gress TW, Nieto FJ, Shahar E, et al. The Atherosclerosis Risk in Communities Study. Hypertension and antihypertensive therapy as risk factors for type 2 diabetes mellitus. N Engl J Med. 2000;342(13): 905–912.
80. Verdecchia P, Reboldi G, Angeli F, et al. Adverse prognostic significance of new diabetes in treated hypertensive subjects. Hypertension. 2004;43(5): 963–969.
81. Bakris GL, Sowers JR. When does new onset diabetes resulting from antihypertensive therapy increase cardiovascular risk? Hypertension. 2004;43(5): 941–942.
82. Ard JD, Grambow SC, Liu D, et al. The effect of the PREMIER interventions on insulin sensitivity. Diabetes Care. 2004;27(2):340–347.
83. Cohn JN, Kowey PR, Whelton PK, et al. New Guidelines for Potassium Replacement in Clinical Practice: a contemporary review by the National Council on Potassium in Clinical Practice. Arch Intern Med. 2000;160(16):2429–2436.
84. Mattes R. The taste for salt in humans. Am J Clin Nutr. 1997;65(2):692S–697S.
85. Loria CM, Obarzanek E, Ernst ND. Choose and prepare foods with less salt: dietary advice for all Americans. J Nutr. 2001;131(2S-1):536S–551S.
86. Zhou BF, Stamler J, Dennis B, et al. Nutrient intakes of middle-aged men and women in China, Japan, United Kingdom, and United States in the late 1990s: the INTERMAP study. J Hum Hypertens. 2003;17(9):623–630.
87. Institute of Medicine (U.S.). Panel on Dietary Reference Intakes for Electrolytes and Water. *DRI, Dietary Reference Intakes for Water, Potassium, Sodium, Chloride, and Sulfate.* Washington, DC: National Academies Press; 2004.
88. U.S. Department of Health and Human Services, U.S. Department of Agriculture. Dietary Guidelines Advisory Committee. *Dietary Guidelines for Americans, 2005,* 6th ed. Washington, DC: G.P.O.; 2005 HHS publication; no. HHS-ODPHP-2005-01-DGA-A.
89. Kumanyika SK, Cutler JA. Dietary sodium reduction: is there cause for concern? J Am Coll Nutr. 1997;16(3):192–203.
90. Sacks FM, Svetkey LP, Vollmer WM, et al. Effects on blood pressure of reduced dietary sodium and the Dietary Approaches to Stop Hypertension (DASH) diet. DASH-Sodium Collaborative Research Group. N Engl J Med. 2001;344(1):3–10.
91. Vollmer WM, Sacks FM, Ard J, et al. Effects of diet and sodium intake on blood pressure: subgroup analysis of the DASH-sodium trial. Ann Intern Med. 2001;135(12):1019–1028.
92. Anonymous. Effects of weight loss and sodium reduction intervention on blood pressure and hypertension incidence in overweight people with high-normal blood pressure. The Trials of Hypertension Prevention, Phase II. The Trials of Hypertension Prevention Collaborative Research Group. Arch Intern Med. 1997;157(6):657–667.
93. Appel LJ, Espeland MA, Easter L, et al. Effects of reduced sodium intake on hypertension control in older individuals: results from the Trial of Nonpharmacologic Interventions in the Elderly (TONE). Arch Intern Med. 2001;161(5):685–693.
94. Cutler JA, Follmann D, Allender PS. Randomized trials of sodium reduction: an overview. Am J Clin Nutr. 1997;65(2 Suppl):643S–651S.
95. Hooper L, Bartlett C, Davey Smith G, et al. Systematic review of long term effects of advice to reduce dietary salt in adults. Br Med J. 2002; 325(7365):628.
96. Klatsky A, Friedman G, Siegelaub A, et al. Alcohol consumption and blood pressure Kaiser-Permanente Multiphasic Health Examination data. N Engl J Med. 1977;296(21):1194–1200.
97. Fuchs FD, Chambless LE, Whelton PK, et al. Alcohol consumption and the incidence of hypertension: The Atherosclerosis Risk in Communities Study. Hypertension. 2001;37(5):1242–1250.
98. Puddey IB, Beilin LJ, Vandongen R, et al. Evidence for a direct effect of alcohol consumption on blood pressure in normotensive men. A randomized controlled trial. Hypertension. 1985;7(5):707–713.
99. Klatsky AL. Alcohol-associated hypertension: when one drinks makes a difference. Hypertension. 2004;44(6):805–806.
100. Stranges S, Wu T, Dorn JM, et al. Relationship of alcohol drinking pattern to risk of hypertension: a population-based study. Hypertension. 2004;44(6): 813–819.
101. Trevisan M, Krogh V, Farinaro E, et al. Alcohol consumption, drinking pattern and blood pressure: analysis of data from the Italian National Research Council Study. Int J Epidemiol. 1987;16(4): 520–527.
102. Marques-Vidal P, Arveiler D, Evans A, et al. Different alcohol drinking and blood pressure relationships in France and Northern Ireland: The PRIME Study. Hypertension. 2001;38(6):1361–1366.
103. Zilkens RR, Burke V, Hodgson JM, et al. Red wine and beer elevate blood pressure in normotensive men. Hypertension. 2005;45(5):874–879.
104. Cushman WC, Cutler JA, Hanna E, et al. Prevention and Treatment of Hypertension Study (PATHS): effects of an alcohol treatment program on blood pressure. Arch Intern Med. 1998;158(11): 1197–1207.
105. Xin X, He J, Frontini MG, et al. Effects of alcohol reduction on blood pressure: a meta-analysis of ran-

domized controlled trials. Hypertension. 2001; 38(5):1112–1117.

106. World Health Organization. *Obesity: Preventing and Managing the Global Epidemic: Report of a WHO Consultation.* Geneva: World Health Organization; 2000.
107. Mulrow CD, Chiquette E, Angel L, et al. Dieting to reduce body weight for controlling hypertension in adults. Cochrane Database Syst Rev. 2000;2: CD000484.
108. Staessen J, Fagard R, Amery A. The relationship between body weight and blood pressure. J Hum Hypertens. 1988;2(4):207–217.
109. Anonymous. The effects of nonpharmacologic interventions on blood pressure of persons with high normal levels. Results of the Trials of Hypertension Prevention, Phase I. JAMA. 1992;267(9):1213–1220.
110. Stevens VJ, Obarzanek E, Cook NR, et al. Long-term weight loss and changes in blood pressure: results of the Trials of Hypertension Prevention, Phase II. Ann Intern Med. 2001;134(1):1–11.
111. Neter JE, Stam BE, Kok FJ, et al. Influence of weight reduction on blood pressure: a meta-analysis of randomized controlled trials. Hypertension. 2003;42(5):878–884.
112. Stevens VJ, Corrigan SA, Obarzanek E, et al. Weight loss intervention in phase 1 of the Trials of Hypertension Prevention. The TOHP Collaborative Research Group. Arch Intern Med. 1993; 153(7):849–858.
113. Aucott L, Poobalan A, Smith WC, et al. Effects of weight loss in overweight/obese individuals and long-term hypertension outcomes: a systematic review. Hypertension. 2005;45(6):1035–1041.
114. Moore LL, Visioni AJ, Qureshi MM, et al. Weight loss in overweight adults and the long-term risk of hypertension: the Framingham Study. Arch Intern Med. 2005;165(11):1298–1303.
115. Whelton PK, He J, Cutler JA, et al. Effects of oral potassium on blood pressure. Meta-analysis of randomized controlled clinical trials. JAMA. 1997; 277(20):1624–1632.
116. Allender PS, Cutler JA, Follmann D, et al. Dietary calcium and blood pressure: a meta-analysis of randomized clinical trials. Ann Intern Med. 1996; 124(9):825–831.
117. Bucher HC, Cook RJ, Guyatt GH, et al. Effects of dietary calcium supplementation on blood pressure. A meta-analysis of randomized controlled trials. JAMA. 1996;275(13):1016–1022.
118. Sacks FM, Brown LE, Appel L, et al. Combinations of potassium, calcium, and magnesium supplements in hypertension. Hypertension. 1995;26(6): 950–956.
119. Sacks FM, Rosner B, Kass EH. Blood pressure in vegetarians. Am J Epidemiol. 1974;100(5):390–398.
120. Sacks FM, Obarzanek E, Windhauser MM, et al. Rationale and design of the Dietary Approaches to Stop Hypertension trial (DASH). A multicenter controlled-feeding study of dietary patterns to lower blood pressure. Ann Epidemiol. 1995;5(2):108–118.
121. Karanja NM, Obarzanek E, Lin PH, et al. Descriptive characteristics of the dietary patterns used in the Dietary Approaches to Stop Hypertension Trial. DASH Collaborative Research Group. J Am Diet Assoc. 1999;99(8 Suppl):S19–S27.
122. Appel LJ, Moore TJ, Obarzanek E, et al. A clinical trial of the effects of dietary patterns on blood pressure. DASH Collaborative Research Group. N Engl J Med. 1997;336(16):1117–1124.
123. Svetkey LP, Simons-Morton D, Vollmer WM, et al. Effects of dietary patterns on blood pressure: subgroup analysis of the Dietary Approaches to Stop Hypertension (DASH) randomized clinical trial. Arch Intern Med. 1999;159(3):285–293.
124. Obarzanek E, Sacks FM, Vollmer WM, et al. Effects on blood lipids of a blood pressure-lowering diet: the Dietary Approaches to Stop Hypertension (DASH) Trial. Am J Clin Nutr. 2001;74(1):80–89.
125. Appel LJ, Miller ER III, Jee SH, et al. Effect of dietary patterns on serum homocysteine: results of a randomized, controlled feeding study. Circulation. 2000;102(8):852–857.
126. Plaisted CS, Lin PH, Ard JD, et al. The effects of dietary patterns on quality of life: a substudy of the Dietary Approaches to Stop Hypertension trial. J Am Diet Assoc. 1999;99(8 Suppl):S84–S89.
127. Ard JD, Svetkey LP. Diet and blood pressure: applying the evidence to clinical practice. Am Heart J. 2005;149(5):804–812.
128. Nowson CA, Worsley A, Margerison C, et al. Blood pressure change with weight loss is affected by diet type in men. Am J Clin Nutr. 2005;81(5): 983–989.
129. Appel LJ, Champagne CM, Harsha DW, et al. Effects of comprehensive lifestyle modification on blood pressure control: main results of the PREMIER clinical trial. JAMA. 2003;289(16): 2083–2093.

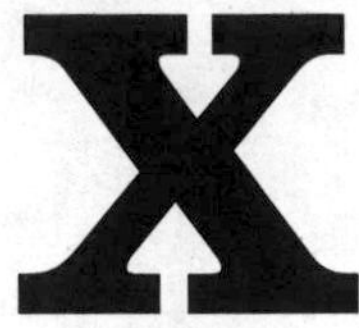

Diet, Food, and Nutrition

57
Food Composition

Joanne M. Holden, James M. Harnly, and Gary R. Beecher

Introduction

"A knowledge of the chemical composition of foods is the first essential in dietary treatment of disease or in any quantitative study of human nutrition."

—McCance and Widdowson,[1] 1940

Human nutrition programs encompass many aspects of science and education, including metabolic and epidemiological research, dietary treatment of disease, dietary guidance for healthy individuals, and planning and implementation of national nutrition policy. Programs oriented toward dietary guidance and disease prevention[2-4] have encouraged consumer demand for healthful foods. Worldwide food-labeling programs have brought information on the composition of foods into every household. New research relating minor, non-nutrient components to the risk reduction of many chronic diseases has brought foods and dietary supplements closer together. The result is an increasing demand by researchers, health professionals, policy makers, and the general public for reliable information on the composition of foods.

The US Department of Agriculture (USDA) has had the responsibility of characterizing and providing information on the nutrient content of the US national food supply for over 100 years. The first US food composition tables were published in 1891 by Atwater and Woods,[5] who assayed the refuse, water, fat, protein, ash, and carbohydrate content of about 200 different foods in their laboratory at the Connecticut Agricultural Experiment Station. Since that first publication, food composition tables for US foods have continuously expanded in both the number and type of foods and the number of food components. Today, food composition data are electronically stored and disseminated, placing an even larger demand on the extent and completeness of this information.[6]

"Food composition" is an all-inclusive term. In the broadest sense, food components may refer to traditional nutrients and other health-related components, as well as radionuclides, pesticide residues, direct and indirect additives, and other constituents that may provide functional properties. Historically, "nutrient" composition databases have been compiled. These databases listed only those components considered to be essential nutrients. Today, many nonnutrient dietary components are recognized to have a positive effect on human health. These components, primarily in fruits and vegetables, have been called "phytonutrients," "secondary metabolites," or "environmental compounds."[7] Examples include carotenoids, flavonoids, isoflavones, proanthocyanidins, and an ever-growing list of previously ignored compounds. As a result, food composition databases now include nutrients and other health-promoting components. Although the concentration of such components as radionuclides, pesticide residues, and heavy metals are routinely monitored, these data are not tabulated as part of food composition databases in the United States.

Development of food composition databases is a difficult and complex undertaking. In addition to the increased number of components described previously, there are the continuous introduction of new foods, product-line expansions, and the increasing complexity of food matrices. New analytical technology offers the advantages of improved speed, sensitivity, and accuracy, but may render previous data obsolete. Foods are a biological phenomenon. The concentration of any component in a specific food can vary from sample to sample depending on plant breed, cultivar, geographical location, and climate. Variability may be exacerbated with prepared foods in that composition can vary with brand name, product formulation, and changes in fortification. Finally, variations can be introduced by the analytical process; variability and bias can be affected by sample selection, sample handling, operator expertise, analytical methodology, and instrumentation.

Food composition data are estimates for levels of components in foods; when these estimates are statistical estimates derived from analytical data, the variance can be as informative as the mean. When appropriately used, food composition data can support nutrition assessment, nutrition research, and policy development for large groups and populations. Although values obtained from nationally representative databases may be used for preliminary planning for studies of individuals, they are not appropriate for use as definitive estimates of an individual's nutrient intake in metabolic or clinical settings.

This chapter is an overview of the status of knowledge on the composition of foods. A discussion of the elements, approaches, and programs that are in place for the assurance of this important national resource is also presented.

Food Composition Data Products

The Nutrient Data Laboratory (NDL) of the Agricultural Research Service, USDA, is responsible for maintaining the National Nutrient Data Bank (NDB) in the United States. The NDB, as the national reference for authoritative food composition data, maintains the considerable documentation related to the acquisition of data for individual foods and components, including the source and quality of the data, individual observations, analytical and statistical methods, algorithms, and factors for generating and calculating values. The NDB is used to produce the Nutrient Database for Standard Reference (SR) as well as small, special-interest databases for specific components.[6,8-11] In addition, NDL uses the data to calculate values for other foods, especially formulated foods. The data are largely based on the chemical analysis of representative food samples, and are acquired from the food industry, scientific literature, other government programs, and USDA-initiated contracts.

Nutrient Database for Standard Reference

The SR database is the primary source of food composition data for the United States. It contains data for over 7100 food items and more than 130 food components. The SR is updated annually; SR-Release 18 was distributed in 2005.[6] The SR is available from NDL at a website (http://www.ars.usda.gov/nutrientdata) maintained and supported by the National Agriculture Library. Latest statistics indicate that the website is being accessed at a rate of about 100,000 user sessions each month. More than 1500 other websites link to the NDL site. The SR is also released on CD-ROM, which is available from the government printing office. Data in the SR are used as the foundation for virtually all other food composition databases within the United States, including those in other government agencies, the food industry, and health care sectors. The SR has come to be regarded as the "benchmark" for values for many foods. The SR is also used to develop the nutrient values for all US nutrition monitoring programs, especially the National Health and Nutrition Examination Survey: What We Eat in America.[31]

Special Interest Databases

The special interest databases are developed for single components (e.g., fluoride) or classes of components (e.g., individual flavonoids) from a limited number of foods to provide seminal databases for research, education, and nutrition policy applications. The data are collected from the literature or generated by state-of-the-art analytical methods in government, industry, or academic laboratories. For example, interest in phytonutrients stimulated the development and release of databases for individual flavonoids and isoflavones. Also, databases for choline, proanthocyanidins, fluoride, and omega-3 fatty acids (update) have been recently completed or are under development.[8-11] As data for specific components accumulate, the databases may be moved directly into the SR database. More information about specific databases is available at http://www.ars.usda.gov/nutrientdata. Since their introduction in the 1990s, data for individual carotenoids, selenium, and vitamin K have been expanded sufficiently to permit their migration into the SR.

Global Databases

Countries all over the world have come to recognize the necessity of developing and maintaining food composition data for national and regional food supplies. The International Network of Food Data Systems of the Food and Agriculture Organization of the United Nations was created in 1984 to encourage the development of worldwide food composition databases.[13] The International Network of Food Data Systems coordinates the training and research to support this effort and maintains a website (http://www.fao.org/infoods) that includes a directory of national and international food composition databases. Unfortunately, the scientific and public interest in food composition has not been matched by funding levels in many countries. Today, over one-half of the food composition data entries in international food composition applications are still adopted from the databases of the United States or United Kingdom. This, however, is rapidly changing. In recent years, many other countries (e.g., Thailand, South Africa, Brazil, People's Republic of China) and regions (e.g., Latin America, Asia) have recognized the importance of having unique food composition data for their own foods and have initiated the development of their own databases.

Status of Food Composition Data

Sources of Data

Food composition data for the United States are obtained primarily from five sources: the food industry, USDA-initiated contracts, other government programs, scientific literature, and imputed data. The data for a specific food can vary significantly between and within sources with respect to quantity and quality.

The food industry and trade associations represent an important source of data for the USDA. Manufacturers typically collect data for up to 14 nutrients, as required by the US Nutrition Labeling and Education Program.[14] Additional data may be collected as part of internal quality assurance programs and research to characterize the content of their own and their competitors' products. Trade associations often collect data or contract for analyses to promote their members' products. Completeness of the data may be an issue; for example, some manufacturers may be willing to share mean values but not variance or specific procedures used to generate the data. These shortcomings not withstanding, the source of data is especially important because food product formulations change often and quickly.

The most direct way for NDL to collect food composition data is to contract for the analysis of specific components in individual or mixed foods. This approach is dependent on the existence of appropriate analytical methodology (Figure 1). Using this approach, NDL designs a nationally representative sampling plan, contracts for the sample pickup, and oversees the sample handling, including homogenization of the samples and analysis of desired constituents (see discussion of National Food and Nutrient Analysis Program later in chapter). This approach is the most expensive method, but it offers maximum control over sampling, sample handling, quality assurance, and statistical treatment of the data.

Other government agencies produce food composition data that can be incorporated into the USDA database. The Food Composition Laboratory, which develops analytical methods and works closely with NDL to acquire needed data for the database, performs limited analyses to validate methods and produces more extensive data as requested by NDL. Food composition data are also produced by the US Food and Drug Administration (Total Diet Survey)[15] and by the Food Safety and Inspection Service of USDA (validation of content of meat and meat products).

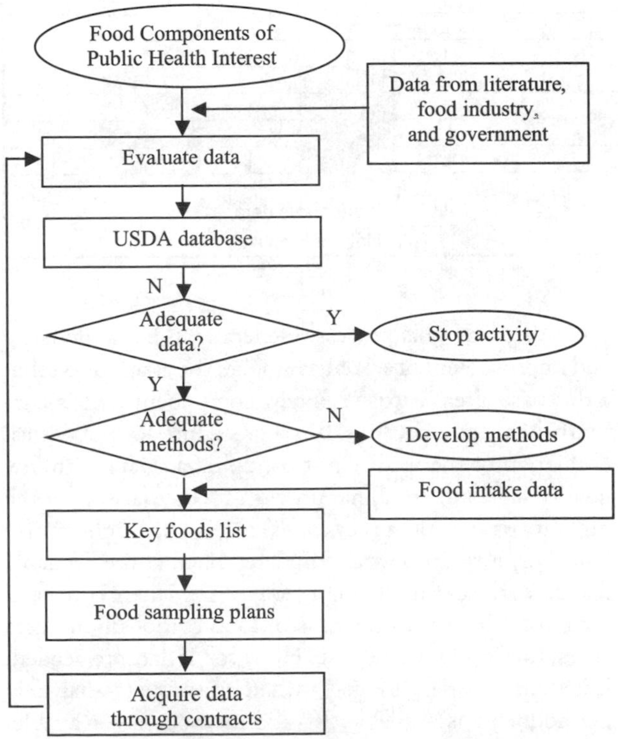

Figure 1. Critical steps in the development of new and updated existing food composition databases.

The scientific literature for research conducted in such disciplines as natural product chemistry, horticulture, pharmacology, animal production, food science, and food technology has been a source of considerable food composition data. These data can be seminal, offering the first recognition of specific components, and are almost always obtained for a purpose other than supporting a database. Consequently, the fact that many of these data are obtained for a very limited number and type of samples is not surprising. The data are often problematic with respect to sampling, sample handling, analytical methodology, quality assurance, and statistical treatment.

Data for some foods and nutrients may be imputed by calculation using standardized procedures. This may be necessary for formulated, multi-ingredient foods, for highly similar foods, for foods made according to recipes, for foods fortified to meet federal standards, or for foods of limited economical impact.

Current Status of Food Composition Data

The staff of NDL reviewed the status of data for each of 24 food types. The food categories correspond to the groupings used in the NDB. Critical elements of the status of data include: 1) the currency of the data, 2) the nature and extent of any food changes, 3) the extent or representativeness of the initial sampling program, and 4) the use of new or modified methods to measure those nutrients and other components in foods. The results of this evaluation are shown in Tables 1 to 4. The food components include the traditional nutrients and newly recognized components that may have health-promoting effects. Although such tables generate considerable discussion as to the accuracy of the evaluation, they provide a broad overview for assessing completeness of the database and establishing program priorities.

For the most part, data for many components of basic foodstuffs, that is, vegetables, cereal grains, and various meats (beef, pork, and lamb), were found to be current. In view of the more extensive food sampling plans that have been instituted, data for the basic foodstuffs are being examined to determine whether the mean values are still representative. Specifically, nutrient data for meat cuts have been revised three to four times since 1975 to reflect the decreasing proportion of fat trim. However, new data for poultry products are needed. Nutrient data for the myriad of processed meat and poultry products are needed. Formulated foods change quickly in the marketplace, and much of the data for these foods, collected only a few years ago, is being replaced. Because many of these values represent samples analyzed over 15 years ago, new values are needed to monitor the existing values, and,

Table 1. Protein, Lipid, Carbohydrate, and Fiber Contents of Common Foods

Food type	Sub-type	Total protein	Total fat	Fatty acids	Individual sugars	Starch	Dietary fiber	Choles-terol	Other sterols	Trans fatty acids	Common amino acid
Baby foods		S	S	L	L	L	S	L	I	I	S
Baked products	Bread	S	S	L	I	L	L	I	I	L	L
	Sweet goods	L	L	L	I	I	I	I	I	I	I
	Cookies/crackers	L	L	L	I	I	I	I	I	I	I
Beverages		I	I	I	I	I					I
Breakfast cereals		S	S	L	I	I	S	I	I	I	I
Candies		I	I	I	I	I	I	L	I	I	I
Cereal grains	Whole	S	S	L	L	I	L		L		S
	Flour	S	S	L	L	I	L		L		S
	Pasta	S	S	L	L	I	L		I		S
Dairy products		S	S	S	S			S			S
Eggs/egg products		S	S	S				S			S
Fast foods		L	L	I	I	I	I	I	I	L	L
Fats and oils			S	S				L	L	L	
Fish and shellfish	Raw	S	S	S				S	L		S
	Cooked	S	S	S				S	L		I
Frozen dinners		I	I	I	I	I	I	I	I	I	I
Fruits	Raw	S	S	L	S	I	L		L		I
	Cooked	L	L	I	L	I	L		I		I
	Frozen/canned	S	S	I	L	I	L		I		I
Infant formula		S	S	L	L	I	L	L	I	I	S
Institutional food		I	I	I	I	I	I	I	I	I	I
Legumes	Raw	S	S	S	I	I	L		L		S
	Cooked	S	S	S	I	I	L		I		S
	Processed	S	S	S	I	I	L				S
Meat	Beef	S	S	S				S	I	I	S
	Lamb	S	S	S				S		I	S
	Pork	S	S	S				S		I	S
	Processed*	S	S	L	I			S		I	L
	Veal	S	S	S				S		I	S
Mixed dishes	Commercial	I	I	I	I	I	I	I	I	I	I
	Home prepared	I	I	I	I	I	I	I	I	I	I
Nuts and seeds		S	S	S	L	I	L	S	L		L
Poultry**		L	L	L		L	L	L		I	L
Restaurant food		I	I	I	I	I	I	I	I	I	I
Snack foods		S	S	L	L	L	L	L	L	I	L
Soups		I	I	I	I	I	I	I	I	I	I
Vegetables	Raw	S	S	L	L	I	L		L		I
	Cooked	S	S	I	L	I	L		I		I
	Frozen	S	S	I	L	I	L		I		I
	Canned	S	S	I	L	I	L		I		I

* Under revision
** Needs revision

S Substantial data
L Limited data
I Inadequate data
(shaded) Not applicable

when necessary, the existing values will be replaced. Since folate fortification of cereal grains, pasta, and rice was initiated in 1998, NDL has been analyzing folic acid and food folate levels in foods to generate current values for many foods that contain grains as ingredients, as well as the foods themselves.[16] However, some values for related foods may be calculated because available resources do not permit the analysis of all foods.

Maintenance and Improvement of Food Composition Databases

The design of programs to complete and systematically update food composition databases is complex and iterative. Figure 1 illustrates several critical steps of a logical progression for this process. Generally, the maintenance and improvement of a database makes the assumption that a database already exists. A new component that is currently being added to NDB is a procedure for the critical evaluation of the quality of existing data. Data with low quality scores in combination with foods that supply the majority of a nutrient (key foods) receive the highest analytical priority for new and updated data. If the available database is assessed as being adequate, then there is no need for improvement. In the case of food composition databases, this is seldom the case. However, if data are needed, it is then necessary to assess whether adequate analytical methodology is available. If valid methods are available, then analyses of representative food samples can be purchased from commercial laboratories or obtained through

Table 2. Vitamin Contents of Common Foods

Food type	Sub-type	Vit A	Thiamin	Riboflavin	Vit B12	Folate	Vit D	Vit E	Pantothenic acid
Baby foods		S	S	S	L	L	L	L	I
Baked products	Bread	I	L	L	L	L	I	I	L
	Sweet goods	I	L	L	L	L	I	I	L
	Cookies/crackers	I	L	L	L	L	I	I	L
Beverages		I	I	I	I	L			L
Breakfast cereals		S	S	S	S	L	L	L	I
Candies		L	L	L	I	L		I	L
Cereal grains	Whole	L	S	S		L		L	L
	Flour		S	S		L		L	L
	Pasta		S	S		L		L	L
Dairy products		S	S	S	S	L	L	L	S
Eggs/egg products		S	S	S	S	L	I	S	S
Fast foods		I	L	L	I	I	I	I	I
Fats and oils		I					L	L	
Fish and shellfish	Raw	L	L	L	L	L	L	L	L
	Cooked	I	I	I	I	L	L	L	L
Frozen dinners		I	I	I	I	I	I	I	I
Fruits	Raw	S	S	S		L		L	L
	Cooked	L	L	L		L		I	L
	Frozen/canned	L	S	L		L		I	L
Infant formula		S	S	S	S	S	L	S	L
Institutional food		I	I	I	I	I	I	I	I
Legumes	Raw	L	S	S		S		S	S
	Cooked	I	S	S		S		S	S
	Processed	L	L	L		I		L	I
Meat	Beef	S	S	S	S	L	L	L	L
	Lamb	L	S	S	S	L	L	L	L
	Pork	L	S	S	S	L	L	L	L
	Processed*	L	S	S	L	L	L	L	L
	Veal	L	S	S	S	S	L	L	L
Mixed dishes	Commercial	I	I	I	I	I	I	I	I
	Home prepared	I	I	I	I	I	I	I	I
Nuts and seeds		L	L	L		L	L	L	L
Poultry**		L	L	L	L	L	L	L	L
Restaurant food		I	I	I	I	I	I	I	
Snack foods		L	L	L	L	L	L	L	L
Soups		I	I	I	I	I		I	I
Vegetables	Raw	S	S	S		L		L	L
	Cooked	L	L	L		L		L	L
	Frozen	S	S	S		L		I	L
	Canned	S	S	S		L		I	L

* Under revision
** Needs revision

S Substantial data
L Limited data
I Inadequate data
(shaded) Not applicable

collaboration with academia, government agencies, or the food industry. USDA scientists have developed procedures for the selection of the most highly qualified analytical contractors. If analytical methods are not available, then it is necessary to initiate the development of appropriate methodology.

Evaluation of Data

Several factors have been recognized as contributing to the quality of food composition data.[17,18] As a result, systematic protocols have been developed. First, manual procedures were devised,[17,18] but ultimately a multifaceted, computer-driven expert system approach was developed.[19] The general approach included the development of categories to evaluate sampling, sample handling, number of samples, analytical methodology, and analytical quality control. The manual system was initially used to evaluate the available data on selenium.[18] Later, an expert system, SELEX, was created using artificial intelligence technology to automate the evaluation process.[19] It has been demonstrated that this system can be tailored to any specific nutrient or component in foods. This system has been applied to copper, carotenoid, and vitamin K data.[20-23] More recently, data for flavonoids, proanthocyanidins, and fluoride have been evaluated by a modified system that evolved from the original approach.[8-11]

Table 3. Mineral Contents of Common Foods

Food type	Sub-type	Ca	Fe	P	Zn	Cu	Mn	Se	Co, Ni, Si, Sn, V
Baby foods		S	S	S	L	L	I	L	I
Baked products	Bread	L	L	L	I	I	I	I	I
	Sweet goods	L	L	L	I	I	I	I	I
	Cookies/crackers	L	L	L	I	I	I	I	I
Beverages		L	L	L	L	L	L	I	I
Breakfast cereals		S	S	S	S	S	I	I	I
Candies		L	L	L	L	L	I	I	I
Cereal grains	Whole	S	S	S	S	S	L	L	I
	Flour	S	S	S	S	S	L	L	I
	Pasta	S	S	S	S	S	L	L	I
Dairy products		S	S	S	S	L	L	I	I
Eggs/egg products		S	S	S	S	S	S	S	I
Fast foods		L	L	I	I	I	I	I	I
Fats and oils		I	I	I	L	L	I	S	I
Fish and shellfish	Raw	S	S	S	S	L	L	I	I
	Cooked	S	S	S	S	L	L	I	I
Frozen dinners		I	I	I	I	I	I	I	I
Fruits	Raw	S	S	S	L	L	L	L	I
	Cooked	L	I	I	I	I	I	L	I
	Frozen/canned	S	S	S	L	L	I	L	I
Infant formula		S	S	S	L	L	L	L	I
Institutional food		I	I	I	I	I	I	I	I
Legumes	Raw	S	S	S	S	S	S	L	I
	Cooked	S	S	S	S	S	S	L	I
	Processed	L	L	L	I	I	I	I	I
Meat	Beef	S	S	S	S	S	S	S	I
	Lamb	S	S	S	S	S	S	S	I
	Pork	S	S	S	S	S	S	S	I
	Processed*	S	S	S	S	S	S	L	I
	Veal	S	S	S	S	S	S	S	I
Mixed dishes	Commercial	I	I	I	I	I	I	I	I
	Home prepared	I	I	I	I	I	I	I	I
Nuts and seeds		S	S	S	S	S	S	S	I
Poultry**		S	S	S	S	S	S	S	S
Restaurant food		I	I	I	I	I	I	I	I
Snack foods		S	S	S	L	L	I	L	I
Soups		I	I	I	I	I	I	I	I
Vegetables	Raw	S	S	S	S	S	S	I	I
	Cooked	L	L	L	L	L	L	L	I
	Frozen	S	S	S	S	S	I	I	I
	Canned	S	S	S	S	S	I	I	I

* Under revision
** Needs revision

S — Substantial data
L — Limited data
I — Inadequate data
Not applicable

As part of ongoing upgrades to the NDB, the expert system is being expanded to address many nutrients.[24] Analytical experts drawn from the large global community of scientists engaged in food composition research have been asked to contribute an assessment and ranking of critical methodological steps for specific nutritional components. This input will provide the questions and point ratings to be used to evaluate published scientific literature reports of food composition results. Eventually, all analytical data for food components will be rated to provide relative scores of data quality for values disseminated from the NDB. Quality scores (confidence codes) can be used to set new research priorities for method development and analysis. The confidence codes can also be used by authors, editors, and reviewers to improve the quality of documentation for food composition data that appear in the scientific literature.

Availability of Analytical Methods

Appropriate analytical methods are critical to the development of reliable food composition databases. These methods must not only meet technical specifications for accuracy and precision, but also must be fast, economical, and user-friendly to permit the number of analyses necessary to characterize the many foods that exist nationally and internationally. Unfortunately, appropriate methods

Table 4. Food Components of Recent Interest

Food type	Sub-type	Choline	Heme Fe	Inositol PO_4	Phenolics	Se-Methionine	Gluco-sinolates	Thiosul-finates	Flavon-oids
Baby foods		S	I	I	I	I			I
Baked products	Bread	L	I	I	I	I			I
	Sweet goods	L	I	I	I	I			I
	Cookies/crackers	I	I	I	I	I			I
Beverages		L	I	I	I	I			L
Breakfast cereals		L	I	I	I	I			I
Candies		L	I	I	I	I			I
Cereal grains	Whole	S		I	I	I			I
	Flour	L		I	I	I			I
	Pasta	L		I	I	I			I
Dairy products		L	I	I	I	I			I
Eggs/egg products		S	I	I	I	I			
Fast foods		S	I	I	I	I	I	I	I
Fats and oils		L	I	I	I	I			I
Fish and shellfish	Raw	I	I	I	I	I			
	Cooked	I	I	I	I	I			
Frozen dinners		I	I	I	I	I	I	I	I
Fruits	Raw	S		I	I	I	I	I	L
	Cooked	L		I	I	I			L
	Frozen/canned	L		I	I	I			I
Infant formula		I	I	I	I	I			I
Institutional food		I	I	I	I	I			I
Legumes	Raw	L		I	I	I	I	I	I
	Cooked	L		I	I	I	I	I	I
	Processed	L		I	I	I	I	I	I
Meat	Beef	L	I	I	I	I			
	Lamb	I	I	I	I	I			
	Pork	S	I	I	I	I			
	Processed*	I	I	I	I	I			
	Veal	L	I	I	I	I			
Mixed dishes	Commercial	I	I	I	I	I	I	I	I
	Home prepared	I	I	I	I	I	I	I	I
Nuts and seeds		L		I	I	I	I	I	L
Poultry**		L	I	I	I	I			
Restaurant food		I	I	I	I	I	I	I	I
Snack foods		L	I	I	I	I			I
Soups		I	I	I	I	I			I
Vegetables	Raw	S		I	I	I	I	I	L
	Cooked	S		I	I	I	I	I	L
	Frozen	L		I	I	I	I	I	I
	Canned	L		I	I	I	I	I	I

* Under revision
** Needs revision

S Substantial data
L Limited data
I Inadequate data
(shaded) Not applicable

are lacking for a large number of the food components, especially those newly recognized as having potential health-promoting properties. In fact, scientific interest in the newly recognized components, for example, proanthocyanidins, is more intense than the interest in many traditional nutrients. Although significant progress has been made in the development of methods for proanthocyanidins, analytical methods for other components are in the preliminary stages of development.[25,26]

Development of analytical methods is a complex task for various reasons. The number of foods available to the world population is enormous, varied, and increasing. The demand for data on new, previously ignored food components is escalating. The development of new technology offers increased analytical capabilities, but frequently renders existing data inaccurate or incomplete. Changes in government regulations and reports by expert panels, such as the National Academy of Sciences, create demands for the report of more specific nutrient forms, for example, folic acid, food folate, and dietary folate equivalents as specific forms of folate.[27] Finally, there is the difficulty of the analysis itself. Foods constitute some of the most difficult and varied chemical environments at the macro (ranging from high-fat to high-protein to high-carbohydrate) and micro levels (e.g., there are over 4000 flavonoids found in the plant world, of which only a dozen or so are found in significant concentration in any particular species). Given all of these factors, the lack of appropriate methods for many foods and components is understandable.

Table 5 provides an assessment of the current status of analytical methodology for those food components of current interest for database development. This table was compiled by the scientists of the Food Composition Laboratory at USDA. Obviously, an evaluation of this nature is highly subjective. It must be remembered, however, that this evaluation focused on the usefulness of the methods for producing the large numbers of analyses necessary to populate a database.

The methodologies for the food components shown in Table 5 have been rated as robust, limited, or inadequate. This assessment is based on the evaluation of a list of criteria that can be conveniently grouped as qualitative, quantitative, and economical factors. The yardstick for each factor is the ability of the method to meet the intended purpose. For this assessment, the intended purpose is to generate data on food components for incorporation into food composition databases. A method is judged to be robust if it meets all three criteria, limited if it satisfies two of the three criteria, and inadequate if less than two of the criteria are met.

We define a method as qualitative if it is capable of separating the target food components and detecting a useful signal from each component. The number of target components depends on the specific compound. For example, six naturally occurring forms of folate (or vitamers) are known that differ by functional groups at two sites and exhibit varying degrees of biological activity. Applying our definition, a method is qualitative for folates if it is capable of separating and obtaining individual signals for each of the six vitamers. The qualitative suitability of a method may change with time. As research reveals more compounds with biological activity, new or modified methods may become necessary.

A method is defined as quantitative if it is capable of providing the accuracy, precision, and detection limits required for the target food components at their naturally occurring levels in commonly consumed foods. Specifications that meet the intended purpose will depend on each nutrient and on the frequency of food consumption (i.e., lower detection limits are required for foods of low concentration consumed in higher quantities). In most cases, a method cannot be judged to be quantitative without the availability of an appropriate reference material (a representative sample matrix characterized with respect to the concentration of the component of interest). Determination of accuracy is difficult without a target or reference value. Additional factors, such as stability of a specific nutrient vitamer over time, have a major impact on the ability to quantify levels in foods.[28] The better the chemistry of the nutrient and the food matrix are understood, the more likely that interferences can be anticipated and corrected.

Finally, we define a method as economical if determinations can be made at a high rate with low cost. The analysis rate is determined by the time duration of the sample preparation and the analytical procedure and the user-friendliness of the method and instrumentation. The cost per analysis is determined by the cost of instrumentation, the cost of purchase and disposal of reagents, and the skill level of the operator. The number of determinations per run will also affect both rate and cost. This last factor is most obvious with trace element determinations, where multi-element determinations reduce the cost and time per determination. Obviously, the economical criteria can be fairly subjective. In general, economical factors are of considerable importance in determining the use of a method for large-scale analytical projects and their widespread adoption by analytical laboratories. However, if the data are badly needed, more time-consuming and costly methods may become acceptable.

The evaluation in Table 5 reveals that a considerable number of food components exist for which the methods are limited or inadequate. In general, methods are inadequate for those components that are of most recent interest, for example, resistant starch, folates, and most phytonutrients. Many methods exist for total trace element determinations but almost none for organo-metallic species. Most microbiological assays for the vitamins were considered limited because they were not qualitative; the assays fail to provide information on different vitamers. Also, a number of methods are rated as limited because of the lack of reference materials, that is, quality assurance materials with well-characterized and accepted values, which is particularly true for the organic components. The lack of a robust method does not necessarily mean that there is a lack of data in databases. It does mean that the existing data was expensive to acquire, usually in terms of time and equipment. With robust methods, more cost-effective analyses would be expected and, consequently, more data.

Selection of Key Foods

The staff at NDL has developed a method called the key foods approach, which is based on the premise that a relatively small number of foods contribute to the majority of the intake of a particular nutrient or component for the US population.[29] Data on the content of these relatively few foods, combined with food-intake data, provide reasonably accurate estimates of total intake of the component. Initially, NDL combined national survey data on food consumption with the USDA-SR to identify and rank the "key foods" that are the major contributors to intake for more than 50 components. The primary source of food consumption data is the HHS-USDA National Health and Nutrition Examination Survey: What We Eat in America.[12] For any new components not included in the SR, a preliminary key foods list is developed using the Special Interest Databases. If these databases or food survey data do not exist, panels of experts use

Table 5. State of Method Development Appropriate for the Determination of Food Components for Composition Databases

Nutrient Category	Robust*	Limited†	Inadequate‡
Phytonutrients	Carotenoids	Flavonoids	Thiosulfinates
		Isoflavones	Indoles
		Lignans	Isothiocyanates
		Phytosterols	Inositol phosphates
		Proanthocyanidins	Phenolics
			Protease inhibitors
			Saponins
			Thiols
Carbohydrates	Starch	Oligosaccharides	Resistant starch
	Monosaccharides	Total dietary fiber	Amylose/amylopectin
	Disaccharides	Pectins/uronic acids	Polysaccharides
	Trisaccharides	β-glucan	Lignins
Proteins	Total nitrogen	Tryptophan	
	Amino acids (most)	Cysteine	
		Total protein	
Lipids	Total fat	*Trans*-fatty acids	Tocotrienols
	Saturated fatty acids	Conjugated linolela acid	Oxidized fatty acids
	Cis fatty acids		Oxidized cholesterol
	n-3 fatty acids		Aldehydes
	n-6 fatty acids		
Vitamins	Tocopherols (E)	Vitamin D	Cobalamins (B_{12})
	Vitamin C	Vitamin K	Folates
	Vitamin A	Pantothenic acid	Biotin
		Choline	
		Niacin	
		Thiamin	
		Riboflavin	
		Vitamin B_6	
Minerals	Total Na	Total Si	Heme/nonheme Fe
	Total K	Total Li	Selenomethionine
	Total Ca	Total As	
	Total Mg	Total S	
	Total Fe	Total B	
	Total Cu	Total Co	
	Total Mn	Total Se	
		Fluoride	
		Iodine	

*Satisfies all three criteria: qualitative, quantitative, and economical (see text).
†Satisfies two of the three criteria.
‡Fails to meet more than one criterion.

food production data and/or composition databases "borrowed" from countries with similar foods to develop a key foods list.

Food Sampling and Analysis Program

In 1997, NDL developed the National Food and Nutrient Analysis Program, a research project that is achieving long-sought improvements to the NDB. This project is a partnership for funding, planning, and implementing between the USDA, 17 institutes of the National Institutes of Health, and several associations and companies of the food industry. The primary goal of the program is to review and update as necessary mean nutrient values for 1000 key foods and ingredients to ensure representative and accurate estimates of today's food supply. This program was renewed in 2005, with an emphasis on the continuation of updating USDA's food composition databases; the five linked components (specific aims) include the following: 1) institute a monitoring program for key foods and critical nutrients; 2) conduct a comprehensive analysis of selected key foods; 3) develop databases for high priority foods consumed by US ethnic subpopulations; 4) develop and expand databases for selected bioactive compounds, such as vitamin D, glucosinolates and isothiocyanates, trans fatty acids, conjugated linoleic acids, and fluoride; and 5) develop a validated database for ingredients in dietary supplements. The new data generated under this program will be migrated into successive versions of the SR. This program incorporates the approach outlined in Figure 1 and the specific components discussed in the previous section.

Since 2002, a nationwide probability model, covering the United States and up to 48 locations, was developed and expanded to guide the sampling and selection of foods to be analyzed.[30] Using this sampling frame, foods can be selected from grocery chains, restaurants and fast-food outlets, production sites, etc. Units of foods are selected according to type and market share (or volume consumed) to provide a representative sample mix. Food samples may be analyzed indvidually or composited according to specific criteria to achieve efficient use of resources. Samples of more than 750 foods have been selected. Analysis of nutritional components has been conducted under USDA-initiated contracts. Components include individual carotenoids, choline, folate, flavonoids, fluoride, vitamin K, and α-tocopherol, as well as the conventional proximates, vitamins, and minerals. Following statistical analysis, the data are being added to the NDB to provide accurate estimates for nutrients in foods.

Selection of Analytical Contractors

The NDL process for awarding contracts for the analysis of foods includes: 1) submission of a technical proposal by prospective contractors, 2) evaluation of proposals, and 3) evaluation of results of test samples.

The proposals focus on the technical approach and include: 1) analytical methods and procedures that will be used to complete each task, 2) precautionary measures to prevent contamination and deterioration, 3) sample handling and storage, 4) discussion on the ability of the lab to do the work, and 5) a description of the laboratory. To monitor accuracy and precision of data, quality conrol procedures, including information on the use of certified reference materials and in-house quality control materials, are used. Comparisons with other definitive methods, spikes, recoveries, blanks, blind duplicates, standard curves, internal standards, and validation of methods are also included. The certification and résumés of key administrative personnel and other personnel who will be directly involved in conducting recipe preparation, sample purchase, sample preparation, and analytical methods are included for evaluation on qualifications, expertise, and previous experience.

The evaluation of the proposals is performed by a panel consisting of NDL staff members and other government experts in the area of food composition and analysis. The previously mentioned criteria are scored according to how well the prospective contractors have addressed the items, and those contractors whose proposals are deemed technically acceptable proceed to the next step.

Test samples or reference materials procured from various sources are sent to the contractor for analysis. Sources of these materials include the National Institute of Standards and Technology, American Association of Cereal Chemists, National Food Association, and others. The analytical results are then evaluated against acceptable ranges for each nutrient, which are prepared by NDL staff. Nutrients for which results are in the acceptable ranges are included in the contract awards.

Databases for the New Millennium

Many components of foods and diets, in addition to "traditional" nutrients, alter biological activities in mammalian systems. Interest is currently focused on plant foods and the many compounds (phytonutrients) that they contain. Nearly a dozen classes of these compounds have been associated with biological activities that directly relate to reducing the risk and incidence of chronic diseases.[31] Previously, the lack of comprehensive databases of values for the phytonutrients had greatly hampered the assessment of any direct association of the intake of these specific minor components or families of components with the incidence and/or risk of chronic disease(s). As a result, substantial efforts have been focused toward the development of these databases.

Selection of Food Components

Selection of food components to be included in a database should be guided by the review of various sources of information regarding public health problems. These include authoritative reviews of scientific literature by professional societies and expert committees, as well as by national food and nutrition policy guidelines. Examples are the Third Report on Nutrition Monitoring in the United States by the Interagency Board for Nutrition Monitoring and Related Research[32] and Dietary Reference Intakes released by the Food and Nutrition Board of the National Academy of Sciences.[27,28,33] Traditionally, databases include the fundamental nutrients listed in Tables 1 to 3. Recently, a much larger number of food components have been identified that have biological activities associated with health promotion. They include some components for which Dietary Reference Intakes have only recently been established (e.g., choline), as well as some components for which additional research is needed, such as the phytonutrients identified in Table 4.[27] Additional components must be considered as new research is reported.

Databases for several food components have been developed and are available on the NDL website, for example, choline, flavonoids, and proanthocyanidins. Earlier databases were developed because of the scientific interest in the potential promotion of health by the respective components; for example, carotenoids because of the interest in β-carotene as an anticancer nutrient. However, some of the earlier databases have now been expanded and migrated into the SR.

Partnerships in the Development of Databases

The sampling, analysis, and compilation of nutrient data are time-consuming and costly. Traditionally, scientists at government agencies and land-grant academic institutions conducted nutrient analysis, and USDA scientists compiled and published data in official USDA food composition tables. However, many more food constituents have possible health importance than the "traditional" nutrients. Priorities vary, money for performing food compositional analysis is limited, and the workload involved is great. For many of these components, analytical methodology must be developed, which adds additional cost and further delays in the analysis of foods and the development of a database.

Because of the health relationship for many of the components, food companies have shown interest in knowing the concentration and biological activity of specific compounds in their foods with the potential of acquiring a health claim. Epidemiologists in academia, the food industry, and government seek food composition data so that they can investigate associations between individual food components and the incidence of disease. As a result of these interests, several partnerships have been built to reduce the financial burden, to hasten the analysis of foods, and to speed the development of specific databases. For example, the National Food and Nutrient Analysis Program partnership between USDA, National Institutes of Health, and other government agencies has contributed to the improvement of the quality of data in NDB. Additional partnerships are being sought for other components of foods and the food supply.

The partnerships have been invaluable in terms of expediting the acquisition of data for the development and improvement of databases. Also, the analytical expertise and detailed knowledge of food products by food-industry scientists have greatly strengthened the scientific reliability of food composition data that have been generated.

Training Programs

As the global demands for food composition data have increased, the need for training in the production and use of these data have also increased. Training is needed for both developed and emerging regions to establish and/or expand the competence base and to stimulate networking and communication between countries and regions. This leads to the standardization of data generation and data-handling methods and the subsequent interchange of food composition data. The ultimate goal of training is to improve data quality and data access by all users.

In Europe, the International Postgraduate Course on the Production and Use of Food Composition Data (FoodComp) was developed by Dr. David Southgate (retiree of UK Institute of Food Research) and the late Dr. Clive West (of Wageningen Agricultural University, The Netherlands), and was first conducted in 1992 to train data generators, compilers, and users in the production and use of food composition data.[34] Course topics included an overview of the uses of these data, followed by discussions of the analytical methodology, quality assurance techniques, sampling and sample handling procedures, and, finally, computerization, compilation, and data dissemination. This course has been conducted in Wageningen about every other year since 1992, but also has been held in several regions around the world. See website, http://www.fao.org/infoods for schedules and locations of this course.

The value of this training program can be seen in the results achieved since 1992. Approximately 300 data generators, compilers, and users representing almost 50 countries worldwide have been trained. Food composition programs in six countries have been established, and five countries have released food composition tables. Focused analytical courses have been held to train analysts. A reference materials program was developed in Thailand, and interlaboratory comparisons are under way in Latin America and other regions. This program has had a major impact on the production and reliable use of food composition data.

Future Directions

Food composition databases are essential for measuring the consumption of nutrients and food components, and for determining associations between these intakes and health status. In coming years, the demand for accurate and comprehensive data will only increase. The authors foresee questions in several areas that will require attention.

First, maintenance of existing databases must be recognized as a dynamic proposition. Databases must continuously evolve to keep pace with changes in nutrition science, food production, and analytical methodology. Such factors as new cultivars, changing environments, genetic modifications, new food products, new analytical methods and instrumentation, new government regulations and policies, and changes in food consumption patterns limit the useful life of a database. Are we willing to commit to the considerable resources necessary to keep databases current and representative for existing nutrients and components?

Second, what food components are needed in the database; that is, how large of a database do we want or can we afford? Several families of minor food components have been associated with reduced risk of chronic disease(s). Databases of food values for several of these have been assembled (flavonoids, procyanidins).[8,10] This area is the primary focus for the addition of new components to the database system.[31] The assembly of databases for many of these compounds awaits development of robust analytical techniques and generation of reliable data. Development of partnerships with scientists in academia, food industry, and other government laboratories has accelerated generation of data and assembly of values into functional databases and is expected to facilitate data generation in the future. How many food components do we want in our databases?

Third, should authoritative databases for dietary supplements be developed to complement food composition databases? Supplements (vitamin- and mineral-containing pills and capsules) and botanical and herbal preparations have become an increasingly important source of nutrients and biologically active components. Results from the National Health and Nutrition Examination Survey: What We Eat in America[12] have demonstrated that approximately 50% of its participants take a dietary supplement at some frequency. More than 35% take a multivitamin multimineral product on a regular basis. Databases of the content of these formulas and preparations are maintained by other US federal agencies and academic departments.[35] Harmonization of food codes, where applicable, and presentation of data with USDA food composition databases are necessary for the future. The Office of Dietary Supplements, National Institutes of Health, is supporting research at USDA and at the National Center for Health Statistics and other federal and academic centers to assess the impact of dietary supplement intake on the health status of the US population.[35] Basic research in the development of analytical methods and reference materials is ongoing. Do we want authoritative values for dietary supplements in a central database that is accessible by the Internet?

Finally, how should the data in the USDA food composition databases be used? Considering that the data represent the food supply of a large country, the most appropriate application is to estimate intakes of nutrients for large populations, subpopulations, or study cohorts, for example, national nutrition surveys and the national school lunch program, where menus are well established. Although food composition data have been used in software packages for menu planning and nutrient intake assessment for individuals, the results that are generated are only starting points and estimates. In the case of planning menus for research studies, the final composition of meals must be established through chemical analysis. Similarly, nutrient intakes of individuals are only estimates when calculated from these data, and definitive intakes must be derived from chemical analysis of duplicate plates of meals or other samples of the foods that are consumed. Do we have the resources to properly conduct this research? As health research becomes more specific and sophisticated, food and dietary supplement databases will need to be updated on a continuous basis to support future needs for data. Parallel efforts in analytical methods development and the development of reference materials will be needed to ensure the accuracy and precision of measurements. Private-public partnerships will be critical to generating sound and representative estimates for dietary components.

References

1. McCance RA, Widdowson EM. The chemical composition of foods. Med Res Counc Spec Rep Ser. 1940;235. London: His Majesty's Stationery Office.
2. *Dietary Guidelines for Americans*. USDHHS Pub. No. HHS-ODPHP-2005-01-DGA-A and the USDA Home and Garden Bulletin No. 232. US GPO, Washington DC: 2005. Available at http://www.healthierus.gov/dietaryguidelines.
3. MyPyramid.gov. Steps to a Healthier You. U.S. Department of Agriculture, Center for Nutrition Policy and Promotion. Alexandria, VA: CNPP-15; April 2005. Available at http://www.mypyramid.gov.
4. Shaw GM, Carmichael SL, Yang W, et al. Preconceptional dietary intake of choline and betaine and neural tube defects in offspring. Am J Epidemiol. 2004;160(2):102–109.
5. Atwater WO, Woods CD. *Investigations Upon the Chemistry and Economy of Foods.* Report of the Storrs School Experiment Station for 1891. Storrs, CT: U.S. Department of Agriculture; 1891.
6. U.S. Department of Agriculture, Agricultural Research Service. USDA Nutrient Database for Stan-

dard Reference, Release 18. Beltsville, MD: Nutrient Data Laboratory; 2005.

7. Steinmetz KA, Potter JD. Vegetables, fruit, and cancer prevention: a review. J Am Diet Assoc. 1996;96: 1027–1039.
8. Holden JM, Bhagwat SA, Haytowitz D, et al. Development of a database of critically evaluated flavonoid data: application of USDA's data quality evaluation system. J Food Comp Anal. 2005;18: 829–844.
9. U.S. Department of Agriculture, Agricultural Research Service, Nutrient Data Laboratory. USDA database for the choline content of common foods. Beltsville, MD: Nutrient Data Laboratory; 2004. Available at http://www.ars.usda.gov/ba/bhnrc/ndl.
10. U.S. Department of Agriculture, Agricultural Research Service, Nutrient Data Laboratory. USDA database for the proanthocyanidin content of selected foods. Beltsville, MD: Nutrient Data Laboratory; 2004. Available at http://www.ars.usda.gov/ba/bhnrc/ndl.
11. U.S. Department of Agriculture, Agricultural Research Service, Nutrient Data Laboratory. National fluoride database. Beltsville, MD: Nutrient Data Laboratory; 2004.
12. National Center for Health Statistics (NCHS), CDC, DHHS. NHANES 2001–2002 Data Files: Data, Docs, Codebooks, SAS Code. Hyattsville, MD: NHANES; 2004.
13. The International Network of Food Data Systems (INFOODS). Rome, Italy: INFOODS; 2000.
14. U.S. Congress Public Law 101-445. Nutrition Labeling and Education Act of 1990. Washington, DC: U.S. Government Printing Office; 1990.
15. Egan SK, Tao SS, Pennington JA, et al. U.S. Food and Drug Administration's total diet study: intake of nutritional and toxic elements, 1991–96. Food Addit Contam. 2002;19(2):103–125.
16. Chun J, Martin JA, Chen L, et al. A differential assay of folic acid and total folate in foods containing enriched cereal-grain products to calculate μg dietary folate equivalents (μg DFE). J Food Comp Anal. 2006;19(2–3):1182–1187.
17. Exler J. Iron Content of Food. Home Econ Res Report No. 45. Hyattsville, MD: Consumer Nutrition Division, Human Nutrition Information Service, U.S. Department of Agriculture; 1983.
18. Holden JM, Schubert A, Wolf WR, et al. A system for evaluating the quality of published data: selenium, a test case. In: Rand WM, ed. *Food Composition Data: A User's Perspective.* Tokyo: The United Nations University; 1987; 177–193.
19. Bigwood DW, Heller SR, Wolf WR, et al. Selex: an expert system for evaluating published data on selenium in foods. Anal Chim Acta. 1987;200: 411–419.
20. Lurie DG, Holden JM, Schubert A, et al. The copper content of foods based on a critical evaluation of published analytical data. J Food Comp Anal. 1989;2: 298–316.
21. Mangels AR, Holden JM, Beecher GR, et al. Carotenoid content of fruits and vegetables: an evaluation of analytic data. J Am Diet Assoc. 1993;93: 284–296.
22. Booth SL, Sadowski JA, Weihrauch JL, et al. Vitamin K, phylloquinone content of foods: a provisional table. J Food Comp Anal. 1993;6:109–120.
23. Weizmann N, Peterson JW, Haytowitz D, et al. Vitamin K content of fast foods and snack foods in the U.S. diet. J Food Comp Anal. 2004;17:379–384.
24. Holden JM, Bhagwat SA, Patterson KY. Development of a multi-nutrient data quality evaluation system. J Food Comp Anal. 2002;15(4):339–348.
25. Gu L, Kelm MA, Hammerstone JF, et al. Concentration of proanthocyanidins in common foods and estimations of normal consumption. J Nutr. 2004; 134(3):613–617.
26. Gu L, Kelm MA, Hammerstone JF, et al. Screening of foods containing proanthocyanidins and their structural characterization using LC-MS/MS and thiolytic degradation. J Agric Food Chem. 2003;51: 7513–7521.
27. Standing Committee on the Scientific Evaluation of Dietary Reference Intakes, Food and Nutrition Board, Institute of Medicine. *Dietary Reference Intakes for Thiamin, Riboflavin, Niacin, Vitamin B_6, Folate, Vitamin B_{12}, Pantothenic Acid, Biotin, and Choline.* Washington, DC: National Academies Press; 1998; 451.
28. Phillips KM, Wunderlich KM, Holden JM, et al. Stability of 5-methyltetrahydrofolate in frozen fresh fruits and vegetables. Food Chem. 2005;92:587–595.
29. Haytowitz DB, Pehrsson PR, Holden JM. The identification of key foods for food composition research. J Food Comp Anal. 2002;15(2):183–194.
30. Perry CR, Pehrsson PR, Holden J. *A Revised Sampling Plan for Obtaining Food Products for Nutrient Analysis for the USDA National Nutrient Database.* Proceedings of the American Statistical Association, Section on Survey Research Methods (CD-ROM). Alexandria, VA: American Statistical Association; 2003.
31. Beecher, GR. Phytonutrients role in metabolism: Effects on resistance to degenerative processes. Nutr. Rev. 1999, 57 (Pt2), 53–6.
32. Interagency Board for Nutrition Monitoring and Related Research. Third Report on Nutrition Monitoring in the U.S. Prepared by the Life Sciences Research Office, Federation of American Societies for Experimental Biology, Bethesda, MD; 1995.
33. Standing Committee on the Scientific Evaluation

of Dietary Reference Intakes, Food and Nutrition Board, Institute of Medicine. *Dietary Reference Intakes for Calcium, Phosphorus, Magnesium, Vitamin D, and Fluoride.* Washington, DC: National Academy Press; 1997; 432.

34. Greenfield H, Southgate DAT. Food composition data: production, management and use. Food Agric Org; United Nations, Rome 2003.

35. Dwyer J, Picciano MF, Raiten DJ, Members of the Steering Committee. Food and dietary supplement databases for What We Eat in America—NHANES. J Nutr. 2003;133:624S–634S.

58
Estimation of Dietary Intake

Wija A. van Staveren and Marga C. Ocké

Estimations of dietary intake always focus on food consumption for individuals or groups, but the underlying purpose may vary. For instance, socioeconomic surveys are conducted for national food planning and administration, toxicologic studies investigate the exposure to biochemicals via foods, metabolic studies focus on the fate of nutrients in the body, and public health studies examine the adequacy of the diet and the relation between food consumption and health.

Various study designs exist for each objective, and approaches are possible at different levels: national accounts of annual food availability per head of the population (food balance sheets), family budget and household consumption surveys, and individual food intake or dietary surveys. In the context of this book, individual dietary surveys are most relevant, so we will concentrate on these methods.

Several dietary assessment tools directed at the individual are available. They differ in the time frame used, method of administration, assessment of the foods eaten, and conversion into food components. Moreover, the immediate goals (information on meals, food groups, and specific nutrients or compounds), underlying assumptions, and cognitive approaches to acquiring dietary intake information vary among dietary assessment methods (Table 1).[1,2]

This chapter describes the main dietary assessment methods and the strengths and weaknesses of each. The concept of these methods has not changed much since the first edition of this book, but a wider range of suitable equipment and related resources for field use are now available. New technology includes the use of computers, databanks, and data-processing facilities. More use is made of epidemiologic studies, and the development and use of biomarkers have led to more information on sources of variation and errors inherent to these methods.[3] These sources have to be taken into account in study design, data treatment, and interpretation of results to give a greater internal and external validity to the study conclusions.[4] Because the main causes of death are nutrition-related diseases,[5] more valid knowledge about dietary patterns is of the utmost importance.

Dietary Assessment Methods

In general, methods can be divided into two basic categories: those that record data at the time of eating (so-called weighed and estimated records methods) and those that collect data about foods eaten in the recent past or over a longer period of time (interview methods).

Interview methods may refer to current diet (24-hour food recalls) or habitual diet (dietary history and food frequency methods). The three methods differ in many

Table 1. Dimensions in Dietary Survey Methods

Observation unit	• Individual • Household • Other groups

Mode of administration	• Double portion collection
	• Record by mail, with or without check
	• Interview
	  ○ Telephone
	  ○ Face to face
	  ○ Computerized
	  ○ Video

Time frame	• Usual • Current
Measurement amounts of food	• Weighing • Estimation with or without models
Conversion into nutrients	• Nutrient databases • Direct chemical analyses

aspects, but some practical aspects in conducting the interview are similar for all. Interviewers should have a thorough knowledge of the purpose of the method; dietary components of interest; nutrient database to be used (so that interviewers can recall dietary detail appropriate for coding); details of the standardized protocol, including a quality control system to minimize errors; and foods available in the marketplace (including prevalent regional or ethnic foods), local names for foods, and preparation practices. The location of the interview may affect respondents' willingness and ability to report their diets. It is recommended that all interviews be conducted in the same type of location and that no third person be present. The location should allow for a relaxed atmosphere.[6]

The success of the interview relies on the respondents' ability to remember and adequately describe their diets. Because memory of these events is based on cognitive processes, it is important to take advantage of what is known about how respondents remember dietary information and how that information is retrieved and reported to the interviewer.[7] Although probing is useful, the questions asked in an interview should be as neutral as possible (e.g., questions such as "Did you eat before you left home?" and "What did you eat?" rather than "Did you have cereal for breakfast?").

In collaborative research, all interviewers must have had the same training and must be visited regularly during fieldwork. Checks should be made to detect systematic differences among interviewers in data collecting and coding. Standardization of interviewers is enhanced when the interview is administered with the aid of a computer.[8]

Dietary Records

Principles. In the weighed record technique, the subject is taught to weigh and record the food and its weight immediately before eating and to weigh any leftovers. In most surveys, not all items are weighed. When weighing would interfere with normal eating habits, describing the quantity of food consumed is acceptable. For example, for snacks eaten between meals or meals eaten in a restaurant, the nutritionist investigator will estimate weights from the description. The weighed method differs from the estimated record, for which subjects do not use a scale but keep records of portion sizes of all the food they eat on 1 or more days. The portion sizes are described in natural units (household measures) by using the utensils commonly found in homes.

Practical Aspects. The number of days needed to record food intake depends on the aim of the survey and the expected between- and within-individual variation in intake of the nutrients of interest. However, in practice, no more than 3 or 4 consecutive days are included because of respondent fatigue. The form used to record intake is kept in a record book and may be closed or open. A closed form is a precoded list of all of the commonly eaten foods in units of specified portion size and grouped by nutrient composition. This list allows for rapid coding but may be less adequate because it requires subjects to describe the foods eaten in defined units that may be unfamiliar. A semi-open form may be meal based and preconstructed with many foods and amount options listed, but include sufficient space for other nonlisted foods and amounts. Precoded forms should be pretested in small pilot studies. In general, an open form is used more often. If habitual diet is being assessed, it must be stressed that usual diet is being investigated and that the subject must not use the opportunity, for example, to restrict energy intake. To avoid bias in response, it is advantageous not to disclose the nutrient being studied. Dietary records may be completed by someone other than the subject. For example, children under 10 years of age will not supply adequate records, and the caretaker (often the mother) might help.

Respondents must be trained to record the level of detail needed to adequately describe the foods and amounts consumed, including the name of the food (brand names if possible), preparation methods, and recipes. At the end of the recording period, the record should be checked in detail and the subject thanked. The records should be coded for computer calculation as soon as possible so that the subject can be contacted again if necessary.

Strengths and Uses. Strengths include that 2 or more days of recording provide data on within- and between-individual variation in dietary intake, which allows the estimation of the population distribution of usual intake;[9] multiple days of recording may allow individuals to be classified according to their usual intakes;[10] and 1- or 2-day records kept intermittently over the year may provide an estimate of usual intake by an individual. In the latter situation, open-form records may provide data on less frequently eaten foods in a defined time period. Portions can be measured or weighed to increase accuracy.

Weaknesses. In general, respondents must be literate and highly cooperative. This requirement may lead to response bias as a result of overrepresentation of more highly educated individuals who are interested in diet and health. Other weaknesses include: food consumed away from home may be less accurately reported; the usual eating pattern may be influenced or changed by the recording process[11]; record keeping increases respondent burden, which may adversely affect response rates; accuracy of records may decrease as the number of days increases; and moderate underreporting often occurs and substantial underreporting is suspected in specific groups of the population (e.g., obese persons).[12]

Twenty-Four-Hour Food Recall

Principles. During an interview, an individual recalls actual food intake for the immediate past 24 or 48 hours or for the preceding days. The 24-hour food recall is the most common recall used. Food quantities are usually assessed by use of household measures, food models, or photographs. Information is obtained by the interviewer during a personal interview or by telephone using either an open form or a precoded questionnaire, tape recorder, or computer program.

Practical Aspects. The recall is traditionally conducted by a personal interview with open forms, but computer-assisted interviews are becoming more common.[13,14] Well-trained interviewers are crucial in administering 24-hour recall interviews because this information is obtained by asking probing questions. Most commonly, the recalled day is defined as the time when the respondent gets up 1 day until the time the respondent gets up the next day. The 24-hour recall is often structured with specific probes to help the respondent remember all foods consumed throughout the day. Sometimes at the end of the interview there is a checklist with foods or snacks that might be easily forgotten.[13] Computer-assisted 24-hour recalls usually consist of multiple steps.[13,14] The five-pass method currently used in the National Health and Nutrition Examination Survey has five steps: 1) the quick list, which is an uninterrupted listing of the food and beverages consumed; 2) the forgotten food list, which queries the subject on categories of food that have been documented as frequently forgotten; 3) time and occasion during which food was consumed; 4) the detail cycle, which elicits descriptions of food and amounts; and 5) the final probe review.[14]

Because the recall method depends on the subjects' ability to remember and adequately describe their diets, this method is not suitable for children younger than approximately 7 years or for many older adults ≥ 75 years. The 24-hour recall method is appropriate for describing the mean intake of groups of individuals. Days of the week must be equally represented and, because this is not always possible, the distribution of recalls according to the days of the week—and sometimes the season—should be reported.[15]

It is advised that no prior notification be given to the subjects about whether or when they will be interviewed about their food intake. Although notification could help the memory of some subjects, others might change their usual diet in some way for the occasion.[16]

Strengths and Uses. The design of the method is appropriate for describing the mean intake of a group[17]: 2 or more days provide data on within- and between-individual variation, which allows for estimation of the distribution of usual intake; open interviews provide data on less frequently eaten foods; administration time is short; the time period is well defined; literacy is not required; and the open form is not culture specific. Response rates are usually rather high for recalls. Administration by a dietitian allows for probing for incomplete information and requires fewer callbacks.

Weaknesses. Weaknesses are that respondents' recall depends on short-term memory; portion size is difficult to estimate accurately; and, compared with other methods, intake tend to be underreported. A 1-day intake for each subject does not supply information on within-individual variation, will overestimate between-individual variation, and the method is vulnerable to variability among interviewers.

Dietary History

Principle. The dietary history assesses an individual's total daily food intake and usual meal pattern over varied periods of time. In theory, the history may cover any period in the past, but more usually it covers the past 1 month, 6 months, or 1 year. Originally, Burke[18] developed the dietary history technique in three parts. The first was an interview about the subject's usual daily pattern of food intake with quantities specified in household measures. The second was a cross-check using a detailed list of foods to verify and clarify the overall eating pattern. Finally, the subject recorded food intake at home, in household measures, for 3 days. Today, the diet history is applied in many ways. The meal pattern and checklist of food are considered as essential for the method, but the 3-day record is often omitted.

Practical Aspects. In an open interview, the subject is questioned about a typical day's eating pattern, or the interview may start with a 24-hour recall. The purpose of the study must be so well known to the interviewer that it is easy for him or her to judge how much detailed information should be collected for each food group. For example, if a study is focused on the intake of macronutrients and dietary fiber is not an issue, then for most surveys there is no need to distinguish between brown and white bread. Usual portion sizes are estimated with standard household measures, and food models or replicas are checked by weighing.

Because a dietary history is a more abstract interview than the 24-hour recall, it is difficult for a non-nutritionist to carry out this interview. An exception may be diet histories that are guided and controlled by a precoded interview form or computer software.[19]

The diet history is also more demanding for the subject. Because it asks for a habitual dietary pattern, it is more liable to evoke socially desirable answers and is not appropriate for individuals with a large day-to-day variation in their diet. A satisfactory history is not usually obtained from young children, people preoccupied with weight problems, and mentally retarded people.

A short version of this method with a limited checklist of foods is often used in the clinical setting for diagnosis and as a basis for therapeutic dietary guidelines.

Strengths and Uses. The dietary history is used for assessment of usual meal patterns and details of food intake.[20] The data can be used to characterize individuals according to their food and nutrient intake, to classify them in categories (e.g., quantiles) of intake,[21] and to assess the relative average intakes of groups of people and the distribution of intakes within these groups.[22] Respondent literacy is not required for an interviewer-administered dietary history.

Weaknesses. Respondents are asked to make many judgments about their usual food intake and the amounts of those foods, and the recall period is difficult to conceptualize accurately—higher estimates are observed in methods covering a longer period.[23] Respondents need to have a regular dietary pattern and a good memory, which may hamper getting a representative sample of the population. Highly trained nutritionists with well-developed social skills are required to conduct the interview, and the interview is liable to evoke socially desirable answers.

Food Frequency Method

Principle. The first food frequency questionnaires were developed for large epidemiologic studies, for example, on the relationship between diet and chronic disease. In such studies, the diet history puts too heavy a burden on subject and investigator.

The questionnaire is a preprinted list of food on which subjects are asked to estimate the frequency and often also amount of habitual consumption during a specified period. The types of food vary depending on whether the researcher is interested in specific nutrients or the total diet. A nutrient value must be assigned to each food item listed. The value is based most often on weighting each food in a group by usage.[24] The first questionnaires did not include quantitative estimates other than servings or portions per day, week, or month. The data from these questionnaires are based on the assumption that total intake is more determined by variations in consumption frequency than by variations in portion size, and that consumption frequency is related to consumed quantities. These are gross assumptions, and therefore some investigators have built a quantitative aspect into the technique and called their method a semiquantitative food frequency method. Not all investigators advocate the inclusion of portion sizes because errors made by the estimation may outweigh the variance in intake of most food.[25]

Practical Aspects. Food frequency questionnaires vary in the food listed, length of the reference period, response intervals for specifying frequency of use, procedure for estimating portion size, and manner of administration. It is therefore necessary to validate the method as applied in specific situations or population groups. The development of the method is crucial to success and may take a lot of time when the evaluation is included. Block et al.[26] and later Cade et al.[25] described the development of this method based on a nationwide database approach.

If the food frequency method is administered by an interviewer, all requirements mentioned for the diet history and 24-hour recall have to be taken into account (setting and training), but nutritionists are not necessarily required for the interview. The advantage of the food frequency method is that it is standardized, which reduces between-interviewer variation. Because the questionnaire is usually self-administered, the accompanying instructions are important.

Strengths and Uses. The food frequency method estimates the usual food (group) intake of an individual. When portion sizes are included or when certain assumptions are made, individuals can be ranked according to nutrient intake. A self-administered questionnaire may require little time to complete and to code; the response burden is generally low and therefore, response rates, are high. The method can be automated easily and is not very costly.[27]

Weaknesses. Weaknesses of this method include that memory of food use in the past is required and that the respondents' burden is governed by the number and complexity of foods listed and the quantification procedure. The quantification of portion sizes might be less accurate, as in other methods.[28,29] Also, the development and testing of the food list takes much time, no information on day-to-day variation is provided, and the suitability is questionable for groups in the population who consume culture-specific food not on the list. Longer food lists and longer reference periods often lead to overestimation of intake,[30] and the cognitive process for answering questions about food frequency may be more complex than those about a daily food pattern.[7]

Combined Methods

Sometimes a combination of two or more methods provides greater accuracy. As described above and summarized in Table 2, each method has specific strengths and weaknesses and a combination might balance the shortcomings of one method with the strengths of another. For example, a 2-day record combined with a food frequency list may provide valid absolute mean intakes of groups, including within- and between-individual variation and a classification of high-risk groups for low (e.g., iron) or high (e.g., cholesterol) intake. This approach might be too expensive for small-scale studies, but is often done in large multicenter studies[31,32] or nationwide surveys.[33,34] Combined methods are more time consuming for respondents and field-workers. Table 3 gives an estimation of the time required for field-workers for interviewing, checking, and coding.

Assessment of Specific Food Components and Dietary Supplements

Bioactive Components

For many diseases, research interest has now shifted to the bioactive components of food, such as carotenoids, flavonoids, glucosinolates, allyl compounds, and phytoestrogens. Dietary measurement tools often need to be adapted specifically to the bioactive component of interest. Moreover, dietary assessment of these components requires good data about the content of the bioactive components in food, which are often not available in food composition tables, necessitating chemical analyses in individual foods or replicate portions. It is important that the analysis values in foods are published with sufficient detail so others can benefit from them.

Table 2. Sources of Error in Techniques Estimating Food Consumption

Sources of Error	Weighed Record	24-Hour Recall	Diet History	Food Frequency
Variation with time	+	+	−	−
Response errors				
Omitting foods	+	+	+	−
Including foods	−	+	+	+
Estimation of weight of foods	−	+	+	+
Estimation of frequency of foods consumed	NA	NA	+	+
Changes in real diet	+	+/−	−	−
Errors in conversion into nutrient				
Food conversion tables	+	+	+	+
Coding	+	+	+	−

+, error is likely; −, error is unlikely; NA, not applicable.
Adapted from Cameron and van Staveren, 1988.[1]

Dietary Supplements, Fortified Foods, and Functional Foods

In North American and western European populations, the use of dietary supplements, fortified foods, and functional foods is substantial. These products can contribute more than 50% of micronutrient intake for an individual. Failure to include such important sources of nutrient intake can result in estimates of intake that bear little relation to biochemical status, which is often the ultimate parameter of interest.[35] Supplement users may take supplements irregularly.[36] Therefore, to take a measure of supplement use at 1 or a few days as a proxy for long-term intake incorporates measurement error that attenuates measures of association with status parameters.[37] The same conclusions are probably true for fortified and functional foods.[34]

In large-scale studies focusing on diet-disease relationships, the frequency and number of supplements taken seems to be much more important than precision about content. Distinction between single and multiple vitamin supplements is essential; distinction between 1-a-day and high-dose types is desirable. Within each of these subtypes, the exact brand name or exact content does not seem to be necessary because assumptions about the amount will be approximately correct.[35] For assessment of actual intake—in contrast to usual intake—and for quantitative assessment of the distribution of intake for a population, brand name and dose information are relevant.

An approach similar to that used for dietary supplements will probably work for foods marketed in a fortified or functional version as well as the ordinary version. Examples of such foods are milk products when calcium is the component of interest: consumers will probably know whether they buy the fortified version, and amounts of added calcium will not vary substantially. Usual intake of milk can then be questioned separately for calcium-fortified milk as a generic term. However, for many other types of functional foods, information at the brand name level and subtype will be required. This may be the case because the consumer is unaware of consuming a fortified or functional product, or does not know the specific content of the product, or the amounts of added components in some products vary enormously.

For fortified foods, functional foods, and dietary supplements, obtaining the nutrient content for brand names

Table 3. Estimation of Time to be Spent for an Interview by a Field-worker

	Administration/ Explanation (minutes)	Check Completeness/ Interview (minutes)	Coding (minutes)
Weighted record: 3 days face-to-face interview (excluding travel time)	30	30	60
24-hour recall	25	5	30
Diet history	45–90	–	60
Scannable food frequency questionnaire	30	5	5–10 (scan)

via nutrient databases or food tables is difficult. Products are often only on the market for a few years, and manufacturers tend to change the content of their products. These products are included in regular food composition tables only after they have been marketed for a long time.

Alcohol

The assessment of alcohol intake should also be conducted carefully because alcohol is not always considered a normal food substance. On a population level, alcohol intake might be assessed by using official data such as food balance sheets collected by the Food and Agriculture Organization of the United Nations or sales statistics. The advantage of using these statistics is that the population is not aware of the registration and socially desirable answers—a big problem in individual-based approaches—are thus avoided. However, these statistics do not provide data on manner and amount of alcohol consumption of specific groups or individuals and are not very useful for epidemiologic purposes. Most individual-based dietary assessment methods described here will include questions on alcohol intake. In addition, specific frequency questionnaires have been developed to assess alcohol intake. Altogether, according to the literature, there are five main approaches:[38] the quantity frequency method (includes simple questions on intake of glasses of alcoholic drinks in a specific period), the extended quantity frequency (includes questions on specific drinks—wine, beer, liquor—and variability during the week and weekends), prospective and retrospective diaries, and repeated 24-hour recall.

The mean level of intake may differ by 20% by these methods. Intake data yielded higher estimates for beer, wine, and liquor consumption than did sales information. Nevertheless, underestimation is common to all methods, and heavy drinkers seldom will participate in a survey on alcohol intake, which leads to selection bias. Ranking participants according to alcohol intake may distinguish among those who consume small and large quantities sufficiently for epidemiologic purposes.

There has been some discussion about including alcohol intake in research on estimating daily energy intake. On one hand, if energy from alcohol is not included, the proportions of macronutrients contributing to the daily energy supply are incorrect. On the other hand, high alcohol intake may mask relatively high fat intake contributing to the daily energy supply.

Variation and Error

An experimental study of the function of food components in the body requires relatively few people in a metabolic ward. The study of diet adequacy or the relationship between nutrition and health often requires the use of a population-based observational study (cross-sectional or longitudinal). The choice of the most appropriate assessment tool depends on purpose and design, type of information required (in statistic terms, such as means, medians, distribution), and practical issues (e.g., available funding, time, skilled staff, characteristics of the subjects). There is a tendency to consider results from experimental designs to be more accurate than results from population-based observations. However, for the study of nutrition and health, these different designs have different purposes, limitations, and strengths. To select the most appropriate dietary method to answer a research question, it is important to understand the potential sources of variation and error for each method and their effects on the results of the study.

Sources of Variation

At the level of the individual, dietary intake is characterized by daily variation superimposed on an underlying consistent pattern.[27] Factors such as day of the week or season often contribute to daily variation in a systematic way, whereas other factors are random. Dietary data collected on multiple days incorporate these kinds of variations. In food frequency questionnaires and the dietary history method, participants are asked to filter out the underlying consistent dietary pattern themselves. This is more difficult in the case of a large random daily variations (i.e., in the absence of a regular dietary pattern). All dietary data include variations due to measurement error, but measurement error can also result in losing some of the real variance. Measurement error usually consists of random and systematic components.

The degree of random and systematic variation in dietary data differs across nutrients. For example, total energy and macronutrient intake have relatively little random variation, whereas intake of some nutrients such as retinol and marine fatty acids is characterized by large random variation resulting from the large variation in their daily intake. Within- and between-subject variation in nutrient intake is illustrated in Table 4 with data from a Dutch validation study for 24-hour recalls repeated 12 times and food frequency questionnaires repeated three times.[39] The findings are, however, culturally determined because they depend on dietary pattern.

Measurement Error

From a methodologic point of view, four types of measurement error exist: random within-person error, systematic within-person error, random between-person error, and systematic between-person error.[27] Systematic error is also called bias. The type and size of errors vary with the particular dietary assessment method and probably also with the population in which it is applied. The four types of error and their effects on the parameters to be estimated are discussed here, along with examples and references to the various types and aspects of dietary assessment. (See also Table 2.)

Random within-person error may be due to day-to-day variation in an individual's daily intake when habitual intake is estimated. Thus, error in this methodologic sense does not mean mistake in the data collection sense,

Table 4. Within- (CV_w) and Between-Subject (CV_b) Coefficients of Variation in Nutrient Data Collected by Repeated 24-Hour Dietary Recalls and Food Frequency Questionnaires*

	24-Hour Dietary Recalls				**Food Frequency Questionnaires**			
	Men		**Women**		**Men**		**Women**	
Nutrient	CV_w	CV_b	CV_w	CV_b	CV_w	CV_b	CV_w	CV_b
Energy	26%	18%	24%	18%	12%	23%	11%	20%
Protein	27%	16%	26%	17%	13%	20%	12%	18%
Fat	38%	26%	37%	24%	16%	28%	14%	25%
Carbohydrates	26%	24%	22%	22%	14%	27%	12%	25%
Cholesterol	56%	29%	52%	23%	17%	29%	15%	24%
Retinol	259%	35%	155%	44%	32%	41%	41%	50%
Vitamin C	65%	33%	68%	36%	26%	37%	32%	33%
Calcium	40%	29%	32%	31%	24%	32%	18%	31%

* Data are based on 12 24-hour recalls and three food frequency questionnaires in 63 Dutch men and 59 Dutch women
From Ocké et al., 1997[39]; used with permission from Oxford University Press.

but rather, a mismatch in timeframe. Random within-person error also includes errors in the measurement of intake on any occasion that are not systematic. Examples of this type of error are foods that are omitted or included falsely in dietary records or recalls, portion sizes that are estimated inaccurately, and coding mistakes. When random within-person error is the only type of error present, the precision of the estimated mean value for an individual depends on the within-subject variation and the number of replicate measurements, as shown in Equation 1. This equation can also be rearranged to calculate the number of days required to estimate mean intake for an individual given the size of the random variation and the precision that is needed[17]:

$$(1) \qquad D_o = Z_\alpha(CV_w)(n^{-1/2})$$

Where D_o is the greatest deviation from the mean (as a percentage of long-term true intake), Z_α is the normal deviate for the percentage of times the measured value should be within a specified limit (1.96 for 95% confidence), CV_w is the within-subject coefficient of variation, and n is the number of days for the person. When replicate measurements are available, it is also possible to estimate the distribution of usual intake from the data on actual short-term intake that include day-to-day variations.[9]

Systematic within-person error may be caused when a person consciously or unconsciously underestimates or exaggerates his food intake. An important food for an individual that is not included in a questionnaire or a question that is systematically misunderstood by an individual will also lead to systematic within-person error. If the dietary assessment method is repeatedly administered, the error will occur again. Consequently, the estimation of mean intake for an individual is not improved by repeated measurements and remains biased. Increasing evidence suggests that most dietary assessment methods, recalls, and records are likely to be flawed with systematic person-specific biases.[40]

Random between-person errors may be due to random and systematic within-person error if they are distributed randomly across individuals; an overestimation by some individuals is counterbalanced by an underestimation by others. The estimated mean intake is consequently not biased, but the precision is affected and the distribution of measured intake is artificially widened. Estimates for the percentage of subjects below or above a certain cutoff level (e.g., recommended dietary allowances) are therefore not valid. Also, the validity of measures of associations with health parameters is hampered, and the validity for univariate association is attenuated. In Equation 2, it is shown that the precision of the estimate of the mean group intake can be improved by increasing the number of subjects or the number of replicate measurements[17]:

$$(2) \qquad D_t = Z_\alpha(CV_b/g + CV_w/gn)^{1/2}$$

Where D_t is the greatest deviation from the mean (as a percentage of long-term true intake), Z_α is the normal deviate for the percentage of times the measured value should be within a specified limit (1.96 for 95% confidence), CV_b is the between-subject coefficient of variation, CV_w is the within-subject coefficient of variation, g is the number of persons, and n is the number of days per person.

Systematic between-person error is caused by systematic within-person error that is not randomly distributed across individuals. Questionnaires that fail to include important foods for a population, incorrect standard portion sizes used in algorithms for food frequency questionnaires, food photographs that systematically give rise to overestimation of portion sizes, socially desirable answers given by groups of people, recalls or records that do not include weekend days, and large errors in food composition tables will all result in systematic between-person error. As a result, the mean intake and the percentage of persons above or below a certain cutoff level are not estimated correctly. The standard deviation may or may not be correct depending on whether the systematic between-person error applies equally to all subjects. Testing whether an association with a health parameter exists is not affected by a systematic between-person error that applies equally to all subjects. However, this error may be associated with a variable for which the relationship with dietary intake is the topic of study, and a misleading conclusion might be drawn. A well-known example of a parameter related to systematic underreporting is body mass index: subjects with a higher body mass index underreport their energy intake more than do subjects with lower body mass index.[12]

The effects of random and systematic between-person measurement errors on various parameters to be estimated is summarized in Table 5. Formulas that correct for the effects of random measurement errors are now available for many outcome measures, such as the distribution of intake and measures of associations with other variables such as correlation coefficients, regression coefficients, and relative risks.[27] Information on the size of random measurement error can be obtained from dietary reproducibility and validity studies. The former only gives information on part of the total random between-person error (i.e., not that based on systematic within-person error). In theory, validity studies supply information on the total error. However, in practice this is limited by the lack of a true gold standard—that is, dietary assessment methods without errors or with completely independent errors. The Observing Protein and Energy Nutrition study is an example of a study that gives insight to the error matrix for 24-hour diet recalls and food frequency questionnaires because of the use of biomarkers with independent errors.[40]

Table 5. The Effects of Random and Systematic Between-Person Error in Dietary Intake on Parameters to be Estimated*

Parameter to be Estimated	Type of Between-Person Error	
	Random	Systematic
Mean intake	↓ Precision	↓ Validity
Variation of intake	↓ Validity	No effect
% of Subjects below recommended dietary allowanc	↓ Validity	↓ Validity
Association with health outcome	↓ Validity	no effect

* Prepared by Jan Burema, Division of Human Nutrition, Wageningen University, The Netherlands.

Quality control checks can indicate systematic measurement error. An often-used check for underestimation is the ratio of energy intake to estimated basal metabolic rate. If this ratio is below a certain cutoff value, energy intake is very likely underreported.[27] Techniques for adjustments are not well developed for systematic measurement error associated with parameters of interest.

Assessment in Specific Situations

Clinical Settings

Diet might be assessed in a clinical setting for diagnostic purposes, as a screening tool for probable dietary risk, or as a basis for dietary advice. The required accuracy of the collected information depends on the purpose of the data collection. However, because dietary treatments should be evidence based rather than experience based, a reproducible estimate—standardized for the specific purposes of the assessment—is required so that the results of treatment can be evaluated and compared. When current diet is the information of interest, structured questionnaires based on the meal pattern of the clinic may be effective.[16]

Remote Areas

Food consumption surveys in remote areas can be important for two reasons: the diet available to the inhabitants may be monotonously restricted, and health care facilities and other services may be limited or nonexistent. Survey data can be used to document the particular situation so that the program and services needed are introduced, monitored, and evaluated. The main deterrents to surveying remote areas are the cost and time involved in fielding survey teams. Mail, telephone, and Internet services can be inexpensive alternatives to face-to-face interviewing. Special sampling techniques and procedures can be used to limit the geographic scatter of the sample selected from remote areas. Cluster sampling, for example, can reduce the number of such locations selected without affecting the representativeness of the sample, substantially reducing the logistic demands and operating costs of the survey.[1,41]

Season of the Year

The season of the year has large effects on the food supply in non-industrialized areas and some effects in industrialized countries.[15,41] After-harvest and dry-season food intakes can be remarkably different in quantity, variety, and quality from before-harvest and wet-season intakes. Therefore, the timing of surveys describing and evaluating food patterns is important. Seasonal variations other than climate—such as cultural and economic events—also have to be considered. Because of the likelihood of higher consumption of food on market day or the day after, surveys in rural areas should be organized

so that these days are not overrepresented. If food frequencies are sought, the respondents may describe them more easily in relationship to agricultural or local calendars rather than in terms of weeks or months, which are commonly used in urban areas. The logistics of travel are also influenced by season. The accessibility of roads, bridges, and rivers may be an important seasonal consideration in scheduling surveys.

Assessment in Specific Populations

Individuals with Disabilities

Disabilities affecting sight, hearing, speech, memory, or the ability to write are particular problems in the collection of all kinds of data, including dietary intake data from affected individuals. If only one faculty is affected, survey methods relying on other faculties provide a good solution. For example, carefully prepared, self-explanatory written instructions and questionnaires are required when the subject of a study is deaf. Interviews can be conducted, but they take more time. The process can be helped by using printed instructions, questionnaires, and probing techniques or a sign language interpreter. Replica models or pictures can help with the identification of the food and the quantity consumed. If speech is impaired, provision should be made for written responses.

Individuals Unable to Respond

When respondents are unable to respond, surrogate responders may be used. Individuals who know the most about a subject's lifestyle (e.g., caretakers) are assumed to be the best surrogate responders. Although the accuracy of surrogate reports has not been examined, some studies have compared information from surrogates and subjects. Mean frequencies of food group use reported by subjects and surrogates are more or less similar depending on the type of food (e.g., frequencies are better for drinks than for other foods).[42] Furthermore, although subjects reporting themselves at an extreme of the distribution seldom are reported by their surrogate to be at the other extreme, many are reported to be in the middle of the distribution.[42] This limits the usefulness of surrogate information for analyses that rely on proper ranking of people. When surrogates are included in a study, analyses should also be conducted after the surrogates are excluded to examine the sensitivity of reported associations to possible biases in the surrogates' reports.[2]

Young Children

Young children up until the age of 7 years have insufficient abilities to cooperate in dietary assessment procedures. Therefore, parents or other caretakers often function as surrogate respondents. Studies comparing direct observations with recalls by parents suggest that the latter are reliable reporters of food intake at home.[43] However, the concern is the reliability of recalls on out-of-home consumption. Solutions for this problem are culturally dependent, and no publications give very satisfactory answers. Out-of-home consumption is a major limiting factor in dietary studies in young children.[44]

From the age of 8 years forward, there is a rapid increase in the ability to self-report food intake. Issues to take into account are limited memory, concept of time, attention span, and knowledge of foods and food preparation. Food preference and the rapidly changing food habits affect the reliability of the recall of food consumption. Of key importance in designing questionnaires is to understand how food-related information is organized in memory and subsequently retrieved in dietary recall. Baranowski and Domel[45] developed a model that showed that the usual retrieval mechanism categories employed by children were: visual imagery (appearance of the food: color, shape, consistency), usual practice (familiarity with eating the food previously), behavior chaining (linking foods to other food items or activities during the meal), and food preference.[46] By adolescence, cognitive abilities should be fully developed; limiting problems for that age are issues of motivation and body image. An attractive short picture-sort method has been shown to be very helpful in this age group.[47,48]

The Elderly

When people become older, the risk for disabilities increases. Up until the age of 70, the participation of older adults in dietary assessment studies does not differ significantly from younger adults. Some of the techniques reported in the previous sections may help the elderly to report reliably on their food intake. Because memory fades with age, surveying the elderly requires particular care. The 24-hour recall and food frequency method are inappropriate, but adaptations of record methods and diet histories have resulted in valid reports for older adults.[49] Similar to adolescents, a picture-sort technique, including a cognitive processing approach, helps elderly people to remember what they usually eat by allowing them to select foods in pictures.[50]

Ethnic Populations

Structured questionnaires or records need to be adapted when populations with a strong ethnic identity are included. People in minority groups should be con- tacted through their own organizations, if possible, an should use interviewers with the same background. Foo tables or nutrient databases should be checked on com pleteness regarding ethnic foods, and recipes should b checked carefully (dishes may look similar but conta different ingredients). Photo books often are necessary identifying foods.[41]

Equipment for Dietary Surveys

Mode of Administration and Survey Form

Interviews may be conducted by telephone, n computer, or face-to-face meeting at home or in a sp

setting. Each mode has advantages and disadvantages. For example, mailed and telephone interviews have the advantage of lower costs because no costs and time for traveling have to be included. However, the response rates are in general lower with these types of interviews. Instructions with mailed questionnaires must be clear, and portion sizes, as in telephone interviews, are difficult to assess.[1] Computerized interviews are highly standardized, and errors in coding are minimized, but the development is costly and takes time. Face-to-face interviews require highly skilled and trained interviewers.

All interviews must include a survey form that is easy to complete. The form should include clear instructions for the interviewer and subject and have a logical layout. Information should be recorded sequentially by the subject or field-worker, and there should be adequate space for recording information to facilitate computer entry. It is helpful to look at examples and do a trial run before beginning the survey.

Scales and Models

The quantities consumed can be assessed in various ways, although, as explained earlier, not all approaches are suitable for all dietary assessment methods. Equipment for quantifying portion sizes is not always necessary because foods can be expressed in household measures, natural or commercial units, or typical serving sizes.[51] Examples of this approach are the amount of coffee expressed as the number of cups of coffee, the quantity of egg in the number of eggs, the quantity of fish fingers in the number of fish fingers, and the amount of green salad in the number of cups of standard salad. This approach is suitable for many but not all foods. This type of quantification seems less accurate for vegetables and meats. Information on the weight of the reported units and serving sizes and the volume of typical household measures are required for portions to be converted to weight.

Scales. If calibrated weighing scales of good quality are used, this method is most accurate for obtaining the quantity of a food. However, the weighed quantity does not necessarily represent the quantity that would have been eaten if the weighing process were not necessary. When scales are used, they should be robust, be accurate to at least 5 g, and weigh up to 1.5 kg so that a normal plate can be used when weighing the food to be eaten. The weight of foods need not be recorded by hand but can be done verbally, for example, by using a scale with an audiocassette.[52]

Food Photographs. During the past decade, food photographs have been used increasingly for estimating portion sizes. In most cases, a series of photographs representing different quantities is offered to the subject, who is asked to identify the photograph that most resembles the quantity consumed. Sometimes only one photograph is available for each food, and the quantity is indicated as a fraction or multiple of the amount shown. This latter approach gives rise to larger systematic error than does a series of food photographs.[53] Several studies have examined the validity of this type of portion size estimation or the added value of food photographs versus standard methods. The angle at which the photographs are taken, as well as the number and range of depicted quantities, are important for the perception of the shown quantities.[54]

Food Models. Food replicas are three-dimensional models representing specific foods. They are lifelike in size and color and are often made of plastic. Portion-size models are more abstract and represent sizes of portions (mounds, cubes, balls, etc.) rather than specific foods. Drawings are an alternative way to help estimate amounts of food. The validity of the various food models seems highly dependent on the specific model and the culture of the subjects.[51]

Computer Software

Many computer packages for data processing and converting foods to nutrients include a nutrient database as well as software to convert subjects' food consumption into intake of energy, nutrients, and other bioactive compounds. The quality of the food composition data is critically important; the quality of the data for nutrients and other food components important for answering the research questions of the survey should be checked as soon as possible. Software should be chosen on the basis of the research needs and hardware and other software programs already available for the research team. Automation has been incorporated into dietary surveys to various degrees.[8]

Summary

In this chapter we have described the different dietary assessment methods, their strengths and weaknesses, and the importance of examining the sources of error and variation. There is no best method for all purposes, and therefore the investigator has to select the method appropriate for the purpose and target group of the survey. In selecting a dietary method, it is important to answer several basic questions. Who are the subjects, and is group-based or individual information wanted? What information is wanted on which foods, nutrients, or other food compounds? Is the focus usual or current diet? Are special times of the day, days of the week, or seasons of the year of interest? Where is the food is consumed? (e.g., it may be important whether the food was consumed at home or at a restaurant.) Why is the study being conducted? The aim of the study determines the type of information of interest, such as mean intake of groups and distribution and characterization of individuals. It also determines how accurate the data have to be to adequately answer the research question. In addition, it may be beneficial to know which method has been used in studies with a similar research question. Results of the study can be compared more reliably when similar methods have been used. This information, plus consideration of practical issues such as available time, trained staff, and funding,

will direct a researcher to the most efficient method for answering specific research questions.

References

1. Cameron ME, van Staveren WA. *Manual on Methodology for Food Consumption Studies*. New York: Oxford University Press; 1988; 284 pp.
2. Thompson FE, Byers T. Dietary assessment resource manual. J Nutr. 1994;124:2245–2317.
3. Beaton GH. Approaches to analysis of dietary data: relationship between planned analyses and choice of methodology. Am J Clin Nutr. 1994;59:253S–261S.
4. Taren D, Dwyer J, Freedman L, Solomons NW. Dietary assessment methods: where do we go from here? Public Health Nutr. 2002;5:1001–1003.
5. World Health Organization. Diet, nutrition and the prevention of chronic diseases. Report of a joint WHO/FAO Expert Consultation. Technical report series 916. Geneva: WHO; 2003.
6. Kohlmeier L. *The Diet History Method: Proceedings of the 2nd Berlin Meeting on Nutritional Epidemiology*. London: Nishimura, Smith-Gordon; 1991; 143 pp.
7. Subar AF, Thompson FE, Kipnis V, et al Comparative validation of the Block, Willett and National Cancer Institute food frequency questionnaires: the Eating at America's Table Study. Am J Epidemiol. 2001;154:1089–1099.
8. Feskanich D, Sielaff BH, Chong K, Buzzard IM. Computerized collection and analysis of dietary intake information. Comput Methods Programs Biomed. 1989;30:47–57.
9. Hoffmann K, Boeing H, Dufour A, for the EFCOSUM Group. Estimating the distribution of usual dietary intake by short-term measurements. Eur J Clin Nutr. 2002;56(Suppl 2):S53–S62.
10. Bingham SA, Cassidy A, Cole JT. Validation of weighed records and other methods of dietary assessment using the 24 h urine nitrogen technique and other biological markers. Br J Nutr. 1995;73: 531–533.
11. Goris AHC, Westerterp KR. Underreporting of habitual food explained by undereating in motivated lean women. J Nutr. 1999;129:878–882.
12. Heitmann BL, Lissner L. Dietary underreporting by obese individuals—is it specific or non-specific? BMJ. 1995;311:986–989.
13. Slimani N, Deharveng G, Charrondiere RU, et al. Structure of the standardized computerized 24-h recall interview used as reference method in the 22 centres participating in the EPIC project. European Prospective Investigation into Cancer and Nutrition. Computer Methods Programs Biomed. 1999;58: 251–266.
14. Conway JM, Ingwersen LA, Vinyard BT, Moshfegh AJ. Effectiveness of the US Department of Agriculture 5-step multiple-pass method in assessing food intake in obese and nonobese women. Am J Clin Nutr. 2003;77:1171–1178.
15. van Staveren WA, Deurenberg P, Burema J, et al. Seasonal variation in food intake, pattern of physical activity and change in body weight in a group of young adult Dutch women consuming self-selected diets. Int J Obes. 1986;10:133–145.
16. Ireton-Jones CS, Gottschlich MM, Bell SJ. *Practice-Oriented Nutrition Research: An Outcomes Measurement Approach*. Gaithersburg, MD: Aspen Publishers; 1998; 260 pp.
17. Beaton GH, Milner J, Corey P. Sources of variance in 24-hour dietary recall data: implications for nutrition study design and interpretation. Am J Clin Nutr. 1979;32:2546–2459.
18. Burke B. The dietary history as a tool in research. J Am Diet Assoc. 1947;23:1041–1046.
19. Mensink GB, Haftenberger M, Thamm M. Validity of DISHES 98, a computerised dietary history interview: energy and macronutrient intake. Eur J Clin Nutr. 2001;55:409–417.
20. van Staveren WA, de Boer JO, Burema J. Validity and reproducibility of a dietary history method estimating the usual food intake during one month. Am J Clin Nutr. 1985;42:554–559.
21. Byers T, Marshall J, Anthony E. The reliability of dietary history from the distant past. Am J Epidemiol. 1987;125:999–1011.
22. Hankin JH, Yoshinawa ZN, Kolonel LN. Reproducibility of a diet history in older men in Hawaii. Nutr Cancer. 1990;13:129–140.
23. Hankin JH, Wilkens LR, Kolonel LN, Yoshizawa CN. Validation of a quantitative diet history method in Hawaii. Am J Epidemiol. 1991;133:616–628.
24. Jain M, McLaughin J. Validity of nutrient estimates by food frequency questionnaires based either on exact frequencies or categories. Ann Epidemiol. 2000;10:354–360.
25. Cade J, Thompson R, Burly V, Warm D. Development, validation and utilization of food frequency questionnaires—a review. Public Health Nutr. 2002; 5:567–587.
26. Block G, Hartmann AM, Presser CM. A data based approach to diet questionnaire design and testing. Am J Epidemiol. 1986;124:453–469.
27. Willett WC. *Nutritional Epidemiology*. 2nd ed. New York: Oxford University Press; 1998; 528 pp.
28. Sempos CT. Invited commentary: some limitations of semiquantitative food frequency questionnaires. Am J Epidemiol. 1992;135:1127–1132.
29. Schaefer EJ, Augustin JL, Schaefer MM, et al. Lack of efficacy of a food frequency questionnaire in assessing dietary macronutrient intakes in subjects consuming diets of known composition. Am J Clin Nutr. 2000;71:746–751.
30. Krebs-Smith SM, Heimendinger J, Subar AF, et al. Estimating fruit and vegetable intake using food fre-

quency questionnaires: a comparison of instrument. Am J Clin Nutr. 1994;59:283S.

31. Kaaks R, Plummer M, Riboli E, et al. Adjustment for bias due to error in exposure assessments in multicenter cohort studies on diet and cancer: a calibration approach. Am J Clin Nutr. 1994;59:245S–250S.
32. van Staveren WA, de Groot CPGM, Dirren H, Hautvast JGAJ. Evaluation of the dietary history method used in the SENECA study. Eur J Clin Nutr. 1996;50(suppl 2):47S–55S.
33. Beaton GH, Burema J, Ritenbaugh C. Errors in the interpretation of dietary assessments. Am J Clin Nutr. 1997:65;1100S–1107S.
34. Dwyer J, Piccanio MF, Raiten DJ. Estimation of usual intakes: what we eat in America—NHANES. J Nutr. 2003;133:609S–623S.
35. Block G, Shinha R, Gridley G. Collection of dietary-supplement data and implications for analysis. Am J Clin Nutr. 1994;59:232S–239S.
36. Bates CJ, Prentice A, van der Pols JC, et al. Estimation of the use of dietary supplements in the National Diet and Nutrition Survey: people aged 65 years and over. An observed paradox and a recommendation. Eur J Clin Nutr. 1998;52:917–923.
37. Patterson RE, Neuhouser ML, White E, et al. Measurement error from assessing use of vitamin supplements at one point in time. Epidemiology. 1998;9: 567–569.
38. Feunekes GIJ, van't Veer P, van Staveren WA, Kok FJ. Alcohol intake assessments: the sober facts. Am J Epidemiol. 1999;150:105–112.
39. Ocké MC, Bueno de Mesquita HB, Pols MA, et al. The Dutch EPIC food frequency questionnaire. II. Relative validity and reproducibility for nutrients. Int J Epidemiol. 1997;26:49S–58S.
40. Kipnis V, Subar AF, Midthune D, et al. Structure of dietary measurement error: results of the OPEN biomarker study. Am J Epidemiol. 2003;158:14–21.
41. den Hartog AP, van Staveren WA, Brouwer ID. *Manual for Social Surveys on Food Habits and Consumption in Developing Countries.* Weikersheim, Germany: Margraf Verlag; 1995; 153 pp.
42. Hislop TG, Goldman AJ, Zengh YY, et al. Reliability of dietary information from surrogate respondents. Nutr Cancer. 1992;18:123–129.
43. Baranowski T, Sprague D, Baranowski JH, Harrison JA. Accuracy of maternal recall for preschool children. J Am Diet Assoc. 1991;91:669–674.
44. Livingstone MBE, Robson PJ. Measurement of dietary intake in children. Proc Nutr Soc. 2000;59: 279–293.
45. Domel SB, Thompson WO, Baranowski T, Smith AF. How children remember what they have eaten. J Am Diet Assoc. 1994;94:1267–1272.
46. Domel SB, Thompson WO, Davis HC, Johnson MH. "How do you remember you ate" a Delphi technique study to identify retrieval categories from fourth-grade children. J Am Diet Assoc. 1997;97: 31–36.
47. Yaroch AL, Resnicow K, Davis M, Davis A, Smith M, Khan LK. Development of a modified picture-sort food frequency questionnaire administered to low-income, overweight, African American adolescent girls. J Am Diet Assoc. 2000;100:1050–1056.
48. Rockett HR, Berkey CS, Colditz GA. Evaluation of dietary assessment instruments in adolescents. Curr Opin Clin Nutr Metab Care. 2003;5:557–562.
49. van Staveren WA, de Groot CPGM, Blauw YH, van der Wielen RPJ. Assessing diets of elderly people: problems and approaches. Am J Clin Nutr. 1994;59: 221S–223S.
50. Kumanyika SK, Tell GS, Shemanski L, et al. Dietary assessment using a picture approach. Am J Clin Nutr. 1997;65:1123S–1129S.
51. Cypel YS, Guenther PM, Petot GJ. Validity of portion-size measurement aids: a review. J Am Diet Assoc. 1997;97:289–292.
52. Bingham SA. Limitations of the various methods for collecting dietary intake data. Ann Nutr Metab. 1991;35:117–127.
53. Nelson M, Atkinson M, Darbyshire S. Food photography I: the perception of food portion size from photographs. Br J Nutr. 1994;72:649–663.
54. Nelson M, Atkinson M, Darbyshire S. Food photography II: use of food photographs for estimating portion size and the nutrient content of meals. Br J Nutr. 1996;76:31–49.

59
Taste and Food Selection

Adam Drewnowski and Pablo Monsivais

Food choices are largely guided by taste, cost, and convenience. Concerns with health and variety play a secondary role. The concept of food "taste" includes the sensations of taste, aroma, and texture, as well as the pleasure response to foods. Whereas the chemical senses, taste and olfaction, mediate the orosensory perception of food attributes, the central nervous system determines the perception of food reward. Recent research has linked hedonic response to foods to activity within specific brain pathways. The most palatable foods tend to be energy-dense and high in fat, sugar, or both. Taste preferences for sugar and fat vary with age and gender and can be modulated by anticipation as well as by diverse pathologies of eating behavior, such as anorexia nervosa, obesity, or binge eating. However, innate hedonic responses to sugar or fat do not wholly account for the development of eating habits. Food choices are also the outcome of economic decisions made in response to prices, incomes, wealth, access variables, and time constraints. The notion that a sensory "sweet tooth" leads to obesity through excess sugar consumption is overly narrow. The notion that blocking oral sensitivity to fats can protect the consumer from cardiovascular disease ignores the many intermediate steps between taste functioning, dietary choices, and eventual health outcomes. On the other hand, striking a balance between good nutrition and good taste is important. Strategies for dietary change that ignore taste preferences are bound to fail. Public health programs to improve population diets ought to consider age-specific food preferences and culturally driven eating patterns, as well as a wide range of demographic and socioeconomic variables.

Introduction

Food choices are economic decisions made in response to food prices, income, wealth, time constraints, and a broad variety of socioeconomic and cultural variables.[1] Yet when asked what factors influenced their food purchases, consumers always say that the most important factor is taste.[2] The concept of how foods "taste" is based on the physiological sensations of taste, aroma, and texture,[3] and on the pleasure response to foods.[3,4] As documented later, the best-tasting or most rewarding foods are also energy-dense and can be high in added sugars and fats.[4,5] They are also the foods with the least satiating power and the most potential for overconsumption.[6] To complicate matters, such foods are inexpensive, accessible, and widely distributed in the modern food supply.[7] Insofar as taste preferences for palatable, low-cost, energy-dense foods influence food selection patterns, they will affect eating habits and, potentially, health outcomes.

Humans like sweet and dislike bitter tastes[8,9] and display distinct reactions to these stimuli at birth.[10] Sweet foods and beverages are universally liked across all cultures and by all age groups.[3,4] Growing children equate palatability with sweetness and selectively consume the sweetest and the most energy-dense foods.[8] Because bitter taste signals dietary danger, young children tend to reject bitter-tasting vegetables and fruit,[9] especially those that are devoid of energy. The reason is because the perceived reward value or palatability of foods also depends on energy needs. Whereas adolescents select calorie-laden foods and energy-dense diets, older adults dislike oversweet tastes, no longer favor energy-dense foods, and learn to tolerate bitter taste, especially when accompanied by fat, caffeine, or alcohol.[9]

The establishing of causal links between taste function, food choices, and health outcomes poses several challenges. First, data linking taste responses with actual eating habits are extremely limited, because very few studies have examined taste responses, food preferences, and nutrient intakes in the same subject population. Second, given the likely confounding of eating patterns by age, gender, energy needs, and the economics of food choice, it may prove difficult to link taste-related variables with a particular health outcome.

As a result, some of the hypotheses regarding taste functioning and chronic disease risk have never been supported by epidemiological data. For example, the notion that persons with a sensory "sweet tooth" overconsume sweets and therefore are at greater risk for obesity was never supported by corresponding dietary data on sugar consumption.[11] Similarly, no data on sodium intakes supported the claim that higher salt taste preferences in old age led to a greater risk of hypertension. Likewise, the more recent argument that "super tasters" of 6-N-propylthiouracil were at lower risk for heart disease because of their alleged dislike of the texture of dairy fat[12] was not supported by a shred of epidemiological data on fat consumption. In all of those cases, sensory responses of a handful of subjects tested in the laboratory were taken as predictive of food choices and eventual health status of a population.

In reality, multiple steps exist between taste factors and food selection (Figure 1).[3,4] The factors that influence taste and food preferences operate at multiple levels and can range from molecular biology to economics. Although the individual responsiveness to sweetness or fat texture may depend on physiological variables,[13] little doubt exists that the sugar and fat content of a country's diet is an economically driven function of per capita income.[14] Also, some very complex links are present between eating habits and obesity, cancer, cardiovascular disease, and other health outcomes.[15] The complexity of the diet-disease relationship is brought to light by the current controversy of whether a long-term adoption of a low-fat diet has any impact on disease risk.[16,17] Examining some of these causal pathways linking taste with food selection is the topic of this review.

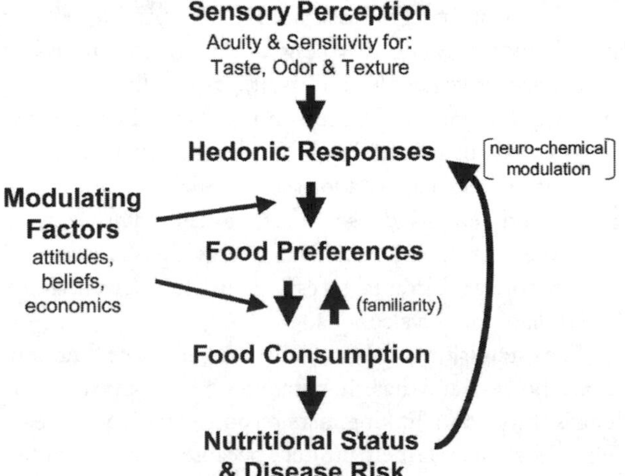

Figure 1. Diagram illustrating hypothesized chain of events between sensory perception and food consumption and nutritional status. At least three steps lie between sensitivity to taste stimuli and nutritional status and disease risk. The strength of some links is modulated by various factors. Note that hedonic responses and food preferences receive feedback from sources indicated in parentheses.

Measuring Taste Responses

Individual taste responses comprise taste perception and taste preferences. Taste perception includes taste acuity, which is determined by using detection and recognition thresholds and taste sensitivity, based on intensity scaling of more concentrated taste stimuli.[18] Most research in nutrition and taste psychophysics has focused on the four basic tastes: sweet, sour, salty, and bitter. The typical stimuli were aqueous solutions of sugars (sweet), sodium chloride (salty), hydrochloric acid (sour), and either caffeine or quinine (bitter). Studies of standard odorants have focused similarly on detection, recognition, and intensity scaling of odors. The food industry has also made use of more complex stimuli that combined taste, texture, and olfaction as well as real foods.

With the exception of bitter taste, the ability to detect extremely low concentrations of a given tastant does not predict preferences for that taste at above-threshold levels. As a result, studies on taste and food choice have focused on intensity scaling of suprathreshold solutions[19] and on hedonic response profiles. Among the methods used for intensity scaling were nine-point category scales, visual analog scales (VAS), the labeled magnitude estimation scale, magnitude estimation, and other ratio scales.[20] Intensity ratings recorded in taste psychophysics are on a logarithmic scale, because taste, like other sensory systems, has sensitivity to stimulus concentration that spans several orders of magnitude.

The measures of taste sensations are distinct from the hedonic preference response, a measure of the acceptability or pleasantness of a given taste stimulus.[21] Laboratory studies have tested hedonic preference ratings for sugar solutions, sweetened lemonade, salted soups or salted tomato juice, or food-like mixtures of milk, cream, and sugar.[21] Studies on the taste acceptability of real foods, conducted in commercial sensory evaluation laboratories, generally asked respondents to rate the acceptability of flavor, color, and texture, as well as the overall acceptability of the food product.[22] The key measure of food preference has been the nine-point hedonic preference scale developed in the 1950s by the US Army Quartermaster Corps.

Sweet Taste Preferences

Intensity and pleasantness ratings for the same taste stimuli follow different psychophysical curves.[21] Although stimuli perceived as more bitter are more strongly disliked,[9] individual ratings of sweetness intensity need not predict sweet taste acceptance or rejection. Hedonic response profiles for increasing concentrations of sugars are highly diverse, ranging from a monotonic rise to an inverse U-shape, or a sharp decline with increasing sweetness. For most people, 10% of sugar in water is the ideal point or "breakpoint."[21]

Despite many attempts, taste response profiles to increasing concentrations of sweet taste have never been linked to body weight, body mass index, or dietary restraint. The only major influence on sweet taste preferences is age. Young children, ages 3 to 5, categorized foods according to whether they were familiar or sweet.[8] Such children did not show the characteristic hedonic optimum or breakpoint for sucrose (around 8%–10% wt/vol) and selected the most intensely sweet solutions in the 20% range. The sweetness breakpoint declined during adolescence, and sweet taste preferences diminished further with age. Although taste functioning is still robust, sugar consumption among adults is less than half of what it is among younger age groups.

A number of influential studies attempted to link the taste preferences for sweetness with obesity and the physiological set-point of body weight. Studies showing that obese persons did not reduce their preferences for sweet taste even after drinking 200 mL of sweet glucose solution[23] were used to support the argument that obese persons were "external," hyperresponsive to sweet taste, and incapable of judging whether they were hungry. However, the externality hypothesis was soon abandoned, because sensory studies demonstrated a wide variety of sensory responses to sweetness among the obese. Studies using sucrose solutions, sweetened soft drinks, or chocolate milkshakes found no connection between sweetness preferences and body weight. These studies, mostly conducted in the 1970s and 1980s, failed to make the case that a "sweet tooth" was the principal cause of human obesity.

Sensory Response to Fats

Fats endow foods with their characteristic taste and texture and contribute to the overall palatability of the diet. The first sensory response to fat involves perception through the nose or mouth of fat-soluble volatile flavor molecules. Oral perception of fat content is largely determined by food texture as sensed by the oral cavity during chewing or swallowing. Other mechanisms involved in signaling the presence of fats in the mouth have been identified in animal studies, including a potassium channel activated by free polyunsaturated fatty acids.[24] The precise type of sensation depends on the food product. In dairy products, fat takes the form of emulsified globules that are perceived as smooth and creamy. Water-binding qualities of fat account for the tenderness and juiciness of steaks and the moistness of cakes and other baked goods. Heat transfer at a high temperature gives rise to food textures that are crispy, crunchy, and brittle. Among textural qualities that depend on the fat content of foods are hard, soft, juicy, chewy, greasy, viscous, smooth, creamy, crunchy, crisp, and brittle. Generally, the high-fat content of foods has been a desirable sensory feature and one that is often linked with higher product quality. Self-reported preferences for fat in foods may be influenced to some extent by the amount of fat in the habitual diet.[25] Rather than eating what they like, consumers like what they already eat.

Fat potentiates the hedonic response to sweetness.[10] A study using 20 different mixtures of dairy products of different fat content and sweetened with different amounts of sugar found evidence for hedonic synergy. Peak hedonic ratings were obtained for stimuli containing 20% fat wt/wt and 8% sucrose wt/wt, corresponding to whipping cream with sugar.[10] These studies made use of response surface methodology and three-dimensional projections of the hedonic response surface. These findings of a hedonic synergy for sugar and fat mixtures were later extended to sweetened cream cheese, fromage blanc, cake frosting, and ice cream.

The hedonic response to sugar and fat mixtures was dependent, to some extent, on the participant's body weight. Massively obese women selected mixtures of milk, cream, and sugar that were less sweet but had a much higher fat content than the mixtures preferred by normal-weight women.[10] Conversely, anorectic women below normal body weight had lower preference ratings overall, tending to select stimuli that were relatively sweet but virtually fat-free. The highest preferences for both sugar and fat were obtained from formerly obese patients who had lost weight and, at the time, were struggling against weight regain.

Since that time, other studies confirmed that preferences for high-fat foods were directly linked to the adult subjects' own percent of body fat. Studies on children ages 3 to 5 later reported that both preferences for and the consumption of fats by children were linked to the body mass indices of their parents.[26,27] Preferences for fat in foods may carry a familial component and may better predict food choices than the universal taste preferences for sugar.

Taste Preferences and Food Choices

Self-reported preferences for pure tastants in solution are often thought to predict food preferences in real life. However, taste preferences for sugar and salt under laboratory conditions were not a good predictor of self-reported preferences for sweet or salty foods.[20] Those measures of food preference were not based on real foods but on the participants' reaction to a checklist of food names. Such data merely reflect attitudes toward a verbal concept of a given food, because the food itself is never presented to the subject and is not available for consumption. Although taste preferences rarely predict actual choices, a closer correspondence between two sets of ratings is obtained when the taste stimulus closely resembles the food product. For example, preferences for sugar solutions in water may predict the same subjects' preferences for cola or fruit juice, but not preferences for other sweet foods, such as doughnuts or candy. So far, sweet taste preferences have not been linked with epidemiological measures of sugar consumption.

Food Choices in Childhood

Studies of preschool children have shown that food preferences in early life are determined by two factors: familiarity and sweetness.[8] Preferences for fat may be acquired early in life, because children learn to prefer those flavors that are associated with high energy density and fat content. Fat and sugar are the chief components of peanut butter and jelly sandwiches, chocolate candy, cookies, and ice cream.

Both sweet taste preference and sugar consumption decline between adolescence and adult life.[28] Whereas children's food preferences are often guided by taste alone,[8] food choices of adults tend to be influenced by nutritional beliefs and attitudes toward weight and dieting.[1] However, all evidence is indirect, because no study has yet examined taste preferences, diet-related attitudes, and food intakes in the same subject group. Surveys of adolescent food habits are typically based on food preference checklists and so reflect food-related attitudes rather than taste preferences. In general, adolescents report liking foods rich in fat, sugar, and salt. Observational studies have confirmed that the most frequently consumed foods include candy, potato chips, sweetened beverages, dry presweetened cereal, cupcakes, doughnuts, and pies.

Children also show an aversion to bitter foods.[29,1] Typical food dislikes are based on taste (bitter), aversive trigeminal stimulation (sharp), and various unpleasant food textures. Acquired preferences for coffee, beer, alcohol, and hot peppers are commonly cited as evidence that food preferences can be learned and modified with age. Indeed, food preferences and aversions are modifiable by growth, maturation, and hormonal status. Both taste preferences and food choices are further shaped by prior experience and associative learning. Preferences for bitter foods (caffeine), alcohol, and hot spices are all said to be the result of associating the often unpleasant taste with the desirable post-ingestive consequences.[1] A previously neutral or even unpleasant taste can become preferred, provided that it is linked with a suitable mechanism of reward.

Taste and Aging

Age-related deficits in taste and smell are reputed to decrease the enjoyment of food and to reduce food consumption, leading, eventually, to malnutrition and ill health. However, little evidence supports this view. Although many elderly people suffer from olfactory and some suffer from taste deficits, their impact on food choices, nutrition, and health is not always clear. No study has demonstrated a causal relationship between sensory impairment, diminished hedonic response, and altered food patterns in the same group of elderly persons.[30]

Most studies on taste and aging have focused on taste acuity and sensitivity rather than hedonic preference. Aqueous solutions of sugar and salt were the stimuli of choice because of the presumed impact on sugar and salt intakes, diabetes, and hypertension. One assumption was that elderly subjects suffering from taste losses would prefer sweeter and saltier stimuli and so consume more sugar and salt. Though some studies reported that hedonic ratings for solutions of sucrose, sodium chloride, and citric acid increased with age, other studies failed to confirm a broad age-related shift in hedonic response.[30] Taste function is relatively robust, and whole-mouth tasting can be normal even into advanced old age. In at least one study, older adults showed no impairments in taste sensitivity or hedonic response profiles for sucrose and sodium chloride solutions.[31] Furthermore, preference profiles for salty taste had no impact on sodium consumption.[31]

Rolls and Drewnowski[30] have argued that sensory losses and a decline in sensory-specific satiety are responsible for reduced dietary variety in old age. Flavor amplification has been suggested as one mechanism to increase food intake.[32] However, although diets of some older persons are indeed monotonous, it is difficult to separate the effects of taste function from those of illness, education, and income.[30] Changed social and economic circumstances, as well as a host of psychological variables, including depression, loneliness, bereavement, and social support, all have a major impact on dietary habits. Although taste and smell deficits do not always have a consistent effect on nutrition and health,[20,32] social and taste factors seem to influence eating habits in old age.

Taste and Food Choices in Obesity

Taste preferences for mixtures of sugar and fat were higher among obese women and patients who had recently lost weight.[10] Obese women selected fat-rich taste stimuli in sensory studies and listed high-fat foods as their favorites on food preference checklists. Obese women, when asked to list their top 10 favorite foods, listed bread, doughnuts, cake, cookies, ice cream, chocolate, pies, and other desserts. In contrast, obese men listed steaks, roasts, hamburgers, French fried potatoes, pizza, and ice cream. Whereas women selected foods that were mixtures of sugar and fat, men selected foods that included fat, protein, and salt. These findings were consistent with a more recent longitudinal study, which found that hedonic response to sweetness was positively associated with subsequent weight gain.[33]

Neurobiology of Pleasure and Reward

Eating is one of life's greatest pleasures. Food can provide pleasure through its sensory qualities and can be the object of cravings and the intense desire for a specific food or foods, independent of hunger.[34] Eating is also a matter of life or death. Like other behaviors that are vital for survival, eating is reinforced. Behavioral, pharmacological, and, more recently, functional brain imaging studies have revealed that the hedonic response to food,

food cravings, and the reinforcement of eating are controlled by specific brain pathways.

Craving and the Hedonic Response to Food

Studies of food cravings have implicated the serotonergic system, endogenous opiate peptides, and endocannabinoids. Serotonergic pathways were first linked to food cravings and intake from studies of clinically depressed individuals.[33] Serotonin is primarily associated with cravings for carbohydrates in what is thought to be a homeostatic regulatory process: low serotonin levels stimulate the ingestion of carbohydrates, which can increase levels of l-tryptophan, the metabolic precursor of serotonin.[34,35]

Endogenous opiates or endorphins are implicated in food cravings for fats and sweets.[36] Opiates act via the μ-type opioid receptor[37] to increase sweet taste in humans and the intake of sweet solutions by rats,[38] whereas antagonists decrease sweet preferences. Fat consumption in rats was likewise increased by the opiate agonists morphine and butorphanol. Endogenous opiates also mediate the hedonic response to preferred foods.[39] Opiate antagonists, such as naloxone, naltrexone, or nalmefene, appear to reduce food intakes by lowering preferences for selected foods. Whereas the consumption of nonpreferred foods remained stable after naltrexone, rated pleasantness of sweet glucose solutions declined.[40] Similar results were obtained with another opiate antagonist, nalmefene.[41]

Plant-derived or synthetic cannabinoids have long been used for alleviating nausea and promoting food intake in cancer and AIDS patients. The discovery of endocannabinoids in the 1990s fostered research on the natural function of these fatty acid-derived neurotransmitters.[42] The orexigenic effect of endocannabinoids is thought to be localized to endocannabinoid receptors in the hypothalamus and limbic forebrain. Endocannabinoid levels are elevated with fasting. Unlike opiate receptor blockade, pharmacological block of CB-1, an endocannabinoid receptor, reduces intake of all food, both preferred and nonpreferred.[42] Malfunction in the metabolism of endocannabinoids has been implicated in obesity. Fatty acid amine hydrolase is the primary enzyme involved in degradation of endocannabinoids. Loss of fatty acid amine hydrolase function associated with genetic polymorphisms in humans was associated with overweight and obesity in a recent cross-sectional study.[43]

Food Reward

Energy intake is regulated by brain circuitry that is linked to reward centers in the striatum,[44] where feeding is thought to be reinforced by dopaminergic projections from the midbrain.[45,46] Unlike opiates and endocannabinoids, dopamine's release is not tied to the reported hedonics of a food stimulus.[47] Abnormalities in reward circuitry have been linked to obesity. Human brain imaging has shown an inverse relationship between levels of the D2-type dopamine receptor in the striatum and subjects' body mass index.[46] Beyond this correlation, identifying the contribution of dopamine to food reward and obesity remains an important goal for future work.

Eating Disorders and Addiction

Obvious parallels have been drawn between binge eating and drug addiction, because both behavioral syndromes involve cravings and loss of control. Endogenous opiate peptides are thought to mediate alcohol cravings, and naltrexone, a long-lasting opiate antagonist, has been used to curb these cravings in alcoholics. Opiate addictions have been associated with an enhanced appetite for sweets, and opiate withdrawal is eased by ice cream and chocolate.[36] Functional imaging studies have found a paucity of available D2 receptors in both obese and drug-addicted subjects.[46] Together, these findings suggest that craving and reward are mediated by distinct neurochemical pathways, and that these pathways provide a common anatomical substrate for behavioral responses to both food and drugs of abuse. These findings also suggest that food palatability does have an underlying neurochemical component.

Palatability and Satiety

Palatability and satiety have opposite effects on food intakes. Although palatability increases appetite and therefore food consumption, satiety limits consumption by reducing meal size or by delaying the onset of the next meal. However, both palatability and satiety tend to be measured in terms of the amount of food consumed. As a result, the foods that are overeaten are, by definition, the most palatable foods and the least satiating.

Standard measures of palatability include the perceived pleasantness of a given food, intent to eat, or the amount of food consumed. Marketing research studies often use palatability as a predictor of purchase intent and actual food use. Among standard measures of satiety are reduced hunger, fullness, reduced intent to consume a meal or snack, or the amount of food consumed. Some investigators have made a distinction between satiety and satiation.[20] Whereas satiation is responsible for the termination of a given meal and reduced meal size, satiety, defined as a state of internal repletion, delays the onset of the next meal and so reduces energy intakes in the long-term.

Increased satiety has also been measured in terms of reduced palatability. Sensory-specific satiety was defined as reduced palatability of the just-consumed food relative to other foods. In other words, given the reciprocal nature of palatability and satiety measures, the most palatable foods are, by definition, the least satiating and vice versa.

The low satiating power of energy-dense sweet and fat-rich foods has been singled out for special scrutiny.[48,49] Some researchers have argued that the palatability of sugar overrode normal satiety signals, leading to overeating and overweight.[50] Others have noted that fat had low satiating power, judging by the "passive overeating" of fat-rich foods.[51] One question is whether palatable fat-rich foods are overeaten because of their high energy density or because of their fat content.[51] If satiety is macronutrient-driven, fat may be overeaten because it affects satiety less than a corresponding amount (in kilocalories) of carbohydrate or protein. The creation of palatable and yet highly satiating foods, the avowed goal of the weight-loss industry, may represent a contradiction in terms.

Food Preferences and Food Use

Food preferences are generally assumed to predict food consumption. However, it is equally possible that self-reported food preferences reflect existing food consumption. In other words, consumers may have positive attitudes toward foods that they frequently eat. This association between food preferences and reported frequencies of food use has major implications for the study of nutritional epidemiology.

In recent years, food frequency questionnaires have become the dominant tool of dietary intake assessment in large-scale survey studies.[52] Food preference checklists and food frequency questionnaires instruments share a number of key features. Both are printed, self-administered surveys that require respondents to form a mental representation of a food item and to generate an appropriate self-report. A typical food frequency questionnaires consists of a list of about 100 or more foods and food groups.[52] Food groups can be very specific (e.g., "raw spinach") or aggregated by groups (e.g., "hamburger, steak, and roast beef"). Respondents are asked to report the usual frequency of consumption of each food using anchored nine-point category scale, in which the categories can range from "never or less than once per month" to "5 + per day." Nutrient intakes are calculated by multiplying the reported frequency of consumption of each food by the amount of nutrients in a specified (or assumed) portion size, and then summing for all foods on the list.[52]

Respondents who complete a food preference checklist are also presented with a long list of food names and are asked to generate an appropriate self-report. Respondents also rate their preferences using anchored nine-point category scales. The hedonic preference scale, which ranges from "1 = dislike extremely" to "9 = like extremely," serves to assess preferences for foods and beverages in sensory evaluation studies.

How respondents estimate the frequency of food use has been a matter of debate.[29] The assumption is that respondents consider the consumption of each item, integrate information over the reference year, and then derive a mean frequency of food use.[52] The frequency score is supposedly a measure of past dietary behavior, based on a combination of memory and retrieval processes.[52] Past efforts at improving food frequency questionnaires instruments have focused on aided recall, cognitive interviewing, and other ways to help the respondents' memory of past food use,[52,53] which is very different from preferences, thought to reflect a subjective attitude or a predisposition toward a mental image of a given food.[20]

Not all researchers agree that the food frequency response is based on memory and food recall.[29,54] Research on the structure of human memory has distinguished between episodic memory—memory for specific events—and recall constructed from general memory and attitudes about foods. With some exceptions, the consumption of common foods over the course of a year is not encoded as a series of discrete episodic events. The implication is that food frequencies are inferred, as opposed to recalled, and are based on some perceived notion of a "usual" or "typical" diet.[29,54] Far from being based on a memory representation, food frequency scores might reflect an individual's accumulated mental image of his or her habitual diet rather than his or her actual diet during the reference period.[29]

Correlations between food preferences (as recorded by the food preference checklist) and consumption frequencies (as measured by the food frequencgy questionnaires) of individual foods have been found to range from 0.04 to 0.56, with food likes and dislikes accounting for 30% of the variance of overall reported food use.[55] Reported food dislike was invariably linked to a food's nonuse, whereas higher preference scores were associated with higher mean frequencies of consumption. This direct relationship was not observed for all foods or in all respondents. Respondents often reported consuming certain preferred foods only rarely, suggesting other factors that modulate the link between preferences and food intake.[20,55]

Economics of Food Choice

As food companies have learned, market research studies based on blinded taste tests do not always predict purchase intent or actual consumer behavior. Although taste is regarded as the deciding factor, consumption patterns are also influenced by price, convenience, safety, and nutritional concerns.[1,2] Other demographic, sociocultural, and economic factors also modulate the connection between taste responsiveness and food choice.

Consumer food choices are economic decisions made in response to prices, incomes, time constraints, and the perceived nutritional value of foods. The monetary cost of food is a dominant factor guiding food selection and a major constraint on the diet quality of individuals. Several economic studies have made the association between the declining monetary and time cost of food and rising obesity rates.[56,57] Those studies pointed to the widespread availability of energy-dense fast foods, the entry of women into the labor force, and lower physical activity associated with work.[57,58] However, as argued by Drewnowski and Specter,[59] not all foods have become less expensive. Rather, there is a growing price disparity between the lower-cost refined grains, added sugars, and added fats and the more expensive lean meats, dairy products, whole grains, and fresh vegetables and fruit.[59] Further, the availability of healthier foods tends to be more limited in economically disadvantaged areas.[60-62] Disparities in access to healthy foods, together with the increasingly limited time devoted to food preparation and consumption, may help to explain some of the observed disparities in health.

The nature of the relationship between diet quality and diet cost at different levels of socioeconomic position has important implications for the study of diets and disease risk. One key question is whether the more nutrient-dense diets are necessarily more expensive. Preliminary data from France suggest that the relationship is asymmetrical. Whereas the more expensive diets are not necessarily high quality or nutrient dense, reducing food costs below a certain limit virtually guarantees that the resulting diet will be nutrient poor.[63] Another question is whether low-cost diets are invariably selected by low-income consumers, or do some low-income groups choose healthier diets, perhaps because of improved nutrition knowledge, education, or culture, or because of participation in food assistance programs? Consumer food choices in response to food prices are very likely modulated by socioeconomic variables.

Perhaps the key question regarding diets and obesity rates is, "Do the consumers of low-cost, energy-dense, and palatable diets tend to consume more energy overall?" In other words, can body mass index values be linked directly to food prices and to diet costs ($/d or $/MJ) after adjusting for covariates? Although some preliminary data on diet quality and diet cost are available,[59,64] the answers to all of these questions are far from clear.

Conclusions

Nutrition education and intervention strategies aimed at improving diet quality have focused almost exclusively on the nutritional quality of foods and not on taste or the pleasure response. Much effort has been spent to persuade consumers to replace palatable, energy-dense foods with less palatable, but, arguably, healthier, starches and grains. Social marketing and other strategies for behavioral change[65,66] are used in an effort to reduce fat and sugar consumption by children, adolescents, and adults. Yet such efforts to change dietary behavior face multiple challenges. Humans have an innate preference for sugar and fat, which is available in an ever-expanding variety of attractive, palatable, convenient, and inexpensive forms. To succeed, dietary intervention strategies aimed at improving diet quality should consider the sensory pleasure response to foods, as well as a wide range of demographic, economic, social, and cultural variables.

References

1. Logue AW. *The Psychology of Eating and Drinking*, 3rd ed. New York: Brunner-Routledge; 2004.
2. Glanz K, Basil M, Maibach E, et al. Why Americans eat what they do: taste, nutrition, cost, convenience, and weight control concerns as influences on food consumption. J Am Diet Assoc. 1998;98:1118–1126.
3. Drewnowski A. Taste preferences and food intake. Annu Rev Nutr. 1997;17:237–253.
4. Drewnowski A. Energy density, palatability, and satiety: implications for weight control. Nutr Rev. 1998;56:347–353.
5. Drewnowski A. The role of energy density. Lipids. 2003;38:109–115.
6. Drewnowski A, Almiron-Roig E, Marmonier C, et al. Dietary energy density and body weight: is there a relationship? Nutr Rev. 2004;62:403–413.
7. Putnam J, Allshouse J, Kantor LS. U.S. per capita food supply trends: more calories, refined carbohydrates and fats. Food Rev. 2002;25:2–15.
8. Birch LL. Development of food preferences. Ann Rev Nutr. 1999;19:41–62.
9. Drewnowski A. The science and complexity of bitter taste. Nutr Rev. 2001;59:163–169.
10. Drewnowski A, Brunzell JD, Sande K, et al. Sweet tooth reconsidered: taste responsiveness in human obesity. Physiol Behav. 1985;35:617–622.
11. Anderson CH. Sugars, sweetness, and food intake. Am J Clin Nutr. 1995;62(1S):195S–201S.
12. Duffy VB. Associations between oral sensation, dietary behaviors and risk of cardiovascular disease (CVD). Appetite. 2004;43:5–9.
13. Mattes RD. Fat taste and lipid metabolism in humans. Physiol Behav. 2005;86:691–697.
14. Drewnowski A, Popkin BM. The nutrition transition: new trends in the global diet. Nutr Rev. 1997; 55:31–43.
15. Willett WC, Leibel RL. Dietary fat is not a major determinant of body fat. Am J Med. 2002; 113(Suppl):47S–59S.
16. Beresford SA, Johnson KC, Ritenbaugh C, et al. Low-fat dietary pattern and risk of colorectal cancer: the Women's Health Initiative Randomized Controlled Dietary Modification Trial. JAMA. 2006; 295:643–654.
17. Howard BV, Van Horn L, Hsia J, et al. Low-fat dietary pattern and risk of cardiovascular disease: the Women's Health Initiative Randomized Controlled Dietary Modification Trial. JAMA. 2006;295: 655–666.
18. Drewnowski A. Genetics of human taste perception. In: Doty RL, ed. *Handbook of Olfaction and Gustation*, 2nd ed. New York: Marcel Dekker; 2003; 847–860.
19. Bartoshuk LM. The biological basis of food perception and acceptance. Food Qual Pref. 1993;4:21–32.
20. Mattes RD, Hollis J, Hayes D, et al. Appetite: measurement and manipulation misgivings. J Am Diet Assoc 2005;105:S87–S97.
21. Moskowitz HR, Kluter RA, Westerling J, et al. Sugar sweetness and pleasantness: evidence for dif-

ferent psychophysical laws. Science. 1974;184: 583–585.
22. Clydesdale FM. Color as a factor in food choice. Crit Rev Food Sci Nutr. 1993;33:83–101.
23. Cabanac M, Duclaux R. Obesity: absence of satiety aversion to sucrose. Science. 1970;168:496–497.
24. Gilbertson TA, Liu L, Kim I, et al. Fatty acid responses in taste cells from obesity-prone and resistant rats. Physiol Behav. 2005;86:681–690.
25. Cooling J, Blundell J. Are high-fat and low-fat consumers distinct phenotypes? Differences in the subjective and behavioral responses to energy and nutrient challenges. Eur J Clin Nutr. 1998;52:193–201.
26. Fisher JO, Birch JL. Fat preferences and fat consumption of 3- to 5-year-old children are related to parent adiposity. J Am Diet Assoc. 1995;95: 759–764.
27. Wardle J, Guthrie C, Sanderson S, et al. Food and activity preferences in children of lean and obese parents. Int J Obes Relat Metab Disord. 2001;25: 971–977.
28. Bowman SA. Diets of individuals based on energy intakes from added sugars. Fam Econ Nutr Rev. 1999;12:31–38.
29. Drewnowski A. Diet image: a new perspective on the food frequency questionnaire. Nutr Rev. 2001; 59:370–374.
30. Rolls BJ, Drewnowski A. *Nutrition and Aging. Encyclopedia of Gerontology.* New York: Academic Press; 1996.
31. Drewnowski A, Henderson SA, Driscoll A, et al. Salt taste perceptions and preferences are unrelated to sodium consumption in healthy older adults. J Am Diet Assoc. 1996;96:471–474.
32. Rolls BJ. Do chemosensory changes influence food intake in the elderly? Physiol Behav. 1999;66: 193–197.
33. Salbe AD, Del Parigi A, Pratley RE, et al. Taste preferences and body weight changes in an obesity-prone population. Am J Clin Nutr. 2004;79: 372–378.
34. Pelchat ML. Of human bondage: food craving, obsession, compulsion, and addiction. Physiol Behav. 2002;76:347–352.
35. Yanovski S. Sugar and fat: cravings and aversions. J Nutr. 2003;133:835S–837S.
36. Drewnowski A, Krahn DD, Demitrack MA, et al. Naloxone, an opiate blocker, reduces the consumption of sweet high-fat foods in obese and lean female binge eaters. Am J Clin Nutr. 1995;61:1206–1212.
37. Kelley AE, Bakshi VP, Haber SN, et al. Opioid modulation of taste hedonics within the ventral striatum. Physiol Behav. 2002;76:365–377.
38. Pecina S, Berridge KC. Hedonic hot spot in nucleus accumbens shell: where do mu-opioids cause increased hedonic impact of sweetness? J Neurosci. 2005;25:11777–11786.
39. Levine AS, Kotz CM, Gosnell BA. Sugars: hedonic aspects, neuroregulation, and energy balance. Am J Clin Nutr. 2003;78:834S–842S.
40. Hetherington MM, Ed. Food cravings and addiction. London: Leatherhead Publishing; 2001.
41. Yeomans MR, Wright P. Lower pleasantness of palatable foods in nalmefene-treated human volunteers. Appetite. 1991;16:249–259.
42. Di Marzo, Matias
43. Sipe JC, Waalen J, Gerber A, et al. Overweight and obesity associated with a missense polymorphism in fatty acid amide hydrolase (FAAH). Int J Obes (Lond). 2005;29:755–759.
44. Lattemann DP. The CNS physiology of food reward: current insights and future directions. In: Stricker E, Woods S, eds. *Neurobiology of Food and Fluid Intake,* 2nd ed. New York: Plenum Publishers; 2004; 43–59.
45. Epstein LH, Leddy JJ. Food reinforcement. Appetite. 2006;46:22–25.
46. Wang GJ, Volkow ND, Thanos PK, et al. Similarity between obesity and drug addiction as assessed by neurofunctional imaging: a concept review. J Addict Dis. 2004;23:39–53.
47. Wang GJ, Volkow ND, Fowler JS. The role of dopamine in motivation for food in humans: implications for obesity. Expert Opin Ther Targets. 2002;6: 601–609.
48. Erlanson-Albertsson C. How palatable food disrupts appetite regulation. Basic Clin Pharmacol Toxicol. 2005;97:61–73.
49. Holt SH, Brand Miller JC, Petocz P, et al. A satiety index of common foods. Eur J Clin Nutr. 1995;49: 675–690.
50. Green SM, Burley VJ, Blundell JE. Effect of fat- and sucrose containing foods on the size of eating episodes and energy intake in lean males; potential for causing overconsumption. Eur J Clin Nutr. 1994; 48:547–555.
51. Blundell JE, Burley VJ, Cotton JR, et al. Dietary fat and the control of energy intake: evaluating the effects of fat on meal size and postmeal satiety. Am J Clin Nutr. 1993;57:772S–778S.
52. Willett WC, ed. *Nutritional Epidemiology,* 2nd ed. New York: Oxford University Press; 1998.
53. Subar AF, Thompson FE, Smith AF, et al. Improving food frequency questionnaires: a qualitative approach using cognitive interviewing. J Am Diet Assoc. 1995;95:781–788.
54. Kristal AR, Peters U, Potter JD. Is it time to abandon the food frequency questionnaire? Cancer Epidemiol Biomarkers Prev. 2005;14:2826–2828.
55. Drewnowski A, Hann C, Henderson SA, et al. Both food preferences and food frequency scores predict fat intakes of women with breast cancer. J Am Diet Assoc. 2000;100:1325–1333.
56. Lakdawalla D, Philipson T. The growth of obesity

and technological change: a theoretical and empirical examination. Natl Bur Econ Res. 2002. Available at http://www.nber.org/papers/w8946.)

57. Philipson T. The world-wide growth in obesity: an economic research agenda. Health Econ. 2001;10: 1–7.
58. Cutler DM, Glaeser El, Shapiro JM. Why have Americans become more obese? Natl Bur Econ Res. 2003; working paper 9446.
59. Drewnowski A, Specter SE. Poverty and obesity: dietary quality, energy density, and energy costs. Am J Clin Nutr. 2004;79:6–16.
60. Chung C, Myers SL. Do the poor pay more for food? An analysis of grocery store availability and food price disparities. J Consum Aff. 1999;33:276–296.
61. Kantor LS. Community food security programs improve food access. Food Rev. 2001;24:20–26.
62. Neault N, Cook JT, Morris V, et al. *The Real Cost of a Healthy Diet: Healthful Foods Are Out of Reach for Low-Income Families in Boston, Massachusetts.* Report published by the Boston Medical Center Department of Pediatrics, Boston, MA, August 2005. Available at http://dcc2.bumc.bu.edu/csnappublic/HealthyDiet_Aug2005.pdf.
63. Darmon N, Ferguson E, Briend A. A cost constraint alone has adverse effects on food selection and nutrient density: an analysis of human diets by linear programming. J Nutr. 2002;132:3764–3771.
64. Andrieu E, Darmon N, Drewnowski A. Low-cost diets: more energy, fewer nutrients. Eur J Clin Nutr. 2006;60:434–6.
65. Ashfield-Watt PA, Welch AA, Day NE, et al. Is "five-a-day" an effective way of increasing fruit and vegetable intakes? Public Health Nutr. 2004;7: 257–261.
66. Contento I, Balch GI, Bronner YL, et al. The effectiveness of nutrition education and implications for nutrition education policy, programs, and research: a review of research. J Nutr Edu. 1995;27:278–418.

60 Energy Intake, Obesity, and Eating Behaviors

Megan A. McCrory

Obesity is one of the leading public health problems of our time. Approximately two-thirds of US adults are overweight (body mass index [BMI] 25 kg/m^2 or more) or obese (BMI 30 kg/m^2 or more),[1] and worldwide the prevalence of obesity is greater than ever.[2] Energy balance is ultimately the result of complex interactions between several lifestyle, metabolic, and genetic factors. Stated simply, however, weight gain ensues when energy intake exceeds energy expenditure.

Trends in Energy Intake and Eating Patterns in the United States

Per-capita energy intake in the United States is on the rise, with Americans consuming anywhere from approximately 150 to 500 kcal/d more than in the 1980s.[3,4] Several food intake patterns may be contributing to this trend. For example, survey data show that snacking, breakfast skipping, and consumption of foods high in energy density and away from home all increased between 1977 and 1998.[3,5-8] Other dietary factors, such as an increasing variety of foods high in energy density[9] and increasingly large portion sizes, may also be important contributors.[10] A recent analysis of eating pattern changes from US Department of Agriculture surveys conducted in 1977–78, 1989–91, and 1994–96 showed that energy intake, snacking frequency and portions, and food away from home (FAFH) increased disproportionately in overweight and obese individuals compared with normal-weight individuals over this period (M. McCrory, S. Roberts, T. Huang, unpublished observations), suggesting that these eating patterns may be particularly important contributors to the US obesity epidemic. Several eating patterns that have been shown to influence appetite regulation in controlled studies are discussed below.

Portions

The portion consumed appears to be an important determinant of BMI and weight change. Recently, positive associations of meal and snack portions with BMI in older children and adults were seen in analyses of data from the Continuing Survey of Intakes by Individuals 1994–96.[11,12] Moreover, consuming reduced portions is key to long-term weight loss success.[13,14] Several controlled feeding studies suggest that cognitive control over portions served and eaten is necessary to limit energy intake, and that the increased portion size of prepackaged foods and restaurant food[10] may make it more difficult than ever to do so. In several single-meal studies, energy intake increased with increasing portion served.[4,15] For example, subjects consumed 30% more energy (162 kcal) from a macaroni-and-cheese entrée when the portion was doubled from 500 g to 1000 g.[16] Similar results have been shown for other foods.

Individuals may rely more on visual cues than on internal satiety signals when determining how much to eat. Wansink et al.[17] suggest that people may have an expectation for how much they will consume that may be based on how much they plan to leave uneaten (rather than how much they will eat per se). In their "bottomless soup bowl" study, subjects consumed tomato soup from either a normal bowl that was refilled by a server when it was 25% full, or from a bowl that was self-refilling from the bottom at a constant rate. The bottomless nature of the bowl was concealed from the subjects. Subjects who ate from the bottomless bowl consumed 73% more soup (113 kcal) than those who ate from the normal bowl. In addition, subjects who ate from the bottomless bowl were not aware that they had consumed more soup, nor were their ratings of hunger and fullness different from the controls. These latter findings are in agreement with other studies,[15] and support the idea that visual cues may be a primary factor people use to determine when to stop eating.

Relying on visual cues for how much to consume may be a learned phenomenon, perhaps from early childhood.[18] The secular trend in larger portions served in restaurants and of prepackaged foods may also have led to certain expectations about how much is "normal" or usual to consume. The fact that sustained weight loss can be in part accomplished by reductions in portions consumed[14] strongly suggests that it is possible to unlearn this reliance on visual cues, or at least to cognitively override it.

Dietary Variety

The variety of foods available on the US market has increased markedly over the past several decades, particularly in nutrient-poor, high-energy-dense categories.[9] As reviewed previously, people consume approximately 25% more calories in a meal when served a variety of foods that differ in sensory properties such as flavor, texture, and appearance than they do when an unlimited amount of single and equally palatable food is served.[4] For example, when sandwiches with three different fillings were served, more calories were consumed than when one sandwich type was served. Similar findings have occurred for several other foods, including yogurts, pasta, and ice cream. The effects of variety on caloric intake and body weight are not limited to humans. Laboratory animals (rats, cats, and hamsters) also consume about 25% more calories and gain more weight when fed different-flavored chows.[4]

The effects of dietary variety on consumption appear to extend beyond a single meal. Adults consuming a greater variety from different food groups over several days or months consumed more energy from each of those groups.[19,20] However, variety may be positively or negatively associated with body weight status, depending on the food group. In a small clinical study[19] and a larger survey sample,[20] more variety consumed from energy-dense groups such as sweets, snacks, condiments, entrées, and carbohydrate-based foods was associated with increased adiposity, whereas more variety consumed from energy-weak vegetable, fruit, and legume foods was associated with leanness.

"Sensory-specific satiety" is thought to be the underlying reason that variety enhances food consumption.[21] Sensory-specific satiety refers to the observation that as a food is consumed, its palatability, or taste pleasantness, decreases, whereas the palatability of unconsumed foods remains high. Thus, when only one or a few foods are available, satiation sets in more quickly than when a higher variety of foods are present. Potentially, having more flavors and textures to choose from allows the palatability of the meal be maintained at an overall high level. Overconsumption at restaurants, buffets, potlucks, and special holiday meals, and underconsumption of leftovers, may be explained in part by sensory-specific satiety and dietary variety.

Reducing energy-dense variety and increasing energy-weak and micronutrient-dense food variety may help to reduce excess body weight and maintain the loss. Recently, Raynor et al.[22] reported a lower variety consumed from all food groups except fruit and mixed items in more than 2200 persons in the National Weight Control Registry who maintained a 30-lb (13.6-kg) weight loss for an average of 6.1 years than people who recently lost 30 over 6 months in a behavioral weight loss program. In another study,[23] subjects undergoing an 18-month standard obesity treatment regimen without specific advice on dietary variety self-selected an increase in variety of vegetable and low-fat bread groups and a decrease in variety of high-fat food and fats/sweets/oils groups.

Restaurant Food, Fast Food, and PrePrepare prepared Food

In 1995, the average American consumed approximately one-third of his or her daily energy intake as FAFH, an increase from 18% of daily energy intake in 1977–78.[3] Roughly 41% of Americans reported consuming three or more commercially prepared meals a week in 1999–2000.[24] Several investigators have reported a positive association between the frequency of consuming fast food, restaurant food, or other take-away food and higher body fatness.[24] Also, more frequent consumption of these foods independently predicts weight change in observational studies and behavioral interventions.[25-27]

More frequent consumption of FAFH has been associated with higher daily energy intakes in observational studies.[24-28] A recent study showed extremely high amounts of energy consumed in a single eating occasion in a food court setting.[29] In this study, lean adolescents consumed 1458 kcal (57% of estimated energy requirements) and obese adolescents consumed 1860 kcal (61% of estimated energy requirements). Also, unscheduled 24-hour dietary recall data showed that obese adolescents consumed more total energy on days in which fast food was consumed, whereas lean adolescents did not. Reasons for overconsumption of FAFH are several and are thought to include the high palatability, variety, energy density, and portions and lower fiber content of FAFH compared with other foods.[28] More food is often consumed in the presence of other people as well, a phenomenon known as "social facilitation of energy intake."[30]

Energy-Containing Beverages

US per-capita soft drink consumption increased by more than 60% between 1977 and 1998.[3] Several lines of evidence suggest that consumption of energy-containing beverages may contribute to excess energy intake and weight gain. Consumption of energy-containing beverages adds to total caloric intake from food compared with consumption of a beverage with no calories or to not consuming a beverage[31,32] over a single eating occasion. Also, energy-containing beverages appear to increase daily energy intake. In an observational study, daily energy intakes of adults 18 to 75 years of age were higher on days in which soda, alcohol, milk, or juice was consumed compared with days in which those items were not consumed.[33] A limited number of short- and long-term studies in children and adults suggest that increased and decreased soft-drink intake is linked with weight gain and weight loss, respectively.[34-37]

Several different mechanisms by which energy-containing beverages may increase total energy intake have been proposed. First, the energy in beverages may simply add to the energy consumed from food.[32] In 1996, Mattes[38] reviewed the literature and concluded that the calories in energy-containing beverages are less compensated for in the next eating occasion compared with when an equal amount of solid food is consumed; however, findings from more recent studies on this topic have been mixed.[39,40] Second, the amount and types of sugars in the beverages may be particularly important. Fructose, a component of high-fructose corn syrup, which is a major ingredient in many sweetened beverages, may have metabolic effects that promote hunger, appetite, and food intake.[41,42] Recently, St. Onge et al.[43] reported that 600 kcal of a sugar-only versus a mixed-nutrient beverage (energy distribution of 17% protein, 67% carbohydrate, 16% fat), both with a 1:1 ratio of sucrose to corn syrup solids, evoked a small but significant reduction in the thermic effect of feeding (23 kcal) and lower satiety ratings 3 to 4 hours after consumption of the beverages.

Eating Frequency and Regularity

US national data show that the total number of eating occasions per day moved from 3.8 in the late 1970s to 4.2 in the mid-1990s;[3] this increase was primarily due to an increase in snacking from 1.1 to 1.6 times per day. Most studies examining relations between reported daily eating frequency and body fatness show either an inverse association or no association[44]; however, positive associations have also been observed.[11,12,45] It has previously been hypothesized that the inverse relation seen between eating frequency and body fatness in observational studies may be an artifact of underreporting of energy intakes.[46] Recent studies in physiologically plausible energy intake reporters compared with the total sample of participants in a US national survey support this suggestion.[11,12]

Controlled laboratory studies have compared frequent, small-portion feeding regimens ("nibbling") with isocaloric, infrequent larger-portion feeding regimens ("gorging"), and found no differential effects on energy expenditure.[46] However, in one single-day study, gorging in the morning led to higher voluntary energy intake at lunch compared with nibbling.[47] Gorging has been shown to result in greater glucose and insulin excursions,[48] which may lead to increased hunger, appetite, and later energy intake.[49] However, findings from a more recent study are in contrast with those above. Farschi et al.[50] conducted a 2-week intervention in which a variable eating frequency (irregular pattern of 3, 6, or 9 times a day) was compared with a regular eating frequency (consistently 6 times a day). Within the variable pattern, increasingly higher ad libitum energy intakes were observed with increasing number of meals a day. Also, a reduced thermic effect of feeding was seen with the irregular pattern compared with the consistent pattern. Overall, strong links between eating frequency, energy intake, and obesity have not been clearly demonstrated, and further well-controlled studies are needed.[51]

Snacking

The relative contribution of snacking to energy intake and obesity has been difficult to determine. Snackers report consuming more energy daily than do non-snackers.[4] A few studies have shown an increase in snacking associated with television viewing; the latter has also been associated with higher adiposity.[52] In contrast, studies show that overweight and obese persons report consuming a lower percentage of their daily energy intake as snacks.[4] The equivocal findings among different types of observational studies may be partly due to selective underreporting of high-energy-dense, snack-type foods.

Interventions show mixed results of the effects of snacking on energy intake,[44,53,54] which may in part be due to short-term versus longer-term effects. In longer study periods, added snacking does not affect energy intake or body weight, perhaps due to reduced intake at other eating occasions.[44]

Breakfast Skipping

Habitually skipping breakfast has been associated with a higher BMI in observational studies in adults[55-57] and children.[58] In addition, intentional weight loss (and maintenance of this loss) is associated with consistently consuming breakfast.[14] However, switching from breakfast eating to breakfast skipping or vice versa did not affect body weight over 2- or 3-week periods.[59,60] Reasons for inconsistencies among studies may in part be due to reverse causation, because overweight persons may attempt to lose weight by skipping breakfast. Another reason may be that intentional weight loss is more easily maintained when coupled with consuming breakfast, whereas simply consuming breakfast or not has no effect on body weight without a deliberate reduction in daily energy intake. Finally, as noted previously, in observational studies, underreporting of energy intake is extremely common,[12] and breakfast foods that are rather dessertlike, such as pastries, muffins, and donuts, may be underreported. Therefore, the relative importance of breakfast over other eating occasions in energy regulation remains to be determined. Recent analysis of the CSFII 1994–96 showed that skipping breakfast or any other meal was not associated with BMI in either the total or plausible samples (Howarth et al., unpublished observations), whereas energy intake at all eating occasions (not just breakfast) was positively associated with BMI. Interestingly, in adults 20 to 90 years old, skipping breakfast was much less common than was skipping lunch. Taken together, these findings suggest that no one eating occasion should be the sole target for interventions for reducing energy intake and body weight.

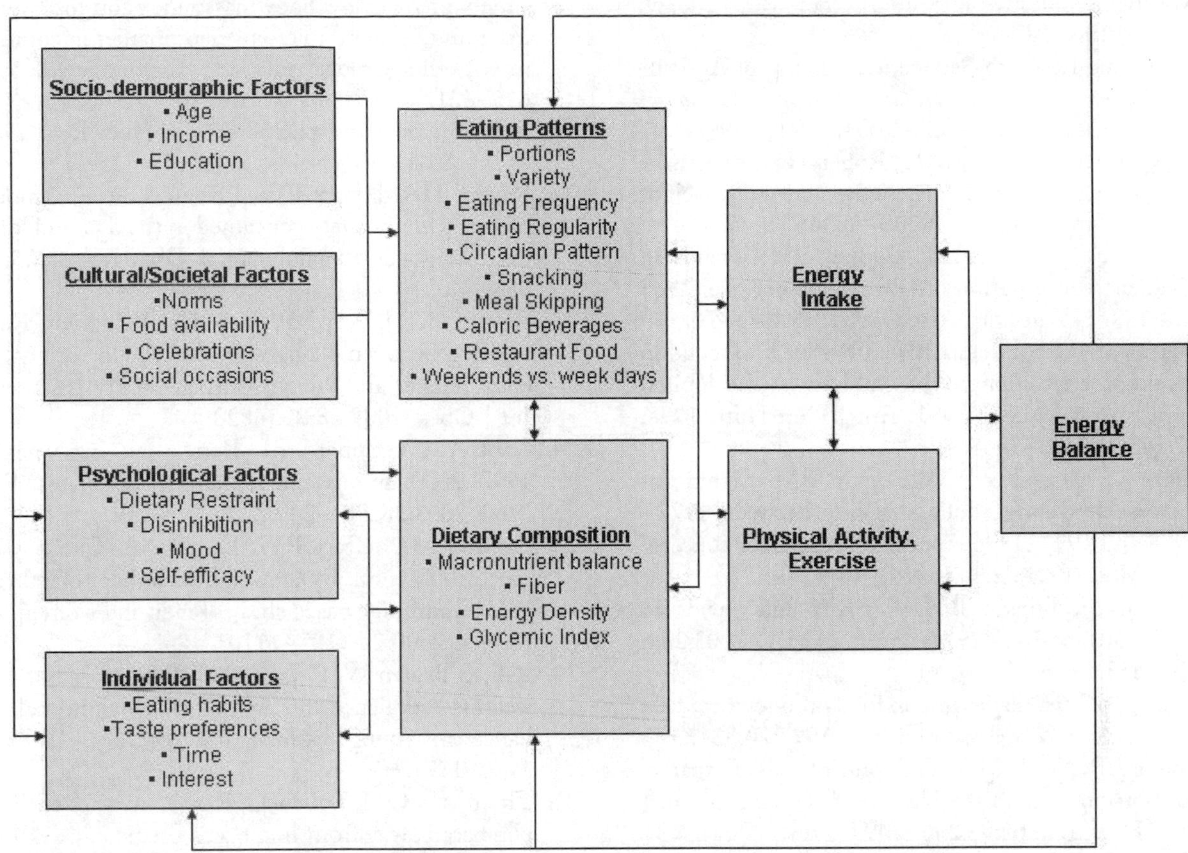

Figure 1. Theoretical model depicting complex interrelationships between psychosocial, dietary, and energy balance factors.

Complex Interrelationships Between Psychosocial, Dietary, and Energy Balance Factors

Although the effects of eating patterns and behaviors on energy intake and weight change can be studied in isolation, they do not occur in isolation in the real world. Figure 1 depicts a theoretical model of several psychosocial, dietary, and energy balance factors interacting. Eating patterns and dietary composition factors such as macronutrient distribution, energy density, and fiber affect energy intake and may also affect physical activity. In turn, physical activity and energy intake not only affect energy balance, but also may influence eating behavior and dietary composition selection. Dietary choices and patterns are also strongly influenced by multiple psychological, sociodemographic, cultural, and individual factors, and vice versa, only some of which are shown here. In short, relations among these variables are complex, and this in part explains why solving the problem of obesity remains elusive.

Future Directions

To date, eating patterns such as increased dietary variety, portion size, consumption of energy-containing beverages, and frequency of FAFH have been consistently demonstrated to be associated with increases in energy intake and, over the long term, body weight. Less clear are the associations of meal timing and frequency with energy balance. Among all eating behaviors studied, there is a lack of well-controlled, longer-term interventions, which contributes to our lack of understanding of the relative importance of different eating patterns in overeating, obesity, or weight loss. Also, it is probable that no single eating pattern or behavior is responsible for weight gain among individuals or for the population-wide obesity epidemic in the United States and now around the world. These behaviors may cluster together, and in fact there are likely to be multiple potential targets for intervention. On the other hand, it is possible that focusing on changing any single eating behavior may be enough to significantly affect energy intake so that weight gain is prevented or weight loss ensues. Research on the role of eating behaviors in energy regulation should examine these issues in both adults and children.

References

1. Hedley AA, Ogden CL, Johnson CL, et al. Prevalence of overweight and obesity among US children, adolescents, and adults, 1999–2002. JAMA. 2004; 291:2847–2850.

2. James PT, Leach R, Kalamara E, Shayeghi M. The worldwide obesity epidemic. Obes Res. 2001;9: 228S–33S.
3. Economic Research Service, U.S. Dept. of Agriculture. *America's Eating Habits: Changes and Consequences.* Washington DC: USDA/ERS, 1999.
4. McCrory MA, Suen VMM, Roberts SB. Biobehavioral influences on energy intake and adult weight gain. J Nutr. 2002;132:3830S–3834S.
5. Haines PS, Guilkey DK, Popkin BM. Trends in breakfast consumption of U.S. adults between 1965 and 1991. J Am Diet Assoc. 1996;96:464–470.
6. Siega-Riz AM, Popkin BM, Carson T. Trends in breakfast consumption for children in the United States from 1965 to 1991. Am J Clin Nutr. 1998; 67(suppl):748S–756S.
7. Zizza C, Siega-Riz AM, Popkin BM. Significant increase in young adults snacking between 1977–1978 and 1994–1996 represents a cause for concern! Prev Med. 2001;32:303–310.
8. Nielsen SJ, Popkin BM. Patterns and trends in food portion sizes, 1977–1998. JAMA. 2003;289: 450–453.
9. Gallo AE. First major drop in food product introductions in over 20 years. Food Rev. 1997;20:33–35.
10. Young LR, Nestle MN. The contribution of expanding portion sizes to the US obesity epidemic. Am J Publ Health. 2002;92:246–249.
11. Huang TT, Howarth NC, Lin BH, et al. Energy intake and meal portions: associations with BMI percentile in U.S. children. Obes Res. 2004;12: 1875–1885.
12. Huang TT, Roberts SB, Howarth NC, et al. Effect of screening out implausible energy intake reports on relationships between diet and BMI. Obes Res. 2005; 13:1205–1217.
13. Ditschuneit HH, Flechtner-Mors M. Value of structured meals for weight management: risk factors and long-term weight maintenance. Obes Res. 2001; 9(Suppl 4):284S–289S.
14. Wing RR, Phelan S. Long-term weight loss maintenance. Am J Clin Nutr. 2005;82(suppl):222S–225S.
15. Ledikwe JH, Ello-Martin J, Rolls BJ. Portion size and the obesity epidemic. J Nutr. 2005;135:905–909.
16. Rolls BJ, Morris EL, Roe LS. Portion size affects energy intake in normal-weight and overwieght men and women. Am J Clin Nutr. 2002;76:1207–1213.
17. Wansink B, Painter JE, North J. Bottomless bowls: why visual cues of portion size may influence intake. Obes Res. 2005;13:93–100.
18. Rolls BJ, Engell D, Birch LL. Serving portion size influences 5-year-old but not 3-year-old children's food intakes. J Am Diet Assoc. 2000;100:232–234.
19. McCrory MA, Fuss PJ, McCallum JE, et al. Dietary variety within food groups: association with energy intake and body fatness in men and women. Am J Clin Nutr. 1999;69:440–447.
20. Roberts SB, Hajduk CL, Howarth NC, et al. Dietary variety predicts low body mass index and inadequate macronutrient and micronutrient intakes in community-dwelling older adults. J Gerontol. 2005;60: 613–621.
21. Rolls BJ. Sensory-specific satiety. Nutr Rev. 1986; 44:93–101.
22. Raynor HA, Jeffery RW, Phelan S, et al. Amount of food group variety consumed in the diet and long-term weight loss maintenance. Obes Res. 2005;13: 883–890.
23. Raynor HA, Jeffery RW, Tate DF, Wing RR. Relationship between changes in food group variety, dietary intake, and weight during obesity treatment. Int J Obes. 2004;28:813–820.
24. Kant AK, Graubard BI. Eating out in America, 1987–2000: trends and nutritional correlates. Prev Med. 2003;38:243–249.
25. Crawford D, Jeffery RW, French SA. Can anyone successfully control their weight? Findings of a three-year community-based study of men and women. Int J Obes. 2000;24:1107–1110.
26. Ball K, Brown W, Crawford D. Who does not gain weight? Prevalence and predictors of weight maintenance in young women. Int J Obes. 2002;26: 1570–1578.
27. Thompson OM, Ballew C, Resnicow K, et al. Food purchased away from home as a predictor of change in BMI score among girls. Int J Obes. 2004;28: 282–289.
28. McCrory MA, Fuss PJ, Hays NP, et al. Overeating in America: association between restaurant food consumption and body fatness in healthy adult men and women ages 19 to 80. Obes Res. 1999;7:564–571.
29. Ebbeling CB, Sinclair KB, Pereira MA, et al. Compensation for energy intake from fast food among overweight and lean adolescents. JAMA. 2004;291: 2828–2833.
30. de Castro JM. Socio-cultural determinants of meal size and frequency. Br J Nutr. 1997;77:S39–55.
31. Holt SH, Sandona N, Brand-Miller JC. The effects of sugar-free vs. sugar-rich beverages on feelings of fullness and subsequent food intake. Int J Food Sci Nutr. 2000;51:59–71.
32. DellaValle DM, Roe LS, Rolls BJ. Does the consumption of caloric and non-caloric beverages with a meal affect energy intake? Appetite. 2005;44: 187–193.
33. de Castro JM. The effects of the spontaneous ingestion of particular foods or beverages on the meal patterns and overall nutrient intake of humans. Physiol Behav. 1993;53:1133–1144.
34. Tordoff MG, Alleva AM. Effect of drinking soda sweetened with aspartame or high-fructose corn syrup on food intake and body weight. Am J Clin Nutr. 1990;51:63–69.
35. Ludwig DS, Peterson KE, Gortmaker SL. Relation

between consumption of sugar-sweetened drinks and childhood obesity: a prospective, observational analysis. Lancet. 2001;357:505–508.

36. James J, Thomas P, Cavan D, et al. Preventing childhood obesity by reducing consumption of carbonated drinks: cluster randomised controlled trial. Br Med J. 2004;328:1237–1242.
37. Schulze MB, Manson JE, Ludwig DS, et al. Sugar-sweetened beverages, weight gain, and incidence of type 2 diabetes in young and middle-aged women. JAMA. 2004;292:927–934.
38. Mattes RD. Dietary compensation by humans for supplemental energy provided as ethanol or carbohydrate in fluids. Physiol Behav. 1996;59:179–187.
39. DiMeglio DP, Mattes RD. Liquid versus solid carbohydrate: effects on food intake and body weight. Int J Obes. 2000;24:794–800.
40. Almiron-Roig E, Flores SY, Drewnowski A. No difference in satiety or in subsequent energy intakes between a beverage and a solid food. Physiol Behav. 2004;82:671–677.
41. Bray GA, Nielsen SJ, Popkin BM. Consumption of high-fructose corn syrup in beverages may play a role in the epidemic of obesity. Am J Clin Nutr. 2004; 79:537–543.
42. Teff KL, Elliott SS, Tschop M, et al. Dietary fructose reduces circulating insulin and leptin, attenuates postprandial suppression of ghrelin, and increases triglycerides in women. J Clin Endocrinol Metab. 2004; 89:2963–2972.
43. St-Onge MP, Rubiano F, DeNino WF, et al. Added thermogenic and satiety effects of a mixed nutrient vs. a sugar-only beverage. Int J Obes Relat Metab Disord. 2004;28:248–253.
44. Kirk TR. Role of dietary carbohydrate and frequent eating in body-weight control. Proc Nutr Soc. 2000; 59:349–358.
45. Forslund HB, Lindroos AK, Sjostrom L, et al. Meal patterns and obesity in Swedish women: a simple instrument describing usual meal types, frequency and temporal distribution. Eur J Clin Nutr. 2002;56: 740–747.
46. Bellisle F, McDevitt R, Prentice AM. Meal frequency and energy balance. Br J Nutr. 1997;77:S57-S70.
47. Speechly DP, Buffenstein R. Greater appetite control associated with an increased frequency of eating in lean males. Appetite. 1999;33:285–297.
48. Jenkins DJA, Wolever TMS, Vuksan V, et al. Nibbling versus gorging: metabolic advantages of increased meal frequency. N Engl J Med. 1989;321: 929–934.
49. Ludwig DS, Majzoub JA, Al-Zahrani A, et al. High glycemic index foods, overeating, and obesity. Pediatrics. 1999;103:E261-E266.
50. Farshchi HR, Taylor MA, Macdonald IA. Decreased thermic effect of food after an irregular compared with a regular meal pattern in healthy lean women. Int J Obes. 2004;28:653–660.
51. Mattson MP. Energy intake, meal frequency, and health: a neurobiological perspective. Annu Rev Nutr. 2005;25:237–260.
52. Foster JA, Gore SA, West DS. Altering TV viewing habits: an unexplored strategy for adult obesity intervention? Am J Health Behav. 2006;30:3–14.
53. Johnstone AM, Shannon E, Whybrow S, et al. Altering the temporal distribution of energy intake with isoenergetically dense foods given as snacks does not affect total daily energy intake in normal-weight men. Br J Nutr. 2000;83:7–14.
54. Marmonier C, Chapelot D, Louis-Sylvestre J. Metabolic and behavioral consequences of a snack consumed in a satiety state. Am J Clin Nutr. 1999;70: 854–866.
55. Cho S, Dietrich M, Brown CJP, et al. The effect of breakfast type on total daily energy intake and body mass index: results from the Third National Health and Nutirtion Examination Survey (NHANES III). J Am Coll Nutr. 2003;22:296–302.
56. Keski-Rahkonen A, Kaprio J, Rissanen A, et al. Breakfast skipping and health-compromising behaviors in adolescents and adults. Eur J Clin Nutr. 2003; 57:842–853.
57. Ma Y, Bertone ER, Stanek EJI, et al. Association between eating patterns and obesity in a free-living U.S. adult population. Am J Epidemiol. 2003;158: 85–92.
58. Rampersaud GC, Pereira MA, Girard BL, et al. Breakfast habits, nutritional status, body weight, and academic performance in children and adolescents. J Am Diet Assoc. 2005;105:743–762.
59. Tuttle WW, Daum K, Myers L, et al. Effect of omitting breakfast on the physiologic response of men. J Am Diet Assoc. 1959;26:332–335.
60. Farshchi HR, Taylor MA, Macdonald IA. Deleterious effects of omitting breakfast on insulin sensitivity and fasting lipid profiles in healthy lean women. Am J Clin Nutr. 2005;81:388–396.

61 Strategies for Changing Eating and Exercise Behavior

Rena R. Wing, Amy Gorin, and Deborah Tate

The leading causes of disease and death in the United States—coronary heart disease and cancer—are related to lifestyle factors. By changing eating and exercise habits and eliminating smoking, the prevalence of these diseases could be markedly reduced. The goal of this chapter is to provide readers with an overview of behavioral strategies that can be used to modify lifestyle behaviors. Although the behavioral principles are applicable to changing any type of health habit, this chapter will focus primarily on obesity and will review strategies that may help in both the treatment and prevention of this disease.

History of Behavioral Weight-loss Programs

The underlying premise of a behavioral approach is the functional analysis of behavior, also known as the "A-B-C" model. A functional analysis involves identifying the behaviors to be changed, which in the case of obesity are eating and exercise behaviors; the antecedent cues in the environment; and the consequences or reinforcers that influence the behaviors. Behaviorists propose that by changing the antecedents and consequences, it is possible to change the behavior.

Antecedent → Behavior ← Consequences
Cues (Reinforcers)

The earliest application of behavioral principles to the problem of obesity occurred in the 1960s and 1970s. With the notable exception of Stuart's initial study of eight overweight women,[1] these early behavioral weight-loss programs were typically conducted in groups with mildly overweight patients and lasted about 10 weeks. The primary "behavior" that was targeted was a change in eating patterns (when and where food was eaten) rather than total calories. Similarly, participants were encouraged to change activity patterns by strategies such as using stairs instead of elevators, but no specific calorie goals for physical activity were prescribed. These early studies produced weight losses of 3.8 kg over an 8- to 10-week treatment program, and were shown to be more effective than alternative approaches, such as nutrition education or psychotherapy.

The next generation of behavioral programs, conducted in the 1980s, placed greater emphasis on caloric intake and expenditure and typically prescribed moderate goals for these behaviors. There was also increased attention given to changing cognitions related to eating and exercise. With a more balanced focus on diet, exercise, and behavior (rather than focusing entirely on behavior), these programs produced average weight losses of 8.5 kg over approximately 15 weeks.

Weight-loss programs conducted in the 1990s continued these trends.[2] Treatments were lengthened still further and often involved weekly meetings for 26 weeks; a few studies used weekly meetings for a full year. The emphasis on nutrition was further expanded, and patients were often taught to monitor fat grams as well as calories. Moreover, the calorie intake goals were often stricter (some studies even used very–low-calorie diets [VLCDs]), and more structured exercise and higher exercise goals were included. Weight losses averaged 9.7 kg over an average of 27 weeks.[2] Typically, treatments were stopped after 26 to 27 weeks, and participants were recontacted 1 year later to determine if the weight loss had been maintained. On average, patients maintained a weight loss of 5.6 kg, or about 60% of their initial weight loss. The most recent studies have even better follow-up results, with patients maintaining about 80% of their weight loss at 1-year follow-up.[3] Few studies have included longer follow-up. It appears, however, that by 3- to 5-year follow-up, patients are back to their baseline weight.[4]

Behavioral Strategies

This section provides a brief description of the key behavioral strategies used in weight-loss programs. These same basic strategies are applicable to changing any type of nutrition behavior.

Identifying the Behaviors to Be Changed

The first step of a behavioral intervention is to clearly identify the specific behaviors to be modified. For example, for weight loss, the key behaviors that are targeted are those related to energy balance (calories consumed and calories expended). In applying behavioral principles to reduction of cholesterol levels, the key behaviors would include reductions in saturated fat intake and cholesterol intake. Similarly, in an intervention to reduce blood pressure levels, reducing sodium intake would be an additional behavioral focus.

Setting Goals

In changing behaviors, it is helpful to set specific goals that can be achieved by the participant. Often, both behavioral and physiologic (outcome) goals are identified. For example, participants in weight-loss programs may aim to consume no more than 1200 kcal/d (5023 kJ/d) or to expend at least 1000 kcal/week (4186 kJ/week) in exercise; a weight-loss goal of 2 pounds/week is often used. Short-term goals have been shown to be more effective than long-term goals in promoting behavior change.[5] Often behaviors are "shaped," by setting easier goals initially and then increasing the goal as the participant progresses. An example of shaping is seen in physical activity, in which participants are first helped to increase their activity to 250 kcal/week (1046 kJ/week) or 500 kcal/week (2093 kJ/week) before attempting the 1000-kcal/week (4186-kJ/week) goal.

Self-monitoring

A key strategy in the behavioral treatment of obesity is teaching participants to observe and record their own eating- and activity-related behaviors, a technique known as self-monitoring. A variety of information can be recorded through self-monitoring, including the type and amount of food eaten, the number of calories in each food, the number of fat grams, and other eating-related items such as eating situation and premeal mood. Similarly, types and amounts of physical activity can be recorded in minutes or calories. Participants are instructed to record their daily intake and bring their self-monitoring books to group meetings, providing an opportunity for feedback from group leaders and other participants. Self-monitoring is usually done on a daily basis for the initial 6 months of treatment and then on a periodic basis during maintenance. Several studies support the utility of self-monitoring, suggesting a strong association between the completeness and consistency of self-monitoring and weight loss.[6]

Stimulus Control

As mentioned earlier, a central tenet of behavior modification is that individuals' behaviors are influenced by their environments. Thus, by manipulating their surroundings, participants can change the likelihood of behavioral outcomes. Participants in behavioral treatment programs are thus taught to restructure their environments to decrease cues for inappropriate food consumption and increase cues for appropriate diet and exercise.[1] For example, participants are instructed to limit their purchases of high-fat foods and, if purchased, to store these foods out of sight. Conversely, participants are encouraged to purchase more fruits and vegetables and to increase the visibility of these items by storing them in prominent locations. Similarly, they are encouraged to put items related to exercise in places where they will be seen on a frequent basis. Other stimulus-control strategies such as restricting eating to a designated place and eliminating the pairing of eating with other activities (e.g., watching television, reading) may also be effective means for altering antecedents that influence eating behavior. Likewise, stimulus-control techniques can be used to change other types of dietary behaviors; for example, individuals attempting to reduce their blood pressure might be instructed to remove salt shakers from the table.

Problem Solving

When attempting to make permanent lifestyle changes, participants face many hurdles and obstacles. To help participants successfully navigate this process, training in problem-solving skills is included in behavioral treatment programs. Participants are taught to: 1) identify a specific problem that is hindering their weight-loss effort, 2) generate as many solutions as possible to the problem, 3) evaluate the possible solutions and select one, 4) implement the chosen solution, and 5) evaluate the outcome and repeat the problem-solving process if necessary. Problem-solving techniques are used for individually identified problems; for example, one participant may have difficulty with overeating while preparing dinner and another may focus on the difficulty of eating out in restaurants.

Cognitive Restructuring

A more recent addition to behavioral weight-loss treatment is cognitive restructuring. Cognitive restructuring involves identifying and modifying maladaptive thoughts contributing to overeating and physical inactivity. These thoughts can take several forms, such as dichotomous thinking (e.g., "If I can't exercise for 30 minutes, I might as well not do it all") and rationalization (e.g., "I've had a stressful day so I deserve a piece of cake"). Participants are often unaware of the impact that thoughts have on behavior. Cognitive restructuring serves to highlight this process by having participants identify and challenge maladaptive thoughts and develop more positive self-statements to assist in behavior change.

Relapse Prevention

Helping participants prepare and plan for lapses or slips in the weight-loss process is also included in behaviorally based programs. An extension of Marlatt and Gordon's work with addictions,[7] relapse prevention in behavioral weight-control programs involves teaching participants to anticipate problematic situations that might result in overeating and to develop specific strategies for overcoming these lapses. Participants are encouraged to have plans in place so that one overeating slip or lapse does not develop into a full-blown relapse.

Changing Eating Behavior

As noted above, the behaviors that must be targeted to produce weight loss are the behaviors related to energy balance. However, the best way to accomplish these changes, and to optimize long-term adherence, remains unclear. In fact, there is little information about very basic aspects of these behaviors, such as what level of caloric intake is best to prescribe and what types of macronutrient composition of the diet should be recommended. In the following sections, we will describe some of the behavioral research that has addressed these issues. Readers interested in more information about behavior changes to reduce saturated fat or sodium or to increase intake of fiber and fruits and vegetables are referred to the review by Kumanyika et al.[8]

Calorie Intake

Behavioral weight-loss programs typically utilize low-calorie diets of approximately 1200 to 1500 kcal/d (5023–6278 kJ/d) that are designed to produce weight losses of 1 to 2 lb/week. However, several years ago there was a great deal of interest in the use of VLCDs during the initial phase of a behavioral program.[9,10] VLCDs are diets of 400 to 800 kcal/d (1674–3348 kJ/d), typically given as liquid formula or lean meat, fish, and fowl. The advantage of these regimens is that they produce large initial weight losses, averaging 20 kg over 12 weeks. The thought was to combine VLCDs with behavioral strategies so that the VLCD would increase initial weight loss and the behavioral techniques would help maintain the weight loss long term.

Several trials have been conducted to compare low-calorie diets with VLCDs used in combination with behavioral techniques.[4,10-13] In all of these studies, the VLCDs were clearly effective in increasing initial weight loss. However, despite providing ongoing weekly contact with patients and even using a second 12-week period of VLCD, the initial large weight losses produced by the VLCD were followed by large weight regains.[11,13] Thus, by the 1-year follow-up, there were no significant differences in weight loss for VLCD compare with low-calorie diet groups.

Macronutrient Composition

A second issue relates to the macronutrient composition of the diet. In the past, behavioral researchers focused primarily on calories and paid less attention to the types of foods consumed. However, based on epidemiologic and metabolic studies showing an association between dietary fat intake and body weight,[14] researchers began to examine whether restricting fat intake would improve long-term weight-loss outcome. Jeffery et al.[15] compared the effect of restricting calories against restricting fat intake. They studied 122 women, half of whom were given a 20-g/d fat goal (and no restriction on calories) and the other half were given a 1000- to 1200-kcal/d (4186- to 5023-kJ/d) goal (and no restriction on fat). No differences in weight loss between the two groups were observed at the end of the 6-month program or at the 18-month follow-up.

The combination of restricting calories and dietary fat intake was examined by Schlundt et al.[16] (compared with a group that restricted fat only) and by Pascale et al.[17] (compared with a group that restricted calories only). In both studies, there was some evidence that the combination of calorie plus fat restriction was most effective. Weight losses of 4.6 kg versus 8.8 kg at 20 weeks and 2.6 kg versus 5.5 kg at the 9- to 12-month follow-up were observed, both favoring the combination condition.[16] A large dropout rate limited the conclusiveness of these findings. Type 2 diabetics lost 4.6 kg versus 7.7 kg at the end of 16 weeks and 1.0 kg versus 5.2 kg at 1 year, again favoring the combination of fat and calorie restriction; however, the nondiabetics in this study had no differences in weight loss on the two dietary regimens.[17]

Recently, there has been tremendous interest in low-carbohydrate, high-protein diets (e.g., the Atkins diet). These diets limit the amount of carbohydrate that is consumed, without restricting dietary fat or protein or overall caloric intake. A 1-year randomized trial was conducted to compare this low-carbohydrate approach with a traditional low-calorie, low-fat approach in 63 obese men and women. Both interventions were conducted with minimal professional contact, and participants were given self-help books outlining the principles of each approach. Adherence to both diets was poor, and attrition was quite high (only 37 participants completed the 1-year assessment). Although the high attrition limits the conclusions that can be drawn, it appears that weight losses were better on the low-carbohydrate diet than the low-calorie, low-fat approach at 3 months (−6.8% vs. −2.7% of body weight) and at 6 months (−7.0% vs. −3.2%), but there were no significant differences at 12 months (−4.4% vs.

−2.5%). Other studies have suggested similar benefits to the low-carbohydrate diet at 6 months, but again have been marked by high attrition.[19,20] The advantage of the low-carbohydrate approach appears to derive from its effect on limiting overall caloric intake; for example, one study reported that patients on the low-carbohydrate diet decreased their overall caloric intake by 460 kcal/d, whereas the low-fat group reduced by 271 kcal/d.[19] Thus, although patients on the low-carbohydrate diet are not told to limit their overall intake, such changes occur, perhaps due to the monotonous quality of the diet or to the satiating effects of the high-fat, high-protein regimen.

It is also important to consider the impact of other aspects of the diet on long-term weight loss; for example, the effect of energy density and/or the amount of variety in the diet. McCrory et al.[21] reported that a large variety of sweets, snacks, condiments, entrees, and carbohydrates, in combination with a low variety of vegetables, was associated with increased intake and greater body weight. These results fit within the laboratory data on "sensory-specific satiety," showing that individuals will satiate on one food item but suddenly find "room" to eat more if offered a different type of food.[22] Recently, the relationship between food group variety and outcome was examined in a behavioral weight-loss program.[23] Participants (N = 122) were followed at 6-month intervals using a food frequency questionnaire to assess food group variety and dietary intake and obtaining direct measures of body weight. Over the course of treatment, participants reported increased variety in low-fat breads and vegetables and decreased variety in high-fat foods and fats, oils, and sweets. Decreases in the variety of high-fat foods and increased variety in low-fat breads were related to weight loss at 18 months.[23]

Food Provision and Structured Meal Plans

Behaviorists have long recognized the importance of modifying the home environment as a means of influencing eating behaviors. Stimulus control techniques, in which patients are taught to rearrange their home environment to make cues for healthy behaviors more prominent and to reduce cues for unhealthy behaviors, are an important component of behavioral programs, as noted above. Recently, behavioral researchers suggested that it might be possible to make even greater changes in the home environment by actually providing patients with the food they should eat in appropriate portion sizes. Jeffery et al.[24] tested this in a two-center study with 202 overweight patients. Patients were randomly assigned to one of five groups: 1) no treatment control, 2) standard behavioral program, 3) standard behavioral program plus food provision, 4) standard behavioral program plus financial incentives, or 5) standard behavioral program plus food provisions and financial incentives. Groups 2 through 5 all received the same 18-month behavioral program and were given comparable goals for fat and calorie intake and for physical activity. In addition, groups 3 and 5 were given a box of food each week for 18 months; this food box contained all the food they were to eat for five breakfasts and five dinners each week. The foods provided were quite simple (cold cereal, milk, fruit for breakfast; chicken breast, rice, and peas or a frozen entree for dinner). Providing food to participants increased their weight losses at 6, 12, and 18 months. The food provision groups lost 10.1 kg, 9.1 kg, and 6.4 kg at 6, 12, and 18 months, respectively; the groups given the behavioral intervention without food lost 7.7, 4.5, and 4.1 kg at the three time points. There was no effect of the financial incentives on weight loss.

It is clearly expensive to provide food to patients, so a follow-up study examined whether weight losses would be similar if participants shared the cost for the food or received meal plans and grocery lists for the five breakfasts and five dinners (without actually receiving the food). Overweight women (N = 163) were randomly assigned to either a standard behavioral program, standard behavioral program plus meal plans and grocery lists, standard behavioral program plus food with the costs of the food shared, or standard behavioral program plus free food.[25] The three groups that were given either meal plans or food all had significantly better weight losses than the standard behavioral program group, with no differences among these three groups (8.0, 12.0, 11.7, and 11.4 kg for groups 1–4, respectively). These superior weight losses appeared to reflect differences in eating behavior. Groups 2 through 4 all reported increases in the frequency of eating breakfast and lunch and a decrease in snacking, whereas group 1 did not report such changes. Likewise, groups 2 through 4 reported greater increases than group 1 in the number of fruits/vegetables, low-fat and medium-fat meats, breads/cereals, and low-calorie frozen entrees stored in their home. Groups 2 to 4 also reported less difficulty finding times to plan meals, having appropriate foods available, estimating portion size, and controlling eating when not hungry.

Positive results have also been obtained in several other recent studies in which patients were given prepared meals[26] or in which Slim-Fast[27] was used for 1 or 2 meals/d along with a healthy low-fat dinner meal. One of the most convincing studies on the benefits of such structured meals included randomizing 53 obese women to one of three groups: a group assigned to use weight-loss medication (sibutramine), a group assigned to medication plus participation in a standard behavioral weight-loss program (drug + lifestyle), or a group assigned to medication plus the standard behavioral program plus a prescribed 1000-kcal/d, portion-controlled diet (combined treatment). For the first 16 weeks, this latter group consumed 4 servings/d of a nutritional supplement with an evening meal of a frozen entree, fruit, and salad. Results are shown in Figure 1 and clearly illustrate that the portion-controlled diet improved weight losses over the standard behavioral program. These studies suggest that simplifying eating for patients by providing them with structure

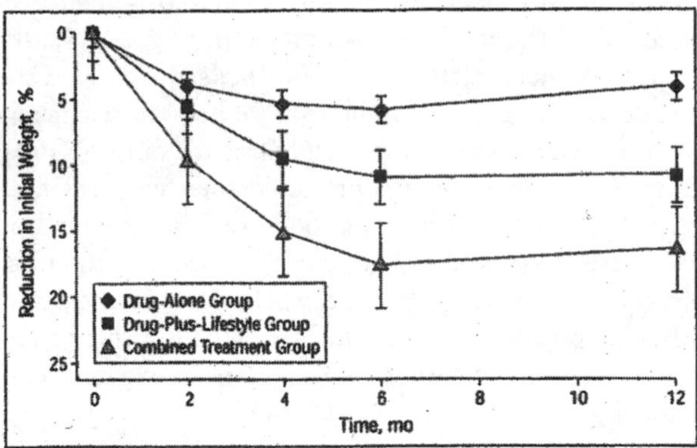

Figure 1. Percentage reduction in initial body weight for women treated with sibutramine hydrochloride alone (drug alone), sibutramine plus group lifestyle modification (drug + lifestyle), and sibutramine and lifestyle modification group (combined treatment), as assessed by a last observation carried forward analysis. All three groups differed significantly ($P < 0.05$ for all) from each other at month 6. At month 12, the 19 women in the drug-alone group lost significantly ($P < 0.05$) less weight than women in the other two groups (which did not differ significantly from each other). (Used with permission from Wadden et al., 2001[28], copyright 2001, American Medical Association. All rights reserved.)

and models of appropriate meals may promote adherence to weight-loss regimens.

Changing Exercise

The single best predictor of long-term maintenance of weight loss is physical activity.[29] Individuals who continue to exercise long term are the ones who are the most successful at maintaining their weight loss. The challenge for behavioral researchers is to get overweight individuals to adopt and maintain an exercise program.

Home Based vs. Supervised

Having patients exercise under supervised conditions allows researchers to better quantify the activity, to adjust the intensity or dose of activity over time, and to teach participants about warming up, cooling down, etc. However, traveling to a supervised site adds an extra burden for the participant and may discourage continued adherence. Several researchers have compared long-term participation in supervised activity with home-based activity. In Project Active,[30] 235 nonobese (<140% of ideal weight), sedentary men and women, 35 to 60 years of age, were randomly assigned to a lifestyle physical activity program or to a structured activity program. The activity goal for both groups was to increase activity by 3 kcal/kg (which is approximately 1500 kcal/week (6278 kJ/week) for a 75-kg individual) during the first 6 months of the program, and to maintain an increased exercise level of 2 kcal/kg (approximately 1000 kcal/week [4186 kJ/week]) throughout the remainder of the 18-month intervention. Participants in the structured exercise program were asked to exercise at a supervised facility for the first 6 months. The lifestyle group, which was encouraged to "accumulate" at least 30 minutes of moderate-intensity activity on "most or preferably all days in the week," met weekly as a group for 16 weeks and then biweekly through week 24 to learn cognitive and behavioral skills to increase physical activity. Both groups attended occasional meetings and received newsletters to help them maintain their activity over the 18-month follow-up. Increases in physical activity were comparable in the two groups over the first 6 months, but the supervised group had greater increases in fitness. At 24 months, the two groups had similar increases in activity and fitness. Neither group experienced changes in weight, but both groups reduced their percentage of body fat. Thus, this study suggested that both lifestyle and supervised activity may be options for increasing activity level and fitness in sedentary adults.

Two weight-loss studies have likewise compared structured versus lifestyle activity programs. Andersen et al.[31] assigned participants in a standard behavioral weight-loss program to either a supervised exercise group, which attended three aerobic dance classes/week for the first 16 weeks, or to a lifestyle group, which exercised on their own and aimed to increase moderate or vigorous activity by 30 min/d on most days of the week. Weight losses in the lifestyle and supervised groups were comparable at week 16 (7.9 kg vs. 8.3 kg); from week 16 to the 1-year follow-up, the aerobic group regained 1.6 kg vs. 0.08 kg in the lifestyle group ($P = 0.06$).

A similar comparison of lifestyle versus supervised (group) activity in the treatment of obesity resulted in comparable weight losses from months 1 to 6 in the two conditions.[32] However, from month 6 forward, exercise participation and weight losses were better in the home exercise group than in the supervised group. At month 15, the home-based program had an average weight loss of 11.65 kg, whereas the supervised group had a mean weight loss of 7.01 kg. Taken together, these two weight-loss studies suggest that home-based exercise may be more effective than supervised exercise for long-term weight loss maintenance.

Short Bouts vs. Long Bouts

The supervised versus lifestyle programs described above may have differed not only in location but also the way in which the activity occurred. In the studies cited above, participants in the supervised exercise conditions completed their activity in one bout on each of 3 to 5 d/wk. The participants in the lifestyle conditions were told to "accumulate" 30 minutes of exercise each day. These participants may likewise have done this exercise in one bout or alternatively completed several short bouts each day. Since lack of time is considered the greatest barrier to exercise, it may be easier for participants to exercise in multiple short bouts (e.g., four 10-minute bouts), rather than one full-length bout (e.g., one 40-minute bout). To test this hypothesis, Jakicic et al.[33,34] completed two weight-loss studies comparing programs that prescribed the same amount of lifestyle exercise in either one 40-minute bout or four 10-minute bouts 5 days/week. The first study found better exercise adherence over 6 months and somewhat greater weight losses in the short-bout condition.[33] The second study again found greater exercise participation in the short bout group for the first several weeks of the study; however, from 6 to 18 months of the program, no differences between the short bout and long bout groups were observed.[34] These two groups had comparable exercise participation, initial and long-term weight losses (−3.7 kg and −5.8 kg) and long-term improvements in fitness. Thus, short-bout prescriptions of exercise may be particularly helpful during the initial phase of a weight-loss program; for long-term changes, these two different types of exercise formats appear to provide alternative, equally effective approaches to physical activity.

Providing Home Exercise Equipment

Another approach to promoting adherence to exercise is to provide patients with home exercise equipment. Although it is often noted anecdotally that such equipment receives little use over time, there has been little empirical investigation of this strategy. A correlation was observed between the number of pieces of activity equipment in the home and activity level.[35] Conceptually, it would appear that providing exercise equipment to participants (like providing food) would help two cue the appropriate behavior and reduce barriers related to access, cost, etc. Jakicic et al.[34] recently examined this strategy in a study of overweight women participating in a behavioral weight-loss program. As described above, one group of women in this study was asked to complete their exercise in short bouts. Another group was given the same exercise prescription and provided with a home treadmill. The group given the exercise equipment maintained a higher activity level from months 13 to 18 of the program and had significantly better weight loss over the 18-month study (−7.4 vs. −3.7 kg). Thus, this study supports the use of this strategy for improving long-term exercise adherence and weight loss.

Decreasing Sedentary Activities

Several studies have attempted to decrease sedentary activity, rather than increase exercise, as a way to influence overall activity level and either treat or prevent obesity. To date, this approach has been used only with children, although it should be applicable to adults as well. Various approaches have been studied for the treatment of obesity in children 8 to 12 years of age and the effects of decreasing sedentary activities (TV, video games) and increasing physical activity, and the combination of both have been compared.[36] The group that focused on decreasing sedentary activities had the greatest decreases in percent overweight at 4 months and at 1 year (−18.7% in sedentary; −10.3% in combined, and −8.7% in increased physical activity group). The group that was instructed to decrease sedentary activity also reported the greatest increases in their liking for vigorous activity. All groups showed comparable improvements in fitness level.

Reducing television viewing as a means to prevent obesity was also examined in a school-based study with 192 children (mean age = 9 years).[37] One school was randomly assigned to an 18-lesson, 6-month curriculum designed to decrease TV viewing. The children in that school self-monitored their television, video game, and videotape use and attempted a 10-day "turnoff" during which they watched no TV or video games. Subsequently, they attempted to decrease these sedentary activities to 7 hours/week. Electronic devices were attached to home television sets to monitor and budget viewing time. The control school received no intervention. Children in the intervention school had statically significant decreases in television viewing and meals eaten in front of the TV. The intervention children also had smaller increases in body mass index (18.38 to 18.67) than the control children (18.10 to 18.81) over the 7-month study.

Amount of Physical Activity

Behavioral weight-loss programs have traditionally encouraged participants to gradually increase their physical activity until they achieve a 1000-kcal/week (4186-kJ/week) goal. (A 150-pound individual can achieve this caloric expenditure by walking 10 miles/week or 2 miles on each of 5 days in the week.) Recently, researchers have begun to question whether this amount of activity is really optimal for weight-loss maintenance. The notion that higher levels of activity may be associated with better long-term weight-loss maintenance was first suggested by data collected in the National Weight Control Registry. This registry is a database of more than 2500 individuals who have lost at least 30 pounds (mean = 66 pounds) and kept it off for at least 1 year (mean = 6 years). Data from the first 784 subjects in the registry (629 women and 155 men) indicated that, on average, these individuals were expending 2829 kcal/week (11,841 kJ/week) in physical activity.[38] They expended approximately 1100 kcal/week (4604 kJ/week) in walking, 200 kcal/week (827 kJ/week) in stair climbing, and 200 (1837 kJ), 500 (2093 kJ), and 800 (3348 kJ) kcal/week, respectively, in light, medium, and heavy sports activities.

A similar finding emerged in a recent study of physical activity and weight loss.[39] Post hoc analyses were done in this study to compare self-reported exercise level at 18 months and long-term weight-loss maintenance. Subjects (N = 196) were divided into quartiles according to their self-reported activity level at 18 months. Quartiles 1 through 3, which reported expending 250 to 1300 kcal/week (1046–5441 kJ/week), did not significantly differ from each other in long-term weight-loss maintenance (−3.0 to −4.8 kg). However, the top quartile, which reported an average of 2550 kcal/week (10,673 kJ/week) of activity, maintained a 7.6-kg weight loss, significantly greater than the other three conditions. This high-exercise quartile also reported a pattern of activity quite similar to the registry participants. The top quartile exercisers reported approximately 1125 kcal/week (4709 kJ/week) in walking, 250 kcal/week (1046 kJ/week) in stairs, and 170, 400, and 600 kcal/week (712, 1674, and 2511 kJ/week, respectively) in light, medium, and heavy activity, respectively.

On the basis of these data, Jeffery et al.[40] recently conducted a randomized clinical trial with 202 overweight participants comparing the weight-loss effects of a 1000-kcal/week (4186-kJ/week) exercise prescription with a group prescribed a 2500-kcal/week (10,464-kJ/week) level of activity. To help the participants in the high-exercise group achieve their goal, they were encouraged to recruit two to three friends to join the program with them, were given additional coaching from an exercise physiologist, and were given small monetary incentives. Both groups received the same dietary intervention and behavioral treatment program with weekly meetings for the first 6 months, then biweekly meetings for 6 months, and then monthly meetings for 6 months. The high-exercise intervention was effective in increasing physical activity levels to approximately 2300 kcal/week at 6, 12, 18 months compared with approximately 1675 kcal/week in the standard condition. The high-activity group also achieved significantly greater weight losses at 12 and 18 months (Figure 2). At the 18-month point, participants in the 1000-kcal exercise group maintained a weight loss of 4.1 ± 7.3 kg compared with 6.7 ± 8.1 in the high-exercise condition.

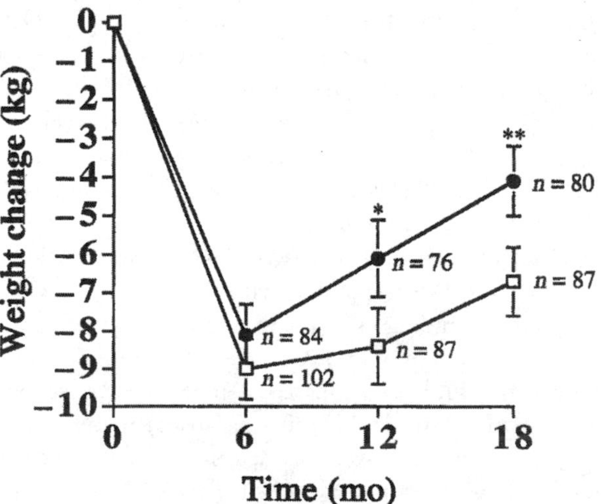

Figure 2. Mean (± SEM) weight change over time by treatment group (●, standard behavior therapy group; □, high physical activity treatment group). *, ** Significantly different from the high physical activity treatment group (SAS general linear modeling procedure): *P = 0.07; ** P = 0.04. (From Jeffery et al., 2003.[4] Used with permission from *The American Journal of Clinical Nutrition*. Copyright Am J Clin Nutr. American Society for Nutrition.)

Support for Healthy Eating and Exercise Behavior

Behavioral weight-loss programs were initially designed with weekly meetings for 10 weeks. As noted above, these treatment programs were gradually lengthened to 16 weeks and then to 20 or 24 weeks. After this phase of weekly meetings, treatment is typically stopped and there is no further contact until 1 year later. Although researchers were surprised to observe weight regain over this year, this finding should have been anticipated based on the behavioral model. It is difficult to change eating and exercise behaviors and maintain these new, healthier habits if the environment is not supportive of the new behaviors.

Several approaches have been utilized in an effort to provide ongoing support for long-term behavior change. One approach is to continue treatment and therapist contact over longer periods of time. Perri[41] compared a 20-week behavioral program with a 40-week program. At the end of 20 weeks, weight losses were comparable in the two conditions. When the program ended for the 20-week treatment group, these individuals began to regain weight, whereas patients in the extended program continued to lose weight from week 20 to 40. At week 40, weight losses averaged 6.4 kg in the 20-week program and 13.6 kg in the 40-week program. When treatment was stopped at week 40, both groups regained; however, at week 72, there continued to be significant differences in weight loss favoring the longer program (9.8 kg vs. 4.6 kg). Other behavioral programs providing a full year of weekly treatment contact have also obtained excellent weight-loss results (14.4 kg[11]and 10.5 kg[13]).

Reducing treatment contact to biweekly sessions during maintenance also appears effective. Perri et al.[42] found that biweekly contact produced better maintenance of weight loss than no contact. The specific nature of the contact (i.e., whether the sessions included exercise and/or social support) had less effect on the outcome. The ideal contact schedule, the nature of that contact, and whether the contact must be made by a therapist (vs. a peer or research assistant) remains unclear.

Another approach to providing ongoing support is to include the spouse or friends in the treatment process. Several studies have evaluated the effects of spouse support, with mixed results; a meta-analysis of this literature suggested a small positive effect for spouse involvement.[43] Wing et al.[44] developed a spouse support intervention in which participants and their spouses were treated together in a weight-loss program. Both were given goals for intake and exercise, both were instructed to self-monitor, and both attended all treatment meetings. In addition, the couples were taught strategies to help each other with weight loss, such as good listening skills and ways to offer or request support. This spouse intervention was compared with a standard behavioral program focused on the patient only. No overall differences in weight loss were found at the end of the treatment program or at the 1-year follow-up. A significant interaction effect did emerge, however, in which women in the spouse support intervention and men in the standard behavioral program achieved the best weight-loss results.

Recently, Wing and Jeffery[45] evaluated two new approaches to social support. These investigators recruited participants for a weight-loss program and asked them to identify three overweight friends who would also like to be in the program and work with them as a team to lose weight. Individuals who identified three friends were compared with individuals who were unable or unwilling to identify three friends or were not asked to recruit others (i.e., this aspect of the study was not randomized). This natural social support intervention was crossed with an experimental manipulation of social support in a 2 × 2 research design. The experimental manipulation of social support included intergroup cohesiveness activities and intragroup competitions in which patients competed for money that was returned contingent on maintenance of weight loss. Those participants who were recruited with friends and given the social support manipulation had the best outcome. Whereas 95% of these individuals completed the 10-month study, only 76% of the standard behavioral group (those recruited alone and not given the social support intervention) completed the study. Moreover, 66% of participants recruited with others and given the social support intervention maintained their weight loss in full from month 4 of the program to month 10; only 24% of the standard behavioral group maintained their weight loss in full over the same time frame.

A recent examination of the impact of involving support partners in obesity treatment suggests that merely bringing support partners to treatment is not enough to improve weight-loss success. Rather, support partners have to lose weight themselves for participants to benefit from their attendance.[46] Participants in this study were encouraged but not required to invite up to three partners to attend treatment. The number of partners that participants voluntarily brought to treatment (range, 0–3) was not associated with weight-loss outcomes over 18 months. However, participants with at least one successful partner (defined as losing ≥10% of initial weight after 6 months of treatment) lost significantly more weight themselves over 18 months than participants with no partners or unsuccessful partners, suggesting that participants in weight-loss programs should be encouraged to invite support partners who are also motivated to lose weight.

Tailoring Treatment to Individual Subgroups

Given the difficulty in maintaining weight loss long term, clinicians and researchers have begun to tailor interventions to specific subgroups of the obese population in hopes of improving treatment response. Some examples of tailoring include modifying treatment based on a participant's ethnicity and adapting treatment to address binge-eating disorder (BED).

Ethnicity

Several studies have suggested that African Americans achieve less weight loss than white participants in behavioral weight loss programs.[47,48] This may be due to physiologic differences that impede weight loss in African Americans[49] or to the fact that behavioral weight-loss programs are not culturally sensitive to the issues affecting African Americans. Several programs have been developed to be more appropriate to the needs of African Americans. Perhaps the most successful is a program developed specifically for inner-city black women with type 2 diabetes.[50] The program was based on an active problem-solving approach; program materials were carefully reviewed by a minority panel and included a food guide with ethnic and regional food items. Ten of the 13 participants in this study completed the 18-week program and the 1-year follow-up. Average weight losses were 4.1 kg during treatment and 4.4 kg at the 1-year follow-up. Further research is needed to determine how best to tailor programs to make them more appropriate for minority populations. The ethnicity of the other group members, ethnicity of the therapist, locations used for treatment meetings, and specific treatment materials might all influence outcome for minority participants.

BED

It is estimated that 30% to 50% of overweight patients seeking weight-loss treatment meet the diagnostic criteria for BED.[51,52] Consequently, it may be important to develop treatments specifically designed for this group of overweight patients.

BED is characterized by the presence of binge eating, loss of control over eating, and the absence of purging. It is included in the *Diagnostic and Statistical Manual of Mental Disorders*, 4th ed, as a diagnosis of further study and as an example of eating disorder not otherwise specified. The overall prevalence of BED in the general population is approximately 2%, and BED is evenly distributed among men and women.[51] The *Diagnostic and Statistical Manual of Mental Disorders*, makes no reference to weight in the BED diagnostic criteria; however, it is recognized that there is considerable overlap between obesity and BED and 50% of individuals with BED are overweight.

Obese individuals with BED differ from the obese individuals without BED on several physical and psychological dimensions. Specifically, binge eating is associated with depression, low self-esteem, and poor body image.[52,53] Binge eating is also associated with higher rates of attrition from behavioral weight-control programs.[48,54] Given these factors, many have argued that binge eating should be addressed prior to weight loss to enhance treatment outcome.

BED treatment has largely focused on the role of dietary restraint and negative affect in the binge-eating cycle. Presently, cognitive-behavioral therapy is considered the treatment of choice for this population. Cognitive-behavioral treatment for BED is typically offered in 10 to 12 weekly group sessions and produces binge abstinence rates of 40% to 50%.[55] The importance of binge abstinence prior to weight-loss treatment has been emphasized in the literature. In a review of three Stanford-based cognitive-behavioral treatment studies, Agras et al.[56] reported that participants who achieved binge abstinence prior to weight-loss treatment evidenced small weight losses at 1 year post-treatment (4.0 kg) compared with a small weight gain in participants who continued to binge eat (3.6 kg). Based on this finding, they concluded that binge-eating cessation is a necessary precursor to long-term weight loss.

Another study, however, questioned the position that binge eating needs to be addressed independently of weight control.[57] Overweight binge eaters were randomly assigned to either a behavioral weight-loss treatment, cognitive-behavioral treatment program for binge eating, or a no-treatment control group. Participants in both active treatments decreased their binge-eating frequency; however, only participants in behavioral weight-loss treatment lost a significant amount of weight. This study suggests that binge eaters might be better served by attending treatment programs that are focused on weight loss rather than binge-eating cessation. A retrospective examination of 444 women who participated in behavioral weight-loss treatment that included no discussion of binge eating supports this conclusion; binge eaters and non-bingers had comparable short- and long-term weight loss.[58]

A second, related question is whether participation in a weight-loss program causes binge eating. To examine this, Wadden et al.[59] recruited 123 overweight and obese individuals who had no problems with binge eating and randomly assigned them to either a weight-loss intervention with a 1000-kcal/d diet based on liquid meal replacement products, a 1200- to 1500-kcal/d balanced deficit diet of conventional foods, or a non-dieting approach that discouraged calorie restriction. At no time during this study did any participant in the three conditions meet criteria for binge eating. Thus, for overweight individuals, there is no evidence that weight loss, achieved by an appropriate program of diet, exercise, and behavior modification, causes eating disorders.

Increasing the Audience for Behavioral Interventions

Traditionally, behavioral weight-loss programs have been offered in face-to-face meetings with health professionals. However, recent research has focused on developing treatment approaches that involve little or no personal contact. Behavioral interventions have been developed for different forms of media including telephone, television, and, more recently, the Internet and e-mail. Such programs have the potential to be more cost effective, more convenient for participants, and offered to a larger portion of the population.

Telephone calls have been used as part of traditional clinic-based programs, often during the maintenance phase of treatment. Phone calls enable therapists to maintain contact with participants, but also gradually reduce the number of in-person contacts. The purpose of these calls is to monitor weight, food intake, and exercise. Anecdotal evidence suggests that these calls are helpful. However, in a study in which telephone calls were the primary mode of intervention (after two initial group meetings), weekly calls did not produce greater weight losses than no contact.[60]

Television broadcasts have also been used to deliver behavioral weight-loss interventions. In the first study using this approach, a behavioral diet intervention was delivered during a local television broadcast and produced an average weight loss of 0.7 to 1.0 kg/wk.[61] In another study, a series of eight 1-hour broadcasts of a behavioral group intervention produced weight losses of slightly greater than 0.45 kg/wk.[62] One of the advantages of this approach over the weekly clinic meeting is that television programs were rebroadcast throughout the week, giving participants multiple opportunities to view the program. Alternatively, the broadcast could be recorded by the participant for later viewing or reviewing.

Television broadcasts are a passive mode of intervention, as the viewer does not participate in the program. However, interactive television changes this one-way communication into a two-way "interactive" process. In interactive TV technology, participants can see and hear the therapist and all other participants. The disadvantage of this approach is that participants must go to an interactive television studio; however, this technology is rapidly advancing and this or other variations of this approach (e.g., Internet) will be available in our homes in the near future. Interactive television for delivery of a behavioral weight-loss program was found to perform as well as a standard, therapist-led "in-person" program producing average weight loss of 0.45 to 1.0 kg/wk in 12 weeks.[63]

Computer-assisted therapies for obesity began with the development of powerful, lightweight portable computers. These approaches offered a new means for patients to record self-monitoring information and the ability to provide quick feedback and reinforcement for incremental steps toward weight loss—often with less direct contact from the therapist. Burnett et al.[64] reported one of the initial studies using this method for behavioral treatment of obesity. Twelve subjects were randomly assigned either to use an interactive computer to enter self-monitoring data, receive feedback about caloric values, and receive praise or further instructions to modify eating contingent on performance or to use pencil and paper self-monitoring techniques and to look up caloric values themselves. Participants lost an average of 3.7 kg after 8 weeks in the computer-assisted condition compared with 1.5 kg in the control condition.

Computerized treatment approaches have evolved into programs offered via the Internet. The Internet can reduce barriers to care such as geographic access and may be more convenient for participants. Early research in this area has focused on initial efficacy of this approach. Tate et al.[65] found that combining behavioral procedures with informational websites produced significantly better weight losses compared with informational websites alone. Participants were randomly assigned to receive Internet behavior therapy or an Internet education program. Participants in the Internet education program were given an initial face-to-face meeting and directed to weight-loss–related websites they could use to develop their own weight-loss program, but were given no further help to do this. Participants in the Internet behavior therapy program received this meeting, access to the same website resources plus additional behavioral procedures, all delivered via the Internet and e-mail, including a sequence of weekly behavioral weight-loss lessons, prompting for submission of weekly online self-monitoring diaries, personalized feedback, and an online bulletin board for social support. Weight losses measured at 6 months were significantly greater for the Internet behavior therapy program than for the Internet education program (4.1 kg vs. 1.6 kg). A second study of a 1-year intervention for adults at increased risk for type 2 diabetes was conducted to isolate the effects of weekly e-mail behavioral counseling in an Internet program.[66] This study showed that Internet behavioral weight-loss programs with weekly structured behavioral lessons, self-monitoring, and peer support produced significantly more weight loss when the program included e-mail counseling from a behaviorally trained weight-loss counselor (Figure 3). Although numerous commercial programs for weight loss are available on the Internet, few have been studied. One study of these programs found a commercial online program to be less effective than a structured weight-loss manual.[67] Both groups received four (quarterly) face-to-face visits with a behavioral psychologist and 11 in-person weigh-ins during the year. The authors hypothesized that the Internet program lacked some of the structure offered by the manual.

A series of studies using the Internet for maintenance of weight loss following initial weight loss were conducted via either face-to-face[68] or interactive TV interventions.[69] The first study compared Internet maintenance programs with face-to-face maintenance programs and found the Internet to be a feasible means of delivering a behavioral maintenance program; however, participants randomly assigned to Internet maintenance did not appear to maintain weight loss as well as those in the face-to-face programs. The second study found interactive TV and Internet maintenance programs to be equally effective for weight maintenance. This second study was important from a public health perspective, given the increased reach and accessibility of these methods.

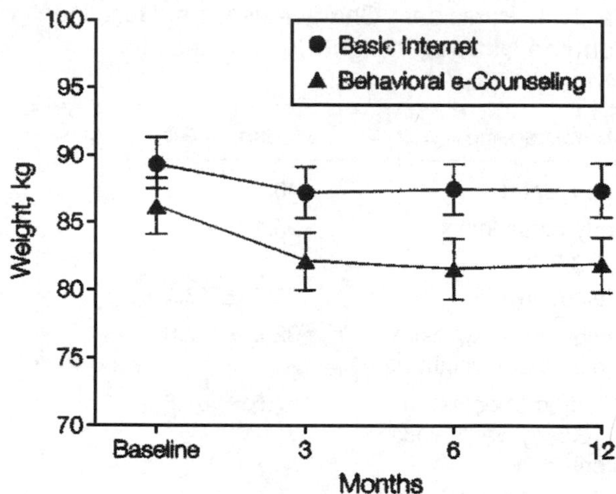

Figure 3. Pattern of change in body weight. Each data point represents the mean value for all participants randomized with missing data assuming no change from baseline ($P < 0.05$ at 3, 6, and 12 months). Error bars indicate SEM. (Used with permission from Tate et al., 2003[66]; copyright 2003, American Medical Association. All rights reserved.)

The National Weight Control Registry

Another approach to understanding the behaviors associated with weight loss and maintenance is to study those individuals who have been successful in accomplishing these goals. In 1993, James Hill, PhD, and Rena Wing, PhD, established the National Weight Control Registry to begin to study successful weight losers. To enter the registry, individuals must have lost at least 30 pounds and kept them off for at least 1 year. Registry members complete questionnaires at entry into the registry and then annually thereafter.[70]

There are now more than 4000 members in the registry, and they far exceed these minimum criteria. As shown in Table 1, registry members report having lost an average of 70 pounds, which they have kept off for 5.5 years. They have reduced from a body mass index of 36.6 to 25.1. Thus, by any criterion one would suggest, these individuals are clearly successful.

Several limitations should be kept in mind when considering findings from the registry. First, the registry is a self-selected group of successful weight losers. As shown in Table 1, the registry members are disproportionately female, white, and educated. This likely reflects characteristics of the population that is interested enough in their weight to complete the questionnaires and join the registry, rather than necessarily reflecting the characteris-

Table 1. Participant Characteristics at Baseline from the National Weight Control Registry, January 2005 (N = 4643)*

Characteristic	Mean ± SD	%
Age (years)	46.7 ± 12.5	
Body mass index (kg/m^2)	25.1 ± 4.7	
Weight (kg)	71.8 ± 16.1	
Weight loss (kg) from maximum weight	32.9 ± 17.8	
Duration (months) at 13.6-kg weight-loss criterion	67.5 ± 87.8	
Gender (% female)		76.9
Ethnicity (% white)		95.3
Marital status (% married)		64.5
Education (% completed)		
High school		10.9
Some college		31.0
College		26.9
Graduate or professional		31.2

*Actual sample size may vary slightly for each variable.

tics of successful weight losers. A second caveat is that all data are self-reported. We have, however, conducted a validation study on a subset of registry members in which their self-reported weights were compared with weights provided by their physician or weight-loss counselor. This validation study found that registry members provide very accurate information about their current and maximum weights. We have also collected information from a national sample of successful weight losers identified by random-digit dialing,[71] and found that the weight-loss maintenance behaviors reported by the National Weight Control Registry are very similar to those seen in this nationally representative sample of successful weight losers.

Registry members report having tried to lose weight many times before—unsuccessfully. They note that this time their successful efforts were characterized by greater commitment to behavior change and weight loss and by greater emphasis on physical activity. Perhaps these differences were responsible for their long-term success. Although more than 90% of registry members used the combination of diet plus physical activity to lose weight, the specific diet and exercise approaches varied tremendously.[38] In fact, about half of the registry members reported receiving some type of help with weight loss (from a physician, nutritionist, or commercial weight-loss program), whereas the other half reported doing it entirely on their own.

In contrast to the variety of approaches used for weight loss, there are certain common themes in the area of weight-loss maintenance. National Weight Control Registry members report that to maintain their weight loss, they continue to consume a low-calorie, low-fat diet, they maintain high levels of physical activity, and they monitor their weight regularly. Registry members complete the Block Food Frequency Questionnaire[72] at entry into the registry. Based on their reports, registry members are consuming approximately 1400 kcal/d (Table 2). Since dietary reports typically underestimate actual intake by approximately 30%, we estimate that National Weight Control Registry members are consuming approximately 1800 kcal/d. Registry members also report eating a low-fat diet; however, with the recent popularity of low-carbohydrate approaches (e.g., the Atkins diet), there has been a slight increase in average daily fat intake. In the initial year of the registry, members reported eating 26% of calories from fat; in 2001 to 2003, they averaged 30% of calories from fat. Another common dietary characteristic in the registry is regular consumption of breakfast. Seventy-eight percent of registry members report eating breakfast daily, with breakfast typically being cold cereal and fruit.[73]

Registry members also report high levels of physical activity, averaging approximately 2700 kcal/week.[38] We estimate that achieving this level requires approximately 60 min/d. The most common physical activity is walking, followed by activities such as weight lifting, cycling, and aerobic dance.

A final common characteristic is frequent monitoring of weight. More than 44% of registry members report weighing themselves at least once a day, and 31% report weighing themselves at least once a week. This frequent monitoring of weight appears to be part of a restrained dietary style in which individuals exert conscious control over their eating behaviors and weight. By weighing themselves frequently, registry members are in a position to identify small weight gains and make corrective behavior changes.

Table 2. Behavioral and Psychological Characteristics of Members of the National Weight Control Registry (N = 4643)*

Block calories consumed/d	1395.8 ± 599.2
% kcal from fat	28.4 ± 12.3
% kcal from carbohydrates	51.1 ± 14.0
% kcal from protein	18.9 ± 4.3
No. of meals or snacks/d	4.7 ± 1.6
No. of fast food meals/week	0.8 ± 1.6
No. of other restaurant meals/week	2.3 ± 2.4
Paffenbarger kcal/week	2603.5 ± 2469.1

*Actual sample size may vary slightly for each variable.

Thus, registry members confirm the message obtained from randomized clinical trials and outlined earlier in this chapter. Namely, the most effective approach for long-term maintenance of weight loss appears to involve the combination of a low-fat, low-calorie diet; high levels of physical activity; and behavioral strategies such as self-monitoring of weight.

Environmental Interventions

The behavioral techniques described thus far are strategies that are used to change an individual's behavior. This individual level approach to weight-control treatment is inconsistent with the growing recognition of the environment's contribution to the obesity epidemic,[74-76] and given the staggering prevalence rates of overweight and obesity, may not be a cost-effective solution. Drawing on ecologic models of health promotion (Figure 4),[77-79] there is increasing interest in identifying and modifying influences on weight-regulating behaviors at several different environmental levels. To date, community- and societal-level variables have received the most attention, with trends such as increased number of meals away from home, supersized portions, increased exposure to food advertising, greater availability of sedentary leisure-time activities, and more reliance on labor-saving devices all commonly implicated as contributing to the rising obesity rates.[80-83]

Specific strategies that have shown success in modifying environmental-level influences on eating behaviors include decreasing the cost and increasing the availability of healthier food items. Jeffery et al. have examined these environmental manipulations in a cafeteria setting[84] and in vending machines.[85] Cafeteria purchases of salad items and fresh fruit were analyzed from cash receipts for a 3-week baseline. The investigators then increased the number of fruit and salad choices that were offered and halved their price. Analyses of cashier receipts over the subsequent 3 weeks showed that these interventions were effective in increasing salad and fruit consumption approximately three-fold over baseline levels. When these interventions were terminated, consumption of these items decreased. A similar study was done to test an intervention in which prices of low-fat snacks in vending machines were decreased by 50%.[85] During baseline, 25.7% of the snacks purchased were low-fat; this increased to 45.8% during the 3-week period of intervention and returned to baseline (22.8%) after the intervention. There were no differences over time in total purchases of snack items.

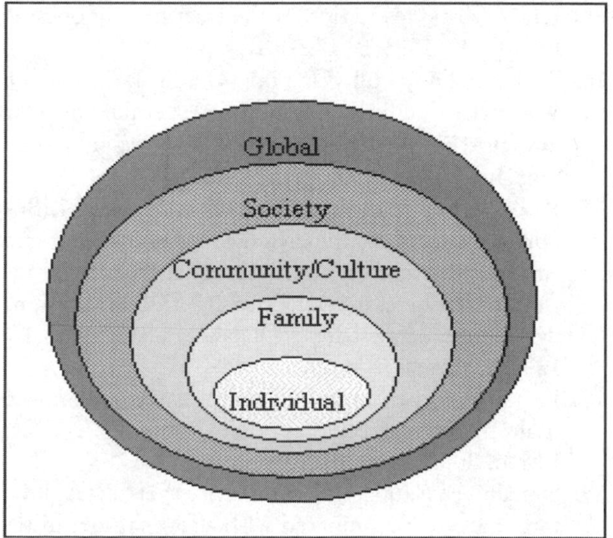

Figure 4. Ecologic model of behavior. (From Bronfenbrenner 1989.[77])

A longer-term study recently conducted in secondary school cafeterias had similar positive effects on healthy food purchases.[86] Simply increasing the number of low-fat food items available in a la carte areas and encouraging student purchases of low-fat items through peer-based promotions (e.g., taste tests, media campaigns) increased students' low-fat food purchases by 10% over 1 year and resulted in a significantly higher percentage of low-fat food sales at year 2 in intervention schools compared with control schools. This line of research consistently suggests that increasing the availability and decreasing the cost of healthier food items is a viable strategy for improving eating choices.

Specific strategies that have shown success in modifying environmental-level influences on physical activity include encouraging stairs rather than escalators through visual prompts, structuring communities to facilitate increased physical activity, and using media campaigns to increase daily walking.[87-89] In terms of increasing stair usage, Brownell[87] investigated this first in 1980 and showed that a sign encouraging use of stairs rather than escalators increased stair use. A replication of this study used two different signs, promoting either the health or weight benefits of using stairs.[88] These signs were placed in a shopping center beside escalators with adjacent stairs. Overall, stair use increased from 4.8% to 6.9% and 7.2% with the health and weight control signs, respectively. Interestingly, however, the signs were only effective with white customers; neither sign was effective in promoting stair use in African Americans. A more recent study by Kerr et al.[90] found that using motivational signs to promote stairs use in combination with environmental changes designed to enhance the sensory appeal of the stairs (e.g., new carpeting, paint, artwork, and stereo system) resulted in even greater increases in stair use by workplace employees.

On a larger environmental level, the effects of creating an entire community conducive to physical activity was studied by building bicycle paths, improving gym facilities, and forming exercise clubs.[89,90] Compared with control communities that did not receive these environmental manipulations, individuals in the modified community had significantly greater improvements in fitness levels over 12 months of study. More recently, Colorado has initiated a statewide campaign to encourage residents to accumulate 10,000 steps each day through the formation of walking groups and the use of shopping discounts and other types of incentives. This campaign has now been extended as a national initiative,[91] with ongoing research studies examining the impact of this type of environmental manipulation on physical activity.

In general, community- and societal-level interventions targeting the cost and availability of food and the promotion of physical activity through environmental modifications have shown promise in changing eating and exercise behaviors, leading to calls for more policy-wide changes in areas such as food pricing, tax structures, and urban planning.[75,80,92]

Conclusions

Behavioral treatments have been shown to be effective in producing significant initial weight losses. Currently, attention is focused on developing more effective maintenance interventions and on investigating ways to prevent the development of obesity. While we know that both eating and exercise behaviors are related to body weight, we lack very basic information regarding the specific diet and exercise recommendations that are most effective for long-term weight control. Further research is needed on ways to improve weight-loss outcome by increasing support for habit change, tailoring treatment to specific patient groups, and developing stronger techniques for changing both the home and the outside environment. Behavioral strategies that are helpful in the treatment of obesity, such as stimulus control, relapse prevention, and self-monitoring, may also be useful in modifying other dietary habits and may thus be applied to the treatment and prevention of hypertension, hyperlipidemia, and some forms of cancer.

References

1. Stuart RB. Behavioral control of overeating. Behav Res Ther. 1967;5:357–365.
2. Wing RR. Behavioral approaches to the treatment of obesity. In: Bray G, Bouchard C, James P, eds. *Handbook of Obesity*. New York: Marcel Dekker; 1998; 855–873.
3. Bray G, Bouchard C, eds. *Handbook of Obesity: Clinical Applications*. 2nd ed. New York: Marcel Dekker; 2004.
4. Wadden TA, Sternberg JA, Letizia KA, Stunkard AJ, Foster GD. Treatment of obesity by very low calorie diet, behaviour therapy, and their combination: A five-year perspective. Int J Obes. 1989;13: 39–46.
5. Bandura A, Simon KM. The role of proximal intentions in self-regulation of refractory behavior. Cognit Ther Res. 1977;1:177–193.
6. Wadden TA, Letizia KA. Predictors of attrition and weight loss in patients treated by moderate and severe caloric restriction. In: Wadden TA, VanItallie TB, eds. *Treatment of the Seriously Obese Patient*. New York: Guilford Press; 1992; 383–410.
7. Marlatt GA, Gordon JR. *Relapse Prevention: Maintenance Strategies in Addictive Behavior Change*. New York: Guilford Press; 1985; 558 pp.
8. Kumanyika SK, Van Horn L, Bowen D, et al. Maintenance of dietary behavior change. Health Psychol. 2000;19(1 Suppl):42–56.
9. National Task Force on the Prevention and Treatment of Obesity. Very low-calorie diets. JAMA. 1993;270:967–974.
10. Wadden TA, Stunkard AJ. Controlled trial of very low calorie diet, behavior therapy, and their combination in the treatment of obesity. J Consult Clin Psychol. 1986;54:482–488.
11. Wadden TA, Foster GD, Letizia KA. One-year behavioral treatment of obesity: comparison of moderate and severe caloric restriction and the effects of weight maintenance therapy. J Consult Clin Psychol. 1994;62:165–171.
12. Wing RR, Marcus MD, Salata R, Epstein LH, Miaskiewicz S, Blair EH. Effects of a very-low-calorie diet on long-term glycemic control in obese type 2 diabetic subjects. Arch Int Med. 1991;151:1334–1340.
13. Wing RR, Blair E, Marcus M, Epstein LH, Harvey J. Year-long weight loss treatment for obese patients with type II diabetes: does inclusion of an intermittent very low calorie diet improve outcome? Am J Med. 1994;97:354–362.
14. Tucker LA, Kano MJ. Dietary fat and body fat: a multivariate study of 205 adult females. Am J Clin Nutr. 1992;56:616–622.
15. Jeffery RW, Hellerstedt WL, French SA, Baxter JE. A randomized trial of counseling for fat restriction versus calorie restriction in the treatment of obesity. Int J Obes. 1995;19:132–137.
16. Schlundt DG, Hill JO, Pope-Cordle J, Arnold D, Virts KL, Katahn M. Randomized evaluation of a low fat ad libitum carbohydrate diet for weight reduction. Int J Obes. 1993;17:623–629.
17. Pascale RW, Wing RR, Butler BA, Mullen M, Bononi P. Effects of a behavioral weight loss program stressing calorie restriction versus calorie plus fat restriction in obese individuals with NIDDM or a family history of diabetes. Diabetes Care. 1995;18: 1241–1248.
18. Foster G, Wyatt HR, Hill JO, et al. A randomized trial of a low-carbohydrate diet for obesity. N Engl J Med. 2003;348:2082–2090.
19. Samaha FF, Iqbal N, Seshadri P, et al. A low-carbohydrate as compared with a low-fat diet in severe obesity. N Engl J Med. 2003;348:2074–2081.
20. Yancy WS, Olsen MK, Guyton JR, Bakst RP, West-

man EC. A low-carbohydrate, ketogenic diet versus a low-fat diet to treat obesity and hyperlipidemia. Ann Intern Med. 2004;140:769–777.

21. McCrory MA, Fuss P, McCallum J, et al. Dietary variety within food groups: association with energy intake and body fatness in men and women. Am J Clin Nutr. 1999;69:440–447.
22. Rolls BJ. The role of sensory-specific satiety in food intake and food selection. In: Capaldi ED, Powley TL, editors. *Taste, Experience, and Feeding*. Washington, DC: American Psychological Association; 1990; 197–209.
23. Raynor HA, Jeffery RW, Wing RR. Relationship between changes in food group variety, dietary intake, and weight during obesity treatment. Int J Obes. 2004;28:813–820.
24. Jeffery RW, Wing RR, Thorson C, et al. Strengthening behavioral interventions for weight loss: a randomized trial of food provision and monetary incentives. J Consult Clin Psychol. 1993;61:1038–1045.
25. Wing RR, Jeffery RW, Burton LR, Thorson C, Sperber Nissinoff K, Baxter JE. Food provision vs. structured meal plans in the behavioral treatment of obesity. Int J Obes. 1996;20:56–62.
26. Pi-Sunyer F, Maggio C, McCarron D, et al. Multicenter randomized trial of a comprehensive prepared meal program in type 2 diabetes. Diabetes Care. 1999;22:191–197.
27. Ditschuneit HH, Flechtner-Mors M, Johnson TD, Adler G. Metabolic and weight-loss effects of a long-term dietary intervention in obese patients. Am J Clin Nutr. 1999;69:198–204.
28. Wadden TA, Berkowitz RI, Sarwer DB, Prus-Wisniewski R, Steinberg C. Benefits of lifestyle modification in the pharmacologic treatment of obesity. Arch Int Med. 2001;161:218–227.
29. Pronk NP, Wing RR. Physical activity and long-term maintenance of weight loss. Obes Res. 1994;2: 587–599.
30. Dunn AL, Marcus BH, Kampert JB, Garcia ME, Kohl HW, Blair SN. Comparison of lifestyle and structured interventions to increase physical activity and cardiorespiratory fitness: a randomized trial. JAMA. 1999;281:327–334.
31. Andersen R, Frankowiak S, Snyder J, Bartlett S, Fontaine K. Effects of lifestyle activity vs. structured aerobic exercise in obese women: a randomized trial. JAMA. 1998;281:335–340.
32. Perri MG, Martin AD, Leermakers EA, Sears SF, Notelovitz M. Effects of group- versus home-based exercise in the treatment of obesity. J Consult Clin Psychol. 1997;65:278–285.
33. Jakicic JM, Wing RR, Butler BA, Robertson RJ. Prescribing exercise in multiple short bouts versus one continuous bout: effects on adherence, cardiorespiratory fitness, and weight loss in overweight women. Int J Obes. 1995;19:893–901.
34. Jakicic J, Wing R, Winters C. Effects of intermittent exercise and use of home exercise equipment on adherence, weight loss, and fitness in overweight women. JAMA. 1999;282:1554–1560.
35. Jakicic JM, Wing RR, Butler BA, Jeffery RW. The relationship between presence of exercise equipment in the home and physical activity level. Am J Health Promot. 1997;11:363–365.
36. Epstein LH, Valoski AM, Vara LS, et al. Effects of decreasing sedentary behavior and increasing activity on weight change in obese children. Health Psychol. 1995;14:109–115.
37. Robinson T. Reducing children's television viewing to prevent obesity. JAMA. 1999;282:1561–1567.
38. Klem ML, Wing RR, McGuire MT, Seagle HM, Hill JO. A descriptive study of individuals successful at long-term maintenance of substantial weight loss. Am J Clin Nutr. 1997;66:239–246.
39. Jeffery RW, Wing RR, Thorson C, Burton LC. Use of personal trainers and financial incentives to increase exercise in a behavioral weight-loss program. J Consult Clin Psychol. 1998;66:777–783.
40. Jeffery RW, Wing RR, Sherwood NE, Tate DF. Physical activity and weight loss: does prescribing higher physical activity goals improve outcome? Am J Clin Nutr. 2003;89:684–689.
41. Perri MG, Nezu AM, Patti ET, McCann KL. Effect of length of treatment on weight loss. J Consult Clin Psychol. 1989;57:450–452.
42. Perri MG, McAllister DA, Gange JJ, Jordan RC, McAdoo WG, Nezu AM. Effects of four maintenance programs on the long-term management of obesity. J Consult Clin Psychol. 1988;56:529–534.
43. Black DR, Gleser LJ, Kooyers KJ. A meta-analytic evaluation of couples weight-loss programs. Health Psychol. 1990;9:330–347.
44. Wing RR, Marcus MD, Epstein LH, Jawad A. A "family-based" approach to the treatment of obese type II diabetic patients. J Consult Clin Psychol. 1991;59:156–162.
45. Wing R, Jeffery R. Benefits of recruiting participants with friends and increasing social support for weight loss and maintenance. J Consult Clin Psychol. 1999; 67:132–138.
46. Gorin AA, Phelan S, Tate D, Sherwood N, Jeffery R, Wing RR. Involving support partners in obesity treatment. J Consult Clin Psychol. 2005;73:341.
47. Kumanyika SK, Obarzanek E, Stevens VJ, Hebert PR, Whelton PK. Weight-loss experience of black and white participants in NHLBI-sponsored clinical trials. Am J Clin Nutr. 1991;53:1631–1638.
48. Yanovski SZ, Gormally JF, Leser MS, Gwirtsman HE, Yanovski JA. Binge eating disorder affects outcome of comprehensive very-low-calorie diet treatment. Obes Res. 1994;2:205–212.
49. Jakicic JM, Wing RR. Differences in resting energy

expenditure in African-American vs Caucasian overweight females. Int J Obes. 1998;22:236–242.
50. McNabb WL, Quinn MT, Rosing L. Weight loss program for inner-city black women with non-insulin-dependent diabetes mellitus: PATHWAYS. J Am Diet Assoc. 1993;93:75–77.
51. Spitzer RL, Devlin M, Walsh BT, et al. Binge eating disorder: a multisite field trial of the diagnostic criteria. *Int J Eat Disord.* 1992;11:191–203.
52. Yanovski SZ. Binge eating disorder: current knowledge and future directions. Obes Res. 1993;1:306–324.
53. Marcus MD. Binge eating in obesity. In: Fairburn CG, Wilson GT, eds. *Binge Eating. Nature, Assessment, and Treatment.* New York: Guilford Press; 1993; 77–96.
54. Marcus MD, Wing RR, Hopkins J. Obese binge eaters: affect, cognitions, and response to behavioral weight control. J Consult Clin Psychol. 1988;56:433–439.
55. Smith DE, Marcus MD, Kaye W. Cognitive-behavioral treatment of obese binge eaters. Int J Eat Disord. 1992;12:249–256.
56. Agras WST, Telch CF, Arnow B, Eldredge K, Marnell M. One-year follow-up of cognitive-behavioral therapy for obese individuals with binge eating disorder. J Consult Clin Psychol. 1997;65:343–347.
57. Marcus MD, Wing RR, Fairburn CG. Cognitive treatment of binge eating v. behavioral weight control in the treatment of binge eating disorder [abstract]. Ann Behav Med. 1995;17:S090.
58. Sherwood NE, Jeffery RW, Wing RR. Binge status as a predictor of weight loss treatment outcome. Int J Obes. 1999;23:485–493.
59. Wadden TA, Foster GD, Sarwer DB, et al. Dieting and the development of eating disorders in obese women: results of a randomized controlled trial. Am J Clin Nutr. 2004;80:560–568.
60. Hellerstedt W, Jeffery R. The effects of a telephone-based intervention on weight loss. Am J Health Promot. 1997;11:177–182.
61. Frankel AR, Birkimer JC, Brown JH, Cunningham GK. A behavioral diet on network television. Behav Counsel Commun Interventions. 1983;3:91–101.
62. Myers A, Graves T, Whelan J, Barclay D. An evaluation of television-delivered behavioral weight loss programs: are the ratings acceptable? J Consult Clin Psychol. 1996;64:172–178.
63. Harvey-Berino J. Changing health behavior via telecommunications technology: using interactive television to treat obesity. Behav Ther. 1998;29:505–519.
64. Burnett KF, Taylor CB, Agras WS. Ambulatory computer-assisted therapy for obesity: a new frontier for behavior therapy. J Consult Clin Psychol. 1985;53:698–703.
65. Tate DF, Wing RR, Winett RA. Using Internet technology to deliver a behavioral weight loss program. JAMA. 2001;285:1172–1177.
66. Tate DF, Jackvony EH, Wing RR. Effects of Internet behavioral counseling on weight loss in adults at risk for type 2 diabetes. JAMA. 2003;289:1833–1836.
67. Womble LG, Wadden T, McGuckin BG, Sargent SL, Rothman RA, Krauthamer-Ewing ES. A randomized controlled trial of commercial Internet weight loss programs. Obes Res. 2004;12:1011–1018.
68. Harvey-Berino J, Pintauro S, Bulzzell P, et al. Does using the Internet facilitate the maintenance of weight loss? Int J Eat Disord. 2002;26:1254–1260.
69. Harvey-Berino J, Pintauro S, Buzzell P, Gold EC. Effect of Internet support on the long-term maintenance of weight loss. Obes Res. 2004;12:320–329.
70. Wing RR, Hill JO. Successful weight loss maintenance. Annu Rev Nutr. 2001;21:323–341.
71. McGuire MT, Wing RR, Klem ML, Hill JO. Behavioral strategies of individuals who have maintained long-term weight losses. Obes Res. 1999;7:334–341.
72. Block G, Hartman AM, Dresser CM, Carroll MD, Gannon J, Gardner L. A data-based approach to diet questionnaire design and testing. Am J Epidemiol. 1986;124:453–469.
73. Wyatt HR, Grunwald GK, Mosca CL, Klem M, Wing RR, Hill JO. Long-term weight loss and breakfast in subjects in the National Weight Control Registry. Obes Res. 2002;10:78–82.
74. Hill J, Peters J. Environmental contributions to the obesity epidemic. Science. 1998;280:1371–1374.
75. Nestle M, Jacobson MF. Halting the obesity epidemic: a public health policy approach. Public Health Rep. 2000;115:12–24.
76. Swinburn B, Egger G, Raza F. Dissecting obesogenic environments: the development and application of a framework for identifying and prioritizing environmental interventions for obesity. Prev Med. 1999;29:563–570.
77. Bronfenbrenner U. Ecological systems theory. Ann Child Devel 1989;22:723–742.
78. Breslow L. Social ecological strategies for promoting healthy lifestyles. Am J Health Promot. 1996;10:253–257.
79. Stokols D. Social ecology and behavioral medicine: implications for training, practice, and policy. Behav Med. 2000;26:129–139.
80. French SA, Story M, Jeffery RW. Environmental influences on eating and physical activity. Annu Rev Public Health. 2001;22:309–335.
81. McCrory MA, Fuss PJ, Hays NP, Vinken AG, Greenberg AS, Roberts SB. Overeating in America: association between restaurant food consumption and body fatness in healthy adult men and women ages 19 to 80. Obes Res. 1999;7:564–571.

82. Nielsen SJ, Popkin BM. Patterns and trends in food portion sizes, 1977–1998. JAMA. 2003;289:450–453.
83. Owen N, Leslie E, Salmon J, Fotheringham MJ. Environmental determinants of physical activity and sedentary behavior. Exerc Sport Sci Rev. 2000;28:153–158.
84. Jeffery RW, French SA, Raether C, Baxter JE. An environmental intervention to increase fruit and salad purchases in a cafeteria. Prev Med. 1994;23:788–792.
85. French S, Jeffery R, Story M, Hannan P, Snyder M. A pricing strategy to promote low-fat snack choices through vending machines. Am J Public Health. 1997;87:849–851.
86. French SA, Story M, Fulkerson JA, Hannan P. An environmental intervention to promote lower-fat food choices in secondary schools: outcomes of the TACOS study. Am J Public Health. 2004;94:1507–1512.
87. Brownell KD, Stunkard AJ, Albaum JM. Evaluation and modification of exercise patterns in the natural environment. Am J Psychiatry. 1980;137:1540–1545.
88. Andersen R, Franckowiak S, Snyder J, Bartlett S, Fontaine K. Can inexpensive signs encourage the use of stairs? Results from a community intervention. Ann Intern Med. 1998;129:363–369.
89. Linenger JM, Chesson CV, Nice DS. Physical fitness gains following simple environmental change. Am J Prev Med. 1991;7:298–310.
90. Kerr NA, Yore MM, Ham SA, Dietz WH. Increasing stair use in a worksite through environmental changes. Am J Health Promot. 2004;18:312–315.
91. America on the Move. Available at: http://www.americaonthemove.org. Accessed March 26, 2006.
92. Hill JO, Wyatt HR, Reed GW, Peters JC. Obesity and the environment: where do we go from here? Science. 2003;299:853–855.

62

Nutrition Monitoring in the United States

Ronette R. Briefel

Nutrition monitoring has been defined as "an ongoing description of nutrition conditions in the population, with particular attention to subgroups defined in socioeconomic terms, for purposes of planning, analyzing the effects of policies and program on nutrition problems, and predicting future trends."[1] This chapter provides a brief history of the National Nutrition Monitoring and Related Research Program (NNMRRP) in the United States, uses of nutrition monitoring data, monitoring activities since the mid-1990s, and nutrition monitoring research to meet challenges in the future.

The NNMRRP is composed of interconnected federal and state activities that provide information about the dietary and nutritional status of the US population, conditions existing in the United States that affect the dietary and nutritional status of individuals, and relationships between diet and health.[2-5] A general conceptual model representing the relationship between food and health among the five NNMRRP measurement components is presented in Figure 1. The five components are: nutrition and related health measurements; food and nutrient consumption; knowledge, attitudes, and behavior assessments; food composition and nutrient databases; and food supply determinations. The US nutrition monitoring program is a model for integrating national and state data from many sources to understand the relationship between food and health and to improve nutrition in the population.

History and Milestones

Major legislation to increase federal efforts to coordinate nutrition surveys has been described in detail elsewhere[2-5] and is summarized in Table 1, beginning with the formal establishment of a monitoring system in 1977. The National Nutrition Monitoring and Related Research Act (Pub. L. 101–445) was signed into law on Oct. 22, 1990, after several attempts during 1984 to 1990 had failed.[2] The Act established several mechanisms to ensure the collaboration and coordination of federal agencies as well as state and local governments involved in nutrition monitoring. These included the formation of an inter-agency board to coordinate the preparation of an annual budget report on nutrition monitoring, biennial reports on progress and policy implications of scientific findings, and periodic scientific reports to describe the nutritional and related health status of the US population. A National Nutrition Monitoring Advisory Council provided scientific and technical guidance to the board and made important contributions to improving information dissemination and bringing attention to issues such as the coverage of high-risk population subgroups, assessment

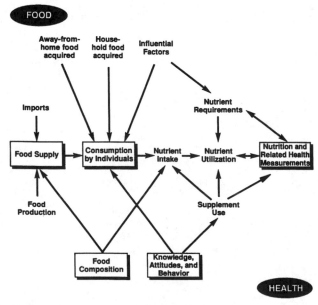

Figure 1. Relationship of food to health.

Table 1. Milestones of the National Nutrition Monitoring and Related Research Program

1977	Food and Agriculture Act (Pub. L. 95-113) passed
1978	Proposal for a comprehensive nutritional status monitoring system submitted to Congress
1981	Joint Implementation Plan for a Comprehensive National Nutrition Monitoring System
1983	Joint Nutrition Monitoring Evaluation Committee formed
1987	Operational Plan for the National Nutrition Monitoring System
1988	Interagency Committee on Nutrition Monitoring (ICNM) formed
1990	National Nutrition Monitoring and Related Research Act (Pub. L. 101-445) passed[2]
199	Interagency Board for Nutrition Monitoring and Related Research (IBNMRR) established through incorporation and expansion of the ICNM
1992	National Nutrition Monitoring Advisory Council formed
1993	Ten-Year Comprehensive Plan (1992–2002) for the NNMRRP published[3]
1998	Memorandum of Understanding to integrate NHANES and CSFII signed by NCHS/CDC and Agricultural Research Service/USDA Expert Panel on Survey Integration formed to review survey integration and dietary methodology research plans
1999	National Academy of Sciences' Symposium on the Future of Nutrition Monitoring
2002	Full integration of NHANES and CSFII in the "What We Eat in America," as a part of data collection in NHANES Stakeholder Workshop on the integrated CSFII-NHANES[6] American Society for Nutritional Sciences Working Group on Nutrition Monitoring[7]
2004	Institute of Medicine Panel on Enhancing the Data Infrastructure in Support of Food and Nutrition Programs, Research, and Decision Making[8,9]

of the needs of data users, and integration of federal, state, and private data needs.

The *Ten-Year Comprehensive Plan* served as the strategy to guide federal actions for nutrition monitoring during the period 1992 to 2002.[3] The plan identified three national objectives critical to the success of the overall goal of a coordinated, comprehensive nutrition monitoring program: 1) provide for a comprehensive program through continuous and coordinated data collection; 2) improve the comparability and quality of data across the program; and 3) improve the research base for nutrition monitoring.[3-5] During the period 1992 to 1997, federal efforts were focused on improving survey coordination and survey methods, conducting research, and increasing nutrition information dissemination.[4-10] To meet one of the research objectives, an 18-item food security measure was developed to track the prevalence of hunger and food insecurity in the population and high-risk subgroups.[11]

During the period 1997 to 2002, the high-priority issues included the survey integration of the two national nutrition surveys (the National Health and Nutrition Examination Survey [NHANES] and the US Department of Agriculture's (USDA) Continuing Survey of Food Intakes by Individuals [CSFII]), welfare reform and nutrition data needs, and food composition data needs. The National Center for Health Statistics (NCHS) and the Agricultural Research Service (ARS) of the USDA signed an agreement in 1998 to integrate NHANES and CSFII, which was fully integrated in 2002 as the *What We Eat in America* survey as part of the NHANES data collection.[6,12] An expert panel reviewed the scope of the proposed research and provided recommendations to the two agencies to strengthen the overall integration plan and the dietary research and evaluation component. In 2002, a workshop was held with nutrition monitoring stakeholders to develop recommendations on how best to meet data needs for policy and research with the integrated survey.[6] In 2004, an Institute of Medicine panel was formed to make recommendations to improve the data infrastructure on food consumption to support food and nutrition programs and policies within the USDA.[8,9]

Nutrition monitoring has also been the focus of scientific and professional organizations. In 1999, the National Academy of Sciences sponsored a symposium on the future of nutrition monitoring because the 1990 legislation was up for reauthorization in 2002. The purpose of the meeting was to draw attention to the federal, research, industry, media, and consumer uses of NNMRRP data and to discuss the future challenges for the program. Despite this symposium, a report by the American Societies for Nutritional Sciences Working Group,[7] and other efforts to gain support for reauthorization, the nutrition monitoring legislation was not renewed in 2002. Monitoring activities are continuing, but without the coordinated guidance of an inter-agency board or legislative mandate. There is a continued need for congressional support to ensure that there is a sound NNMRRP in the future with steady financial resources for national nutrition monitoring.

Scientific and Technical Reports

Table 2 lists the methodologic reports, inventories of activities, and coordinated data reports from the

Table 2. Major National Nutrition Monitoring Reports and Publications

Date	Report	Source	Purpose and Content
Methodologic Reports			
1984	Nutrient Adequacy: Assessment Using National Food Consumption Data	National Academy of Sciences	Funded by USDA and DHHS to facilitate wider application of national dietary survey data
1992	Improving Comparability in the National Nutrition Monitoring and Related Research Program: Population Descriptors	IBNMRR Survey Comparability Working Group	Recommended categories for collecting and reporting data for several sociodemographic descriptors; provided statistical guidelines for reporting nutrition program data
1994	Consensus Workshop on Dietary Assessment: Nutrition Monitoring and Tracking the Year 2000 Objectives	National Center for Health Statistics	Recommended guidelines for the selection of dietary methods, the interpretation of dietary intake data, and data collection methodologies for assessing intakes of fruits and vegetables, fat, calcium, and alcohol
Inventories/Directories of Nutrition Monitoring Activities			
1989	The Directory of Federal Nutrition Monitoring Activities	Interagency Committee on Nutrition Monitoring	Summary of federal nutrition surveys, activities, and contacts for the five measurement components in the program
1992	The Directory of Federal and State Nutrition Monitoring Activities	IBNMRR	Updated the 1989 directory; expanded to include state surveillance activities and contacts
1999 (updated in 2000)	The Directory of Federal and State Nutrition Monitoring and Related Research Activities	IBNMRR	Updated the 1992 directory; expanded to include a summary of nutrition monitoring research; converted from printed form to electronic form available on the Internet
Integrated Data Reports			
1986	A Progress Report from the Joint Nutrition Monitoring Evaluation Committee	Joint Nutrition Monitoring Evaluation Committee	First progress report; provided overview of dietary and nutritional status of the population and recommendations for future nutrition monitoring
1989	An Update Report on Nutrition Monitoring	Life Sciences Research Office	Second progress report; updated information on the dietary and nutritional status of the population with in-depth study of cardiovascular disease risk factors and iron nutriture
1993	Chartbook I: Selected Findings from the National Nutrition Monitoring and Related Research Program	IBNMRR	Provided user-friendly graphs and figures of select nutrition findings available since the second progress report
1995	Third Report on Nutrition Monitoring in the United States	Life Sciences Research Office	Third progress report; provided a comprehensive update of available nutrition data with emphasis on the low-income population and high-risk population groups

DHHS, Department of Health and Human Services; IBNMRR, Inter-Agency Board for Nutrition Monitoring and Related Research; USDA, US Department of Agriculture.

program. Complete citations and report descriptions are available in published sources.[4,5,7,13,14] The 2000 *Directory of Federal and State Nutrition Monitoring and Related Research Activities* was a comprehensive summary of program activities;[13] however, it has not been updated due to lack of resources. In the 1990s, major improvements were made to standardizing the collection and reporting of key socioeconomic variables[15] and the assessment of dietary intake.[16]

In 2005, the Institute of Medicine published a review of the infrastructure to support food and nutrition programs, research, and decision making and provided recommendations to improve the data for such purposes. This report provides more recent information on the nutrition monitoring activities but does not cover the entire program to the extent of the *Directory*.[8,13] Another report by Logan et al.[17] summarizes the types of data available from national surveys and surveillance systems that can be used to assess the relationship between food assistance program participation and nutrition and health outcomes. The inter-agency board most recently published an integrated scientific report of data from across the program in 1995.[14] In 2005, the major sources of nutrition monitoring data are single government agency reports and journal articles, with little attention paid to coordinated reports that synthesize data from across the program.

Purposes and Uses of Nutrition Monitoring Data

Nutrition monitoring is vital to policy making and research.[1-5,7,18] Monitoring provides information and a database for establishing public policy and identifying research priorities.[4-10,18-21] Nutrition research provides data for policy making and for identifying nutrition monitoring needs for data.[3-6,10,18] Table 3 provides examples of uses of nutrition monitoring data for public policy and scientific research purposes. Monitoring provides information for public policy decisions related to nutrition education programs such as the *Dietary Guidelines for Americans*;[22] 5-A-Day for Better Health;[23] public health programs such as the National Cholesterol Education Program[25] and the National High Blood Pressure Education Program;[26] federally supported food service and food assistance programs[8,9,27] such as the National School Lunch Program,[28] the Special Supplemental Nutrition Program for Women, Infants, and Children (WIC),[29] and the Thrifty Food Plan;[30] and food production and marketing, such as the development of reduced-fat or reduced-calorie food products.

Monitoring data are used to evaluate progress toward meeting the Year 2010 Health Objectives[21] and guidelines for prevention, detection, and management of nutritional conditions,[25,26,31] and to identify areas of nutrition research that are needed to increase the knowledge base and revise the standards of human nutrient require-

Table 3. Uses of Nutrition Monitoring Data

Public Policy

Monitoring and Surveillance

- Identify high-risk groups and geographic areas with nutrition-related problems to facilitate implementation of public health intervention programs and food assistance programs
- Evaluate changes in agricultural policy that may affect the nutritional quality and healthfulness of the US food supply
- Track trends in dietary behavior, nutritional status, and health to assess progress toward achieving the nutrition and health objectives in *Healthy People 2010* and the Dietary Guidelines
- Evaluate the effectiveness of nutritional initiatives for military feeding systems
- Recommend guidelines for prevention, detection, and management of nutrition and health conditions
- Develop reference standards for nutritional status
- Monitor food production and marketing

Regulatory

- Develop food labeling policies
- Document the need for, and monitor, food fortification policies
- Establish food safety guidelines

Nutrition-Related Programs

- Develop nutrition education and dietary guidance (e.g., *Dietary Guidelines for Americans* and 5-A-Day)
- Plan and evaluate food assistance programs
- Plan and assess nutrition intervention programs and public health programs

Scientific Research

- Establish nutrient requirements through the life cycle (e.g., *Dietary Reference Intakes* and assess nutrient adequacy and excess)
- Study diet-health relationships and the relationship of knowledge and attitudes to dietary and health behavior
- Develop biomarkers of diet and health behaviors and nutritional status
- Foster and conduct nutrition monitoring research, national and international
- Conduct food composition analysis
- Study the economic aspects of food consumption
- Assess the contribution of dietary supplements to usual nutrient intake

ments.[24] National data on the population's dietary intakes and serum nutrient levels have been used extensively for the investigation of nutrient requirements throughout the life cycle and the development of the *Dietary Reference Intakes* by the National Academy of Sciences.[24]

Data have been used by regulatory agencies such as the Food and Drug Administration (FDA) to examine US food fortification policies[4-6,18-20,32] and dietary supplement usage,[33,34] as a basis for food labeling,[35] and by the FDA and the Environmental Protection Agency (EPA) to provide dietary exposure estimates for nutrient and non-nutrient food components.[36,37] For example, nutrition monitoring data collected in the third National Health and Nutrition Examination Survey (NHANES III) were used to assess folate status and the relationship between serum determinations, diet, and other nutrition and health variables before and after the FDA made rules about folate food fortification.[32,38]

National nutrition monitoring data have been used for biomonitoring of environmental exposures by measuring substances in blood, urine, and hair. In addition to the assessment of nutrient status and the measurement of blood levels of vitamins and minerals, NHANES data have also been used to assess levels of metals, including lead, cadmium, and mercury.[37,39] The data have been used to determine the prevalence of elevated blood levels of nutrients, metals, and environmental chemicals; to establish reference ranges for determining high exposures; to assess the effectiveness of public health efforts to reduce exposures; to track trends in exposure levels; and to set priorities for research on the human health effects of environmental exposures.[36,37,39]

Industry uses nutrition monitoring data for marketing purposes and research.[4-6,18-20,34] The food industry has used national food consumption data to assess brand name loyalty, to target marketing practices, and to study the relationship of a particular food commodity, such as soup or iron-fortified cereals, to overall intake and nutritional status. Pharmaceutical companies have used NHANES data to estimate the proportion of the population taking a particular drug, to estimate treatment of various health conditions with drugs, and to conduct cost-benefit analysis of the use of cholesterol-lowering drugs and cardiovascular risk. National survey data on the population's use of dietary supplements have been used by trade associations to study the characteristics of users and the nutritional effects of supplements[40] and to develop growth charts to assess children's growth and weight status.[41] Consumers and practitioners also use national nutrition data to learn about diet and health[22]; the effects of supplements on diet, nutrition, and health[6,18-20,33,34,40,41]; and the effectiveness of weight loss practices.[42]

Nutrition monitoring data have also been used to identify food and nutrition research priorities of significance to public health[4-6,18-21] and to evaluate the impact of nutrition initiatives for military feeding systems.[43] Trends in energy and food and nutrient intake based on national dietary data have been used to understand the relationship between changes in dietary intake and the population's increase in overweight and health status.[14,21,44,45] State-level data have been used to plan health and nutrition education programs. For example, New York used Behavioral Risk Factor Surveillance System (BRFSS) data on the consumption of whole milk to plan a state campaign to encourage people to drink low-fat milk, and Arkansas used BRFSS data on physical activity and hypertension to design interventions and education programs to target African-American women.[4,46]

Nutrition Monitoring Measurement Components in the United States

The first national dietary surveys were carried out in the 1930s. Since then, more than 40 surveys and surveillance systems have evolved in response to the information needs of federal agencies and other nutrition monitoring data users. Chronological listings of past nutrition monitoring surveys and activities have been published.[3-5,14,47] Table 4 lists the major survey and surveillance activities, sponsoring agencies, dates conducted, and coverage of target populations since the mid-1990s, organized by the five measurement component areas. Brief descriptions of these activities are summarized below; more detailed information is available at the agency websites listed in the references.

Nutrition and Related Health Measurements

Nutrition and related health data have a wide variety of policy, research, health and nutrition education, medical care practices, and reference standards applications. The cornerstone of this NNMRRP measurement component, NHANES, provides national data on the nutritional status, dietary intake, and health of the US population.[2-9,18-21,47,48] It also provides national population reference distributions, national prevalence rates of diseases and risk factors, and trends in nutritional and health status over time. The survey includes a household interview followed by a physical examination and personal interviews in a mobile examination center. Physical measures such as body measurements, blood pressure, dental examinations, and biochemical and hematologic tests allow researchers to study the relationship between dietary, nutritional, and related health status. NHANES follow-up studies allow epidemiologic investigations of the relationships of nutrition and health to risk of death and disability. The current NHANES, which began in 1999, has a continuous, annual sample design.[6,18,19,47,48] The design includes oversampling of Mexican Americans, African Americans, older persons, adolescents, and pregnant women, and, beginning in 2000, targeted sampling of low-income whites to provide reliable estimates for these population groups and for comparisons of differ-

Table 4. Federal Nutrition Monitoring Surveys and Surveillance Activities

Date (initiated)	Dept.	Agency	Survey	Target U.S. Population	Sample Size	Response Rate(s)	Comments
Nutrition and Related Health Measurements							
Annual since 1999 (1971–74)	HHS	CDC/NCHS	National Health and Nutrition Examination Survey (NHANES)	Civilian, non-institutionalized individuals. Oversampling of blacks, Mexican Americans, adolescents, persons age 60 yr and older, and pregnant women	21,004 interviewed and 19,759 examined in 1999–2002; 10,122 interviewed and 9643 examined in 2003–04	76%	2003–04 examination response rate
Annual (1957)	HHS	CDC/NCHS	National Health Interview Survey (NHIS)	Civilian, non-institutionalized household population	94,460 individuals; 36,579 households	87% household 79% children 73% adults	2004 survey
Annual (1997)	HHS	CDC/NCHS	State and Local Area Integrated Telephone Survey (SLAITS)	National and state estimates of target populations	Varies		
Continuous (1979)	HHS	CDC/ NCCDPHP	Pregnancy Nutrition Surveillance System (PNSS)	Low-income, high-risk pregnant and postpartum women; primarily drawn from the WIC program	727,815 records	–	2002; coverage reflects # of women participating in programs in 22 states and 3 Indian tribal governments
Continuous (1973)	HHS	CDC/ NCCDPHP	Pediatric Nutrition Surveillance System (PedNSS)	Low-income, high-risk children, birth to 20 yr	>8 million records age 0–20 yr; >5 million records 0–5 yr	–	2003; coverage reflects the # of clinic visits in participating programs in 36 states and D.C., Puerto Rico, and 6 tribal governments
Annual (1965)	HHS	CDC/NCHS	National Health Care Survey (comprised of separate surveys of hospitals, ambulatory medical care providers, nursing homes, hospice agencies, and ambulatory surgery providers since 1992)	Record-based healthcare provider surveys including visits to hospitals and ambulatory surgical centers; office visits to nonfederal physicians; home health agencies; and nursing homes	500 hospitals and 270,000 patient records; 1500 nursing homes; 120,000 visits to 500 ambulatory facilities in a 3-yr period; 1800 home health and hospice agencies	Ranges from 70–97% across surveys	
Periodic 2002 (1973)	HHS	CDC/NCHS	National Survey of Family Growth	Men and women, 15–44 yr	12,571 men and women	79%	2002 survey
Continuous (1915)	HHS	CDC/NCHS	National Vital Registration System	Total US population; complete coverage	All births and deaths in the US	–	

(*continues*)

Table 4. Continued

Date (initiated)	Dept.	Agency	Survey	Target U.S. Population	Sample Size	Response Rate(s)	Comments
1988–94 (1971–74)	HHS	CDC/NCHS	Third National Health and Nutrition Examination Survey (NHANES III)	U.S. non-institutionalized, civilian population, 2+ mo; oversampling of blacks and Mexican Americans, children 0–5 yr, and individuals 60+ yr	33,994 31,311	86% 79%	Interviewed Examined
Continuous (1992)	HHS	CDC/NCHS	NHANES III Mortality Follow-up Survey	Individuals interviewed and examined in NHANES III, 20+ yr at baseline (1988–94)	NA	–	
Food and Nutrient Consumption							
1999-annual (1971–74)	HHS	CDC/NCHS	National Health and Nutrition Examination Survey (NHANES)	Civilian, non-institutionalized individuals. Oversampling of blacks, Mexican Americans, adolescents, older persons, and pregnant women in the first 3 yrs	See listing above	74%	Dietary interview response rate in 2001–02
Periodic 2005 (1992)	USDA	FNS	School Nutrition Dietary Assessment Study III	School-aged children in grades 1–12 in 48 conterminous states and D.C.	Approx. 300 schools and 2500 students in 2005; 1576 schools in 2002	80% for schools and 88% for menu survey in 2002	2002 survey focused on meals offered and interviews of 1,075 cafeteria managers for the menu survey
Annual supplement (1995)	BLS;CB; USDA	FNS	Current Population Survey (CPS), Supplement on Food Security	Civilian, non-institutionalized US population age 16 yr and older	Approx. 55,500 households in CPS	85%	Response rate is for 2003 supplement
Annual (1980)	DOL	BLS	Consumer Expenditure Survey (expenditures on food purchases)	Civilian, non-institutionalized, population and a portion of the institutionalized population	7500 households/quarter 6000 individuals/year	85% 87%	Quarterly interview survey of consumer units Diary survey of consumer units kept for 2 consecutive 1-week periods
Continuous (1983)	DOC	CB	Survey of Income and Program Participation (SIPP)	Civilian, non-institutionalized population (households) of the US; age 15 yr and older	14,000–36,700 households (36,7000 in 2001 panel)	–	Continuous series of panels with duration of 2.5–4 years
Continuous (1917)	DOD	USARIEM	Nutritional Evaluation of Military Feeding Systems and Military Populations	Enlisted personnel of the Army, Navy, Marine Corps, and Air Force	20–240 individuals depending on study focus	90–99%	

Continuous laboratory monitoring, periodic surveys (1996)	HHS USDA	CDC; FDA; FSIS	FoodNet (surveillance of foodborne illnesses)	Surveys of physicians (1996–97 and 2000–01) and population (2002–03) in target areas (10 Emerging Infections Program sites)	5074 physicians in 1996–97 and 1347 in 2000–01; 8624 individuals in 1996–97	43% for physicians in 2000–01 71% for population	
1994–96, annual and 1998 (1985–86)	USDA	ARS	Continuing Survey of Food Intakes by Individuals (CSFII) and Supplemental Children's Survey	Individuals of all ages residing in households nationwide in 1994–96 and children 0–9 yr in 1998; oversampling of individuals in low-income households; individuals 2+ yr from CSFII 1994–96	15,303 in 1994–96 and 5000 in 1998	76%	1994–96 CSFII
Biennial 2004 (1992)	USDA	FNS	Study of WIC Participants and Program Characteristics	WIC participants using mail surveys of state and local WIC agencies, record abstractions at local WIC service sites	8,016,918 records in 2002	–	Near Census of WIC participants
1995	USDA	FNS	Early Childhood and Child Care Study	Child care sponsors, providers, and children participating in the CACFP	566 1962 1951 2174	74% 87% 82% 59%	Sponsors Providers Households Child-day observations
1988–94	HHS	CDC/NCHS	NHANES III and Supplemental Nutrition Survey (SNS) of Older Americans	See NHANES III listing above. Individuals ages 50+ yr examined in NHANES III with telephones in SNS	2261 (ages 50+ yr) in SNS	65% in SNS	Completed two additional 24-hr recalls by telephone in SNS
Knowledge, Attitudes, and Behavior Assessments							
Continuous (1984)	HHS	CDC/ NCCDPHP	Behavioral Risk Factor Surveillance System	Individuals 18+ yr residing in households with telephones in participating states, D.C., Puerto Rico, Virgin Islands, and Guam	2000–4000 per state	80%	

(*continues*)

Table 4. Continued

Date (initiated)	Dept.	Agency	Survey	Target U.S. Population	Sample Size	Response Rate(s)	Comments
Biennial (1991)	HHS	CDC/ NCCDPHP	Youth Risk Behavior Survey (YRBS) National survey of 32 states and 20 school districts in 2003 (38 states and 19 major cities in 2001); State and local surveys	Youths attending school in grades 9–12 and 12–21 yrs of age in households in 50 states, D.C., Puerto Rico, and Virgin Islands	15,240 in 2003 for national study; average 1800 per state in 2001	67% overall (81% school, 83% student)	2003 response rates
Periodic 2004 (1982)	HHS	FDA;NIH/ NHLBI	Health and Diet Survey	Civilian, non-institutionalized individuals in households w/telephones, 18+ yr, 50 states and D.C.	2743 in 2002; 1798 in 2004	41% 34%	2002 response rate 2004 response rate
Continuous (1987)	HHS	CDC/ NCCDPHP	Pregnancy Risk Assessment Monitoring System (PRAMS)	Women with a recent live birth (sample of birth certificates)	1300–3400 per state	70–85%	2001 response rate
Periodic 2004–05 (1993–94)	HHS	FDA	Infant Feeding Practices Survey II	Pregnant women and new mothers and healthy, full-term infants 0–1 yr	3500 pregnant women (expect 2250 to be surveyed in later infant ages)	NA	
Periodic 2001 (1988)	HHS	FDA	Food Safety Survey	Individuals in households w/ telephones, 18+ yr	4482 in 2001	61%	Food handling, food allergies, consumption of potentially unsafe foods
1994–96 (1989–91)	USDA	ARS	Diet and Health Knowledge Survey	Main meal-planner/ preparers in households participating in 1989–91 and 1994–96 CSFII	5765	74%	1994–96 survey
Food Composition and Nutrient Databases							
Continuous (1892)	USDA	ARS	National Nutrient Data Bank Food Composition Laboratory	–	1000 key foods; 3000 foods in the Primary Nutrient Data Set; 80 nutritional components; 65 nutrients in Standard Reference File	–	
Continuous (1977)	USDA	ARS	Food and Nutrient Data Base for Dietary Studies and Survey Nutrient Data Base for Trends Analysis; Pyramid Servings and Servings Data Base	Used for CSFII and NHANES and other dietary studies	–	–	

Annual (1982)	HHS	FDA	Total Diet Study	Representative diets of specific age-sex groups	280 foods	–	2003 market basket survey
Continuous (1999)	HHS USDA	NIH ARS	Dietary Supplement Ingredient and Labeling Data Base	Dietary supplements	–	–	
Periodic 1995–96 (1977)	HHS	FDA	Food Label and Package Survey	–	1250 food brands	–	
Food Supply Determinations							
Annual (1909)	USDA	ERS, ARS, CNPP	US Food and Nutrition Supply Series: Estimates of Food Available; Estimates of Nutrients	–	400 commodity foods	–	100 key foods, energy and 60 nutrient/components
Annual (1909)	DOC	NOAA/ NMFS	Fisheries of the United States	Civilian resident US population	–	–	
Continuous (1985)	USDA	ERS, CNPP	AC Nielsen SCANTRACK (scanned data in supermarkets) and Homescan Consumer Panel	Supermarkets in 52 major markets for SCANTRACK; households in 23 major markets for the consumer panel	4800 supermarkets; 61,500 households (15,000 for fresh foods)	85% for households in Homescan	

ARS, Agricultural Research Service; BLS, Bureau of Labor Statistics; CB, Census Bureau; CDC, Centers for Disease Control and Prevention; CNPP, Center for Nutrition Policy and Promotion; DOC, Department of Commerce; DOD, Department of Defense; DOL, Department of Labor; FDA, Food and Drug Administration; ERS, Economic Research Service; FNS, Food and Nutrition Service; FSIS, Food Safety Inspection Service; HHS, Department of Health and Human Services; NCCDPHP, National Center for Chronic Disease Prevention and Health Promotion; NCHS, National Center for Health Statistics; NIH, National Institutes of Health; NA, not applicable; NMFS, National Marine Fisheries Service; NOAA, National Oceanic and Atmospheric Administration; USARIEM, US Army Research Institute of Environmental Medicine; USDA, US Department of Agriculture.

– = Not applicable

ences in health conditions and the prevalence of risk factors between racial/ethnic groups.

The National Health Interview Survey provides information about self-reported health conditions annually and about special nutrition and health topics periodically, such as vitamin/mineral supplement usage, youth risk behavior, aging, food program participation, diet and nutrition knowledge, cancer, and disability and food preparation.[49] Other special supplements relate to tracking progress in meeting national health objectives. National Health Interview Survey data collected in 2004 included information on obesity based on self-reported height and weight, diagnosed diabetes, and alcohol consumption.[49] Large sample sizes enable data to be reported for the major racial/ethnic subgroups in the US population in addition to age group, gender, and income level.

The State and Local Area Integrated Telephone Survey was developed to supplement national data with state and regional data. This survey uses a telephone methodology and draws its sample from the same frame as the National Immunization Survey. Previous topics include a child well-being and welfare survey module that included questions on food security in 1997 and a national study on early childhood health.[50]

A number of surveillance systems, primarily conducted by the Centers for Disease Control & Prevention (CDC), also contribute nutrition-related health information (height, weight, hemoglobin, and hematocrit), particularly for low-income pregnant women, infants, and children who participate in publicly funded health, nutrition, and food assistance programs in participating states. The Pregnancy Nutrition Surveillance System monitors nutrition-related problems and behavioral risk factors associated with low birth weight in high-risk prenatal populations, primarily drawn from the WIC program.[51] The Pediatric Nutrition Surveillance System monitors key indicators of nutritional status in low-income infants and children.[51,52] Information on anemia, weight status, birth weight, breast-feeding, and TV/video watching are collected primarily from children in the WIC program.[51,52]

The National Center for Health Statistics conducts a number of other monitoring activities, including tracking deaths due to nutrition-related conditions and monitoring alternative health care settings' availability and utilization of dietary and nutritional services and hospitalizations resulting from nutrition-related diseases (see Table 4). The National Health Care Survey collects nutrition-related information on physician-reported hypertension and obesity, and counseling services for diet, weight reduction, and cholesterol reduction for hospital outpatient department visits.[53] The National Survey of Family Growth collects information on maternal and child health such as breast-feeding and prenatal care.[54] The surveys and surveillance systems that continuously collect nutrition and health measurements are important for monitoring trends over time, for tracking progress toward achieving national health objectives, and for generating reference distributions.

Food and Nutrient Consumption

Food and nutrient consumption measurements include estimates of individuals' intake of foods and beverages (nonalcoholic and alcoholic) and nutritional supplements, as well as levels of nonessential nutrients such as dietary fiber. The NHANES and the CSFII provide national estimates of food and nutrient intakes in the general US population and population subgroups.[6-8,12,13,18,44,47,55,56] Sampling strategies to oversample high-risk groups, such as pregnant women, low-income people, and particular racial/ethnic groups, are used to provide reliable estimates for these groups in addition to the total US population.

The CSFII emphasized the food and nutrient intake of the general population and subgroups of the population as it relates to various socioeconomic factors.[4-9,18-20,47,55,56] The CSFII was most recently conducted in 1994–96, with a supplemental sample in 1998 of children age birth through 8 years to assess pesticide exposures in the diets of infants and young children. CSFII 1994–96 collected 2 days of dietary recall per sample person using an in-person, interviewer-administered methodology.[47,55,56] The ARS developed a multiple-pass approach to collecting 24-hour dietary recalls that was pilot-tested and then integrated into the 2002 NHANES.[47,57]

In NHANES, dietary intake is related to health status in the same individuals, with emphasis on racial determinants of health. In NHANES III, interviewers collected 24-hour dietary recalls in the examination center; a subsample had a second recall to produce estimates of usual nutrient intake in the population.[18,47,58] Following a period of field testing, the second day's intake by telephone to assess response rates and the impact of the data collection mode on dietary intake estimates, NHANES and CSFII were fully integrated in 2002, and the CSFII is no longer conducted.[6,9,12,47,55] Instead, NCHS/CDC and ARS/USDA collaborate to collect 2 days of dietary intake per sample person in NHANES in an integrated dietary survey called *What We Eat in America.*[12,19,47,57,58] The first day's interview is conducted in person, the second day's by telephone.

These surveys, along with the Total Diet Study, provide the potential to assess levels of additives and pesticides in diets. For example, CSFII 1994–96 and 1998 data were used to assess the exposure of children to pesticides in the diet for EPA,[18] and NHANES III data were used to prepare methylmercury intake estimates for an EPA report to Congress assessing human exposure to mercury from fish and shellfish intake.[37] NHANES III data were also used to assess the usual nutrient intake of the lowincome population, school-age children, older adults, and participants in WIC and the Food Stamp program for USDA.[59] Dietary intake data on food program participants will be used as a baseline to monitor the characteristics and intake of these groups over time and to identify priorities for future research.

Evaluations of USDA's nutrition and food assistance programs are routinely conducted.[17-20,27] A number of studies have been conducted to evaluate the nutrition and health effects of participating in WIC and to provide current participant and program characteristics of the WIC program.[29,59] The School Nutrition Dietary Assessment study first assessed the diets of American schoolchildren and the contribution of the National School Lunch Program to overall nutrient intake in 1992. A second study was conducted in 1998 to compare changes in the food and nutrient content of USDA school meals and food service operations,[28] and a third study was conducted in 2005. The most recent study measured schoolchildren's heights and weights and usual nutrient intake and food intake and collected information on school food service operations, the quality of meals offered, and foods and beverages available in vending machines, school stores, and a la carte lines.

Periodic assessments of food and nutrient consumption of specific subgroups of the population not adequately covered in national surveys have been conducted for military populations, American Indians, children, low-income populations, and pregnant and lactating women. FDA's Infant Feeding Study II assesses the diets of pregnant women and new mothers and their infant feeding practices.[60] Since 1995, a special yearly supplement to the Current Population Survey conducted by the US Census Bureau has been devoted to measuring the extent of food insecurity and hunger among people living in low-income households.[11,60] The 18-item food security measure is under review by an expert panel of the Institute of Medicine.[60,61]

FoodNet is a cooperative surveillance effort between CDC's Emerging Infections Program, FDA, and the Food Safety and Inspection Service, USDA, to monitor foodborne illness and to conduct epidemiologic research on illnesses attributable to foodborne pathogens.[62] FoodNet includes laboratory analysis and surveys of physicians and the population. Twelve-month cycles of the population survey are conducted to assess diarrheal disease and exposure.

Knowledge, Attitudes, and Behavior Assessments

National and state surveys that measure knowledge, attitudes, and behavior about diet and nutrition and how these relate to health were added to the nutrition monitoring program in the early 1980s and have expanded in scope and number. Surveys have addressed specific topics such as infant feeding practices, weight loss practices, diet and health knowledge, food handling practices, and progress toward achieving nutrition-related national health objectives.

The focus of the BRFSS, initiated in 1984 as a telephone survey of adults, is on personal health practices such as dietary intake, physical activity, weight control practices, and health screening practices.[46] BRFSS data have been used by state health departments to plan, initiate, and guide health promotion and disease prevention programs and to monitor their progress over time.[46,63] BRFSS collects self-reported height and weight for estimates of overweight and includes optional modules on dietary habits that states can collect periodically. Topics include the consumption of fruits and vegetables and high-fat and cholesterol foods, binge drinking, physical activity, and the use of supplements, particularly folic acid. In 2002, BRFSS data began to be used for prevalence estimates for metropolitan and micropolitan statistical areas, allowing CDC to make estimates for counties to assist local public health planners and program evaluators.[63]

The Youth Risk Behavior Surveillance System (YRBSS) includes national school-based surveys of high school students, as well as state, territorial, and local school-based surveys conducted by health and education agencies.[63] Information is collected on students' health risk behaviors such as smoking, dietary intake, weight loss practices, and physical activity.[63,64] Every 2 years, CDC conducts a national survey to produce data representative of students in grades 9 to 12 in the 50 states and the District of Columbia.

In general, the focus of FDA's Health and Diet Survey is on people's awareness of the relationships between diet and risk for chronic disease and on health-related knowledge and attitudes.[65] The survey has studied consumer use of food labels, weight loss practices, and the effectiveness of the National Cholesterol Education Program. The Diet and Health Knowledge Survey, initiated by USDA in 1989 as a telephone follow-up to the CSFII, focused on the relationship of individuals' knowledge and attitudes about dietary guidance and food safety to their food choices and nutrient intakes. The Diet and Health Knowledge Survey was most recently conducted in 1994–96, and there are plans to collect similar information via a future NHANES module.[8,9,19,56] The FDA conducted a study to assess consumer food handling practices and awareness of microbiological hazards, and several studies to evaluate the Nutrition Facts Label features and usability by consumers.[66] The Food Safety Survey tracks consumers' knowledge, behaviors, and perceptions about food safety and consumption of potentially risky foods.[66]

CDC's Pregnancy Risk Assessment Monitoring System is used by 29 states to monitor selected maternal attitudes, behaviors, and experiences related to adverse maternal and infant outcomes.[67] FDA plans to conduct a second Infant Feeding Practices Survey to assess the diets of pregnant and new mothers and to track breastfeeding and other infant feeding practices.[68]

Food Composition and Nutrient Data Bases

Since 1892, USDA has operated the National Nutrient Data Bank to derive representative nutrient values for more than 6000 foods and up to 80 components consumed in the United States. Data are obtained from the food industry, from USDA-initiated analytical contracts, and from the scientific literature, and are updated to reflect changes in the food supply as well as changes in analytical methodology.[69-71] These values are used as the core of most nutrient databases developed in the United States for special purposes, such as those used in the commercially available dietary analysis programs. USDA produces the Food and Nutrient Database for Dietary Studies, which contains data for energy and 60 nutrients/components for each food item for analysis of CSFII and NHANES. A system is in place at USDA to periodically update this database with the most current information available from the National Nutrient Data Bank and to retroactively apply revised or new food composition data to earlier food composition databases for tracking nutrient consumption patterns.[70] USDA also releases special-interest databases (e.g., fluoride, choline).[69]

The National Institutes of Health Office of Dietary Supplements, USDA, and NCHS collaborate to support the development and maintenance of a dietary supplements food composition database.[71] FDA's Total Diet Study provides annual food composition analysis based on the foods consumed most frequently in the CSFII and NHANES. Representative foods are collected from retail markets, prepared for consumption, and analyzed individually for nutrients and other food components at the Total Diet Laboratory to estimate consumption of selected nutrients (e.g., folate) and organic and elemental contaminants such as pesticide residues.[72] The Food Label and Package Survey, sponsored by a number of agencies, was conducted to monitor labeling practices of US food manufacturers.[73,74] The survey also includes a surveillance program to identify levels of accuracy of selected nutrient declarations compared with values obtained from nutrient analyses of products.

Food Supply Determinations

Since the beginning of this century, US food supply estimates have indicated levels of foods and nutrients available for consumption over time, and per capita consumption for about 400 foods based on food disappearance.[75] These data, updated and published by USDA, are used to: 1) assess the potential of the US food supply to meet the nutritional needs of the population; 2) evaluate the effects of technological alterations and marketing changes on the food supply; 3) indicate the relationships between food and nutrient availability and nutrient-disease associations; and 4) facilitate management of federal marketing, food assistance, nutrition education, and food enrichment and fortification policy. Food supply data indicate trends in food available for consumption rather than absolute food consumption estimates. Use of food disappearance data leads to overestimates of consumption because food wastage and food fed to pets are included in the estimates.

Since 1909, the National Marine Fisheries Service has provided annual estimates of per capita consumption of fish and shellfish based on "disappearance" in the food distribution system.[76] Since 1985, monthly and annual proprietary sales data purchased from A.C. Nielsen Company have been used to measure grocery store sales of all scannable packaged food products.[8,13] Supermarket scanner data (SCANTRACK) do not reflect fruits and vegetables or prepared foods from the supermarket, restaurants, or other food outlets. Households participating in the Homescan Consumer Panel transmit data on scanned purchases, including fresh foods, weekly through a telephone line.

Data Set Availability

A great deal of data generated by the NNMRRP are available in published government and peer-reviewed reports.[4,9,14] Progress has been made in using electronic bulletin boards to announce or distribute survey data, survey reports, and nutrition monitoring publications and to distribute data in various electronic forms, such as diskettes and CD-ROMs. In addition, many agencies are making data sets accessible through the Internet, along with documentation on sampling methods, survey design, sample sizes, and survey instruments and questionnaires. Consult the survey websites for agency-specific information on ways to obtain data sets.

Online data tables can also be found at many websites. NCHS releases short reports and Health-E Stats and CDC publishes the *Morbidity and Mortality Weekly Report* (MMWR) online. ARS posts numerous dietary intake data tables on its survey website. The websites for the major surveys and surveillance systems have been included as references in this publication.

Nutrition Monitoring in Other Countries

Nutrition surveillance activities in developing and developed countries include the use of food balance sheets, household budget surveys, individual surveys of dietary intake, consumer expenditure surveys, and periodic assessments of the nutrition and health status of individuals in the population.[77-80] Food balance sheets are commonly used for surveillance in developing countries because they are more available and less costly than other surveillance methods. In developed countries, current monitoring often includes nutritional status measures, although these measures are typically more recent than those in the United States, which began in 1960. For example, the Luxembourg Nutrition Surveillance System focuses on long-term surveillance of dietary intake and household food expenditures based on household budget sheets; a nutritional status and socioeconomic component was added in the mid-1990s.[81] The New Zealand National Nutrition Survey includes a 24-hour dietary recall, anthropometric and blood pressure measurements, serum cholesterol, and iron status.[82] The United Kingdom has collected weighed food records for dietary intake estimates and blood and urine specimens, blood pressure, and anthropometric measures for the assessment of nutritional and health status. In 2001, the United Kingdom initiated the Expenditure and Food Survey to improve estimates of food eaten away from home and improved the method used for dietary exposure in the National Food Survey.[79] School nutrition policies have also been studied using methods similar to those used in the School Nutrition Dietary Assessment studies in the United States.[83]

In many European countries before 2000, health reporting systems had little or no reference to nutrition indicators, even if they had a nutrition surveillance system.[80] In Germany, a system of continuous health reporting dates back to the early 1970s, but nutrition is generally underrepresented in the system.[84] Several states or republics have reported nutrition and health statistics, but there is no national nutrition system in Germany, and nutrition data were not collected continuously or well planned to meet health data needs. To address this issue, the European Union (EU) defined health indicators to share data among EU countries, and analyze and report public health nutrition data. The 2003 report defines nutrition indicators and measurements to standardize data collection of nutrition information on seven topics: breast-feeding, food and nutrient intake, nutrient status, anthropometry, physical activity and fitness, sociodemographic variables, and alcohol intake.[78] This will facilitate the collection and reporting of nutrition data for future nutrition monitoring in the EU.

Comparisons of data across countries have been facilitated by standardizing definitions of nutrition indicators and outcomes. Examples of worldwide monitoring of nutrition outcomes include the World Health Organization (WHO) body mass index database,[85] and the Food and Agriculture Organization of the United Nations' assessment of food insecurity as a follow-up activity to the World Food Summit in 1996.[86]

Nutrition topics of international concern include micronutrient deficiencies (most notably iodine, vitamin A, folic acid, and iron), child growth and malnutrition, breast-feeding, and obesity and chronic disease prevention. The WHO provides technical and financial support to member states for developing, strengthening, and implementing their national nutrition plans of action.[78] Federal agencies in the United States also provide technical consultation on nutrition survey data collection methodologies and interpretation of data to assist other countries' nutrition monitoring and surveillance efforts. For example, CDC provides support for preventing micronutrient deficiencies worldwide[87] and ARS/USDA has shared the dietary intake data collection method with Canada for use in the Community Health Survey.[57]

Nutrition Monitoring Research to Meet Future Challenges

A focused, comprehensive nutrition monitoring program includes improving methodologies for the collection and interpretation of data, timely processing and release of data, expanding coverage of population subgroups, and conducting research to address current nutrition and public health issues. In the early 1990s, the US President's Science Advisor identified the need for human nutrition research "that is ultimately aimed at promoting health, preventing disease, and reducing health care costs."[10] To meet the expanding needs of the monitoring program, current nutrition monitoring research is aimed at: 1) improving data collection, including population coverage and the use of technology; 2) assessing dietary intake, including usual food and nutrient intake; 3) assessing nutritional status using anthropometric, dietary, and laboratory approaches and biomarkers of diet and nutritional status; 4) understanding the behavioral and economic aspects of diet and health; and 5) conducting food composition analysis.

Improving Data Collection

Continuous collection of data in cross-sectional and longitudinal surveys and surveillance systems within NNMRRP is needed to evaluate and monitor the contribution that diet and nutritional status make to the health of the US population, to plan national strategies for encouraging and assisting people to adopt healthy eating patterns, and to avoid duplication of efforts while meeting nutrition monitoring needs. Progress has been made in integrating and merging NHANES and CSFII into one national dietary data collection effort.[47,48,55] Reducing duplication of effort and merging resources to collect improved dietary intake data should produce more timely releases of dietary data; however, the integrated dietary survey cannot meet all of the data needs that both NHANES and CSFII met in the past. Priorities for data will need to be set, with consideration of rotating topical modules every 4 or 6 years for longer-term monitoring, or conducting special targeted surveys to meet short-term data needs or the needs of particular groups not covered in adequate sample sizes in the national surveys (e.g., Native Americans).[8,9] An annual sample design in NHANES allows for continual monitoring and the ability to rotate or add new content to produce policy-relevant nutrition data.

Population Subgroup Coverage. Many surveys of NNMRRP are designed to collect data on various subgroups of the population, such as low-income persons and minorities; however, data are still limited for select subgroups of the population, such as the homeless and Native Americans. Special subnational studies are the most economical way to cover these and other minority groups, such as Asians and Pacific Islanders. Research is also needed on appropriate methods (e.g., questionnaires, interviewing procedures, physical measures, and biologic indicators) for subgroups at increased nutritional risk.

State and Local Monitoring. In addition to expanded coverage of population subgroups, improved geographic coverage is needed to provide nutrition data at the state and local levels.[4,7,46,51,52] National surveys provide data representative of the United States and major geographic regions, but cannot also provide data representative of states, counties, and cities. The CDC surveillance systems provide data for participating states that are complementary to national data, but there is increasing interest in collecting state and local data to address local health and welfare concerns.[46,51,52] Continued improvements to the state surveillance systems, the use of comparable methodologies, and supplemental data collection for defined population groups will be central to meeting this data need in the future.

National surveys often serve as the standard for methods to measure sociodemographic characteristics, dietary behavior, and nutritional status.[15,16,21] The NCHS has an initiative to study smaller, defined population groups using mobile examination vans.[48] In 2004, the New York City Department of Health and Mental Hygiene conducted the New York City HANES with technical assistance from NCHS.[88] National methods were adapted for use in a smaller-scale examination. About 2000 New Yorkers were sampled to receive a health examination to estimate the prevalence of overweight, diabetes, high blood pressure, high serum cholesterol, and exposure to tobacco, pesticides, and heavy metals, and an interview to assess depression and risky behaviors.[88]

Use of Technology. Researchers have been investigating the use of alternative data collection methods to augment in-person and telephone interviews. State and local monitoring systems should also take advantage of new technology for electronic data transfer. BRFSS is exploring the possibility of using Web-based data collection in future surveys.[46] This would take advantage of technology and access to the Internet, but accommodations will still be needed to assess at-risk groups with no telephone or Internet access. Surveys such as NHANES have incorporated the use of self-administered computerized instruments for sensitive topics and adolescents.[48] Research efforts should focus on the identification and development of methods and the utilization of computer technology that will enhance the monitoring of the nutritional status of the US population and support the timely interpretation and release of information to users.

Assessment of Dietary Intake

The release of the Dietary Reference Intakes and information on the appropriate data collection and statistical methods to use to estimate usual intake have led to improved information on energy and nutrient intake based on national survey data. To better estimate total nutrient intake, the methods used to collect dietary supplement usage have been assessed.[20,47] It is recommended that information on dietary supplement use be collected on the same day as the 24-hour dietary recall to estimate usual total nutrient intake. Another area of research is alternative statistical methods of estimating daily nutrient intake from supplements based on frequency-type questions.

Beginning in 2002, the NHANES included 2 days of intake per examined person for the estimation of usual nutrient intake and a food propensity questionnaire for the estimation of usual food intake.[20,47,58] The food propensity questionnaire was developed by the National Cancer Institute to use to assess infrequently consumed foods to augment the two dietary recalls.[20,89]

Short Dietary Methods. Research continues to develop short dietary surveillance instruments that can be used to assess the intake of food components such as fruits and vegetables. The National Cancer Institute compared the diet history questionnaire and two food frequency questionnaires among a representative sample of 1640 adult men and women and assessed "short screeners" to measure fruit and vegetable intake over the day and by meal.[90] A sample of 462 men and women completed a 24-hour recall by telephone, one per season over 1 year, a food frequency questionnaire 1 to 2 months later, and a screener 7 months later.[90] The short screeners were found to be valuable for estimating the median intake of fruits and vegetables, but not for ranking individuals' intakes.[90]

Assessment of Nutritional Status

A minimum set of indicators to measure nutritional status has been outlined in a Life Sciences Research Office report.[91] Progress has been made in delineating nutrition indicators, which include height and weight to assess growth and overweight, household food security, improved methodologies for nutritional status such as folate status, and the development of standardized dietary indicators and analytic techniques. Reliable, valid, and cost-effective measures of nutritional status need to be developed and improved, along with appropriate interpretive criteria, practical and efficient measures of diet and biochemical and clinical parameters, and applied statistical methodologies for the collection and interpretation of NNMRRP data.

Biomarkers. The development and use of biomarkers in surveys such as NHANES that collect biologic samples (i.e., blood, urine, saliva, and hair) is an important research area for nutrition monitoring. Biomarkers are substances within individuals or tissue samples that can be related to exposure, susceptibility to disease, or health outcomes.[92,93] The field of nutritional epidemiology has provided pertinent research on biomarkers of dietary intake and nutritional status.[94,95] Biochemical measures of long-term exposure or nutritional status are not subject to the same inaccuracies or bias as the reporting of long-term dietary intake, but the sensitivity and specificity of biomarkers need to be evaluated for their role in assessing exposure to foods and nutrients and for identifying high-risk population groups.[95]

Biomarkers are also of interest to validate instruments that can be used to assess diet in studies where biologic measures can not easily be obtained, because it is not always possible or practical to collect biologic materials. For some dietary factors, such as total fat intake, no biomarkers are available. For other dietary factors, such as particular fatty acids, there are a few specific biomarkers in serum or adipose tissue.[92,93,96] Research suggests that plasma and adipose tissue biomarkers of nutrients (e.g., carotenoids and tocopherols) are not interchangeable in epidemiologic or dietary validation studies.[97]

Doubly labeled water studies have been used to validate energy intakes assessed with 24-hour recall and other dietary methods, such as food frequency instruments.[98] In general, the 24-hour recall method, which is extensively used to assess diet in national nutrition surveys, has a systematic bias to underestimate total energy intake.[98,99] Doubly labeled water techniques provide a noninvasive method of assessing energy expenditures that allows for interpreting energy intakes derived from dietary survey methods. The National Cancer Institute's Observing Protein and Energy Nutrition study assessed measurement error using two self-reported dietary methods (a 24-hour recall and a food frequency questionnaire) and two unbiased methods: doubly labeled water and urinary nitrogen.[100] The Observing Protein and Energy Nutrition study found that men and women underreported energy and protein on both instruments.[100] About 9% of men and 7% of women underreported energy intake based on the 24-hour recall compared with 35% and 23%, respectively, based on the food frequency questionnaire.[100] Protein intake was underreported by 11% to 12% by the 24-hour recall and 30% to 34% by the food frequency questionnaire.[99] Underreporting of energy and protein was even higher than that for total energy expenditure.[100]

Improved analytic techniques to control for measurement error (e.g., energy adjustments) and for understanding nutrient-nutrient and food-nutrient interactions will facilitate the interpretation of national dietary data. Biomarkers are also useful in studying immune responses and diet-health relationships.[92-95] Further research to develop better biologic indicators of nutritional status and dietary intake as a means of studying nutrition and health is needed to maximize the usefulness of NNMRRP data for nutrition policy making.[95]

Behavioral and Economic Aspects of Diet and Health

Research to develop and standardize questionnaires for valid and reliable estimators of knowledge, attitudes, and behavior will aid in the development of public health strategies at the federal, state, and local levels to improve dietary status, promote health, and prevent nutrition-related disease. Adding questions on dietary or health behaviors to surveys designed to link socioeconomic factors can augment information on diet and health relationships. For example, the American Time Use Survey draws its sample from the Current Population Survey; respondents complete a time diary and report their height and weight. A Food and Eating Module is being planned for the future, in collaboration with USDA. It would include snacking, TV watching, and food preparation behaviors.[101]

Linking data from various sources is a mechanism to increase food safety research and monitoring. For example, FoodNet surveillance data could be used in conjunction with national survey data on food consumption and food safety practices (i.e., food preparation, handling, and storage) to monitor food safety issues in the United States.[9,62,66]

Physical Activity Behavior. The National Cancer Institute has supported the use of a wearable physical activity monitor for use in NHANES beginning in 2003.[89] These monitors will improve the collection of physical activity behavior, which has relied in the past on self-report or parental reports for children. The School Nutrition Dietary Assessment III measurements of the heights and weights among schoolchildren in 2004–05 will provide information on overweight, dietary intake, and school policies such as sales of competitive foods and beverages.

Food Security Measurement. The 18-item food security scale developed in the 1990s under the Ten-Year Plan, and included in several national studies (e.g., NHANES, the Current Population Survey, the Survey of Income and Program Participation, and the Early Childhood Longitudinal Study) is under review by an expert panel of the Institute of Medicine.[10,102] A short form (six items derived from the 18 items) was also developed to meet state and local needs to assess food insecurity.[103] Any recommendations to change the food security measurement, or its short form, will affect future monitoring and interpretation of trends.

Food Composition

Food composition values need to be continually evaluated and periodically updated as analytic methods are improved, as foods change over time, and as new products are marketed. Even though the National Nutrient Data Bank contains thousands of individual food composition values, gaps and deficiencies still exist for some foods, food components, and specific nutrients. This will continue for the foreseeable future because of the cost and the lack of reliable measurement systems for certain food components. The National Food and Nutrient Analysis Program aims to achieve long-sought improvements in the National Nutrient Data Bank through a comprehensive review of the scientific and technical approach to updating and maintaining the database used by the NNMRRP and other users of food composition data.[40]

The national program, directed by ARS/USDA, comprises four activities: 1) evaluate existing data for scientific quality; 2) identify key foods and nutrients for sampling and analysis plans; 3) devise and implement a nationally based sampling plan for foods; and 4) analyze sampled foods under USDA-supervised laboratory contracts.[69,70] Several federal agencies are supporting these efforts to update and improve the scientific quality and representativeness of the food composition data used in the NNMRRP. NCHS and the National Institutes of Health have developed a database on dietary supplements for use with national survey data to estimate the total intake of nutrients from foods and supplements and to assess the impact of nutritional supplements on nutritional status and health.

Public Health Implications

The primary goal of the Ten-Year Comprehensive Plan put forth in the early 1990s—to establish a comprehensive nutrition monitoring and related research program by collecting quality data that are continuous, coordinated, timely, and reliable; using comparable methods for data collection and reporting of results; conducting relevant research; and efficiently and effectively disseminating and exchanging information with data users—is still pertinent.[3,4] Given competing demands for limited national resources and resulting budget limitations, the goals for the NNMRRP will continue to be evaluated against other competing national needs at specific points in time. Efforts and resources are critical to continue progress and research to expand and strengthen the nutrition monitoring program in the United States in an efficient manner.

Nutrition monitoring data are needed to track progress in meeting the prevention agenda for the nation.[21] The nutrition monitoring program must be positioned to answer the major research and policy questions that are relevant in the 21st century: the relationship of diet and health habits (including physical activity) to the increasing prevalence of overweight and obesity; the chronic disease burden and disparities of health across racial/ethnic and socioeconomic groups; food security in an era of welfare reform; consumer behavior; nutrient-gene interactions; and biomarkers of nutrition and health status. The ability to meet the policy needs of the future will depend on research and the availability of reliable, current national nutrition data.

References

1. Mason JB, Habicht J-P, Tabatabai H, Valverde V. *Nutritional Surveillance*. Geneva: WHO, 1984.
2. U.S. Congress. Pub. L. 101–445. National Nutrition Monitoring and Related Research Act of 1990. Washington, DC: 101st Congress, Oct. 22, 1990.
3. U.S. Department of Health and Human Services and U.S. Department of Agriculture. Ten-year comprehensive plan for the national nutrition monitoring and related research program. Federal Register. 58:32752–32806, June 11, 1993.
4. Briefel RR, Bialostosky K. Interpretation and utilization of data from the National Nutrition Monitoring and Related Research Program. Chapter 13 in *Research: Successful Approaches*, 2nd ed. Monsen ER, ed. Chicago: American Dietetic Association, 2003:185–208.
5. Bialostosky K, Briefel RR, Pennington J. Nutrition monitoring in the United States. Chapter 15 in *Handbook of Nutrition and Food*, Berdanier CD, ed. Washington DC: CRC Press, 2001:407–433.
6. Dwyer J, Picciano MF, Raiten DJ. Future directions for the integrated CSFII-NHANES: What we eat in America-NHANES. J Nutr. 2003;133: 576S–581S.
7. Woteki CE, Briefel RR, Klein CJ, et al. Nutrition monitoring: Summary of a statement from an American Society for Nutritional Sciences Working Group." J Nutr. 2002;132:3782–3783. (Data supplement available at http://www.nutrition.org/cgi/data/132/12/3782/DC1/1)
8. National Research Council. Committee on National Statistics. *Summary of Workshop on Food and Nutrition Data Needs.* Casey J, Scholz JK, eds. Washington DC: National Academies Press, 2004.
9. National Research Council. Panel on Enhancing the Data Infrastructure in Support of Food and Nutrition Programs, Research, and Decision Making. *Improving Data to Analyze Food and Nutrition Policies.* Washington DC: National Academies Press, 2005.
10. Office of Science and Technology Policy, Executive Office of the President. *Meeting the Challenge. A Research Agenda for America's Health, Safety, and Food.* Washington DC: Government Printing Office, February 1996.
11. Hamilton WL, Cook JT, Thompson WW, et al. *Household Food Security in the United States in 1995: Summary Report of the Food Security Measurement Project.* Alexandria, VA: U.S. Department of Agriculture, Food and Consumer Service, 1997.
12. National Center for Health Statistics. *DHHS-USDA Dietary Survey Integration—What We Eat in America.* Hyattsville, MD: National Center for Health Statistics; 2005.
13. Interagency Board for Nutrition Monitoring and Related Research. *The Directory of Federal and State Nutrition Monitoring and Related Research Activities.* Bialostosky K, ed. Hyattsville, MD: National Center for Health Statistics, 2000. DHHS Publ. No. 00-1255.
14. Life Sciences Research Office, Federation of American Societies for Experimental Biology. *Third Report on Nutrition Monitoring in the United States: Volumes 1 and 2.* Prepared for the Interagency Board for Nutrition Monitoring and Related Research. Washington DC: U.S. Government Printing Office, 1995.

15. Survey Comparability Working Group. *Improving Comparability in the National Nutrition Monitoring and Related Research Program: Population Descriptors.* Hyattsville, MD: National Center for Health Statistics, 1992.
16. Consensus Workshop on Dietary Assessment. *Nutrition Monitoring and Tracking the Year 2000 Objectives.* Wright J, Ervin B, Briefel R, eds. Hyattsville, MD: National Center for Health Statistics, December, 1994.
17. Logan C, Fox MK, Lin BH. *Effects of Food Assistance and Nutrition Programs on Nutrition and Health, Volume 2.* Food Assistance and Nutrition Research Report Number 19–2. Washington DC: U.S. Department of Agriculture, 2002.
18. Woteki CE. Integrated NHANES: uses in national policy. J Nutr. 2003;133:582S–584S.
19. Murphy SP. Collection and analysis of intake data from the integrated survey. J Nutr. 2003;133: 585S–589S.
20. Dwyer J, Picciano MF, Raiten DJ, Members of the Steering Committee. Estimation of usual intakes: What We Eat in America-NHANES. J Nutr. 2003;133:609S–623S.
21. U.S. Department of Health and Human Services. *Healthy People 2010. Conference Edition in Two Volumes.* U.S. Department of Health and Human Services. Washington DC: U.S. Department of Health and Human Services, January 2000.
22. U.S. Department of Health and Human Services and U.S. Department of Agriculture. *Dietary Guidelines for Americans, 2005.* HHS Publ. No. HHS-ODPHP-2005-01-DGA-A. USDA Home and Garden Bulletin No. 232. Washington DC: U.S. Government Printing Office, 2005.
23. National Cancer Institute. *About the 5-A-Day Program.* Available at: http://www.5aday.gov/about/index/html.
24. Institute of Medicine. *Dietary Reference Intakes: Applications in Dietary Assessment.* Washington DC: National Academy Press, 2000.
25. National Cholesterol Education Program. *Third Report of the National Cholesterol Education Program (NCEP) Expert Panel on Detection, Evaluation, and Treatment of High Blood Cholesterol in Adults (Adult Treatment Panel III).* NIH Publication No. 02-5215. Bethesda, MD: National Heart, Lung, and Blood Institute, 2002.
26. National Heart, Lung, and Blood Institute. *Seventh Report of the Joint National Committee on Prevention, Detection, Evaluation, and Treatment of High Blood Pressure (JNC 7).* DHHS Publ. No. 04-5230. Washington DC: U.S. Department of Health and Human Services, 2004.
27. Fox MK, Hamilton W, Biing-Hwan L. *Effects of Food Assistance and Nutrition Programs on Nutrition and Health. Volume 4, Executive Summary of the Literature Review.* Food Assistance and Nutrition Research Report No. 19-4. Washington DC: Economic Research Service, USDA, 2004.
28. Fox MK, Crepinsek MK, Connor P, et al. *School Nutrition Dietary Assessment Study, II. Final Report.* Alexandria, VA: Food and Nutrition Service, 2001.
29. Kresge J. *WIC Participant and Program Characteristics 2002. Executive Summary.* Alexandria, VA: Food and Nutrition Service, 2003. Available at: http://www.fns.usda.gov/wic/resources/wicstudies.htm.
30. Carlson A, Kinsey J, Nadav C. Revision of USDA's low-cost, moderate-cost, and liberal food plans—Center Reports—United States Department of Agriculture. Family Economics and Nutrition Review. Spring 2003.
31. National Institutes of Health. Clinical guidelines on the identification, evaluation and treatment of overweight and obesity in adults—the evidence report. Obesity Research. 1998;6(suppl 2):51S–209S.
32. Lewis CJ, Crane NT, Wilson DB, et al. Estimated folate intakes: data updated to reflect food fortification, increased bioavailability, and dietary supplement use. Am J Clinical Nutr. 1999;70:198–207.
33. Commission on Dietary Supplements Labels. *Report of the Commission on Dietary Supplements Labels.* Washington DC: Office of Disease Prevention and Health Promotion, November 1997.
34. Heimbach JT. Using the National Nutrition Monitoring System to profile dietary supplement use. J Nutr. 2001;131:1335S–1338S.
35. U.S. Department of Health and Human Services, Food and Drug Administration. Notice of final rule: food labeling: health claims and label statements; dietary fiber and cardiovascular disease; dietary fiber and cancer. Federal Register. 2552–2605; 2537–2552, Jan. 5, 1993.
36. Life Sciences Research Office. *Estimation of Exposure to Substances in the Food Supply.* Anderson SA, ed. Prepared for the Food and Drug Administration. Bethesda, MD: Life Sciences Research Office, 1988.
37. U.S. Environmental Protection Agency. Office of Air Quality Planning & Standards and Office of Research and Development. *Mercury Study Report to Congress.* EPA-452/R-97-003. Washington DC: Environmental Protection Agency, December 1997.
38. Centers for Disease Control and Prevention. Folate status in women of childbearing age—United States, 1999. MMWR. Oct. 27, 2000;49(42): 962–965.
39. Centers for Disease Control and Prevention. *Second National Report on Human Exposure to Environmental Chemicals.* Atlanta, GA: National Center for En-

vironmental Health. NCEH Publ. No. 03-0022. 2003. Available at: http://www.cdc.gov/exposurereport/2nd/public_health_use.htm.
40. Dickinson A. *Optimal Nutrition for Good Health: The Benefits of Nutritional Supplements*. Washington DC: Council for Responsible Nutrition, 1998.
41. Kuczmarski RJ, Ogden CL, Grummer-Strawn LM, et al. *CDC Growth Charts: United States*. Advance data from vital and health statistics; no. 314. Hyattsville, MD: National Center for Health Statistics, 2000.
42. Levy AS, Heaton AW. Weight control practices of U.S. adults trying to lose weight. Ann Intern Med. 1993;119(7 pt 2):661–666.
43. Poos M, Costello R, Carlson-Newberry SJ. Institute of Medicine, Food and Nutrition Board. *Committee on Military Nutrition Research, Activity Report 1994–1999*. Washington DC: National Academy Press, 1999.
44. Briefel RR, Johnson CL. Secular trends in dietary intake in the United States. Ann Rev Nutr. 2004; 24:401–431.
45. Nielsen SJ, Siega-Riz AM, Popkin BM. Trends in energy intake in U.S. between 1977 and 1996 Similar shifts seen across age groups. Obesity Research. 2002;10:370–378.
46. Centers for Disease Control and Prevention. *Health risks in the United States: Behavioral Risk Factor Surveillance System*. At A Glance 2004. Available at: http://www.cdc.gov/nccdphp/aag_brfss.htm.
47. Dwyer J, Picciano MF, Raiten DJ, Members of the Steering Committee. Collection of food and dietary supplement intake data: What We Eat in America-NHANES. J Nutr. 2003;133:590S–600S.
48. National Center for Health Statistics. *National Health and Nutrition Examination Survey*. Available at: http://cdc.gov/nchs/nhanes/htm.
49. National Center for Health Statistics. *National Health Interview Survey*. Available at http://www.cdc.gov/nchs/nhis/htm.
50. National Center for Health Statistics. *State and Local Area Integrated Telephone Survey*. Available at: http://www.cdc.gov/nchs/slaits.htm.
51. Centers for Disease Control and Prevention. *Pediatric and Pregnancy Nutrition Surveillance System*. Available at: http://www.cdc.gov/pednss/.
52. Polhamus B, Dalenius K, Thompson D, et al. *Pediatric Nutrition Surveillance Report 2003*. Atlanta: Department of Health and Human Services, Centers for Disease Control and Prevention, 2004. Available at: http://www.cdc.gov/pednss/pdfs/PedNSS_2003_Summary.pdf.
53. National Center for Health Statistics. *National Health Care Survey*. Available at: http://www.cdc.gov/nchs/nchs.htm.
54. Abma JC, Martinez GM, Mosher WD, et al. *Teenagers in the United States: Sexual Activity, Contraceptive Use, and Childbearing, 2002*. Hyattsville, MD: National Center for Health Statistics. Vital Health Stat 23(24), 2004.
55. Agricultural Research Service, Food Surveys Research Group. *What We Eat in America*. Available at: http://www.barc.usda.gov/bhnrc/foodsurvey/home.html. Accessed April 18, 2005.
56. Tippett S, Enns CW, Moshfegh A. Food consumption surveys in the US Department of Agriculture. Nutr Today. 1999;34(1):33–46.
57. Raper N, Perloff B, Ingwersen L, et al. An overview of USDA's dietary intake data system. J Food Comp Analysis. 2004;17:545–555.
58. Carriquiry AL. Estimation of usual intake distributions of nutrients and foods. J Nutr. 2003;133: 601S–608S.
59. Fox MK, Cole N. *Nutrition and Health Characteristics of Low-Income Populations: Volume III, School-Age Children*. Washington, DC: Economic Research Service, 2004.
60. U.S. Department of Agriculture, Economic Research Service. *Briefing room. Food Security in the United States*. Available at: http://www.ers.usda.gov/Briefing/FoodSecurity/.
61. National Research Council, Committees on National Statistics. *Panel to Review U.S. Department of Agriculture's Measurement of Food Insecurity and Hunger*. Washington DC: National Academies Press, 2005.
62. Centers for Disease Control and Prevention. *FoodNet-Foodborne Disease Active Surveillance Network*. Available at: http://www.cdc.gov/foodnet/surveillance.htm.
63. Centers for Disease Control and Prevention. *Measuring Behaviors That Endanger Health: Behavioral Risk Factor Surveillance System*. Available at: http://www.cdc.gov/nccdphp/bb_brfss_yrbss/index.htm.
64. Centers for Disease Control and Prevention. Methodology of the Youth Risk Behavior Surveillance System. *MMWR*. Sept. 24, 2004;53(RR-12):1–13.
65. Food and Drug Administration. Consumer Research on Nutrition, Diet, and Health. *The FDA Health and Diet Survey: A Data Resource*. Available at: http://vm.cfsan.fda.gov/~lrd/ab-nutri.html.
66. Food and Drug Administration. *Consumer Research on Foodborne Illness*. Consumer Research Studies. Available at: http://www.cfsan.fda.gov/~lrd/ab-foodb.html.
67. Centers for Disease Control and Prevention. *Pregnancy Risk Assessment Monitoring System*. Available at: http://www.cdc.gov/reproductivehealth/PRAMS/index.html.
68. Food and Drug Administration. Submission for Office of Management and Budget Review. Infant Feeding Practices Study II. Federal Register. 2004; 69(190):58915–58928.
69. Agricultural Research Service. ARS Human Nutrition National Program. *Composition of Foods*.

Available at: http://www.ars.usda.gov/research/programs.htm.

70. Anderson E, Perloff B, Ahuja JKC, et al. Tracking nutrient changes for trends analysis in the United States. J Food Comp Analysis. 2001;13:287–294.
71. Dwyer J, Picciano MF, Raiten DJ, Members of the Steering Committee. Food and dietary supplement databases for What We Eat in America-NHANES. J Nutr. 2003;133:624S–634S.
72. Food and Drug Administration. *Total Diet Study*. Available at: http://www.cfsan.fda.gov/~comm/tds-toc.html.
73. O'Brien T. Office of Food Labeling, Center for Food Safety and Applied Nutrition, Food and Drug Administration. *Status of Nutrition Labeling of Processed Foods: 1995 Food Label and Package Survey (FLAPS)*. Washington DC: Food and Drug Administration, 1996.
74. Brecher S. Office of Food Labeling, Center for Food Safety and Applied Nutrition, Food and Drug Administration. *Status of Serving Size in the Nutrition Labeling of Processed Foods: Food Label and Package Survey (FLAPS)*. Washington DC: Food and Drug Administration, 1997.
75. Center for Nutrition Policy and Promotion. *Nutrient Content of the U.S. Food Supply*. Available at: http://www.cnpp.usda.gov/ifs.html.
76. National Marine Fisheries Service. *Per Capita Consumption*. Available at: http://www.st.nmfs.gov/st1/fus03/08_perita2003.pdf.
77. Kohlmeier L, Helsing E, Kelly A, et al. Nutritional surveillance as the backbone of national nutrition policy: Recommendations of the IUNS Committee on nutritional surveillance and programme evaluation in developed countries. Eur J Clin Nutr. 1990; 44:771–781.
78. World Health Organization. Co-ordinating Centres in Sweden and United Kingdom. *Monitoring Public Health Nutrition in Europe; Nutritional indicators and determinants of health status. Final Technical Report*. Available at: http://europa.eu.int/comm/health/ph_projects/2000/monitoring/fp_monitoring_2000_frep_02_en.pdf.
79. Rimmer DJ. An overview of food eaten outside the home in the United Kingdom National Food Survey and the new Expenditure and Food Survey. Public Health Nutrition. 2001;4(5B):1173–1175.
80. Koehler BM, Dowler E, Feichtinger E, et al. Improving Europe's health: The role of nutrition in public health. In: *Public Health and Nutrition: The Challenge*. Koehler BM, Feichtinger E, Dowler E, Winkler G, eds. Berlin: Ed. Sigma, 1999:13–24.
81. Schmitt A. Food and nutrition policy in the Grand Duchy of Luxembourg. In: *Public Health and Nutrition: The Challenge*. Koehler BM, Feichtinger E, Dowler E, Winkler G, eds. Berlin: Ed. Sigma, 1999:107–115.
82. Parnell WR, Wilson NC, Russell DG. Methodology of the 1997 New Zealand National Nutrition Survey. NZ Med J. 2001;114(1128):123–126.
83. Nelson M, Bradbury J, Poulter J, et al. *School Meals in Secondary Schools in England*. London: King's College London, 2004. Research Report RR 557. Available at: http://www.food.gov.uk/multimedia/pdfs/secondaryschoolmeals.pdf.
84. Borgers D. Health reporting with special regard to nutrition in Germany. In: *Public Health and Nutrition: The Challenge*. Koehler BM, Feichtinger E, Dowler E, Winkler G, eds. Berlin: Ed. Sigma, 1999:87–98.
85. World Health Organization. Nutrition Data Banks. *Global Database on Body Mass Index (BMI)*. Available at: http://www.who.int/nut/db_bmi.htm.
86. Food and Agriculture Organization. *Monitoring Progress Towards the World Food Summit and Millennium Development Goals. The State of Food Security in the World, 2004*. Rome: Food and Agriculture Organization, 2004. Available at: http://www.fao.org//docrep/007/y5650e/y5650e00.htm.
87. Centers for Disease Control and Prevention. IMMPaCT. *International Micronutrient Malnutrition Prevention and Control Program: Projects and Tools: CDCynergy for Micronutrients*. Available at: http://www.cdc.gov/nccdphp/dnpa/impact/index.htm.
88. New York City Department of Health and Mental Hygeine. *New York City Health and Nutrition Examination Survey (NYC HANES)*. Available at: http://www.ci.nyc.ny.us/html/doh/html/hanes/hanes.html.
89. National Cancer Institute. *How is NCI Supporting the NHANES?* Available at: http://www.riskfactor.-cancer.gov/studies/nhanes/.
90. Thompson FE, Subar AF, Smith AF, et al. Fruit and vegetable assessment: performance of 2 new short instruments and a food frequency questionnaire. J Am Diet Assoc. 2002;102:1764–1772.
91. Life Sciences Research Office. Core indicators of nutritional state for difficult-to-sample populations. J Nutr. 1990;120(suppl):1554–1600.
92. Nelson M. Biomarkers in the study of diet and disease. Public Health Rev. 1998;26:11–12.
93. Bingham SA. Biomarkers in nutritional epidemiology. Public Health Nutr. 2002;5:821–827.
94. Byers T. The role of epidemiology in developing nutritional recommendations: past, present, and future. Am J Clin Nutr. 1999;69:1304S–1308S.
95. Byers T, Lyle B, Workshop Participants. Summary statement (for the Workshop: The Role of Epidemiology in Determining When Evidence Is Sufficient to Support Nutrition Recommendations). Am J Clin Nutr. 1999;69:1365S–1367S.
96. Arab L, Akbar J. Biomarkers and the measurement of fatty acids. Public Health Nutr. 2002;5:865–871.
97. Lih-Chyun J, Mai Bui S, Kardinaal A, et al. Differ-

ences between plasma and adipose tissue biomarkers of carotenoids and tocopherols. Cancer Epidemiol Biomarkers Prevention. 1998;7:1043–1048.

98. Schoeller DA. Recent advances from application of doubly labeled water to measurement of human energy expenditure. J Nutr. 1999;129:1765–1768.
99. Bingham SA. The dietary assessment of individuals: methods, accuracy, new techniques, and recommendations. Nutr Abst Rev. 1987;57:705–742.
100. Subar AF, Kipnis V, Troiano RP, et al. Using intake biomarkers to evaluate the extent of dietary misreporting in a large sample of adults: the OPEN study. Am J Epidemiol. 2003;158:1–13.
101. Bureau of Labor Statistics, U.S. Department of Labor. *American Time Use Survey*. Available at: http://www.bls.gov/tus/home.htm. Accessed May 14, 2005.
102. National Research Council. Panel to review U.S. Department of Agriculture's Measurement of Food Insecurity and Hunger. *Measuring Food Insecurity and Hunger*. Washington DC: National Academies Press, 2005.
103. Blumberg SJ, Bialostosky K, Hamilton WL, et al. The effectiveness of a short form of the household food security scale. Am J Public Health. 1999;89: 1231–1234.

63 Dietary Standards in the United States

Suzanne P. Murphy

Introduction

Many types of dietary standards may be used by health professionals in the United States and are also appropriate for use by consumers. Nutrient standards have traditionally been set by committees of the Food and Nutrition Board of the Institute of Medicine (IOM). The latest set of nutrient standards is the Dietary Reference Intakes (DRIs), developed jointly by the United States and Canada. Guidance on how to choose a healthy diet is incorporated into the Dietary Guidelines for Americans. These standards are revised every 5 years by the US Department of Agriculture (USDA) and the US Department of Health and Human Services. A food guidance system is available to help consumers translate the Dietary Guidelines into actual food choices. The most recent system is MyPyramid that consists of a logo and a website that individualizes the guidance. The Dietary Guidelines apply to individuals ages 2 and older, but there is no comparable process for setting dietary standards for infants and children under age 2. Recommendations for feeding infants and young children are made by professional organizations such as the American Academy of Pediatrics and the American Dietetics Association. Each of these types of dietary standards is discussed in more detail in the following sections.

Nutrient Standards for the United States: DRIs

Definitions

Recommended Dietary Allowances (RDAs) are nutrient standards that have been set by the Food and Nutrition Board since 1941. New RDAs were issued periodically through 1989. However, in 1994, the Food and Nutrition Board undertook a major revision of the nutrient standards, beginning with a report titled, "How Should the Recommended Dietary Allowances Be Revised?"[1] A process was then established and used to set new nutrient standards, called the DRIs.[2-7] The DRIs extended the traditional RDAs to include several types of nutrient standards, as follows:

Estimated Average Requirement (EAR). The usual intake level that is estimated to meet the requirement of half the healthy individuals in a life stage and gender group. At this level of intake, the other half of the healthy individuals in the specified group would not have their needs met.

Recommended Dietary Allowance (RDA). The usual intake level that is sufficient to meet the nutrient requirement of nearly all healthy individuals in a particular age and gender group (97.5% of the individuals in a group). If the distribution of requirements in the group is assumed to be normal, the RDA can be derived as the EAR plus two standard deviations of requirements.

Adequate Intake (AI). When information is not sufficient to determine an EAR (and thus an RDA), then an AI is set for the nutrient. The AI is a recommended average daily nutrient intake level based on experimentally derived intake levels or approximations of observed mean nutrient intakes by a group (or groups) of apparently healthy people who are maintaining a defined nutritional state or criterion of adequacy.

Tolerable Upper Intake Level (UL). Many nutrients have a UL, which is the highest level of usual nutrient intake that is likely to pose no risks of adverse health effects to individuals in the specified life stage group. As intake increases above the UL, the risk of adverse effects increases. The absence of a UL does not imply that the nutrient does not have a tolerable upper intake level, but, rather, that the available evidence at this time does not permit its estimation.

Estimated Energy Requirement (EER). An adult EER is defined as the dietary energy intake needed to maintain energy balance in a healthy adult of a given age, gender, weight, height, and level of physical activity. In children, the EER is defined as the sum of the dietary energy intake predicted to maintain energy balance for an individual's age, weight, height, and activity level (and gender for children ages 3 and older), plus an allowance for normal growth and development. For pregnant and lactating women, the EER includes energy needs for deposition of tissues or the secretion of milk. An EER is a type of EAR, in that it is the average requirement for healthy individuals. However, no RDA is set for energy intake, because an intake target above the mean requirement would encourage excessive energy intake, eventually resulting in undesirable body weight gain.

Acceptable Macronutrient Distribution Range (AMDR). For fat, protein, and carbohydrate, the AMDR specifies ranges of desirable intakes expressed as a percentage of energy intake.

DRIs are set for 22 life-stage categories of individuals. Two categories each for infants and children are based on age. Individuals ages 9 and older have 12 categories based on age and gender. Women who are pregnant or lactating have six additional categories (three age groups for each).

A nutrient will often have multiple DRIs. For example, many micronutrients have an EAR, an RDA, and a UL. Others have an AI and a UL.

Micronutrient DRIs

DRIs for vitamins, minerals, and electrolytes have been set in five reports published between 1997 and 2005.[2-5,7] Table 1 gives the recommended intake levels of vitamins for individuals, and Table 2 gives the corresponding levels for elements (minerals and electrolytes). The values in these tables are appropriate targets for intakes by individuals. For most nutrients, these are RDAs; because an RDA could not be determined for some nutrients, some of the values in the tables are AIs. Note that AIs are always used as nutrient standards for infants less than age 6 months and for all nutrients except iron and zinc for infants between ages 7 and 12 months. For infants, the nutrient standards generally reflect the average content of breast milk based on the assumption that this is the ideal intake for infants.

ULs for vitamins are shown in Table 3, and those for elements are provided in Table 4. Not all nutrients have a UL, usually because the data were not sufficient to set one. As noted in its earlier definition, the absence of a UL does not mean that the nutrient is safe at any level. Some elements have a UL but do not have an RDA or an AI (e.g., boron, nickel, and vanadium). For some micronutrients, ULs are not set for all of the life-stage categories, again, due to a lack of data, not a lack of possible risk from high intakes. Usual intakes of individuals should not exceed the ULs unless there is medical supervision.

Macronutrient DRIs

DRIs for macronutrients have been set in a report published in 2002.[6] RDAs are available for protein intake (for individuals over age 6 months) and for carbohydrate intake (for individuals over age 12 months). AIs are available for total water intake (including food, beverages, and drinking water), fiber, and linoleic and α-linolenic acids. RDAs and AIs for these macronutrients are given in Table 5.

Average energy needs may be determined using equations for EERs. Equations for all of the life-stage categories are given in the IOM report on macronutrients.[6] For example, the equations for men and women ages 19 and older are:

$$\text{EER (men)} = 662 - (9.53 \times \text{age}) + (\text{PA} \times [15.91 \times \text{weight in kg}] + 539.6 \times \text{height in m})$$

$$\text{EER (women)} = 354 - (6.91 \times \text{age}) + (\text{PA} \times [9.36 \times \text{weight in kg}] + 726 \times \text{height in m})$$

Where PA stands for physical activity level, which varies from 1.0 for sedentary adults to 1.48 for very active men and 1.45 for very active women. Sample EERs for men age 30, 1.6 m in height and 64 kg in weight (body mass index of slightly under 25), would range from 1993 kcal/d if sedentary to 2769 kcal/d if very active. Corresponding values for a woman of the same age, height, and weight would range from 1907 to 2699 kcal/d. Additional equations are available for individuals who are overweight or obese.

AMDRs are given for fat, n-6 and n-3 polyunsaturated fatty acids, carbohydrate, and protein (Table 6). The ranges differ for young children (ages 1–3), older children (ages 4–18), and adults.

Other recommendations for macronutrient intakes are also suggested by the IOM report.[6] Dietary cholesterol, trans fatty acids, and saturated fatty acids should all be as low as possible while consuming a nutritionally adequate diet. Added sugars should be limited to no more than 25% of total energy intake. The recommended maximum added sugar intake is based on the level at which nutrients in reported diets were found to decrease, presumably because nutrient-dense foods were displaced by energy from added sugars. However, as noted in a later section, this ceiling for sugar intake is well above the level that is likely to fit into a nutritionally adequate diet that does not exceed energy requirements.

Uses of DRIs

The DRIs are used for many purposes, but they fall into two broad categories: intake assessment and intake planning. A further subdivision of each category considers applications for individuals and applications for population groups. Each is briefly discussed later and in more detail in two reports from the Subcommittee on Interpretation and Uses of DRIs.[8,9] A new paradigm is used for many of the applications because the distribution of requirements is specified for most nutrients. The distribution is defined by the EAR, which is the mean of the distribution, and a standard deviation of the EAR. For all micronutrients except iron, the distribution of the requirements is assumed to be normal.

Table 1. Dietary Reference Intakes (DRIs): Recommended Intakes for Individuals, Vitamins

Life Stage Group	Vit A (µg/d)[a]	Vit C (mg/d)	Vit D (µg/d)[b,c]	Vit E (mg/d)[d]	Vit K (µg/d)	Thiamin (mg/d)	Riboflavin (mg/d)	Niacin (mg/d)[e]	Vit B_6 (mg/d)	Folate (µg/d)[f]	Vit B_{12} (µg/d)	Pantothenic Acid (mg/d)	Biotin (µg/d)	Choline[g] (mg/d)
Infants														
0–6 mo	400*	40*	5*	4*	2.0*	0.2*	0.3*	2*	0.1*	65*	0.4*	1.7*	5*	125*
7–12 mo	500*	50*	5*	5*	2.5*	0.3*	0.4*	4*	0.3*	80*	0.5*	1.8*	6*	150*
Children														
1–3 y	**300**	**15**	5*	**6**	30*	**0.5**	**0.5**	**6**	**0.5**	**150**	**0.9**	2*	8*	200*
4–8 y	**400**	**25**	5*	**7**	55*	**0.6**	**0.6**	**8**	**0.6**	**200**	**1.2**	3*	12*	250*
Males														
9–13 y	**600**	**45**	5*	**11**	60*	**0.9**	**0.9**	**12**	**1.0**	**300**	**1.8**	4*	20*	375*
14–18 y	**900**	**75**	5*	**15**	75*	**1.2**	**1.3**	**16**	**1.3**	**400**	**2.4**	5*	25*	550*
19–30 y	**900**	**90**	5*	**15**	120*	**1.2**	**1.3**	**16**	**1.3**	**400**	**2.4**	5*	30*	550*
31–50 y	**900**	**90**	5*	**15**	120*	**1.2**	**1.3**	**16**	**1.3**	**400**	**2.4**	5*	30*	550*
51–70 y	**900**	**90**	10*	**15**	120*	**1.2**	**1.3**	**16**	**1.7**	**400**	**2.4**[i]	5*	30*	550*
> 70 y	**900**	**90**	15*	**15**	120*	**1.2**	**1.3**	**16**	**1.7**	**400**	**2.4**[i]	5*	30*	550*
Females														
9–13 y	**600**	**45**	5*	**11**	60*	**0.9**	**0.9**	**12**	**1.0**	**300**	**1.8**	4*	20*	375*
14–18 y	**700**	**65**	5*	**15**	75*	**1.0**	**1.0**	**14**	**1.2**	**400**[i]	**2.4**	5*	25*	400*
19–30 y	**700**	**75**	5*	**15**	90*	**1.1**	**1.1**	**14**	**1.3**	**400**[i]	**2.4**	5*	30*	425*
31–50 y	**700**	**75**	5*	**15**	90*	**1.1**	**1.1**	**14**	**1.3**	**400**[i]	**2.4**	5*	30*	425*
51–70 y	**700**	**75**	10*	**15**	90*	**1.1**	**1.1**	**14**	**1.5**	**400**	**2.4**[h]	5*	30*	425*
> 70 y	**700**	**75**	15*	**15**	90*	**1.1**	**1.1**	**14**	**1.5**	**400**	**2.4**[h]	5*	30*	425*
Pregnancy														
14–18 y	**750**	**80**	5*	**15**	75*	**1.4**	**1.4**	**18**	**1.9**	**600**[j]	**2.6**	6*	30*	450*
19–30 y	**770**	**85**	5*	**15**	90*	**1.4**	**1.4**	**18**	**1.9**	**600**[j]	**2.6**	6*	30*	450*
31–50 y	**770**	**85**	5*	**15**	90*	**1.4**	**1.4**	**18**	**1.9**	**600**[j]	**2.6**	6*	30*	450*
Lactation														
14–18 y	**1200**	**115**	5*	**19**	75*	**1.4**	**1.6**	**17**	**2.0**	**500**	**2.8**	7*	35*	550*
19–30 y	**1300**	**120**	5*	**19**	90*	**1.4**	**1.6**	**17**	**2.0**	**500**	**2.8**	7*	35*	550*
31–50 y	**1300**	**120**	5*	**19**	90*	**1.4**	**1.6**	**17**	**2.0**	**500**	**2.8**	7*	35*	550*

NOTE: This table (taken from the DRI reports, see www.nap.edu) presents Recommended Dietary Allowances (RDAs) in **bold type** and Adequate Intakes (AIs) in ordinary type followed by an asterisk (*). RDAs and AIs may both be used as goals for individual intake. RDAs are set to meet the needs of almost all (97 to 98 percent) individuals in a group. For healthy breastfed infants, the AI is the mean intake. The AI for other life stage and gender groups is believed to cover needs of all individuals in the group, but lack of data or uncertainty in the data prevent being able to specify with confidence the percentage of individuals covered by this intake.

[a]As retinol activity equivalents (RAEs). 1 RAE = 1 µg retinol, 12 µg β-carotene, 24 µg α-carotene, or 24 µg β-cryptoxanthin. The RAE for dietary provitamin A carotenoids is twofold greater than retinol equivalents (RE), whereas the RAE for preformed vitamin A is the same as RE.

[b]As cholecalciferol. 1 µg cholecalciferol = 40 IU vitamin D.

[c]In the absence of adequate exposure to sunlight.

[d]As α-tocopherol. α-Tocopherol includes *RRR*-α-tocopherol, the only form of α-tocopherol that occurs naturally in foods, and the *2R*-stereoisomeric forms of α-tocopherol (*RRR*-, *RSR*-, *RRS*-, and *RSS*-α-tocopherol) that occur in fortified foods and supplements. It does not include the *2S*-stereoisomeric forms of α-tocopherol (*SRR*-, *SSR*-, *SRS*-, and *SSS*-α-tocopherol), also found in fortified foods and supplements.

[e]As niacin equivalents (NE). 1 mg of niacin = 60 mg of tryptophan; 0–6 months = preformed niacin (not NE).

[f]As dietary folate equivalents (DFE). 1 DFE = 1 µg food folate = 0.6 µg of folic acid from fortified food or as a supplement consumed with food = 0.5 µg of a supplement taken on an empty stomach.

[g]Although AIs have been set for choline, there are few data to assess whether a dietary supply of choline is needed at all stages of the life cycle, and it may be that the choline requirement can be met by endogenous synthesis at some of these stages.

[h]Because 10 to 30 percent of older people may malabsorb food-bound B_{12}, it is advisable for those older than 50 years to meet their RDA mainly by consuming foods fortified with B_{12} or a supplement containing B_{12}.

[i]In view of evidence linking folate intake with neural tube defects in the fetus, it is recommended that all women capable of becoming pregnant consume 400 µg from supplements or fortified foods in addition to intake of food folate from a varied diet.

[j]It is assumed that women will continue consuming 400 µg from supplements or fortified food until their pregnancy is confirmed and they enter prenatal care, which ordinarily occurs after the end of the periconceptional period—the critical time for formation of the neural tube.

Table 2. Dietary Reference Intakes (DRIs): Recommended Intakes for Individuals, Elements

Life Stage Group	Calcium (mg/d)	Chromium (µg/d)	Copper (µg/d)	Fluoride (mg/d)	Iodine (µg/d)	Iron (mg/d)	Magnesium (mg/d)	Manganese (mg/d)	Molybdenum (µg/d)	Phosphorus (mg/d)	Selenium (µg/d)	Zinc (mg/d)	Potassium (g/d)	Sodium (g/d)	Chloride (g/d)
Infants															
0–6 mo	210*	0.2*	200*	0.01*	110*	0.27*	30*	0.003*	2*	100*	15*	2*	0.4*	0.12*	0.18*
7–12 mo	270*	5.5*	220*	0.5*	130*	**11**	75*	0.6*	3*	275*	20*	**3**	0.7*	0.37*	0.57*
Children															
1–3 y	500*	11*	**340**	0.7*	**90**	**7**	**80**	1.2*	**17**	**460**	**20**	**3**	3.0*	1.0*	1.5*
4–8 y	800*	15*	**440**	1*	**90**	**10**	**130**	1.5*	**22**	**500**	**30**	**5**	3.8*	1.2*	1.9*
Males															
9–13 y	1300*	25*	**700**	2*	**120**	**8**	**240**	1.9*	**34**	**1250**	**40**	**8**	4.5*	1.5*	2.3*
14–18 y	1300*	35*	**890**	3*	**150**	**11**	**410**	2.2*	**43**	**1250**	**55**	**11**	4.7*	1.5*	2.3*
19–30 y	1000*	35*	**900**	4*	**150**	**8**	**400**	2.3*	**45**	**700**	**55**	**11**	4.7*	1.5*	2.3*
31–50 y	1000*	35*	**900**	4*	**150**	**8**	**420**	2.3*	**45**	**700**	**55**	**11**	4.7*	1.5*	2.3*
51–70 y	1200*	30*	**900**	4*	**150**	**8**	**420**	2.3*	**45**	**700**	**55**	**11**	4.7*	1.3*	2.0*
> 70 y	1200*	30*	**900**	4*	**150**	**8**	**420**	2.3*	**45**	**700**	**55**	**11**	4.7*	1.2*	1.8*
Females															
9–13 y	1300*	21*	**700**	2*	**120**	**8**	**240**	1.6*	**34**	**1250**	**40**	**8**	4.5*	1.5*	2.3*
14–18 y	1300*	24*	**890**	3*	**150**	**15**	**360**	1.6*	**43**	**1250**	**55**	**9**	4.7*	1.5*	2.3*
19–30 y	1000*	25*	**900**	3*	**150**	**18**	**310**	1.8*	**45**	**700**	**55**	**8**	4.7*	1.5*	2.3*
31–50 y	1000*	25*	**900**	3*	**150**	**18**	**320**	1.8*	**45**	**700**	**55**	**8**	4.7*	1.5*	2.3*
51–70 y	1200*	20*	**900**	3*	**150**	**8**	**320**	1.8*	**45**	**700**	**55**	**8**	4.7*	1.3*	2.0*
> 70 y	1200*	20*	**900**	3*	**150**	**8**	**320**	1.8*	**45**	**700**	**55**	**8**	4.7*	1.2*	1.8*
Pregnancy															
14–18 y	1300*	29*	**1000**	3*	**220**	**27**	**400**	2.0*	**50**	**1250**	**60**	**12**	4.7*	1.5*	2.3*
19–30 y	1000*	30*	**1000**	3*	**220**	**27**	**350**	2.0*	**50**	**700**	**60**	**11**	4.7*	1.5*	2.3*
31–50 y	1000*	30*	**1000**	3*	**220**	**27**	**360**	2.0*	**50**	**700**	**60**	**11**	4.7*	1.5*	2.3*
Lactation															
14–18 y	1300*	44*	**1300**	3*	**290**	**10**	**360**	2.6*	**50**	**1250**	**70**	**13**	5.1*	1.5*	2.3*
19–30 y	1000*	45*	**1300**	3*	**290**	**9**	**310**	2.6*	**50**	**700**	**70**	**12**	5.1*	1.5*	2.3*
31–50 y	1000*	45*	**1300**	3*	**290**	**9**	**320**	2.6*	**50**	**700**	**70**	**12**	5.1*	1.5*	2.3*

NOTE: This table presents Recommended Dietary Allowances (RDAs) in **bold type** and Adequate Intakes (AIs) in ordinary type followed by an asterisk (*). RDAs and AIs may both be used as goals for individual intake. RDAs are set to meet the needs of almost all (97 to 98 percent) individuals in a group. For healthy breastfed infants, the AI is the mean intake. The AI for other life stage and gender groups is believed to cover needs of all individuals in the group, but lack of data or uncertainty in the data prevent being able to specify with confidence the percentage of individuals covered by this intake.

SOURCES: *Dietary Reference Intakes for Calcium, Phosphorous, Magnesium, Vitamin D, and Fluoride* (1997); *Dietary Reference Intakes for Thiamin, Riboflavin, Niacin, Vitamin B_6, Folate, Vitamin B_{12}, Pantothenic Acid, Biotin, and Choline* (1998); *Dietary Reference Intakes for Vitamin C, Vitamin E, Selenium, and Carotenoids* (2000); *Dietary Reference Intakes for Vitamin A, Vitamin K, Arsenic, Boron, Chromium, Copper, Iodine, Iron, Manganese, Molybdenum, Nickel, Silicon, Vanadium, and Zinc* (2001); and *Dietary Reference Intakes for Water, Potassium, Sodium, Chloride, and Sulfate* (2004). These reports may be accessed via http://www.nap.edu.

Table 3. Dietary Reference Intake (DRIs):Tolerable Upper Intakes Levels (ULs),Vitamins[a]

Life Stage Group	Vitamin A (μg/d)[b]	Vitamin C (mg/d)	Vitamin D (μg/d)	Vitamin E (mg/d)[c,d]	Vitamin K	Thiamin	Riboflavin	Niacin (mg/d)[d]	Vitamin B_6 (mg/d)	Folate (μg/d)[d]	Vitamin B_{12}	Pantothenic Acid	Biotin	Choline (g/d)	Carotenoids[e]
Infants															
0–6 mo	600	ND[f]	25	ND	ND	ND	ND	ND	ND	ND	ND	ND	ND	ND	ND
7–12 mo	600	ND	25	ND	ND	ND	ND	ND	ND	ND	ND	ND	ND	ND	ND
Children															
1–3 y	600	400	50	200	ND	ND	ND	10	30	300	ND	ND	ND	1.0	ND
4–8 y	900	650	50	300	ND	ND	ND	15	40	400	ND	ND	ND	1.0	ND
Males, Females															
9–13 y	1700	1200	50	600	ND	ND	ND	20	60	600	ND	ND	ND	2.0	ND
14–18 y	2800	1800	50	800	ND	ND	ND	30	80	800	ND	ND	ND	3.0	ND
19–70 y	3000	2000	50	1000	ND	ND	ND	35	100	1000	ND	ND	ND	3.5	ND
> 70 y	3000	2000	50	1000	ND	ND	ND	35	100	1000	ND	ND	ND	3.5	ND
Pregnancy															
14–18 y	2800	1800	50	800	ND	ND	ND	30	80	800	ND	ND	ND	3.0	ND
19–50 y	3000	2000	50	1000	ND	ND	ND	35	100	1000	ND	ND	ND	3.5	ND
Lactation															
14–18 y	2800	1800	50	800	ND	ND	ND	30	80	800	ND	ND	ND	3.0	ND
19–50 y	3000	2000	50	1000	ND	ND	ND	35	100	1000	ND	ND	ND	3.5	ND

[a] UL = The maximum level of daily nutrient intake that is likely to pose no risk of adverse effects. Unless otherwise specified, the UL represents total intake from food, water, and supplements. Due to lack of suitable data, ULs could not be established for vitamin K, thiamin, riboflavin, vitamin B_{12}, pantothenic acid, biotin, carotenoids. In the absence of ULs, extra caution may be warranted in consuming levels above recommended intakes.

[b] As preformed vitamin A only.

[c] As α-tocopherol; applies to any form of supplemental α-tocopherol.

[d] The ULs for vitamin E, niacin, and folate apply to synthetic forms obtained from supplements, fortified foods, or a combination of the two.

[e] β-Carotene supplements are advised only to serve as a provitamin A source for individuals at risk of vitamin A deficiency.

[f] ND = Not determinable due to lack of data of adverse effects in this age group and concern with regard to lack of ability to handle excess amounts. Source of intake should be from food only to prevent high levels of intake.

SOURCES: *Dietary Reference Intakes for Calcium, Phosphorous, Magnesium, Vitamin D, and Fluoride* (1997); *Dietary Reference Intakes for Thiamin, Riboflavin, Niacin, Vitamin B_6, Folate, Vitamin B_{12}, Pantothenic Acid, Biotin, and Choline* (1998); *Dietary Reference Intakes for Vitamin C, Vitamin E, Selenium, and Carotenoids* (2000); and *Dietary Reference Intakes for Vitamin A, Vitamin K, Arsenic, Boron, Chromium, Copper, Iodine, Iron, Manganese, Molybdenum, Nickel, Silicon, Vanadium, and Zinc* (2001). These reports may be accessed via http://www.nap.edu.

Table 4. Dietary Reference Intake (DRIs):Tolerable Upper Intakes Levels (ULs),Elements[a]

Life Stage Group	Arsenic[b]	Boron (mg/d)	Calcium (g/d)	Chromium	Copper (μg/d)	Fluoride (mg/d)	Iodine (μg/d)	Iron (mg/d)	Magnesium (mg/d)[c]	Manganese (mg/d)	Molybdenum (μg/d)	Nickel (mg/d)	Phosphorus (g/d)	Potassium	Selenium (μg/d)	Silicon[d]	Sulfate	Vanadium (mg/d)[e]	Zinc (mg/d)	Sodium (g/d)	Chloride (g/d)
Infants																					
0–6 mo	ND[f]	ND	ND	ND	ND	0.7	ND	40	ND	ND	ND	ND	ND	ND	45	ND	ND	ND	4	ND	ND
7–12 mo	ND	ND	ND	ND	ND	0.9	ND	40	ND	ND	ND	ND	ND	ND	60	ND	ND	ND	5	ND	ND
Children																					
1–3 y	ND	3	2.5	ND	1000	1.3	200	40	65	2	300	0.2	3	ND	90	ND	ND	ND	7	1.5	2.3
4–8 y	ND	6	2.5	ND	3000	2.2	300	40	110	3	600	0.3	3	ND	150	ND	ND	ND	12	1.9	2.9
Males, Females																					
9–13 y	ND	11	2.5	ND	5000	10	600	40	350	6	1100	0.6	4	ND	280	ND	ND	ND	23	2.2	3.4
14–18 y	ND	17	2.5	ND	8000	10	900	45	350	9	1700	1.0	4	ND	400	ND	ND	ND	34	2.3	3.6
19–70 y	ND	20	2.5	ND	10,000	10	1100	45	350	11	2000	1.0	4	ND	400	ND	ND	1.8	40	2.3	3.6
>70 y	ND	20	2.5	ND	10,000	10	1100	45	350	11	2000	1.0	3	ND	400	ND	ND	1.8	40	2.3	3.6
Pregnancy																					
14–18 y	ND	17	2.5	ND	8000	10	900	45	350	9	1700	1.0	3.5	ND	400	ND	ND	ND	34	2.3	3.6
19–50 y	ND	20	2.5	ND	10,000	10	1100	45	350	11	2000	1.0	3.5	ND	400	ND	ND	ND	40	2.3	3.6
Lactation																					
14–18 y	ND	17	2.5	ND	8000	10	900	45	350	9	1700	1.0	4	ND	400	ND	ND	ND	34	2.3	3.6
19–50 y	ND	20	2.5	ND	10,000	10	1100	45	350	11	2000	1.0	4	ND	400	ND	ND	ND	40	2.3	3.6

[a] UL = The maximum level of daily nutrient intake that is likely to pose no risk of adverse effects. Unless otherwise specified, the UL represents total intake from food, water, and supplements. Due to lack of suitable data, ULs could not be established for arsenic, chromium, silicon, potassium, and sulfate. In the absence of ULs, extra caution may be warranted in consuming levels above recommended intakes.

[b] Although the UL was not determined for arsenic, there is no justification for adding arsenic to food or supplements.

[c] The ULs for magnesium represent intake from a pharmacological agent only and do not include intake from food and water.

[d] Although silicon has not been shown to cause adverse effects in humans, there is no justification for adding silicon to supplements.

[e] Although vanadium in food has not been shown to cause adverse effects in humans, there is no justification for adding vanadium to food and vanadium supplements should be used with caution. The UL is based on adverse effects in laboratory animals and this data could be used to set a UL for adults but not children and adolescents.

[f] ND = Not determinable due to lack of data of adverse effects in this age group and concern with regard to lack of ability to handle excess amounts. Source of intake should be from food only to prevent high levels of intake.

SOURCES: *Dietary Reference Intakes for Calcium, Phosphorous, Magnesium, Vitamin D, and Fluoride* (1997); *Dietary Reference Intakes for Thiamin, Riboflavin, Niacin, Vitamin B_6, Folate, Vitamin B_{12}, Pantothenic Acid, Biotin, and Choline* (1998); *Dietary Reference Intakes for Vitamin C, Vitamin E, Selenium, and Carotenoids* (2000); *Dietary Reference Intakes for Vitamin A, Vitamin K, Arsenic, Boron, Chromium, Copper, Iodine, Iron, Manganese, Molybdenum, Nickel, Silicon, Vanadium, and Zinc* (2001); and *Dietary Reference Intakes for Water, Potassium, Sodium, Chloride, and Sulfate* (2004). These reports may be accessed via http://www.nap.edu.

Table 5. Dietary Reference Intakes (DRIs): Recommended Intakes for Individuals, Macronutrients

Life Stage Group	Total Water[a] (L/d)	Carbohydrate (g/d)	Total Fiber (g/d)	Fat (g/d)	Linoleic Acid (g/d)	α-Linolenic Acid (g/d)	Protein[b] (g/d)
Infants							
0–6 mo	0.7*	60*	ND	31*	4.4*	0.5*	9.1*
7–12 mo	0.8*	95*	ND	30*	4.6*	0.5*	**11.0**[c]
Children							
1–3 y	1.3*	**130**	19*	ND	7*	0.7*	**13**
4–8 y	1.7*	**130**	25*	ND	10*	0.9*	**19**
Males							
9–13 y	2.4*	**130**	31*	ND	12*	1.2*	**34**
14–18 y	3.3*	**130**	38*	ND	16*	1.6*	**52**
19–30 y	3.7*	**130**	38*	ND	17*	1.6*	**56**
31–50 y	3.7*	**130**	38*	ND	17*	1.6*	**56**
51–70 y	3.7*	**130**	30*	ND	14*	1.6*	**56**
> 70 y	3.7*	**130**	30*	ND	14*	1.6*	**56**
Females							
9–13 y	2.1*	**130**	26*	ND	10*	1.0*	**34**
14–18 y	2.3*	**130**	26*	ND	11*	1.1*	**46**
19–30 y	2.7*	**130**	25*	ND	12*	1.1*	**46**
31–50 y	2.7*	**130**	25*	ND	12*	1.1*	**46**
51–70 y	2.7*	**130**	21*	ND	11*	1.1*	**46**
> 70 y	2.7*	**130**	21*	ND	11*	1.1*	**46**
Pregnancy							
14–18 y	3.0*	**175**	28*	ND	13*	1.4*	**71**
19–30 y	3.0*	**175**	28*	ND	13*	1.4*	**71**
31–50 y	3.0*	**175**	28*	ND	13*	1.4*	**71**
Lactation							
14–18 y	3.8*	**210**	29*	ND	13*	1.3*	**71**
19–30 y	3.8*	**210**	29*	ND	13*	1.3*	**71**
31–50 y	3.8*	**210**	29*	ND	13*	1.3*	**71**

NOTE: This table presents Recommended Dietary Allowances (RDAs) in **bold** type and Adequate Intakes (AIs) in ordinary type followed by an asterisk (*). RDAs and AIs may both be used as goals for individual intake. RDAs are set to meet the needs of almost all (97 to 98 percent) individuals in a group. For healthy infants fed human milk, the AI is the mean intake. The AI for other life stage and gender groups is believed to cover the needs of all individuals in the group, but lack of data or uncertainty in the data prevent being able to specify with confidence the percentage of individuals covered by this intake.

[a] Total water includes all water contained in food, beverages, and drinking water.

[b] Based on 0.8 g/kg body weight for the reference body weight.

[c] Change from 13.5 in prepublication copy due to calculation error.

Assessment of Individuals. Many uses of the DRIs involve assessing the diets of individuals, including dietary counseling and nutrition education. Because the distribution of requirements is given for most nutrients, it is possible to estimate the probability of adequacy (or the probability of inadequacy) for a given intake, assuming that the intake represents an individual's "usual" intake (i.e., what is usually consumed over a long period of time). For example, usual intake at the EAR would have a 50% probability of inadequacy, because, by definition, half of the people in the age-sex category have requirements below the EAR and half have requirements above it. Usual intake at the RDA would have a 97% to 98% probability of adequacy, because the RDA is set to cover the needs of 97% to 98% of the individuals in the category. Using a simple statistical algorithm, it is possible to calculate the probability of adequacy for any usual intake level. However, intakes that are reported or observed are not usually long-term usual intakes due to the effect of day-to-day variations in intake. Thus, the configidence that these probability estimates are correct is reduced if only a few days of intake are observed. An adjustment for this reduced configidence is possible and allows an evaluation of the confidence of adequacy, as well as the probability of adequacy.[8] Before the availability of DRIs, individual assessment was based on the percent of the RDA in a usual diet, but, unlike the probability and confidence of adequacy, the percent of the RDA could not be easily interpreted.

Table 6. Dietary Reference Intakes (DRIs): Acceptable Macronutrient Distribution Ranges

Macronutrient	Range (percent of energy)		
	Children, 1–3 y	Children, 4–18 y	Adults
Fat	30–40	25–35	20–35
n-6 polyunsaturated fatty acids* (linoleic acid)	5–10	5–10	5–10
n-3 polyunsaturated fatty acids* α-linolenic acid)	0.6–1.2	0.6–1.2	0.6–1.2
Carbohydrate	45–65	45–65	45–65
Protein	5–20	10–30	10–35

* Approximately 10% of the total can come from longer-chain n-3 or n-6 fatty acids.
Use with permission from Food and Nutrition Board, Institute of Medicine.[6]

For nutrients with an AI rather than an EAR/RDA, usual intakes of the individual may be evaluated by determining whether the intake is above the AI. If so, the intake is likely to be adequate. However, if the intake is below the AI, the probability of adequacy is unknown. Because an AI is usually higher than an RDA (if one were known), intakes below the AI may still have a high probability of adequacy. An individual's usual intake also may be compared with the UL for a nutrient. Usual intakes above the UL are at risk of being excessive.

In summary, several DRIs are used to assess an individual's usual intake: the EAR to estimate the probability of adequacy; the AI, if an EAR is not available, to determine whether the probability of adequacy is high; and the UL to estimate whether the intake is at risk of being excessive.

Planning for Individuals. The DRIs are often used to plan diets for individuals. For example, food guides and dietary guidelines are based on obtaining adequate nutrient intakes. The Nutrition Facts and Supplement Facts labels on consumer products use nutrient standards, although they have not yet been updated to reflect the current DRIs. Also, both consumers and health professionals may use the DRIs to plan diets with a high probability of adequacy and a low probability of being excessive. For all of these uses, the RDA is the appropriate target for an individual's intake, and when an RDA is not available, the AI may be used for the same purpose. If an individual's usual intake is at or above the RDA or AI, the probability of adequacy is high. Likewise, if usual intake is below the UL, the risk of adverse effects is low.

Assessment of Population Groups. The DRIs may be used to assess the intakes of groups of people, such as those participating in a survey or nutrition study. This type of assessment is used for national nutrition surveys (such as the National Health and Nutrition Examination Survey) and to evaluate food assistance programs (such as the National School Lunch Program). Several statistical assumptions are involved in both assessing and planning intakes of population groups, and these assumptions can be made only if the group contains a minimum number of people. For most of the methods discussed later, a reasonable minimum is 100 people in the group.

Assessing the intakes of groups is conceptually more complex than assessing the intakes of individuals, although in practice, computer algorithms can greatly simplify this process. The goal of this type of assessment is to estimate the prevalence of inadequacy within the group, as well as the prevalence of intakes at risk of being excessive. The prevalence of inadequacy may be calculated as the average of the probabilities of inadequacy for each individual in the group. For many nutrients, an even easier estimate of the prevalence of inadequacy is possible; the proportion of the group with usual intakes below the EAR is approximately equal to the proportion of the group with inadequate intakes. This EAR "cut-point" approach may be used for nutrients with a normal distribution of requirements, which is thought to be the case for all nutrients except iron. The cut-point approach also assumes that the variation of usual intakes is greater than the variation of requirements within the group, which is true for most intake distributions. The cut-point method of estimating the prevalence of inadequacy is valid for statistical reasons, but should not be interpreted as implying that the EAR may be used to identify in the group those specific individuals with inadequate intakes. As noted earlier, individuals with usual intakes at the EAR still have a 50% probability of inadequacy. Although iron has an EAR, the cut-point method may not be used because requirements are not normally distributed. This is particularly true for the requirements for menstruating women, but additional evidence shows that requirements for other age-sex categories are also not normal. Thus, tables in Appendix I of the IOM report on iron requirements[5] should be used to calculate the probability of inadequacy for each individual in the group, and then the prevalence of inadequacy should be estimated as the average of the probabilities.

For nutrients with an AI, it is not possible to estimate the prevalence of inadequate intakes. If the median intake of a group is at or above the AI, a low prevalence of inadequacy within the group is likely. However, if the median intake is below the AI, it is still possible that the prevalence of inadequacy is low. Thus, no statement about the prevalence of inadequacy can be made for groups with median intakes below the AI.

The prevalence of excessive intakes may be estimated as the proportion of usual intakes that is above the UL.

Ensuring that the effect of day-to-day variations in intake has been removed from the intake distribution is important before calculating either the prevalence of inadequacy or the prevalence of excess. Computer algorithms are available to make this type of adjustment to the distribution of intakes and may be implemented using the information in Appendix E of the IOM report on planning diets[9] or by using existing software.[10]

In summary, several of the DRIs are used to assess the intakes of groups: The EAR is used to estimate the prevalence of inadequacy, and the UL is used to estimate the prevalence of excessive intakes. Adjusting intake distributions to reflect usual intakes is important before estimating these prevalences. For nutrients without an EAR, the AI may be used to determine whether the prevalence of inadequacy is likely to be low. The RDA is not used to assess the intake of groups.

Planning for Groups. Numerous uses of the DRIs exist for planning intakes of population groups, including planning for institutional feeding, food assistance programs, and military rations. Planning intakes for population groups relies on the same concepts as assessing intakes of groups. The goal of the planning activity is to minimize the prevalence of inadequate intakes and also the prevalence of excessive intakes within the group of interest. Planning and assessment are closely linked, because it is not usually possible to predict the actual outcome of the planning activity.

The first step in a planning group intakes is to identify the nutrients of interest, as well as the acceptable prevalences of inadequacy and excess. Although 2% to 3% have often been used as an acceptable prevalence for both of these indicators, such targets may not always be feasible or even desirable. The next step is to examine the current usual intake distribution for a nutrient and decide whether the distribution needs to be shifted up or down to improve the prevalences of adequacy and excess. As with assessment, adjusting the current intake distribution to reflect usual intakes is important. The third step is to determine the amount of the shift that is needed; this information can be approximated using the EAR and the UL as cutpoints. For example, if 30% of the group has usual intakes of zinc below the EAR, then intakes need to be increased by an amount that will shift the distribution so that only 2% to 3% have zinc intakes below the EAR (if that is the target that was chosen). Such a shift would require that all intakes increase by a specific amount (e.g., 3 mg of zinc) if the shape of the distribution is unchanged. Determining whether the shift would cause an undesirable increase in the prevalence of intakes above the UL is important, again, assuming that the shape of the intake distribution does not change. Because assuming that the distribution's shape will not change is likely to be unrealistic, it is crucial that an assessment activity take place after the new feeding plan is implemented.

In some cases, it may be desirable (or necessary) to try to change the shape of the distribution as part of the planning activity. This might be accomplished, for example, by trying to target those with the lowest intakes. Nutrition education programs could be designed for these individuals, or specific foods or supplements could be provided to them. Once the group is subdivided so that particular individuals are targeted, they would theoretically now fall into the methodology described earlier for planning intakes for individuals. The group planning activity would now apply to the remainder of the group, with these individuals removed.

The AI may be used as the target for the median intake of the group, if an EAR is not available. For nutrients with an AI, the goal is to increase the median intake to at least the level of the AI, without increasing the prevalence of excessive intakes.

Planning intakes for groups is not a simple exercise. The steps described earlier need to be undertaken for each nutrient of interest, and then the results need to be translated into foods to be provided and menus for actual meals. This activity also requires assumptions about the amount of food that will be chosen and consumed by individuals in the group. Again, given the many assumptions involved, an assessment activity should follow implementation of the feeding plan.

A further complexity to planning for groups is that the individuals in the group may not be homogeneous. That is, a mix of life-stage categories will be present within the group, such as boys and girls in a school feeding program. If the EAR and UL for boys are used for the planning activity, then the prevalences of inadequacy and excess may not be acceptable for the girls. Thus, an iterative process may be necessary to set appropriate planning goals for heterogeneous groups. One approach is to determine in advance which category within the group has the greatest prevalence of inadequacy, and then plan intakes to reduce this prevalence to an acceptable level. Theoretically, the intakes of the other categories within the group will also improve to an acceptable level. One concern, of course, is that the prevalence of excessive intakes will become unacceptably high for some life-stage categories at the same time that the prevalence of inadequacy becomes acceptably low. In this case, compromises may be necessary in setting the targets.

Other Issues to Consider When Using the DRIs

An important issue to address is whether the units used to measure intakes match those used for the nutrient standards. In particular, the units for vitamin E, vitamin

A, and folate requirements are different from those used in the past and may not match those available for calculating intakes.[11,12]

Vitamin E as α-Tocopherol. The DRIs for vitamin E (EARs and RDAs) are for milligrams of α-tocopherol and not for milligrams of α-tocopherol equivalents, as have been used in the past. Furthermore, they apply only to RRR-α-tocopherol, the form of α-tocopherol that occurs naturally in foods, and the 2R-stereoisomeric forms, a portion of the α-tocopherol used in most fortified foods and dietary supplements. Thus, vitamin E intakes in α-TE will be higher than intakes in α-T and should not be used to evaluate intakes relative to the DRIs.

Folate in Dietary Folate Equivalents. The DRIs for folate are given as micrograms of Dietary Folate Equivalents (DFE), not in micrograms of folate, as have been used in the past. A microgram of food folate is equal to a microgram of DFE, but a microgram of folic acid (from fortification or supplements) is equal to 1.67 DFE. Thus, folate intakes in micrograms will be lower than folate intakes in micrograms of DFE and should not be used to evaluate intakes relative to the DRIs.

Vitamin A as Retinol Activity Equivalents. The DRIs for vitamin A are given in micrograms of Retinol Activity Equivalents (RAE), rather than in micrograms of Retinol Equivalents. The new unit reflects current bioavailability studies showing a lower conversion of pro-vitamin A carotenoids to vitamin A. The conversion factors are now one-half of those used previously so that intake of vitamin A in RAE will be lower than intake in Retinol Equivalent if any pro-vitamin A carotenoids are in the diet. Thus, intakes in Retinol Equivalents should not be used to evaluate vitamin A intakes relative to the DRIs.

A related issue is that the units for the requirements may differ from the units for the ULs. For example, the magnesium UL is only for pharmacological forms of magnesium (such as magnesium salts), whereas the RDA is for magnesium from food and water. This leads to the possibility of an RDA being above the UL; for men, the magnesium RDA is 400 to 420 mg/d, whereas the UL is 350 mg/d. For several vitamins, the UL applies only to synthetic forms of the nutrient used for fortification and dietary supplements (folic acid, α-tocopherol, niacin). The UL for vitamin A applies only to preformed vitamin A (retinol).

Appropriate uses of the DRIs are discussed in more detail in the IOM reports on using the DRIs for dietary assessment and planning[8,9] and also in several published journal articles.[10-17]

Dietary Guidelines for Americans (2005)

The *Dietary Guidelines for Americans* were first published in 1980 and are meant to provide advice on food choices that promote health and reduce risk of chronic diseases for Americans ages 2 and older. Unlike the DRIs, which provide nutrient guidelines, the Dietary Guidelines provide primarily food-based guidelines.

By law, the Dietary Guidelines must be reviewed every 5 years and updated if necessary. The most recent set of guidelines, the sixth edition, was issued in 2005.[18] The science-based review is conducted by a Dietary Guidelines Advisory Committee (DGAC), whose members are appointed by the US Department of Health and Human Services and the USDA. After its deliberations are concluded, the DGAC issues a report to the secretaries of the USDA and the US Department of Health and Human Services.[19] This report then forms the basis of the guidelines issued by the secretaries. All federal food, nutrition education, and information programs must be based on the Dietary Guidelines.

In 2005, a number of publications and websites resulted from the Dietary Guidelines process. The report by the DGAC is available at http://www.health.gov/dietaryguidelines/dga2005/report/. The report suggested nine guidelines, as shown in Table 7. The very detailed DGAC report has been summarized into a shorter report for policy makers, nutrition educators, nutritionists, and health care providers.[18] Key recommendations within each of the nine focus areas of the DGAC report were made and are summarized in Table 7. Because both of these reports are too detailed for consumers, a more consumer-friendly brochure was also issued.[20] All of the Dietary Guidelines materials are available at http://www.healthierus.gov/dietaryguidelines. As discussed in the next section, the Food Guide Pyramid (now called MyPyramid) is meant to help consumers apply the guidelines to their food choices.

USDA Food Guide/MyPyramid

The USDA Food Guide Pyramid (FGP) was released in 1992 and was intended to help consumers apply the Dietary Guidelines (from 1990) to their diets.[21] Although new Dietary Guidelines were issued in 1995, and again in 2000, no revisions were made to the FGP. However, concurrently with the release of the 2005 Dietary Guidelines, a new pyramid, called MyPyramid, was developed.[22]

The original FGP has become a familiar icon to both health professionals and the public (Figure 1). The FGP was based on several nutritional concepts, including moderation, proportionality, and variety.[23] It was extensively reviewed and tested before release.[24] Although known primarily to health professionals, the FGP was supported by a specific dietary profile for each food group.[24] The nutrient profiles were based on reported consumption of the foods within each of the major food groups and allowed an estimation of the nutrient intake that will result from following the FGP recommendations. Although many alternate "pyramids" have been proposed, few are based on the detailed nutrient analyses that provided the foundation of the FGP.

Table 7. Dietary Guidelines for Americans, 2005

Focus Areas	Guidelines from DGAC*	Key Recommendations†
Adequate Nutrients within Calorie Needs	Consume a variety of foods within and among the basic food groups, while staying within energy needs.	• Consume a variety of nutrient-dense foods and beverages within and among the basic food groups while choosing foods that limit the intake of saturated and *trans* fats, cholesterol, added sugars, salt, and alcohol. • Meet recommended intakes within energy needs by adopting a balanced eating pattern, such as the USDA Food Guide or the DASH Eating Plan.
Weight Management	Control calorie intake to manage body weight.	• To maintain body weight in a health range, balance calories from foods and beverages with calories expended. • To prevent gradual weight gain over time, make small decreases in food and beverage calories and increase physical activity.
Physical Activity	Be physically active every day.	• Engage in regular physical activity and reduce sedentary activities to promote health, psychological well-being, and a healthy body weight. ○ To reduce the risk of chronic disease in adulthood: Engage in at least 30 minutes of moderate-intensity physical activity, above usual activity, at work or at home on most days of the week. ○ For most people, greater health benefits can be obtained by engaging in physical activity of more vigorous intensity or longer duration. ○ To help manage body weight and prevent gradual, unhealthy body weight gain in adulthood: Engage in approximately 60 minutes of moderate- to vigorous-intensity activity on most days of the week while not exceeding caloric intake requirements. ○ To sustain weight loss in adulthood: Participate in at least 60 to 90 minutes of daily moderate-intensity physical activity while not exceeding caloric intake requirements. Some people may need to consult with a healthcare provider before participating in this level of activity. • Achieve physical fitness by including cardiovascular conditioning, stretching exercises for flexibility, and resistance exercises of calisthenics for muscle strength and endurance.
Food Groups to Encourage	Increase daily intakes of fruits and vegetables, whole grains, and reduced-fat milk and milk products.	• Consume a sufficient amount of fruits and vegetables while staying within energy needs. Two cups of fruit and 2 1/2 cups of vegetables per day are recommended for a reference 2000-calorie intake, with higher or lower amounts depending on the calorie level. • Choose a variety of fruits and vegetables each day. In particular, select from all five vegetable subgroups (dark green, orange, legumes, starchy vegetables, and other vegetables) several times a week. • Consume 3 or more ounce-equivalents of whole-grain products per day, with the rest of the recommended grains coming from enriched or whole-grain products. In general, at least half the grains should come from whole grains. • Consume 3 cups per day of fat-free or low-fat milk or equivalent milk products.
Fats	Choose fats wisely for good health.	• Consume less than 10% of calories from saturated fatty acids and less than 300 mg/d of cholesterol, and keep *trans* fatty acid consumption as low as possible. • Keep total fat intake between 20% to AAP, 1999[35]% of calories, with most fats coming from sources of polyunsaturated and monounsaturated fatty acids, such as fish, nuts, and vegetable oils. • When selecting and preparing meat, poultry, dry beans, and milk or milk products, make choices that are lean, low-fat, or fat-free. • Limit intake of fats and oils high in saturated and/or *trans* fatty acids, and choose products low in such fats and oils.
Carbohydrates	Choose carbohydrates wisely for good health.	• Choose fiber-rich fruits, vegetables, and whole grains often. • Choose and prepare foods and beverages with little added sugars or caloric sweeteners, such as amounts suggested by the USDA Food Guide and the DASH Eating Plan. • Reduce the incidence of dental caries by practicing good oral hygiene and consuming sugar- and starch-containing foods and beverages less frequently.
Sodium and Potassium	Choose and prepare foods with little salt.	• Consume less than 2300 mg (approximately 1 tsp of salt) of sodium per day. • Choose and prepare foods with little salt. At the same time, consume potassium-rich foods, such as fruits and vegetables.
Alcoholic Beverages	If you drink alcoholic beverages, do so in moderation.	• Those who choose to drink alcoholic beverages should do so sensibly and in moderation—defined as the consumption of up to one drink per day for women and up to two drinks per day for men. • Alcoholic beverages should not be consumed by some individuals, including those who cannot restrict their alcohol intake, women of childbearing age who may become pregnant, pregnant and lactating women, children and adolescents, individuals taking medications that can interact with alcohol, and those with specific medical conditions. • Alcoholic beverages should be avoided by individuals engaging in activities that require attention, skill, or coordination, such as driving or operating machinery.
Food Safety	Keep foods safe to eat.	• To avoid microbial foodborne illness: ○ Clean hands, food contact surfaces, and fruit and vegetables. Meat and poultry should *not* be washed or rinsed. ○ Separate raw, cooked, and ready-to-eat foods while shopping, preparing, or storing foods. ○ Cook foods to a safe temperature to kill micro-organisms. ○ Chill (refrigerate) perishable food promptly and defrost foods properly. ○ Avid raw (unpasteurized) milk or any products made from unpasteurized milk, raw or partially cooked eggs or foods containing raw eggs, raw or undercooked meat and poultry, unpasteurized juices, and raw sprouts.

*From Dietary Guidelines Advisory Committee. *2005 Dietary Guidelines for Americans.* Accessed September 7, 2004, at http://www.health.gov/dietaryguidelines/dga2005/report.
†From United States Department of Health and Human Services, United States Department of Agriculture. Finding Your Way to a Healthier You: Based on the Dietary Guidelines for Americans. HHS Pub. No.: HHS-ODPDP-2005-01-DGA-B. USDA Pub. No.: Home and Garden Bulletin No. 232-CP. Washington, DC: US Government Printing Office: 2005.

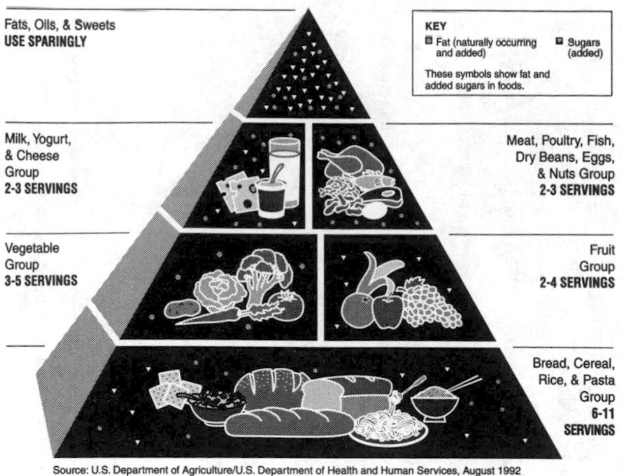

Figure 1. The Food Guide Pyramid. A Guide to Daily Food Choices

Grains are the base of the pyramid, fruits and vegetables are at the next level, followed by meats and meat substitutes and dairy products. At the "tip" of the FGP are fats, oils, and sweets, with a message suggesting that they should be used "sparingly." The appropriate number of servings from each of the food groups was specified for three levels of energy intake: 1600, 2200, and 2800 kcal/d. Thus, a range of servings was specified for each of the food groups: 6 to 11 servings of grains, 3 to 5 servings of vegetables, 2 to 4 servings of fruit, 2 to 3 servings of dairy products, and 2 to 3 servings of meat or meat alternates. The FGP consumer information provided details on what constituted a serving and what types of foods belonged in each of the FGP food groups.

MyPyramid

Revised Icon. After extensive feedback from health professionals, MyPyramid was released in April 2005. It is a companion to the Dietary Guidelines, 2005 and replaces the 1992 Food Guide Pyramid. The new icon is shown in Figure 2. The components of the new pyramid are illustrated by lines that divide the pyramid vertically, rather than horizontally, as in the original FGP. Each vertical section is meant to indicate a food group. The original five food groups are maintained, but an additional "oils" group has been added. As in the past, the icon conveys moderation, proportionality, and variety. The width of the vertical section illustrates proportionality among the food groups (e.g., the grains section is wider than the meat and beans section), whereas the narrowing of each group from bottom to top indicates that moderation is needed for some foods within each group (e.g., those with more solid fats and added sugars should be chosen less often). Variety is symbolized by the six-color bands showing that food from all of the groups are needed each day for good health. An important addition to the MyPyramid logo is the figure of a person climbing the steps of the pyramid, indicating the importance of daily physical activity. A slogan under the icon, "Steps to a healthier you," suggests that gradual improvement is encouraged, and that individuals can benefit by taking small steps to improve their diet and physical activity every day.

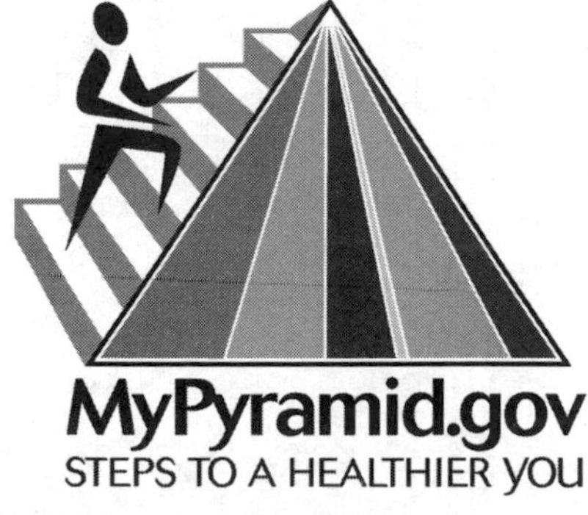

Figure 2. MyPyramid: Steps to a Healthier You

Food Intake Patterns. Rather than try to communicate further details, such as the appropriate amounts to consume from each group, the icon invites consumers to personalize MyPyramid by seeking further information at http://www.MyPyramid.gov. A tailored version of MyPyramid may be obtained at this website, after indicating a person's age, gender, and activity level (sedentary, moderately active, or active). Based on this information, a person is classified in 1 of 12 energy intake groups, ranging from 1000 kcal/d to 3200 kcal/d (Table 8). A version of MyPyramid is available that corresponds to each of these energy intake groups, and the daily amount of food from each food group varies with the energy level (Table 9). For example, the recommended amount of fruit varies from 1 cup/d to 2.5 cups/d, depending on the calorie level. The original FGP specified only three calorie levels (1600, 2200, and 2800 kcal/d), so it was not possible to tailor the dietary guidance as accurately as is now done using the MyPyramid guidelines.

The amount to be consumed from each of the food groups is specified in common measures such as cups and ounce rather than in servings (Table 9). Thus, it should be easier for consumers to determine how much an actual portion contributes to the recommended amount. For example, a person who requires 2000 kcal/d should consume 2 cups of fruit/d, so a 1-cup portion of fruit would meet 50% of this recommendation. Fruits, vegetables, and milk are specified in cups, whereas grains and meat/beans are specified in ounce-equivalents. In general, a cup of fruits and vegetables is equal to two of the FGP servings, whereas an ounce-equivalent of grains is equal to one FGP grain serving. The following are additional details for each food group:

- For the fruit group and the vegetable group, a cup of fresh, frozen, or canned forms (including juices) are equivalent, or one-half cup of the dried form. Two cups of raw leafy green vegetables is equivalent to one cup of other vegetables.
- An ounce-equivalent of grains corresponds approximately to the dry weight of the grain (such as flour

Table 8. MyPyramid Food Intake Pattern Calorie Level*

MALES				FEMALES			
Activity level AGE	**Sedentary***	**Mod. Active***	**Active***	**Activity level AGE**	**Sedentary***	**Mod. active***	**Active***
2	1000	1000	1000	**2**	1000	1000	1000
3	1000	1400	1400	**3**	1000	1200	1400
4	1200	1400	1600	**4**	1200	1400	1400
5	1200	1400	1600	**5**	1200	1400	1600
6	1400	1600	1800	**6**	1200	1400	1600
7	1400	1600	1800	**7**	1200	1600	1800
8	1400	1600	2000	**8**	1400	1600	1800
9	1600	1800	2000	**9**	1400	1600	1800
10	1600	1800	2200	**10**	1400	1800	2000
11	1800	2000	2200	**11**	1600	1800	2000
12	1800	2200	2400	**12**	1600	2000	2200
13	2000	2200	2600	**13**	1600	2000	2200
14	2000	2400	2800	**14**	1800	2000	2400
15	2200	2600	3000	**15**	1800	2000	2400
16	2400	2800	3200	**16**	1800	2000	2400
17	2400	2800	3200	**17**	1800	2000	2400
18	2400	2800	3200	**18**	1800	2000	2400
19–20	2600	2800	3000	**19–20**	2000	2200	2400
21–25	2400	2800	3000	**21–25**	2000	2200	2400
26–30	2400	2600	3000	**26–30**	1800	2000	2400
31–35	2400	2600	3000	**31–35**	1800	2000	2200
36–40	2400	2600	2800	**36–40**	1800	2000	2200
41–45	2200	2600	2800	**41–45**	1800	2000	2200
46–50	2200	2400	2800	**46–50**	1800	2000	2200
51–55	2200	2400	2800	**51–55**	1600	1800	2200
56–60	2200	2400	2600	**56–60**	1600	1800	2200
61–65	2000	2400	2600	**61–65**	1600	1800	2000
66–70	2000	2200	2600	**66–70**	1600	1800	2000
71–75	2000	2200	2600	**71–75**	1600	1800	2000
76 and up	2000	2200	2400	**76 and up**	1600	1800	2000

* MyPyramid assigns Individuals to a calorie level based on their sex, age, and activity level.
The chart below identifies the calorie levels for males and females by age and activity level.
Calorie levels are provided for each year of childhood, from 2–18 years, and for adults in 5-year increments.Calorie levels are based on the Estimated Energy Requirements (EER) and activity levels from the Institute of Medicine Dietary Reference Intakes Macronutrients Report, 2002.
Sedentary, less than 30 minutes a day of moderate physical activity in addition to daily activities. Mod. active, at least 30 minutes up to 60 minutes a day of moderate physical activity in addition to daily activities. Active, 60 or more minutes a day of moderate phyisical activity in addition to daily activities.

or rice) and is equivalent to one slice of bread, one cup of breakfast cereal, or one-half cup of cooked grains.

- For meat and beans, an ounce-equivalent corresponds to an ounce of lean meat, poultry, or fish. One egg, one tablespoon of peanut butter, one-fourth cup of cooked dry beans, and one-half ounce of nuts or seeds counts as an ounce equivalent.
- A cup from the milk group includes fluid milk or yogurt. Two ounces of processed cheese, or 1.5 ounces of natural cheese are equivalent to one cup from this group.

Table 9. MyPyramid Food Intake Pattern Daily Amount of Food From Each Group*

Daily Amount of Food From Each Group

Calorie Level	1000	1200	1400	1600	1800	2000	2200	2400	2600	2800	3000	3200
Fruits	1 cup	1 cup	1.5 cups	1.5 cups	1.5 cups	2 cups	2 cups	2 cups	2 cups	2.5 cups	2.5 cups	2.5 cups
Vegetables	1 cup	1.5 cups	1.5 cups	2 cups	2.5 cups	2.5 cups	3 cups	3 cups	3.5 cups	3.5 cups	4 cups	4 cups
Grains	3 oz-eq	4 oz-eq	5 oz-eq	5 oz-eg	6 oz-eg	6 oz-eq	7 oz-eq	8 oz-eq	9 oz-eq	10 oz-eq	10 oz-eq	10 oz-eq
Meat and Beans	2 oz-eq	3 oz-eq	4 oz-eq	5 oz-eq	5 oz-eq	5.5 oz-eq	6 oz-eq	6.5 oz-eq	6.5 oz-eq	7 oz-eq	7 oz-eq	7 oz-eq
Milk	2 cups	2 cups	2 cups	3 cups	3 cups	3 cups	3 cups	3 cups	3 cups	3 cups	3 cups	3 cups
Oils	3 tsp	4 tsp	4 tsp	5 tsp	5 tsp	6 tsp	7 tsp	8 tsp	8 tsp	8 tsp	10 tsp	11 tsp
Discretionary calorie allowance	165	171	171	132	195	267	290	362	410	426	512	648

* The suggested amounts of food to consume from the basic food groups, subgroups, and oils to meet recommended nutrient intakes at 12 different calorie levels. Nutrient and energy contributions from each group are calculated according to the nutrient-dense forms of foods in each group (e.g., lean meats and fat-free milk). The table also shows the discretionary calorie allowance that can be accommodated within each calorie level, in addition to the suggested amounts of nutrient-dense forms of foods in each group.

- The oils group is specified in teaspoons and includes fats that are liquid at room temperature, as well as foods that are mainly oils, such as mayonnaise, soft margarine, and certain salad dressings.

The amounts recommended for the MyPyramid food groups are generally similar to those for the FGP at equivalent energy intakes, although there are some important changes that need to be incorporated into nutrition education efforts. One is the increased amounts of fruits and vegetables that are part of the new recommendations: For a 2000-kcal diet, 4.5 cups are recommended, or 9 half-cup servings. Formerly, seven servings were recommended for a 2200-kcal/d diet. Furthermore, many consumers remembered only messages such as "five a day" for fruits and vegetables, a level that was previously recommended for a 1600-kcal/d diet and is now the recommended level for only a 1200 kcal/d children's diet. However, a fluid cup of fruit and vegetable juice is now directly equivalent to a cup of fresh fruits and vegetables, rather than requiring six ounces for a half-cup serving (or 12 ounces as equivalent to an 8-fluid ounce serving).

Another change in the recommended amounts is for the milk group, where all adolescents and adults should consume at least 3 cups/d, as should older children. The former FGP recommended 2 to 3 cups/d for adults. Another change is in the equivalents for nuts and beans, which are now smaller than those for the previous FGP, so more must be consumed to meet the recommended intakes for this food group.

As shown in Table 9, the concept of "discretionary calorie allowance" is now included as part of the MyPyramid food intake information. Discretionary calories are those calories that remain after the recommendations for all of the food groups have been met. Discretionary calories include those from added sugars and those from extra fat (beyond the recommendation for oils and the leanest or lowest-fat options within each of the food groups, such as lean meat or nonfat milk). Any fats (other than oils) or sugars that are added to foods are, by definition, counted as discretionary calories. Food intake patterns for diets of 1600 kcal/d or less have less than 200 discretionary calories—enough for approximately one 12-ounce can of carbonated beverages or the fat in one cup of ice cream.

Although the FGP materials made several recommendations about choices within the food groups, these details have been made more explicit by MyPyramid. As shown in Table 10, specific suggestions for types of vegetables (dark green, orange, legumes, starchy, and "other") are now included, in cups per week. Another explicit recommendation is that at least half of the grains consumed should be whole grains.

MyPyramid Tracker. An interactive website, http://www.MyPyramidtracker.gov, is available for consumers who wish to evaluate their diets in comparison to the MyPyramid recommendations. After entering information on age, gender, physical activity, and body weight, the user selects the foods consumed in a day and portion sizes for each. Then the program calculates food group and nutrient intakes and provides an analysis of the one-day diet. Reports include a nutrient analysis, a comparison of food group consumption against the MyPyramid recommendations, and an evaluation of energy intake. An-

Table 10. MyPyramid Food Intake Pattern Vegetable Subgroup Amounts (in Cups Per Week)

Calorie Level	1000	1200	1400	1600	1800	2000	2200	2400	2600	2800	3000	3200
Dark green veg.	1 c/wk	1.5 c/wk	1.5 c/wk	2 c/wk	3 c/wk	3 c/wk	3 c/wk	3 c/wk	3 c/wk	3 c/wk	3 c/wk	3 c/wk
Orange veg.	0.5 c/wk	1 c/wk	1 c/wk	1.5 c/wk	2 c/wk	2 c/wk	2 c/wk	2 c/wk	2.5 c/wk	2.5 c/wk	2.5 c/wk	2.5 c/wk
Legumes	0.5 c/wk	1 c/wk	1 c/wk	2.5 c/wk	3 c/wk	3 c/wk	3 c/wk	3 c/wk	3.5 c/wk	3.5 c/wk	3.5 c/wk	3.5 c/wk
Starchy veg.	1.5 c/wk	2.5 c/wk	2.5 c/wk	2.5 c/wk	3 c/wk	3 c/wk	6 c/wk	6 c/wk	7 c/wk	7 c/wk	9 c/wk	9 c/wk
Other veg.	3.5 c/wk	4.5 c/wk	4.5 c/wk	5.5 c/wk	6.5 c/wk	6.5 c/wk	7 c/wk	7 c/wk	8.5 c/wk	8.5 c/wk	10 c/wk	10 c/wk

Table 11. Dietary Guidance for Infants and Children Under the Age of Two Years[25]

Guidance	Source
Breastfeeding	
Breastfeeding is the preferred method of infant feeding because of the nutritional value and health benefits of human milk.	AAP, 2004[26]; AAP, 2005[27]
Encourage breastfeeding with exclusion of other foods until infants are around 6 mo of age.[a]	AAP, 2005[27]; WHO, 2002[39]
Continue breastfeeding for first year of life.	AAP, 2004[26]; AAP, 2005[27]
Continue breastfeeding into second year of life if mutually desired by the mother and child.	AAP, 2004[26]; AAP, 2005[27]; AAP 1997[30], ADA, 2004[34]; Kleinman, 2000[37]
Formula Feeding	
For infants who are not currently breastfeeding, use infant formula throughout the first year of life.	AAP, 2004[26]; AAP, 2005[27]; Kleinman, 2000[37]
Infant formula used during the first year of life should be iron-fortified.	AAP, 2004[26]; AAP, 2005[27]; AAP, 1999[32]; ADA, 2004[34]
Infants with specific medical conditions may require medical formula and this should be readily available through projects such as the WIC program.	ADA, 2004[34]
Feeding Other Foods to Infants and Young Children	
Introduce semisolid complementary foods gradually beginning around 6 mo of age.[*]	AAP, 2004[26]; AAP, 2005[27]; Kleinman, 2000[37]; WHO, 2001[38]; WHO, 2002[39]
Introduce single-ingredient complementary foods, one at a time for a several day trial.	AAP, 2004[26]
Introduce a variety of semisolid complementary foods throughout ages 6–12 mo.	WHO, 2001[38]
Encourage consumption of iron-rich complementary foods during ages 6–12 mo.	AAP, 2004[26]; AAP, 2005[27]; AAP, 2001[33]
Avoid introducing fruit juice before 6 mo of age.	AAP, 2004[26]; Kleinman, 2000[37]; AAP, 2001[33]
Limit intake of fruit juice to 4–6 oz/d for children ages 1–6 y.	AAP, 2004[26]; AAP, 2005[27]; AAP, 2001[33]; Kleinman, 2000[37]
Encourage children to eat whole fruits to meet their recommended daily fruit intake.	AAP, 2004[26]; AAP, 2001[33]
Delay the introduction of cow's milk until the second year of life.	AAP, 2004[26]; AAP, 2005[27]; AAP, 1992[29]
Cow's milk fed during the second year of life should be whole milk.	AAP, 1992[28]; AAP, 1998[31]
Developing Healthy Eating Patterns	
Provide children with repeated exposure to new foods to optimize acceptance and encourage development of eating habits that promote selection of a varied diet.	ADA, 1999[35]; ADA, 2004[36]
Prepare complementary foods without added sugars or salt (i.e., sodium).	AAP, 2004[26]
Promote healthy eating early in life.	ADA, 1999[35]; ADA, 2004[36]
Promoting Food Safety	
Avoid feeding hard, small, particulate foods up to age 2–3 y to reduce risk of choking.	AAP, 2004[26]; Kleinman, 2000[37]

[*]There is acknowledged disagreement among experts on the subject of timing of introduction of complementary foods (twenty-six, twenty-seven).

AAP, American Academy of Pediatrics; ADA, American Dietic Association; WHO, World Health Organization.

other section of the tracker allows an evaluation of physical activity in comparison to the recommendations. An energy balance summary uses the information on energy intake and physical activity to graphically show energy balance. A user can track up to 1 year of dietary and physical activity data using the tracker. Several educational opportunities are also included for users who wish more information on specific topics. The website replaces the Interactive Healthy Eating Index website that performed similar analyses using the FGP recommendations.

Dietary Guidance for Children Under Age Two

The information about the Dietary Guidelines and MyPyramid, discussed in the previous sections, applies to individuals ages 2 and older. The information is not meant to be used for infants and children under age 2. Although the DRIs include nutrient standards for infants and young children, they are difficult to translate into food-level dietary guidance. A recent report from the IOM[25] filled this gap by summarizing current guidance, primarily from the American Academy of Pediatrics (Table 11). Recommendations cover breast-feeding and formula feeding, the introduction of other foods, healthy eating patterns, and food safety.

Future Directions

Because advances in nutritional science occur rapidly, dietary standards cannot be static. A review of the Dietary Guidelines for Americans is mandated every 5 years, but no such timeline is specified for the nutrient standards. For example, the first DRIs were set in 1997,[2] and there have been many published studies in the past 9 years that could potentially affect the standards specified in this report (for calcium, phosphorus, magnesium, vitamin D, and fluoride). Thus, a systematic review process that allows periodic revisions of the DRIs should be implemented.

Summary

Dietary standards in the United States continue to evolve as the scientific understanding of the relationship between diet and health improves. Recently revised standards for both nutrient and food intakes are now available and provide a platform for consumer education and other intervention efforts to improve the dietary choices of Americans.

References

1. Food and Nutrition Board, Institute of Medicine. *How Should the Recommended Dietary Allowances Be Revised?* Washington, DC: National Academies Press; 1994.
2. Food and Nutrition Board, Institute of Medicine. *Dietary Reference Intakes for Calcium, Phosphorus, Magnesium, Vitamin D, and Fluoride.* Washington, DC: National Academies Press; 1997.
3. Food and Nutrition Board, Institute of Medicine. *Dietary Reference Intakes for Thiamin, Riboflavin, Niacin, Vitamin B_6, Folate, Vitamin B_{12}, Pantothenic acid, Biotin and Choline.* Washington, DC: National Academies Press; 1998.
4. Food and Nutrition Board, Institute of Medicine. *Dietary Reference Intakes for Vitamin C, Vitamin E, Selenium, and Carotenoids.* Washington, DC: National Academies Press; 2000b.
5. Food and Nutrition Board, Institute of Medicine. *Dietary Reference Intakes for Vitamin A, Vitamin K, Arsenic, Boron, Chromium, Copper, Iodine, Iron, Manganese, Molybdenum, Nickels, Silicon, Vanadium, and Zinc.* Washington, DC: National Academies Press; 2001.
6. Food and Nutrition Board, Institute of Medicine. *Dietary Reference Intakes for Energy, Carbohydrate, Fiber, Fat, Fatty Acidss, Cholesterol, Protein, and Amino Acids.* Washington, DC: National Academies Press; 2002.
7. Food and Nutrition Board, Institute of Medicine. *Dietary Reference Intakes for Water, Potassium, Sodium, Chloride, and Sulfate.* Washington, DC: National Academies Press; 2005.
8. Food and Nutrition Board, Institute of Medicine. *Dietary Reference Intakes. Applications in Dietary Assessment.* Washington, DC: National Academies Press; 2000a.
9. Food and Nutrition Board, Institute of Medicine. *Dietary Reference Intakes. Applications in Dietary Planning.* Washington, DC: National Academies Press; 2003.
10. Carriquiry A. Assessing the prevalence of nutrient adequacy. Public Health Nutr. 1999;2:23–33.
11. Murphy SP. Changes in dietary guidance: implications for food and nutrient databases. J Food Compost Anal. 2001;14:269–278.
12. Murphy SP. Dietary reference intakes for the U.S. and Canada: update on implications for nutrient databases. J Food Compost Anal. 2002;15:411–417.
13. Murphy SP, Barr SI, Poos MI. Using the new dietary reference intakes to assess diets: a map to the maze. Nutr Rev. 2002;60:267–275.
14. Murphy SP. Impact of the new Dietary Reference Intakes on nutrient calculation programs. J Food Compost Anal. 2003;16:365–372.
15. Stumbo PJ, Murphy SP. Simple plots tell a complex story: using the EAR, RDA, AI and UL to evaluate nutrient intakes. J Food Compost Anal. 2004;17: 485–492.
16. Barr SI, Murphy SP, Agurs-Collins T, et al. Planning diets for individuals using the Dietary Reference Intakes. Nutr Rev. 2003;61:352–360.

17. Murphy SP, Barr SI. Challenges in using the DRIs to plan diets for groups. Nutr Rev. In press, 2005.
18. US Department of Health and Human Services, US Department of Agriculture. *Dietary Guidelines for Americans 2005,* 6th ed. HHS Pub. No.: HHS-ODPDP-2005-01-DGA-A. USDA Pub. No.: Home and Garden Bulletin No. 232. Washington, DC: U.S. Government Printing Office; 2005.
19. Dietary Guidelines Advisory Committee. *2005 Dietary Guidelines for Americans.* Available at http://www.health.gov/dietaryguidelines/dga2005/report/.
20. US Department of Health and Human Services, US Department of Agriculture. *Finding Your Way to a Healthier You: Based on the Dietary Guidelines for Americans.* HHS Pub. No.: HHS-ODPDP-2005-01-DGA-B. USDA Pub. No.: Home and Garden Bulletin No. 232-CP. Washington, DC: U.S. Government Printing Office; 2005.
21. US Department of Agriculture. *The Food Guide Pyramid.* Home and Garden Bulletin No. 252. Washington, DC: U.S. Government Printing Office; 1992.
22. MyPyramid. Available at http://www.MyPyramid.gov.
23. Cronin FJ, Shaw AM, Krebs-Smith SM, et al. Developing a food guidance system to implement the Dietary Guidelines. J Nutr Educ. 1987;19:281–301.
24. Welsh SO, Davis C, Shaw A. *USDA's Food Guide.* Background and Development. Human Nutrition Information Service Misc. Pub. No. 1514. Beltsville, MD: Human Nutrition Information Service; 1993.
25. Institute of Medicine. *WIC Food Packages. Time for a Change.* Washington, DC: National Academies Press; 2005.
26. American Academy of Pediatrics. *Pediatric Nutrition Handbook,* Kleinman RE (ed.), 5th ed. Elk Grove Village, IL: American Academy of Pediatrics; 2004.
27. American Academy of Pediatrics. Breastfeeding and the use of human milk. Pediatrics. 2005;115(2):496–506.
28. American Academy of Pediatrics. Committee on Nutrition. Statement on cholesterol. Pediatrics. 1992;90(3):469–473.
29. American Academy of Pediatrics. Committee on Nutrition. The use of whole cow's milk in infancy. Pediatrics. 1992;89:1105–1109.
30. American Academy of Pediatrics. Work Group on Breastfeeding. Breastfeeding and the use of human milk. Pediatrics. 1997;100(6):1035–1039.
31. American Academy of Pediatrics. Committee on Nutrition. Cholesterol in childhood. Pediatrics. 1998;101:141–147.
32. American Academy of Pediatrics. Committee on Nutrition. Iron fortification of infant formulas. Pediatrics. 1999;104:119–123.
33. American Academy of Pediatrics. Committee on Nutrition. The use and misuse of fruit juice in pediatrics. Pediatrics. 2001;107(5):1210–1213.
34. American Academy of Pediatrics. Provisional section on breastfeeding. WIC Program. Pediatrics. 2001; 108(5):1216–1217.
35. American Dietetic Association. Position of the American Dietetic Association: dietary guidance for healthy children aged 2 to 11 years. J Am Diet Assoc. 1999;99:93–101.
36. American Dietetic Associatioin. Position of the American Dietetic Association: dietary guidance for healthy children ages 2 to 11 years. J Am Diet Assoc. 2004;104(4):660–677.
37. Kleinman RE. American Academy of Pediatrics recommendations for complementary feeding. Pediatrics. 2000;106:1274.
38. World Health Organization. *Complementary Feeding: Report of the Global Consultation and Summary of Guiding Principles for Complementary Feeding of the Breastfed Child.* Geneva, Switzerland: World Health Organization; 2001. Accessed March 22, 2005, at http://www.who.int/child-adolescent-health/publications/nutrition/report_cf.htm.
39. World Health Organization. *Report of the Expert Consultation on the Optimal Duration of Exclusive Breastfeeding.* Geneva, Switzerland: World Health Organization; 2002. Accessed March 7, 2005, at http://www.who.int/ nut/documents/optimal_duration_of_exc_bfeeding _report_eng.pdf.

64

International Dietary Standards: FAO and WHO[a]

Christine Lewis Taylor, Janice Albert, Robert Weisell, and Chizuru Nishida

Introduction

This chapter focuses on the work of two specialized agencies of the United Nations—the Food and Agriculture Organization (FAO) and the World Health Organization (WHO)—and their efforts internationally to quantify and in turn recommend levels of intake for essential nutrients, and to promote food-based guidelines to encourage healthy eating patterns. It also highlights the work of the Codex Alimentarius Commission in providing guidelines for the presentation of specific nutrition information on the label of food products.

In its most pragmatic sense, knowledge of human nutrient requirements is essential for assessing whether food supplies are adequate to meet a population's nutritional needs. This information can allow estimation of the numbers of persons globally, regionally, or nationally who may be food or nutrient deficient or at nutritional risk. Such knowledge also underpins the ability to plan for agriculture production and for nutrition interventions such as food fortification. More recently, interest has expanded to include concerns about excess consumption of nutrient substances, as well as dietary choices that may reduce disease risk. Food-based dietary guidelines and efforts to provide nutrition information on food labels are designed to both assist consumers in making better food choices and to support the implementation of nutrition-related health programs.

Throughout history, human societies have observed relationships between the consumption of certain foods and the preservation of good health or the avoidance of disease.[1] However, today's concept of nutrition—that human life depends on a steady intake of a variety of specific dietary substances in defined amounts—is less than 200 years old. During the past 50 years, resources available to developed and industrialized countries such as the United States, the United Kingdom, and many countries in Europe have allowed for expert committees to provide scientific advice on topics related to nutrient requirements and other information important to consumers in order to address public health needs in these regions. The US government, for example, became involved in efforts to ensure an adequate, safe, and nutritious food supply as a function of its role in consumer protection and for the purpose of military readiness. Concomitant with this development was the interest in establishing dietary standards such as recommended nutrient intakes that could guide the decision making for such programs. Specifically, in 1940 the US National Defense Advisory Commission drew attention to malnutrition in the country and its ability to undermine the security of the nation, specifically as it related to healthy recruits for the military.[1] The president in 1941 convened the National Nutrition Conference, which resulted in the first set of Recommended Dietary Allowances as issued by the Food and Nutrition Board. Dietary standards in the United States are covered in a separate chapter (Chapter 63).

International efforts to address food and nutrition issues were a component of the work of the League of Nations during the 1930s, but the United Nations' efforts had their start in 1948, when the Standing Advisory

---

[a]The views expressed in this publication are those of the authors and do not necessarily reflect the views of the Food and Agriculture Organization of the United Nations, the World Health Organization, or the US Food and Drug Administration.

Committee to the newly formed FAO considered that "the problem of assessing the calorie and nutrient requirements of human beings, with the greatest possible degree of accuracy, is of basic importance to FAO."[2] Over time, scientific and technical recommendations about nutrient requirements have been made by expert groups established by the FAO and WHO. In the 1949, when FAO and WHO began their collaborative efforts on nutrition, the FAO/WHO Expert Committee on Nutrition was formed to provide technical advice to the directors general of the two organizations in all areas of nutrition on a regular basis.[3] The outcomes of these discussions have been widely used internationally.

Recent FAO/WHO reports on human nutrient requirements can be accessed on the Internet at http://www.fao.org/es/esn/nutrition/requirements_pubs_en.stm. Listings of past and upcoming FAO/WHO expert meetings are also available at http://www.fao.org/es/esn/nutrition/requirements_en.stm.

Recommended Nutrient Intakes

Macronutrients

Energy and Protein: 1950–99. Although a range of nutrition topics has been covered by expert groups convened by FAO and WHO, macronutrients and in particular energy and protein have received the most attention over the years. This is due to the considerable concern about hunger and food insufficiency that predates the 1950s and continues through the present. More recently, micronutrients and concerns for overnutrition (notably energy intake) have received increasing attention.

Reports focusing solely on energy requirements, or "calorie needs," were issued in 1950, 1957, and 2004. Reports concerning protein requirements were made available in 1957 and 1964. Energy and protein intake recommendations were considered together in reports published in 1973 and 1985. Many of the considerations outlined by these first expert meetings are still pertinent today. They noted that requirements set by experts were intended for groups of persons rather than individuals, and specified that an average requirement can never be compared directly with an individual requirement.

By 1985,[4] a protein requirement of 0.75 g/kg/d for adults had been established. For energy, a new methodology for calculating requirements based on total energy expenditure (TEE) was acknowledged. However, the experts were aware of the limited data overall and the growing need to explore and specify protein and energy requirements.

Energy: 2000–Current. By 2000, scientific understanding related to energy requirements and protein and amino acids had advanced to a stage that independent deliberations were needed. To facilitate two expert meetings, one on energy and one on protein, a series of working groups were assigned to address key issues and present their results as background papers.

An expert meeting on energy requirements was convened in 2001 and addressed the following:

- Calculation of energy requirements for all ages, based on measurements and estimates of total daily energy expenditure and on energy needs for growth, pregnancy, and lactation;
- In the light of new data, modification of the requirements and dietary energy recommendations for infants and for older children and adolescents, to correct previous overestimations of the former and underestimations of the latter;
- Proposals for differentiating the requirements for populations with lifestyles that involve different levels of habitual physical activity starting as early as 6 years of age;
- Reassessment of energy requirements for adults based on energy expenditure estimates expressed as multiples of basal metabolic rates;
- Classification of physical activity levels based on the degree of habitual activity consistent with long-term good health and maintenance of a healthy body weight;
- Recommendations for physical activity for children and adults to maintain fitness and health and to reduce the risk of developing obesity and comorbid diseases associated with a sedentary lifestyle;
- An experimental approach for factorial estimates of energy needs during pregnancy and lactation; and
- Particularly for women in developing countries, the distribution of total recommended additional dietary energy needs within the second and third trimesters of pregnancy.

The meeting report, issued in 2004,[5] contains a considerable level of new information, including requirements based on improved data for TEE, most notably for infants and the elderly. Several components of this energy report are highlighted in Table 1.

Following this meeting, a technical workshop was held to discuss the specific issue of "food energy" because recommendations for optimal energy requirements become practical only when they are related to foods that provide the energy to meet these requirements. The gains in understanding of the digestion and metabolism of food and the increasing sophistication of analytic techniques meant that the various options available to express the energy value of foods needed to be standardized and harmonized. The recommendations of this workshop were published in 2003.[6]

Protein and Amino Acids: 2000–Present. A meeting on protein requirements was held in 2002, and the report from this meeting is in preparation.[7] The earlier 1985 report[4] had specified 0.75 g/kg/d of protein as the "safe protein intake" for adults based on both short- and long-term nitrogen balance data, a value that has been adopted by authoritative bodies around the world. The 2002 discussions (R. Weisell, personal communication) therefore focused considerable attention on the more recent use of

Table 1. Highlights: Energy Recommendations, 2004

Definition of energy requirement	• Amount of food energy needed to balance energy expenditure in order to maintain body size, body composition, and a level of necessary and desirable physical activity consistent with long-term good health • Includes energy needed for optimal growth and development of children, for deposition of tissues during pregnancy, and for secretion of milk during lactation consistent with the good health of mother and child • Recommended level of intake for a population group is the mean energy requirement of the healthy, well-nourished individuals who constitute that group.
Population groups specified	• Infants from birth to 12 months • Children and adolescents • Adults • Pregnant Women • Lactating Women
Example: Adults	• Estimated requirements provided on basis of total energy expenditure for three levels of activity • Requirements calculated from factorial estimates of habitual total energy expenditure further specified for gender, age range, mean weight, and mean basal metabolic rate • Noted that growth is no longer an energy-demanding factor and basal metabolic rate is relatively constant among population groups of a given age and gender
Example: Infants from birth to 12 months	• Estimated requirements provided on basis of monthly age and gender • Requirements calculated by adding energy deposited in growing tissues (i.e., energy needs for growth) to total energy expenditure

Used with permission from Food and Agriculture Organization of the United Nations, 2004.[5]

stable isotopic techniques that may replace nitrogen balance in assessing protein, and notably amino acid, requirements. Specific information on the newest protein and amino acid requirements must await the publication of the report, but it can be noted that the approach used during the meeting to estimate requirements: 1) considered all available studies, 2) used 24-hour measurements of amino acid oxidation when such data were available 3) used isotopic studies when 24-hour measurements were not available, and 4) used nitrogen balance and plasma amino acid measures as supportive data. However, the experts were handicapped by the limited nature of the available data for infants and children and could reach no consensus for amino acid requirements for these subpopulations. However, considerable new data for pregnancy and lactation produced significant changes from the 1985 report.

Fats and Oils. Although FAO and WHO have devoted considerable resources to energy and protein requirements, other macronutrients have also been the subject of expert meetings. Nutritional needs for dietary fats and oils were addressed during meetings in 1977[8] and 1993.[9] Both expert groups found it necessary to develop recommendations for poorer populations whose diets may lack sufficient fat and for more affluent populations who may experience health risks related to excessive consumption of fat.

In addition to the key recommendations highlighted in Table 2, the report of the last meeting noted the importance of periodic surveys of adult weight status (as body mass index [BMI]) in all countries to identify trends and specific populations at greatest nutritional risk, as well as the risk, for diet-related noncommunicable diseases.

Carbohydrates. Recommendations concerning carbohydrates in human nutrition were first issued in 1980.[10] A second expert meeting was held and a report issued in 1998.[11] The report continued the discussions begun in 1980, but also focused on the role of carbohydrates in the maintenance of health and in disease reduction. Further, it included a section on goals and guidelines for carbohydrate food choices. Discussions are under way to determine the best approach to update the recommendations on carbohydrates.

Several key points from the 1998 report are listed in Table 3. The report specified terminology and classification nomenclature for carbohydrate components and encouraged the production and consumption of root crops and pulses. Discussions focused not only on the maintenance of health and reduction of disease risk, but also on glycemic index, which was regarded as a potentially useful

Table 2. Highlights: Fats and Oils Recommendations, 1994

Minimum desirable intake: Adults	• For most adults, dietary fat should supply at least 15% of energy intake. • Women of reproductive age should consume at least 20% of energy from fat. • Concerted efforts should be made to ensure adequate consumption of dietary fat among populations where less than 15% of dietary energy supply is from fat.
Infant and young child feeding	• Infants should be fed breast milk if at all possible. • Fatty acid composition of infant formulas should correspond to the amount and proportion of fatty acids contained in breast milk. • During weaning and at least until 2 years of age, a child's diet should contain 30% to 40% of energy from fat and provide similar levels of essential fatty acids as are found in breast milk.
Upper limits for fat/oil intakes	• Active individuals who are in energy balance may consume up to 35% of their total energy intake from dietary fat if their intake of essential fatty acids and other nutrients is adequate and the level of saturated fatty acids does not exceed 10% of the energy they consume. • Sedentary individuals should not consume more than 30% of their energy from fat, particularly if it is high in saturated fatty acids that are derived primarily from animal sources.
Saturated and unsaturated fatty acids and cholesterol	• Intakes of saturated fatty acids should provide no more than 10% of energy. • Desirable intakes of linoleic acid should provide between 4% and 10% of energy. • Intakes in the upper end of this range are recommended when intakes of saturated fatty acids and cholesterol are relatively high. • Reasonable restriction of dietary cholesterol (less than 300 mg/day) is advised.
Other recommendations in the report	• Isomeric fatty acids • Antioxidants and carotenoids • Essential fatty acids

Used with permission from Food and Agriculture Organization of the United Nations, 1994.[9]

indicator of the impact of foods on the blood glucose response. Further, the report text notes there is no evidence of a direct involvement of sucrose, other sugars, or starch in the etiology of lifestyle-related diseases.

Vitamins and Minerals

The human requirements for vitamins, minerals, and trace elements have been the subject of several FAO/WHO expert meetings. Calcium was reviewed in 1956 and 1961. An expert meeting was held in 1965 on vitamin A, thiamin, riboflavin, and niacin, and in 1969 a meeting focused on ascorbic acid, vitamin D, vitamin B_{12}, folate, and iron. Vitamin A, iron, folate, and vitamin B_{12} were reviewed again in 1985, the first two because they were major nutritional public health problems and the latter two because of their close association with anemia. Specific citations for these reports can be found on the Internet at http://www.fao.org/es/esn/nutrition/requirements_en.stm.

WHO convened the first expert group on trace elements in 1973.[12] By 1990, additional information regarding the role and importance of many trace elements had come to light, and a second expert consultation on trace elements was held under the auspices of FAO and WHO as well as the International Atomic Energy Agency.[13] This group attempted to ensure a reasonable degree of uniformity in the analysis and presentation of the many nutrients considered. A notable conclusion was that trace element requirements can change according to the type and amount of food consumed, interrelationships with other nutrients, and the nutritional status of the individual.

In 1998, a joint FAO/WHO expert consultation on human vitamin and mineral requirements was held in Bangkok.[14] This expert group met to deliberate on all vitamins and minerals in the human diet and to derive recommendations about levels of intake that were specified as Recommended Nutrient Intakes (RNIs). These values were based on the available scientific evidence, although a number of issues for various nutrients were left unresolved, largely because of difficulties in data interpretation. The report itself was delayed in publication due

Table 3. Highlights: Carbohydrate Recommendations, 1998

Definition of Carbohydrate	Carbohydrates are polyhydroxy aldehydes, ketones, alcohols, acids, their simple derivatives, and their polymers having linkages of the acetal type. They may be classified according to their degree of polymerization and may be divided initially into three principal groups: sugars, oligosaccharides, and polysaccharides.
Role in Maintenance of Health	Optimal diet of at least 55% of total energy from a variety of carbohydrate sources for all ages except for children under the age of 2. Fat should not be specifically restricted below the age of 2 years. Optimal diet should be gradually introduced beginning at 2 years of age.
Role in Disease Risk Reduction	• The bulk of carbohydrate-containing foods consumed should be those rich in non-starch polysaccharides and with a low glycemic index. Appropriately processed cereals, vegetables, legumes, and fruits are particularly good food choices. • Excess energy intake in any form will cause body fat accumulation, so that excess consumption of low-fat foods, while not as obesity-producing as excess consumption of high-fat products, will lead to obesity if energy expenditure is not increased. Excessive intakes of sugars that compromise micronutrient density should be avoided.

Used with permission from Food and Agriculture Organization of the United Nations, 1998.[11]

primarily to controversy related to final agreement about the recommendations for some of the nutrient substances.

Further, the foreword to the meeting report highlights the question as to whether changes in recommended intakes for vitamins and minerals are due to better scientific knowledge and understanding of the biochemical role of the nutrients, or whether the criteria for setting the levels of the requirements have changed. The report foreword also suggests that while RNIs for vitamins and minerals were initially established on the understanding that they are meant to meet the basic nutritional needs of over 97% of the population, a fundamental criterion in industrialized countries has become one of the presumptive role that these nutrients may play in the "prevention" of an increasing range of disease conditions that characterize these populations. According to the foreword, the latter approach implies the notion of "optimal nutrition" relative to recommended intakes. Further, it notes that questions have been raised as to whether some of the developments in approaches to establishing recommended intakes are applicable to developing country populations. The foreword also acknowledges that from an international perspective, the RNIs for several if not many micronutrients such as folate, vitamin A, and selenium will need to be re-evaluated as soon as significant additional data become available.

The tables listing the RNIs for minerals and for water- and fat-soluble vitamins issued as a result of this meeting, as well as estimated average requirements (EARs) for several nutrients, can be found in the meeting report on the Internet at http://www.fao.org/es/esn/nutrition/requirements_pubs_en.stm.

FAO and WHO are planning efforts to continue work to update the requirements for vitamins and minerals. Moreover, in 2002, FAO provided a report to the Codex Committee on Nutrition and Foods for Special Dietary> Uses (http://www.codexalimentarius.net/web/archives.jsp?year=03; select Alinorm 3/26A at paragraph 119). This committee works under the mandate of the Codex Alimentarius, an international food standards-setting organization. The report responds to an earlier communication from the Commission of Codex Alimentarius on behalf of the Committee requesting that FAO and WHO work, under their mandate to provide scientific advice to Codex committees, to include upper levels of intake for vitamins and minerals in their future efforts to develop recommended nutrient intakes. The FAO report specifies the intent to produce a general technical document outlining the principles to be adopted in addressing the topic of upper levels of intake and the safety of specific vitamins and minerals. In 2004, FAO and WHO announced a joint effort to develop a framework for establishing upper levels of intake of nutrients and related substances, and a report from a workshop on the topic was issued in early 2006 (http://www.who.int/ipcs/methods/en/).

Food-Based Dietary Guidelines

Quantitative recommendations for the intake of nutrient substances provide the nutritional goals needed to ensure the health of populations. However, in a pragmatic sense, it is difficult for consumers to apply this information when selecting foods and planning meals. In short, there is a need to transform such quantitative recommendations into general advice about dietary choices.

However, while international recommendations on nutrient needs provide critical information for the development of dietary guidelines, an international set of dietary guidelines is not feasible or practical. The types of foods available differ among regions and countries, and foods vary in their nutritional content. The vast differences in food availability and accessibility, coupled with differences in lifestyles, cultures, and public health priorities, mean that national authorities are in the best position to establish dietary guidelines suitable for their population and for their food supply. For this reason, international organizations such as FAO and WHO have as their goal the support of national and regional efforts to develop food-based dietary guidelines (FBDGs). The discussion here focuses on guidelines targeted to the general public, but separate dietary guidelines are at times developed for segments of the population with specific nutritional needs, such as infants and young children, as well as for persons with disease conditions such as autoimmune deficiency, hypertension, and diabetes.

In brief, the purpose of FBDG is to assist the targeted population in implementing nutrition and related health recommendations. Such guidelines present information using language and symbols that the public can easily understand. They usually focus on common foods, portion sizes, and behaviors. A complementary objective of developing FBDGs is to provide a tool for nutrition education to be used by health providers, teachers, journalists, extension agents, and others working directly with the public.

FAO and WHO Promotion of FBDGs

FAO and WHO have promoted the concept of FBDGs during the past decade. They jointly sponsored the International Conference on Nutrition (ICN) in 1992.[15] During the ICN, 159 nations endorsed the World Declaration and Plan of Action for Nutrition, which called upon governments to promote appropriate diets and healthy lifestyles. In 1995, FAO and WHO sponsored the "Expert Consultation on the Preparation and Use of Food-Based Dietary Guidelines" in Cyprus,[16] which reviewed experiences and elaborated a process for developing FBDGs. After the consultation, FAO and WHO promoted the development of FBDGs through their regional offices and institutions. In collaboration with the International Life Sciences Institute, FAO held a number of regional workshops on dietary guidelines,[17] and WHO developed several regional FBDGs that countries in those regions could use, adapting to each country's situation. In 2005, FAO and WHO began to assess the status of FBDG development and implementation. The following discussions reflect observations noted during these ongoing assessment activities, as well as experiences of experts in technical assistance projects and regional workshops.

Common Components of the FBDGs

Although existing FBDGs often appear to be similar, they usually have been developed to meet the specific needs of a nation's population and to suit the cultural, social, and economic contexts. The food graphics associated with FBDGs are highly promoted and may become important symbols in a nation's nutrition communication and education strategy.

General Characteristics of FBDGs. Existing FBDGs from countries throughout the world share certain commonalities:

- All promote consumption of a variety of foods.
- All promote maintenance of a healthy weight.
- All encourage increased consumption of fruits and vegetables.
- Most encourage lowering consumption of salt.
- Most encourage lowering consumption of sugar.
- Most encourage physical activity.
- Some specify types of fats and discourage consumption of saturated fats.
- Some specify carbohydrates and encourage consumption of whole grain products.
- Some encourage increased consumption of water.
- Some mention specific nutrients.

In countries where deficiencies in iron, vitamin A, and/or iodine are common, the FBDGs may address these nutritional problems. In some countries, FBDGs contain recommendations that reflect societal values and may be intended to motivate positive behaviors that have an indirect impact on diets and health. For example, some FBDGs encourage meals as social occasions. Some promote the consumption of local or traditional foods. Some emphasize family life, love, and well-being. Many FBDGs contain negative messages such as discouraging smoking. It is common for FBDGs to encourage moderation in alcohol consumption. Some guidelines contain information about food preparation and food safety.

Graphics to Convey the Message of Variety. Although the importance of consuming a variety of foods is easily appreciated by nutritionists, the concept of variety is often misunderstood by consumers. Many countries have used illustrations as part of FBDGs to convey the concept of variety. The graphics attempt to specify types of foods, proportions of foods, and portion sizes organized according to cultural perceptions.[18] Examples of FBDG graphics can be found on the FAO Food and Nutrition website at http://www.fao.org/es/esn/nutrition/education_guidelines_country_en.stm.

As appropriate, the graphics take different forms and usually have social significance for the population; for example, patriotic symbols may be used. Although the text and graphics are designed to be used together, some FBDG graphics appear alone on packages and posters. Therefore, consumer testing should be carried out to ensure that the graphic is interpreted accurately.

Process for Developing FBDGs

FBDGs are usually created through a comprehensive process that includes assurances that the recommendations are understood and feasible for the average consumer and widely supported by the various government agencies, professional societies, and food industry and consumer associations. The development of FBDGs follows a series of steps, each of which requires different types of activities and expertise. The process of developing

FBDGs may take several years and should include the following activities:

- Planning with multisectoral committee,
- Characterization of target group(s),
- Setting nutrition and health objectives,
- Preparing technical guidelines,
- Testing feasibility of recommendations,
- Preparing FBDGs,
- Validation of recommendations and food graphic,
- Implementation, and
- Evaluation.

Some aspects of this process are discussed below.

Multisectoral Planning Committees. Initiatives to establish FBDGs have been taken by government agencies (e.g., health ministry, agriculture ministry, social welfare agency), professional societies (e.g., nutrition society, medical association), universities and nutrition institutes, international agencies, and private organizations sponsored by the food industry.[17] Regardless of the source of the initiative for the FBDGs, all stakeholders must be invited to participate in the process at an early stage.

To ensure support for the FBDGs, a multisector, interdisciplinary committee should be established with representatives from sectors such as agriculture, health, and education, as well as experts in communication and food and nutrition science. Representatives of the food industry and consumer associations may be invited to participate. Failure to involve important stakeholders may cause delays in approval of the guidelines and poor implementation, as has been the case in several countries.

Specifying the Scientific and Health Basis for FBDGs. To be credible, FBDGs should be based on the best scientific evidence available. Data are required to identify nutrition issues that have a significant influence on public health, estimate the magnitude and severity of these problems, distinguish subgroups within the population that face higher risks, and set priorities for interventions in the health, agriculture, and education sectors.

A technical committee should be convened to identify the data needs and compile and analyze the data used to formulate the recommendations for the general population, as well as subgroups within the population. A range of data sources can be consulted to establish the scientific basis for the FBDGs, including health statistics, nutrition surveys, national census data, household expenditure surveys, food consumption surveys, physical activity assessments, nutrient requirement recommendations, food composition tables, and the scientific literature on diet and health relationships.[19,20]

It is not uncommon to find that the data available are not sufficient or that it is difficult to combine data sets from different sources. For example, data collected for a different purpose may be incomplete or too limited in scope. Large data sets, which are time-consuming and costly to acquire, are not collected often and may be out of date. Further, the food supply in some countries may change significantly if food policies and economic and political situations change.

The process of identifying the objectives for the FBDGs can lead to the recognition that more information is needed, and this may stimulate new data collection and research. However, weaknesses in data should not become an obstacle for developing FBDGs or a reason for postponing the process. When local information is not available, observations from similar countries in a region and information from the international scientific literature can be used to initiate the process.

Usability of FBDGs. The proposed FBDGs should be tested to ensure that ordinary people can follow the advice. Recommendations can be evaluated for utility through focus group research and surveys of different audiences to ensure that they are comprehensible, clear, and realistic.

FBDGs are generally most useful if the recommendations are short, simple, uncomplicated, and memorable. Clearly, each set of national recommendations must take into consideration the range of social and economic conditions within the population. Countries with many ethnic groups, languages, and religions should ensure that recommendations are appropriate for all groups within the population. In general, recommendations to encourage the consumption of foods that are more costly, perishable, or seasonal are unlikely to be followed because many households do not have access to the foods. Therefore, FBDGs should offer options so that individuals with different needs and lifestyles find the advice to be relevant. Convenience and food preparation time are often determinants of food choices, especially in urban settings.

Implementation of FBDGs. The most common methods for disseminating the guidelines focus on providing materials and training through the health and education systems. For instance, schoolteachers may incorporate FBDGs into their classroom curricula, and nurses and home economists can make use of them during counseling sessions. FBDGs are also widely distributed to the target population in the form of brochures, posters, or radio or television messages. It is best also to provide related educational materials and programs to elaborate and explain the guidelines to support the FBDGs. Further, messages should be reinforced by using a number of channels of communication. Regional and national mass media campaigns should ensure coordinated and consistent dissemination of the messages.

Common obstacles to promoting FBDGs are lack of expertise in communication strategies and lack of resources for producing materials. Some countries have procedures for obtaining and approving sponsorship of materials and activities by the private sector. This allows for the promotion of nutrition messages and food guides on food packages or through other communication channels.

Evaluation of FBDGs. Clearly, campaigns and educational programs for the promotion and adoption of FBDGs should be monitored and evaluated to determine their reach, frequency, and impact. However, relatively few countries have evaluated the impact of FBDGs, either because the guidelines were developed only recently and it is too early to evaluate their effects or because the resources and methodologies for evaluation are lacking. Nonetheless, more studies on the impact and effectiveness of the guidelines in assisting individuals to change nutrition behaviors are needed.

Status of Worldwide FBDG Development

Although nearly half of the countries in the world have developed some type of dietary guidelines, there is relatively little information about such guidelines in the published literature. Searches of databases and the Internet, as well as an FAO survey and related WHO work, have identified 125 countries that appear to have put in place some type of dietary guidelines or are in the process of developing them. However, limited accessibility and lack of translations make it difficult to assess the exact types of advice being provided. For some countries, information about dietary guidelines may be found on the Internet in the national language, most often within the health authority website. As noted above, examples of FBDGs can be found on the Internet at http://www.fao.org/es/esn/nutrition/education_guidelines_en.stm. FAO and WHO are collecting more information on dietary guidelines, which will be posted on the FAO and WHO websites.

Most western European governments and nutrition societies have provided dietary guidance since the early 1990s.[17,21] Scientists have published articles about different facets of dietary guidelines in Denmark, Greece, Germany, France, Ireland, the United Kingdom, Spain, and the Netherlands. More recently, the Czech Republic, Hungary, Slovenia, Latvia, and Turkey have elaborated national guidelines, and other countries in eastern Europe are preparing guidelines. For some European countries, the guidelines from WHO's Countrywide Integrated Non-communicable Diseases Intervention (http://www.phac-aspc.gc.ca/ccdpc-cpcmc/cindi/index_e.html) have been used as a basis to draft their FBDGs. Another effort, the "Nutrition and Diet for Healthy Lifestyles in Europe" project, also known as "Eurodiet," was conceived to develop and implement a Europe-wide set of dietary guidelines.[22]

In the Americas, most countries have developed dietary guidelines.[17] In North America, Health Canada has produced "Canada's Guidelines for Healthy Eating and Physical Activity" (http://www.hc-sc.gc.ca/fn-an/food-guide-aliment/index_e.html). The US dietary guidelines are described in a separate chapter elsewhere in this publication (Chapter 63). Mexico and Venezuela were among the first Latin American countries to publish FBDGs in the early 1990s. Notably, Chile and Guatemala have conducted substantial research on the impact of FBDGs.[23-26]

In Asia and the Pacific, most countries have national FBDGs, and some countries use regional guidelines. India and the Philippines developed FBDGs in the late 1980s and early 1990s, respectively. Thailand has carried out extensive work in developing and testing FBDGs.[27] Information about the FBDGs in Australia is available on the Internet at http://www.nhmrc.gov.au/publications/synopses/dietsyn.htm. Similarly, Japan has information available in English on the Internet at http://www.dietitian.or.jp/english/jp_health_nutrition/dietary_guidelines-s.html.

Among African countries, Namibia, Nigeria, and South Africa have published FBDGs, and a number of other countries report that guidelines are under preparation. South Africans have also published information about the process of developing their FBDGs.[28]

In the Near East, nutrition assessments have been carried out, but FBDGs have not been completed. In December 2004, experts from Bahrain, Egypt, Iran, Jordan, Kuwait, Lebanon, and Pakistan met and agreed to expedite preparation of FBDGs,[29] particularly in light of updated population nutrient intake goals recommended by a joint WHO/FAO expert consultation,[30] a strengthened commitment for implementing national food and nutrition plans and policies, and a report (as described below) on reducing risks and promoting healthy life[30] and resulting health strategies.

Finally, although it is generally desirable to develop national guidelines, this is not always practical or possible. Therefore, at times, regional guidelines have been created to serve populations with similar public health problems and diets within a geographic area. For example, the Caribbean Food and Nutrition Institute, a specialized center of the Pan American Health Organization, has provided recommendations that are used throughout the English-speaking Caribbean. Extensive health advice and regional guidelines have been developed for the Pacific Island countries by the Secretariat of the Pacific Community.[31]

Role of the WHO Global Strategy on Diet, Physical Activity, and Health

In 2003, a report from a joint expert consultation on diet, nutrition, and the prevention of chronic diseases was released.[30] This report describes how, in most countries, a few major risk factors account for much of the morbidity and mortality. It specifies that unhealthy diets and physical inactivity are thus among the leading causes of the major non-communicable diseases. In response to a request from member states through a resolution of the World Health Assembly held in 2002, WHO developed the Global Strategy on Diet, Physical Activity, and Health. It was endorsed by the World Health Assembly in 2004. Specific information about this activity is available on the Internet at http://www.who.int/dietphysicalactivity/strategy/eb11344/strategy_english_web.pdf.

The strategy specifies recommendations for populations and individuals intended to: 1) assist in reducing the risk factors for non-communicable diseases stemming from diet and physical activity, 2) increase awareness of the influences of diet and physical activity on health, 3) encourage development of appropriate policies, and 4) monitor scientific data and influences on diet and physical activity. The strategy serves the important purpose of encouraging the development of FBDGs but is not itself an FBDG. Rather, as a component of its recommendations on national policies and action plans, it stipulates that governments are encouraged to draw up national dietary guidelines, taking account of evidence from national and international sources.

Population Nutrient Intake Goals

Population nutrient intake goals, as originally formulated by the WHO Study Group,[32] represent the population average intakes of recognized dietary components and certain food categories that are "judged to be consistent with the maintenance of health in a population. Health, in this context, is marked by a low prevalence of diet-related diseases in the population."[30,32] However, it should be noted that the concept of population nutrient intake goals is based on the assumption that the first priority is to ensure the adequacy of the total food supply at the national level and equity of distribution of the available food in accordance with individual needs. The fundamental focus of the approach for developing these goals is the population as an entity. The population nutrient intake goals are designed to address the situation in which the total intake of energy is reasonably appropriate, but the balance of macronutrients is inappropriate and is a major contributing cause of diet-related chronic diseases in a given population.

There is of course no single "best value" for such a goal. Instead, consistent with the concept of a safe range of nutrient intakes for individuals, there is often a range of population averages that would assist with the maintenance of health. Thus, as highlighted in a 1990 report that first identified these dietary goals,[32] the basis for the population nutrient intake goals is the entire distribution of intakes as reflected by the average per-capita intake. The original goals have been recently reviewed and updated.[30,33] These most recent deliberations underscored the differences between population nutrient intake goals and nutrient requirements for groups of individuals, emphasizing that population nutrient intake goals need to be translated into a national and local context.

For these reasons, the population nutrient intake goals presented in Table 4 are expressed as ranges for each dietary factor. They represent, in brief, desirable intakes that support optimal nutrition and health. If existing population averages fall outside this range, or trends in intake suggest that the population average will move outside the range, health concerns are likely to arise. It would be of notable concern if a large proportion of values were outside of the defined goals.

Table 4. Ranges of Population Nutrient Intake Goals

Dietary Factor	Goals (% of total energy,unless otherwise stated)
Total fat	15% to 30%
Saturated fatty acids	<10%
Polyunsaturated fatty acids (PUFAs)	6% to 10%
n-6 Polyunsaturated fatty acids (PUFAs)	5% to 8%
n-3 Polyunsaturated fatty acids (PUFAs)	1% to 2%
Trans fatty acids	<1%
Monounsaturated fatty acids (MUFAs)	By difference*
Total carbohydrate†	55% to 75%
Free sugars‡	<10 %
Protein	10% to 15%§
Cholesterol	<300 mg/d
Sodium chloride (sodium)¶	<5 g/d(<2 g/d)
Fruits and vegetables	≥400 g/d
Total dietary fiber	From foods#
Non-starch polysaccharides (NSP)	From foods#

* Refers to "total fat – (saturated fatty acids + polyunsaturated fatty acids + trans fatty acids)"
† The percentage of total energy available after taking into account that consumed as protein and fat, hence the wide range.
‡ The term "free sugars" refers to all monosaccharides and disaccharides added to foods by the manufacturer, cook, or consumer, plus sugars naturally present in honey, syrups, and fruit juices.
§ The suggested range should be seen in the light of the Joint WHO/FAO/UNU Expert Consultation on Protein and Amino Acid Requirements in Human Nutrition, held in Geneva April 9–16, 2002. (WHO. *Protein and Amino Acid Requirements in Human Nutrition*. Report of a joint FAO/WHO/UNU Expert Consultation. WHO Technical Report Series, Geneva [in press]).
¶ Salt should be iodized appropriately (WHO/UNICEF/ICCIDD. *Recommended Iodine Levels in Salt and Guidelines for Monitoring Their Adequacy and Effectiveness*. Unpublished document, WHO/NUT/96.13. Geneva, 1996).
# Dietary fiber is expressed as non-starch polysaccharides (NSP). The recommended intake of fruits and vegetables (i.e., ≥400 g/d) and consumption of whole-grain foods is likely to provide >20 g/d of NSP (i.e., >25 g/d of total dietary fiber).

Nutrition Labeling of Packaged Foods: Codex Alimentarius

Codex Alimentarius is an international program intended to facilitate international food trade and guide the food industry while also protecting the consumer. It functions under the auspices of its parent organizations, FAO and WHO. Codex's role is expanding for reasons related to agreements established by the World Trade Organization, one of which[34] incorporates Codex food safety standards and guidelines, indicating that Codex documents reflect international consensus. Codex member countries designate delegates to each of the various standing committees operating under Codex; the delegates work to develop the standards and guidelines through a consensus-building process. The resulting Codex documents are not binding on member countries and do not supersede existing regional and national policies, but they are clearly influential. They serve to harmonize activities related to food trade and are widely used by countries that lack resources to develop their policies. The Codex Committee on Food Labelling (CCFL) meets annually and issues documents relevant to the labeling of packaged foods in international trade. The guidelines from this committee include those for the nutrition labeling of foods.

Nutrition labeling is relevant to the Codex mandate in that it serves to "protect" consumers by informing them about the nutritional content of foods, so that in combination with educational efforts, it can promote appropriate and healthy food choices. It also encourages manufacturers to formulate nutritious foods consistent with dietary recommendations. However, guidelines on nutrition labeling also facilitate trade in food by reducing national regulatory barriers relative to the requirements for such labeling. Again, such guidelines do not replace national provisions for such labeling, but instead have been developed to be sufficiently flexible and generalized so as to be harmonious with as many existing national provisions as possible.

CCFL guidelines on nutrition labeling can be found on the Internet at http://www.fao.org/documents/show_cdr.asp?url_file=/DOCREP/005/Y2770E/y2770e06.htm. As specified by Codex Alimentarius, the purpose of the guidelines is to ensure that: 1) nutrition labeling is effective; 2) nutrition labeling does not describe a product or present information about it that is in any way false, misleading, deceptive, or insignificant in any manner; and 3) no nutritional claims are made without nutrition labeling. The guidelines include principles for nutrition and key definitions. Notably, a "nutrient" is defined as any substance normally consumed as a constituent of food that provides energy or that is needed for growth, development, and maintenance of life, or a deficit of which will cause characteristic biochemical or physiologic changes to occur.

Under the current guidelines, nutrient declarations are identified as "should be mandatory" for foods for which nutrition claims are made ("nutrition claim" means any representation that states, suggests, or implies that a food has particular nutritional properties including, but not limited to, the energy value and to the content of protein, fat, and carbohydrates, as well as the content of vitamins and minerals [Section 2.4 of Codex Guidelines on Nutrition Labelling]). Nutrient declarations are regarded as voluntary if no claim is made. Given the growing interest in the use of nutrition labeling to assist in efforts to reduce chronic disease and promote the health of many populations, there have been discussions about changing the provisions so that they are mandatory even without the presence of a claim on the food label. However, CCFL has not specified this change in its existing guidelines.

Those nutrient declarations that constitute the mandatory declaration (i.e., should be present when a nutritional claim is made) are as follows:

- Energy value;
- Amount of protein, available carbohydrate, and fat;
- Amount of any other nutrient for which a claim is made; and
- Amount of any other nutrient considered to be relevant for maintaining a good nutritional status, as required by national legislation.

The guidelines further clarify the methods for determining these substances in food (including relevant components such as types of fatty acids and types of carbohydrates) and prescribe the nature of the listing. They also indicate that vitamins and minerals may be listed according to "the criteria" that only vitamins and minerals for which recommended intakes have been established and/or are of nutritional importance in the country concerned should be declared. It specifies that when nutrient declarations occur, only those vitamins and minerals that are present in significant amounts should be listed (a footnote is included to indicate that, as a rule, 5% of the recommended constitutes a significant amount).

Quantitative declarations on the label are to be made on the basis of portion size for the purposes of providing nutrient information to consumers. The amounts of energy, protein, carbohydrate, and fat (declared numerically as grams or milliters, or as kilojoules per kilometer for energy) are to be listed per 100 g or 100 mL portion on the label, or per package if the package contains only a single portion. In addition, the information may be given "per serving" as specified on the label, provided that the number of servings contained in the package is stated.

Numeric information on vitamins and minerals is to be expressed in metric units and/or as a percentage of the Nutrient Reference Value using the same provisions for portion size or serving as identified above. The Codex guidelines make use of the Nutrient Reference Values established for the purposes of food labeling in 1988 during an expert consultation held in Helsinki.[35] These values are regarded by many as in need of updating, but such activities have not yet begun. The existing Nutrient Reference Values are listed within the guidelines, and include values for protein, vitamin A, vitamin D, vitamin C, thiamin, riboflavin, niacin, vitamin B_6, folic acid, vitamin B_{12}, calcium, magnesium, iron, zinc, and iodine.

Discussions are in progress to revise aspects of the nutrition labeling guidelines, ranging from the numbers and types of nutrients declared to the criteria for "significant amount" of a nutrient. As these revisions are developed, they move through the steps of the Codex process until they are adopted at the highest step and accepted by the Codex Alimentarius Commission. Reports of the CCFL meetings can be found on the Internet at http://www.codexalimentarius.net/web/archives.jsp?year=05.

Relevant to nutrition labeling, CCFL has also issued guidelines for the use of nutrition claims (http://www.fao.org/documents/show_cdr.asp?url_file=/DOCREP/005/Y2770E/y2770e07.htm), including what some have referred to as nutrient content claims. Also, provisions for health claims are under discussion by CCFL. Key aspects of developing such guidelines focus on the scientific basis for health claims and, in turn, the definition for a health claim, given that the approach to this concept differs greatly from one country to another.

References

1. US Department of Health and Human Services. *The Surgeon General's Report on Nutrition and Health.* Public Health Service, Department of Health and Human Services. DHHS No. 88–50210. Washington DC, 1988.
2. Food and Agriculture Organization. *Calorie Requirements.* Report of the Committee on Calorie Requirements. FAO Nutritional Studies No. 5, Washington DC, 1950.
3. World Health Organizatoin. *Report of the First Joint FAO/WHO Expert Committee on Nutrition.* Geneva, 1949.
4. World Health Organization. *Energy and Protein Requirements.* Report of a Joint FAO/WHO/UNU Expert Consultation. WHO Technical Report Series 724, Geneva, 1985.
5. Food and Agriculture Organization. *Human Energy Requirements.* Report of a Joint FAO/WHO/UNU Expert Consultation. FAO Food and Nutrition Technical Report Series No. 1, Rome, 2004.
6. Food and Agriculture Organization. *Food Energy—Methods of Analysis and Conversion Factors.* Report of a Technical Workshop. FAO Food and Nutrition Paper 77, Rome, 2003.
7. World Health Organization. *Protein and Amino Acid Requirements in Human Nutrition.* Report of a joint FAO/WHO/UNU Expert Consultation. WHO Technical Report Series, Geneva (in preparation).
8. Food and Agriculture Organization. *Dietary Fats and Oils in Human Nutrition.* Joint FAO/WHO Report. FAO Food and Nutrition Paper 3, Rome, 1977.
9. Food and Agriculture Organization. *Fats and Oils in Human Nutrition.* Report of a Joint Expert Consultation. FAO Food and Nutrition Paper 57, Rome, 1994.
10. Food and Agriculture Organization. *Carbohydrates in Human Nutrition.* Joint FAO/WHO Report. FAO Food and Nutrition Paper 15, Rome, 1980.
11. Food and Agriculture Organization. *Carbohydrates in Human Nutrition.* Report of the Joint FAO/WHO Expert Consultation. FAO Food and Nutrition Paper 66, Rome, 1998.
12. World Health Orqanization. *Trace Elements in Human Nutrition.* Report of a WHO Expert Committee. WHO Technical Report Series No 532. Geneva, 1973.
13. World Health Organization. *Trace Elements in Human Nutrition.* Report of a Joint FAO/WHO/IAEA Expert Consultation. WHO Technical Report Series, WHO, Geneva, 1996.
14. Food and Agriculture Organization. *Human Vitamin and Mineral Requirements.* Report of a Joint FAO/WHO Expert Consultation. FAO/WHO non-series publication, Rome, 2002.
15. Food and Agriculture Organization/World Health Organization. *World Declaration on Nutrition and Plan of Action for Nutrition.* Final Report of the International Conference on Nutrition. Rome, 1992.
16. World Health Organization. *Preparation and Use of Food-Based Dietary Guidelines.* Report of a Joint FAO/WHO Consultation. WHO Technical Report Series 880, Geneva, 1998.
17. Food and Agriculture Organization. *Food-Based Dietary Guidelines: Review of Countries' Experiences.* Unpublished document, Rome, 2004.
18. Painter J, Rah JH, Lee YK. Comparison of international food guide pictorial representations. J Am Diet Assoc. 2002;102:483–489.
19. Branca F. *Health Information.* Istituto Nazionale della Nutrizione, Rome. Unpublished paper presented at the FAO/ILSI Workshop on the Development of Local Food Based Dietary Guidelines and Education. Nitra, Solvak Republic, 1997.
20. Tontisirin K. Health and nutrition information needed for the preparation of food-based dietary guidelines in WHO (Regional Office for the Eastern Mediterranean). *Report of the FAO/WHO Technical Consultation on National Food-Based Dietary Guidelines*, WHO-EM/Nutr/232/E, Geneva [in preparation].
21. World Health Organization (Regional Office for Europe). *Food-Based Dietary Guidelines in the WHO European Region.* EUR/03/5045414 E79832, WHO, Geneva, 2003.
22. Gibney M. *A Framework for Food-Based Dietary Guidelines in the European Union Working Party 2.* Final Report. Eurodiet. Feb. 22, 2000. Available at: http:// eurodiet.med.uoc.gr.
23. Castillo C, Uauy R, Atalah E, eds. *Guías de Alimentación para la Población Chilena.* Santiago: Ministerio de Salud, Universidad de Chile, INTA y Depto de Nutrición, 1997.
24. Olivares S, Zacarías I, Benavides X, Boj T. *Difusión de las Guías Alimentarias por los Servicios de Salud.* XVI Congreso Chileno de Nutrición, Viña del Mar, 2004.

25. Molina de Palma V. *Lineamientos Generales para la Elaboración de Guías Alimentarias: Una Propuesta del INCAP*. Guatemala: INCAP/OPS [Publicación INCAP ME/070], 1995.
26. Peña M, Molina V. *Food-Based Dietary Guidelines and Health Promotion in Latin America*. INCAP/OPS, 1999.
27. Schneeman BO. Preparation and use of food-based dietary guidelines: lessons from Thailand and the Philippines. Food Nutrition Agriculture. 2001;28:55–64.
28. Vorster HH, Love P, Browne C. Development of food-based dietary guidelines for South Africa: the process. S Afr J CN. 2001;14(3, suppl):S3–S6.
29. World Health Organization (Regional Office for the Eastern Mediterranean). *Report of the FAO/WHO Technical Consultation on National Food-based Dietary Guidelines*. WHO-EM/Nutr/232/E, Geneva [in preparation].
30. World Health Organization. *Diet, Nutrition and the Prevention of Chronic Diseases*. Report of a joint FAO/WHO Expert Consultation. WHO Technical Report Series 916, Geneva, 2003.
31. World Health Organization (Regional Office for the Western Pacific). *Development of Food-Based Dietary Guidelines for the Western Pacific Region—The shift from Nutrients and Food Groups to Food Availability, Traditional Cuisine and Modern Foods in Relation to Emerging Chronic Noncommunicable Diseases*. Non-series publication, WHO, Geneva, 1999.
32. World Health Organization. *Diet, Nutrition, and the Prevention of Chronic Diseases*. Report of a WHO Study Group. WHO Technical Report Series 797, Geneva, 1990.
33. Nishida C, Shetty P. Diet, nutrition and the prevention of chronic diseases: scientific background papers of the joint WHO/FAO Expert Consultation (Geneva, 28 January–1 February 2002). Public Health Nutr. 2004;7(1A):99–250.
34. World Trade Organization. *Agreement on the Application of Sanitary and Phytosanitary Measures*. World Trade Organization, Final Act of the Uruguay Round, Annex A, paragraph 3. Geneva, 1993.
35. Food and Agriculture Organization/World Health Organization/Ministry of Trade and Industry, Finland. *Recommended Nutrient Reference Values for Food Labeling Purposes*. Report of a Joint FAO/WHO Expert Consultation on Recommended Allowances of Nutrients for Food Labeling Purposes. Helsinki, 1988.

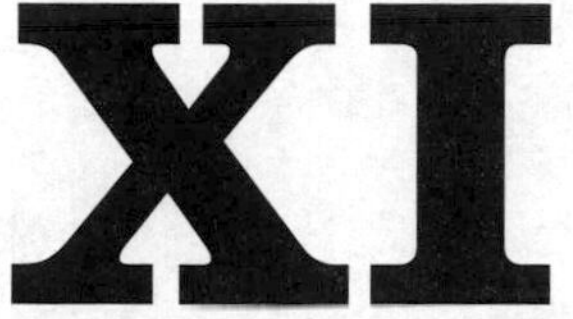

Public Health and International Nutrition

65
The Emergence of Diet-Related Chronic Diseases in Developing Countries

Aryeh D. Stein and Reynaldo Martorell

Introduction

A dual agenda is unfolding. Nutritional deficiencies are receding, but they continue to be important public health problems in sub-Saharan Africa, in the poorest countries in other regions, and for the poorest of the poor in the more developed countries of Latin America and Asia. That today's children are less likely to die from malnutrition and diarrhea than 50 years ago represents a major public health achievement. At the same time, chronic diseases and their related risk factors, such as cancer, cardiovascular diseases, diabetes, obesity, and hypertension, are now major global health concerns. Whereas most people once worried about having too little to eat, today we are becoming increasingly concerned that many around the world, in rich as well as in many developing countries, eat too much. From a nutritional point of view, we are moving away from a dismal past dominated by hunger to an uncertain future of excess consumption and sedentary lifestyles.

This chapter is concerned with the coincidence of these trends in disease and dietary patterns. It is organized into five sections. First, we describe patterns of chronic disease morbidity and mortality, particularly, diabetes, cardiovascular disease, and cancer. We then review levels and trends in diet-related risk factors such as obesity, hypertension, and hyperlipidemia. We describe the epidemiologic, demographic, and nutrition transitions unleashed by the economic forces of industrialization and describe key mechanisms through which these social and economic transformations influence chronic disease epidemiology. As described in the fourth section, these include shifts in the nature of the food supply, in consumption, as well as changes in physical activity. We conclude with a discussion of the implications of the emergence of chronic diseases as a major public health concern in developing countries at a time when undernutrition and infectious diseases still afflict many of the poor in these societies.

Chronic Disease Mortality and Morbidity

Chronic diseases can be defined as conditions that have insidious onset and long preclinical phases, do not spontaneously self-resolve, and result in progressively increasing morbidity.[1] Murray and Lopez[2] analyzed the probabilities of death in 1990 by age and sex across three broad causes (communicable, maternal, perinatal, and nutritional conditions; noncommunicable diseases; injuries) across regions of the world. Total probabilities of death prior to 15 years, between 15 and 60 years, and between 60 and 70 years were greater in developing countries than in industrialized countries. Not unexpectedly, infections explained the much greater total probabilities of death between 0 and 15 years in developing countries relative to developed countries, and infections also contributed to the elevated adult mortality in India and sub-Saharan Africa. Less well appreciated is that the probability of mortality due to noncommunicable diseases was also greater in all developing country regions than in the industrialized countries. As Murray and Lopez[2] note, "[f]or many public health specialists, the higher probability of dying from a noncommunicable disease in high-mortality developing regions contradicts the conventional wisdom that the epidemic of chronic diseases is limited to industrialized countries."

The ratio of age-specific probabilities of deaths from noncommunicable disease to other causes provides a measure of the relative importance of chronic disease across age and by gender in the population. Comparison of these ratios over time allows description of the evolution of chronic disease. Between 1990 and 2020, it is projected that the overall relative rank of infectious disease mortality will decline, with diarrheal diseases, perinatal conditions, measles, and malaria mortality rates expected to decline, while tuberculosis and human immunodeficiency virus (HIV) infections will increase in importance. Noncommunicable disease causes will occupy the top three positions in 2020, with cancers ranking seventh and eighth. Road traffic accidents will move from the tenth to the fifth rank. In industrialized countries, the ratio of noncommunicable to communicable disease deaths is not expected to change between 1990 and 2020, but the ratio will increase dramatically in the former socialist economies.[2] A marked increase is also anticipated in China, from 4.6 in 1990 to 22.0 in 2020. The ratio will rise from less than 2 to 6.9 in Latin America and the Caribbean, to 5.3 in other Asian countries and Oceania, and 4.8 in the Middle Eastern Crescent. Changes are projected to be less extreme in other regions and least in India and in sub-Saharan Africa, in large part because of rising HIV mortality. In 2020, the ratio is projected to be 3.1 in India and below 1 in sub-Saharan Africa.

The accuracy of the national cause-specific death rates from which these estimates were derived, and hence the validity of these patterns and projections, depends mainly on the coverage of physician-certified death registrations and the availability of reliable population denominators. Registration of death may not always occur in many developing countries, and when it does, it may be done by unqualified personnel. Population statistics are also unreliable. An indication of poor quality is that more than 20% of deaths of individuals >60 years are routinely attributed to "signs, symptoms and ill-defined causes" in many developing countries.[3] Many of these deaths probably result from underlying chronic disease, and for this reason, published statistics underestimate the burden of overall and specific chronic diseases. In the rest of this section, we focus on three common chronic diseases that are influenced by diet: type 2 diabetes mellitus, cardiovascular disease (CVD) (especially ischemic heart disease and stroke), and cancer. A recent World Health Organization (WHO) report highlighted these conditions, as well as osteoporosis and dental caries, as emerging nutrition-related concerns in developing countries.[4]

Diabetes Mellitus

The dominant form of diabetes is type 2 (formerly known as non-insulin-dependent) diabetes mellitus (DM). Type 2 DM is characterized by slow onset and is due, at least in part, to an inability of the body to respond appropriately to circulating lipids. Imbalances in the secretion and absorption of insulin result in increased deposition of fat into visceral adipose tissue and elevated circulating glucose levels.[5] Type 2 DM can be diagnosed from elevated fasting glucose levels or from an impaired response to an oral glucose load. Automated analyzers using finger-prick samples are reliable and readily available, although regular calibration is required and there are costs associated with expendable supplies.

There is extensive evidence of epidemic emergence of type 2 DM in developing countries and among migrants from these to industrialized countries.[5-7] Age at diagnosis of type 2 DM reflects prevalence of screening, diagnostic criteria current at the time, and the incidence. In developing countries, most cases of the type 2 DM are diagnosed between 45 and 64 years of age. As the risk of complications is directly proportional to the amount of time a person lives with DM, diabetics in developing countries are at elevated risk of developing long-term complications of the disease, including blindness, kidney failure, and heart disease.[8] WHO estimates that 63% of persons with diabetes in 1997 were from developing countries and that this figure will rise to 76% by 2025.[8] By that year, the worldwide total will be 300 million persons. Then, as today, China, India, and the United States will be the three countries with the largest number of persons with diabetes.

Obesity (especially central obesity) is probably an underlying cause of the metabolic imbalances that result in type 2 DM.[5] Most studies show that successful weight management results in improvement of the glucose profile, while changes in physical activity result in simultaneous changes in both overweight and insulin function. The prevalence of type 2 DM worldwide, therefore, can be expected to track the prevalence of obesity.

Two hypotheses have been developed to attempt to explain the epidemic of type 2 DM in developing countries. Both consider type 2 DM to be an inevitable result of improved food security. The "thrifty genotype" hypothesis posits that over an evolutionary timescale of multiple generations, chronic adverse nutritional circumstances selected for individuals better able to deposit excess energy as fat.[9] In societies that have a plentiful food supply, this adaptation produces excess obesity and type 2 DM due to imbalances in the glucose-insulin axis. Thus, type 2 DM represents a genetic trait that is unmasked in the presence of surplus food. An alternative (but not mutually exclusive) hypothesis argues that the tendency to accrue fat is a phenotypic, epigenetic adaptation to poor nutrition or other adverse circumstances in utero, resulting in programmed metabolic changes that favor deposition of dietary energy as fat.[10,11] This "developmental origins" hypothesis has been extended to explain the emergence of a range of vascular and metabolic diseases in transitional societies as a multigenerational, phenotypic response to the nutrition transition.[10]

Cardiovascular Disease

A substantial fraction of the high levels of CVD in developed countries may be preventable by dietary change.[12,13] Much of this effect can be expected to be mediated through physical activity, overweight, elevated blood pressure, dyslipidemia, and impaired glucose tolerance and diabetes. Thus, adverse changes in these risk factors can be expected, over time, to result in increased rates of CVD incidence and mortality.

In 1985, CVD accounted for 50% of all deaths in economically developed countries and 19% of deaths in developing countries.[14] By 2015, it is projected that circulatory disorders will be the leading cause of death in both the developed (53% of deaths) and developing (35% of deaths) worlds.[14]

The scope of CVD includes two broad groupings that often have diverging trends, namely ischemic heart disease and cerebrovascular disease or stroke. The highest death rates for ischemic heart disease and stroke were recorded for the former socialist economies of Europe and western Asia. Death rates for ischemic heart disease were higher in the industrialized countries than in all developing country regions, and in the latter, the highest rates occurred in India and the Middle Eastern Crescent. Death rates from stroke varied within a narrow range for all developing country regions except China, which had the highest rates, even exceeding those for the industrialized countries.

Death rates for ischemic heart disease and stroke were projected to increase between 1990 and 2000 in all regions except sub-Saharan Africa. Ischemic heart disease and cerebrovascular disease or stroke occupied the second and third spots, respectively, on the 1990 list of causes of death in developing countries; by 2020, these two causes will move to first and second, respectively.[2] Worldwide, the age-adjusted death rate for ischemic heart disease is expected to rise from 118.8 per 100,000 to 129.9 per 100,000 population, an increase of 9.3%. For stroke, the increase in age-adjusted death rate is expected to be 8.9% (83.2 to 90.6 per 100,000 population in 1990 and 2000, respectively).

A limitation of intercountry comparisons of CVD rates is the reliability of classification of causes of death, especially among older people. Specifically, inconsistency in the coding of ischemic heart disease, dysrhythmia, and congestive heart failure is common. Thus, comparisons of large disease groupings are likely to be less subject to error than are finer divisions, and comparisons that focus on individuals under 65 are more likely to be complete.

Cancer

Cancers of several sites (especially cancers of the digestive tract, breast, lung, bladder, and liver) have been strongly linked to dietary factors.[15] It has been estimated that 30% to 40% of cancer mortality is related to dietary exposures, with 22% of all cancers preventable by increasing the consumption of fruits and vegetables from 250 g/d to 400 g/d.[15] As is true for most chronic disease research, etiologic investigations have been concentrated in developed countries, where concerns about obesity, high fat density, and low fruit, vegetable, and fiber intake predominate. Issues related to food preparation, preservation, and storage (pickling, aflatoxin contamination, etc.) have not been stressed, even though in developed countries food preparation methods have been found to explain variation in cancer risk.[16,17]

All Cancers. Cancer was responsible for 4.8 million deaths in 1990, 9.6% of all deaths worldwide.[15] Of these, 2.16 million were in developed countries (representing 18% of developed country deaths), and 2.65 million were in developing countries (7% of all deaths). Over the ensuing 30 years, it is projected that cancer deaths will increase more than two-fold, to 9.3 million.[15] Most of the increase is expected to occur in the developing world, where cancer will account for 14% of all developing country deaths.

Site-specific Cancers. WHO has estimated the incidence of cancer in developed and developing countries.[8] For some cancers (e.g., stomach, liver and esophagus, mouth-pharynx, cervix), the total incidence is greater in developing countries, while the reverse is true for others (e.g., breast, colon and rectum, prostate, lung). The variation across countries in age-adjusted death rates for selected cancers in 1990 is striking. In general, death rates for all but liver and prostate cancers were higher in the established market economies and the former socialist economies than in developing countries. Relative to other developing country regions, China had unusually high death rates from stomach, liver, and lung cancers, while Latin America and the Caribbean had high breast and prostate cancer rates and sub-Saharan Africa had the highest death rates from prostate cancer. Death rates from prostate cancer in sub-Saharan Africa were greater than those in the formerly socialist economies but lower than those in the established market economies. Rates of stomach, liver, and esophageal cancers are declining worldwide, while death rates of breast, colon and rectal, prostate, and lung cancers (especially among women) appear to be increasing.[15] Much of the increase in lung cancer mortality is attributable to the increased prevalence and acceptability of smoking among women. In addition, it has recently been suggested that women are genetically more susceptible than men to lung cancer regardless of exposure to tobacco.[17]

In 1990, the 10 leading causes of death in developing countries did not include cancer. By 2020, cancer of the trachea, bronchus, and lung will occupy the seventh spot, and stomach cancer will follow in the eighth position.[2]

As with CVD, establishing reliable data on cancer incidence and mortality requires comprehensive registration of all events and reliable population denominators for defined populations. Neither is available in most parts of the developing world. Several cancer registries have been set up and maintained in sites from around the world; however, the populations being monitored are overwhelmingly urban. Furthermore, mortality rates are influenced both by incidence rates and by cure rates. In areas where cancers are detected at later stages and are therefore less treatable, mortality rates approximate incidence rates more closely. Where access to high-quality, comprehensive screening, diagnostic, and therapeutic services is available, mortality rates underestimate cancer incidence rates.

Metabolic Risk Factors for Chronic Disease

Obesity

Most of the deleterious consequences of obesity (an excess of adipose tissue) on health are mediated through effects on the cardiovascular and endocrine systems.[18] The altered metabolism that results from obesity includes hyperglycemia, hyperinsulinemia, insulin resistance, hypercholesterolemia, hypertriglyceridemia, and elevated rates of fatty acid synthesis.[18] As a result of these metabolic alterations, obesity contributes to the development of many diseases, including type 2 diabetes, hypertension, stroke, CVD, gallstones, and certain types of cancer.[19] Obesity increases the risk of death from all causes, including CVD, cancer, and other diseases.[4] The health risks associated with obesity have been studied mostly in adults; however, important consequences are known to occur among children. Childhood obesity is predictive of adult obesity and adult mortality and has metabolic and psychosocial consequences on child health.[20]

According to WHO, obesity appears to be increasing worldwide at an alarming rate.[4,21] However, there is limited availability of nationally representative data on which to base these claims, because most studies about obesity are of specific subpopulations, that are not always selected at random. The available information is also limited by the use of different definitions of obesity, the selection of different age groups for study, and the use, in some studies, of reported rather than measured heights and weights. All of these features limit comparisons across countries or time.

Women. Martorell et al.[22,23] analyzed nationally-representative surveys conducted since 1987 in developing countries. Most of the surveys were demographic health surveys that provided data on anthropometry, urban/rural residence, and education for women 15 to 49 years of age and for their children less than 5 years of age. Data were not generally available from these surveys for school-age children, men, and the elderly. Women from 38 developing countries (weighted by population estimates of women 15–49 years for 1996) were compared with women in the United States (1988–1994). The number of countries represented was 18 for sub-Saharan Africa, three for the Middle East and north Africa, two for south Asia, 12 for Latin America and the Caribbean, and three for central eastern Europe/Commonwealth of Independent States. Levels of overweight (body mass index = 25.0 to 29.9 kg/m^2) and obesity (body mass index ≥30 kg/m^2) were extremely low in south Asia, represented by Bangladesh and Nepal. The levels were relatively rare in sub-Saharan Africa, but nearly as common in most other regions of the world as found in the United States, a country in which obesity is deemed to be a major public health problem. Extremely high levels of obesity were reported for some of the islands of Micronesia. Levels of obesity in China were low, similar to levels found in sub-Saharan Africa. While information about trends over time was limited, it was concluded that levels of obesity among women are increasing.[22]

In very poor countries, such as those in sub-Saharan Africa, obesity was concentrated among urban and more highly educated women. In more developed countries, such as those in Latin America and the central eastern Europe/Commonwealth of Independent States region, obesity was more equally distributed in the general population. In Mali, for example, the prevalence of obesity was 9.0 times greater for urban than for rural women, and 6.3 times greater for women with at least 1 year of secondary schooling, compared with women who did not attend secondary school. In Brazil, the relative prevalence of obesity in both of these comparisons was 1.0, and in Mexico the relative prevalence of obesity was 0.9 for urban women and 0.6 for more educated women. In other words, obesity has ceased to be a distinguishing feature of high socioeconomic status in Brazil, and in Mexico, obesity is beginning to be a marker of poverty, as it is in developed countries such as the United States.[22]

Children. Based on an analysis of 71 national nutrition surveys from 50 countries that provided data for children 12 to 60 months of age, overweight among children does not yet appear to be a public health problem in most developing countries, although there are some countries with prevalence similar to or greater than that of the United States.[23] In that analysis, overweight was defined as weight-for-height values greater than one standard deviation above the mean and obesity as greater than two standard deviations above the mean, using the National Center for Health Statistics/WHO reference population.[24] By definition, the prevalence of obesity in the reference population is 2.3%; in the United States it was 3.1% in 1988 to 1994. Out of 50 developing countries represented, 32 had obesity prevalence lower than 2.3%. These results need to be interpreted with caution, because the reference population used is derived from measurements of US children, who may have higher than desired levels of fatness. Also, there is no consensus on how best to measure obesity in children, and the interpretation of weight-for-height indices such as the body mass index in populations with significant levels of stunting has been called into question.[23]

Repeat surveys were available for 17 countries. The prevalence of obesity and overweight appear not to have changed in seven countries in sub-Saharan Africa. In Latin America, on the other hand, prevalence increased in most of the nine countries with data. In Egypt, the prevalence of overweight and obesity has decreased slightly but remains among the highest in developing countries. We note, however, that the age group of children more likely to show problems, and for which few nationally representative data are as yet available, is that of schoolchildren.

Hypertension

Blood pressure level is a strong determinant of coronary heart disease and stroke, with no clear threshold below which risk of disease is no longer related to level.[25] The absolute risk of future disease is related to additional factors (smoking, lipid levels, and genetic predisposition are examples) and can vary by a factor of three across individuals with similar blood pressure levels living in diverse populations.[26] Nevertheless, the relationship between increases in blood pressure and enhanced risk of future disease is remarkably consistent across populations.[26]

Blood pressure levels are very sensitive to body fat,[27] somewhat sensitive to variations in sodium intake,[28] and favorably responsive to a diet rich in low-fat dairy products and fiber-rich fruits and vegetables, even if sodium and total energy are not restricted.[29] Thus, trends in obesity and in dietary patterns away from low-fat, high-fiber foods towards a more energy-dense diet can be expected to result in trends toward higher blood pressure.

It is only recently that blood pressure data from developing countries have become more available. One key study was the International Clinical Epidemiology Network (INCLEN), a collaborative effort conducted in 12 settings in seven countries.[30] In this study conducted in the late 1980s, samples of men 35 to 65 years were drawn from defined populations (not nationally representative) and a CVD risk factor screen administered. There were marked differences in social class and occupation among the various samples. Mean systolic blood pressure ranged from a low of 117 mmHg in Bogotá to a high of 132 in Manila. Diastolic blood pressure ranged from a low of 76 mmHg in rural Thailand to 86 in São Paulo and Santiago. More than 20% of men from urban areas in Thailand, Indonesia, the Philippines, Brazil, and Chile were hypertensive (systolic blood pressure ≥160 mmHg and/or diastolic blood pressure ≥95 mmHg). The urban samples from China had lower blood pressures: 13% of the general population of Shanghai were hypertensive, and the rate was only 5% among factory employees in Chengdu. Only 6% of men were found to be hypertensive in the sample from Bogotá, Colombia, compared with approximately 20% for four other South American cities included in the study. Finally, only approximately 5% of men from rural Thailand were hypertensive.

A second similar study, the WHO Inter-Health Programme, provides additional data from the 1980s for adults 35 to 64 years from developing countries, gives data for men and women, and includes samples from developed countries.[31] While little information is provided about the populations studied, most appear to be from urban areas. In general, the prevalence of hypertension was about twice as high in developed than in developing countries (about 30% vs. 15%) but only slightly greater in men than in women. Blood pressures were as low in the US sample as in the developing countries included. The US samples were from communities near Stanford, California, and might be expected to have lower blood pressures than the US general population. However, US national data from the Third National Health Examination Survey (NHANES III) collected in 1988 to 1994, provide similar values for adults 35 to 64 years. For example, the findings in US men were 125 mmHg for systolic and 79 mmHg for diastolic blood pressures and a prevalence of hypertension of 7%. Blood pressure statistics for Chile and China, which were included in both the INCLEN and Inter-Health studies, were similar.

In summary, the INCLEN and Inter-Health studies suggest that the prevalence of hypertension is higher in developed than in developing countries, in urban compared with rural areas, and only slightly greater in men compared with women. Approximately 15% to 20% of adults in urban areas of developing countries appear to be hypertensive. Estimates of hypertension for rural areas are lower but less certain because of lack of data. Data are not available for estimating trends over time in developing countries.

Hyperlipidemia

The relationship among lifestyle factors, especially diet and physical activity, variation in serum lipid levels, and risk for ischemic heart disease, are well known.[32] Most of the data refer to classes of lipoprotein cholesterol—with elevation of low-density lipoprotein (LDL) conferring additional risk and elevation of high-density lipoprotein (HDL) cholesterol conferring reduced risk. In most populations, LDL cholesterol constitutes the dominant fraction so that overall total cholesterol levels are also directly associated with risk. Ratio measures, such as the ratio of total cholesterol to HDL cholesterol, or the ratio of LDL cholesterol to HDL cholesterol, have been used to better characterize risk.[33]

Cholesterol levels are sensitive to changes in lifestyle. HDL is impacted primarily by physical activity, while LDL is sensitive to dietary fatty acid composition.[34] However, HDL levels are adversely impacted by overall fat restriction and by increased intake of trans fatty acids, a common ingredient in commercial baked goods.[35] Thus, trends in urbanization, changes in employment and activity patterns, and changes in access to foods can be expected to result in changes in serum cholesterol levels.

Measurement of lipids, especially LDL cholesterol, requires a blood sample (venous or capillary) and reagents. Venous samples need to be analyzed in rigorously standardized conditions not available to most field investigations. Even the capillary-blood methods, which can be analyzed on site using portable equipment and standardized kits, require calibration and have significant costs associated with the reagents. Most automated systems provide estimates of total cholesterol, HDL cholesterol, and triglycerides. LDL cholesterol is then calculated using the Friedwald equation.[36] As triglyceride concentrations are sensitive to recent food ingestion, non-fasting samples are not suitable for calculation of LDL cholesterol, the component most sensitive to dietary changes. These factors help to explain why few large-scale studies of serum cholesterol have been conducted in developing countries. Finally, available studies report data for total cholesterol, but only some report HDL values. For this reason, our presentation below focuses on total cholesterol values.

In the United States, mean total cholesterol levels have been declining, probably reflecting changes in diet and increasingly aggressive pharmacologic treatments. Nevertheless, mean total cholesterol is still relatively high. In adults measured in NHANES III (1988–1994), mean total cholesterol was 5.31 mmol/L (205 mg/dL), while more recent data from the 1999 to 2000 NHANES suggest little change since then, with a mean total cholesterol of 5.27 mmol/L (203 mg/dL) (age-adjusted $P = 0.16$). The prevalence of hypercholesterolemia (total cholesterol ≥6.2 mmol/L) was 17.2% in men and 18.4% in women.[37]

The INCLEN study described previously obtained non-fasting venous samples and measured total cholesterol using similar methods across centers.[30] Mean total cholesterol ranged from a low of 3.8 mmol/L in Shanghai, China, to 6.4 mmol/L in Bogotá, Colombia. The percentage of men with high cholesterol values reached a high of 46% in Bogotá and was lowest for China (≤2%), rural Thailand (4%), Manila (7%), and Santiago (10%). For all other samples, which were all taken from urban populations, values were approximately 20%, as in the United States.

Data from the Inter-Health study also suggest low cholesterol values for China and Chile. Cholesterol values were low for Tanzania but not for Mauritius, a small island republic in the Indian Ocean, with higher incomes than most sub-Saharan nations. Cholesterol levels were generally greater in developed compared with developing countries. Between 30% to 50% of adults in Finland, Lithuania, Malta, and Cyprus had high cholesterol values. The prevalence of high cholesterol was approximately 23% in Russia and 15% in the United States. In general, values were similar in men and women.

In summary, there is considerable variability in total cholesterol values across developing and developed countries. Despite the lack of data, some generalizations are possible. Cholesterol values remain low in many areas of the world (e.g., China, rural Thailand), but in some urban areas of Latin America and Asia, the percentage of adults with high cholesterol levels has reached 20%, about the same as in the United States but lower than the figure of 30% to 50% reported for several European countries. Data are not available to assess changes over time in developing countries.

Economic Development and Chronic Disease

As was the case in Europe and North America in the 19th and first half of the 20th centuries, the emergence of diet-related chronic diseases in developing countries in the later 20th century and continuing into the present is driven by improving living standards and rising incomes. The process of worldwide economic development has changed patterns of social organization and livelihood and triggered epidemiologic, demographic, and nutrition transitions. By understanding these transitions and the context in which they typically occur, we can identify the causes of the emerging epidemic of chronic diseases and better plan for present and future needs.

For most of recorded human history, mortality rates were extremely high, fluctuating widely due to wars, famines, and epidemics. However, very high birthrates ensured slow but steady rates of population growth. From about AD 1 to 1750, the human population grew from 300 million to 790 million and reached 1 billion by 1800.[38] Omran[39] has called this period the "Age of Pestilence, and Famine," and proposed it as the first stage of his "epidemiologic transition" theory (Figure 1).

Near the middle of the 19th century the second stage, the "Age of Receding Pandemics," emerged. Epidemics and famines became less frequent in Europe and North America. Living standards improved and mortality rates decreased due to improved nutrition and lower rates of infectious and parasitic decreases, but rapid population growth occurred because birthrates remained high. The European population increased from 203 to 408 million in the 19th century, and that of North America increased from 7 to 87 million, albeit largely as a result of migration from Europe and Africa. The world population reached 1.7 billion in 1900.[38]

In developing countries, mortality rates declined much later, mostly in the second half of the 20th century, and much more rapidly. Advances in public health and medicine such as vaccines, antibiotics, and effective approaches to vector control led to precipitous declines in mortality rates in developing countries and explosive population growth compared with experiences in Europe and North

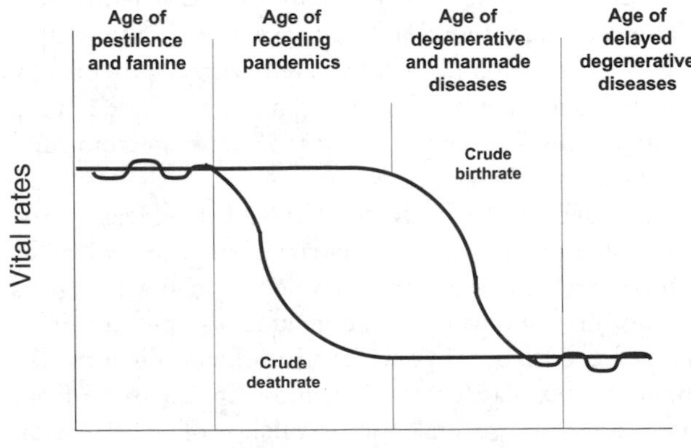

Figure 1. Stages of the epidemiologic transition. (Used with permission from Olshansky et al., 1997.[41])

America. From a population of 2.5 billion in 1950, the world reached 6 billion in 1999.[38]

The third stage, the "Age of Degenerative and Man-made Diseases," is distinguished by falling birthrates. As birthrates decreased in industrialized societies, population growth halted or in some countries reversed. In some industrialized countries, most notably the United States, growth continues due to immigration. Most developing countries are in the third stage of the transition. Birthrates are declining rapidly throughout most of Latin America and Asia, but they have yet to decline appreciably in sub-Saharan Africa. Thus, population growth is slowing in much of the developing world except for sub-Saharan Africa. However, HIV/AIDS has become an important cause of mortality in a number of African countries, reversing gains in life expectancy and slowing population growth.[40] Overall, the epidemiologic transition is occurring at a faster pace in developing countries than it did in Europe and North America.

A fourth stage, the "Age of Delayed Degenerative Diseases," in which healthier lifestyles would prevent or delay the onset of degenerative diseases while medical advances would enhance survival of individuals with cancer, CVD, or other degenerative diseases, has been proposed.[41] Increases in life expectancy in this stage would come from falling death rates among the elderly.

The phenomenon described above is of interest to both demographers and epidemiologists. Demographers focus on the "demographic transition," the shift from high death rates and birthrates (first stage) to low death rates and birthrates (third stage) and on the demographic consequences of these changes (e.g., population growth, aging). Epidemiologists focus on the "epidemiologic transition," changes in the age-specific causes of morbidity and mortality from a pattern dominated by infectious and parasitic diseases in interaction with nutritional deficiencies to a dominance of diet-related, degenerative diseases. Linkages among the stages of the demographic and epidemiologic transitions are shown in Figure 2.

The proportion of people dying from noncommunicable diseases today is greater than it was 100 years ago, largely because fewer people die during early childhood. The effects of an aging population are more pronounced when the demographic transition is completed or well under way (e.g., the industrialized countries, east Asian countries, and Latin America). Between 1990 and 2025, rapid aging will result in increases in the proportion of the population of people ≥65 years of age from 6% to 13.3% in China and from 5% to 15% in the Republic of Korea.[42] Canada and the United States will see large increases in the proportion of people more than 60 years of age, from about 16% in 1995 to more than 25% in 2020.[43] Several Latin American countries will also experience large increases (Cuba from 12% to 21% and Chile from 10% to 16%, for example). Even two of the poorest nations in the region, Honduras and Nicaragua, will see a rise in the proportion of the elderly by 2020, from approximately 5% to more than 7%. Haiti, the poorest, is the only country not expected to experience a rise in the proportion of elderly.

The aging index, the ratio of adults ≥60 years to the population under 15 years multiplied by 100, compares past wage earners to future ones. By 2020, there will be 116 older persons for every 100 youths in the United States. In Canada and Cuba, the corresponding values will be greater, 146 and 130 per 100, respectively. Among the more developed economies of Latin America, the number of older adults will exceed 50 per 100 youths. The poorest countries of the region will remain youthful, with fewer than 30 older adults per 100 youths in Haiti, Bolivia, Paraguay, Guatemala, Honduras, and Nicaragua, although the aging index will double in all of these countries but Haiti.

The Nutrition Transition

Changes in the pattern of disease burden also result from fundamental changes in diet and lifestyle such that age-specific rates of noncommunicable diseases increase. In other words, the epidemiologic transition is driven by both shifts in the denominator (number of adults and their relative proportion in the total population) and in the numerator (proportion of adults with chronic diseases). Popkin,[44] who has written extensively about changes in patterns of risk for noncommunicable diseases, coined the term "nutrition transition" to call attention to changes in diet and physical activity that accompany, and are likely in part to be a cause of the demographic and epidemiologic transitions. The nutrition transition is a shift from a situation in which diets poor in quality and quantity and intensive physical activity predominate (with high rates of undernutrition as a result) to one in which diets become excessive in energy, with a greater proportion as fat and a sedentary lifestyle is the rule (Figure 2).

One of the great achievements of the 20th century was to decrease the threat of famines in developing countries. Due to remarkable increases in food production as a result of the Green Revolution, improved market efficiency, and more responsive government policies, famines have disappeared from many areas where they were endemic, such as India and China, and are now largely confined to areas of armed conflict and political instability. Cases of severe clinical malnutrition, such as kwashiorkor, marasmus, beriberi, and pellagra, which used to be commonly seen in hospital wards around the world, have virtually disappeared. The prevalence of underweight (i.e., a weight-for-age more than two standard deviations below the reference mean) among young children is perhaps the best global indicator of the nutritional status of populations. WHO estimates that since 1980, the prevalence of underweight has declined in Asia and Latin America but has increased in sub-Saharan Africa, reflecting the latter region's economic stagnation.[45] In addition to progress in the elimination of childhood underweight, the United Nations Children's Fund reports worldwide progress in

	Economy	Demographic transition	Epidemiologic transition	Nutrition transition
Preindustrial societies	Agrarian, rural, illiterate, poor	High fertility and mortality	High prevalence of infectious diseases	High prevalence of undernutrition; high levels of physical activity
Developing societies	Modernization of agriculture, urbanization, rising education, improving health services	Reduced mortality, changing age structure	Receding pestilence, declining infectious diseases	Receding famine, improving nutrition
Industrialized societies	Diversified economy, high incomes, urban, literate	Reduced fertility, aging	Chronic diseases predominate	Diet of degenerative diseases predominates, sedentarism
A vision of future societies	Sustainable development, conservation of the environment	Long lifespan	Healthy aging	Healthy diets, increased physical activity

Figure 2. Interrelationships among the demographic, epidemiologic, and nutritional transitions. (Adapted with permission from Popkin 1994.[45])

reducing vitamin A and iodine deficiencies[46]; however, iron deficiency anemia remains more intractable.

The Economic Development Transition

The epidemiologic, demographic, and nutrition transitions are facets of the same phenomenon because they have common causes (Figure 2). We refer to the social and economic changes underpinning the three transitions as the "economic development transition." At the heart of the economic development transition is the shift from a preindustrial society, largely agricultural based and rural in nature, as well as illiterate and poor, to a modern industrial society—literate, largely urbanized, and with a diversified employment sector (i.e., decreased dependence on the agricultural sector and increased importance of industry and services).

By presenting the features of economic development as stages, we do not mean to imply that the process is linear and predestined. The pace of development varies greatly by region, across countries, and through time. Wars, political instability, failed ideologies, natural disasters, financial crises, and many other factors may cause progress to slow or even reverse. As noted by the World Bank, "[t]he evidence of recent decades demonstrates that while development is possible, it is neither inevitable nor easy."[42]

There is no doubt that real incomes have improved around the world.[47] The gross domestic product (GDP) per capita for all developing countries, expressed in 1987 US dollars, increased by 50%, from $600 to $908, between 1975 and 1997. Disappointedly, the poorest or "least developed countries," which includes the poorest nations of sub-Saharan Africa and Asia as well as Haiti, actually lost ground, with the per capita GDP declining from $287 to $245. However, east Asia (which includes China) and southeast Asia (which includes Indonesia) made remarkable gains, as did industrialized countries. A distressing observation is that the overall gap between rich and poor countries has grown. GDP per capita (1987 US dollars) increased from $12,589 in 1975 to $19,283 in 1997 in industrialized countries. Although the percentage increase was more than 50% in both industrialized and developing countries, the gap between them increased from $11,989 in 1975 to $18,375 in 1997.

Increases in GDP per capita, an average measure, will lead to declines in poverty levels to the extent that the new wealth is shared. This was the case in the three largest nations in Asia: China, India, and Indonesia. China and India, each with approximately 1 billion people, combined represent one-third of the world's population. GDP per capita increased in China from $109 to $564 from 1975 to 1997,[47] and this reduced the number of the absolute poor from 270 million in 1978 to 65 million in 1996.[48] In India, GDP per capita increased from $251 in 1975 to $465 in 1997.[48] This resulted in an important reduction in the proportion of people living in poverty, from 55% in the early 1970s to about 35% in 1999.[48,49] In Indonesia, with more than 200 million people, GDP per capita increased from $264 in 1975 to $785 in 1997,[47] and as a result, poverty was reduced significantly from 58% in 1970 to just 8% in 1993, although the recent economic crisis has negated some of these gains.[48]

Urbanization

The process of change, whether measured in economic, epidemiologic, demographic, or nutritional terms, is most expressed in urban areas. According to the World Bank, cities are the dynamic engines of growth and are

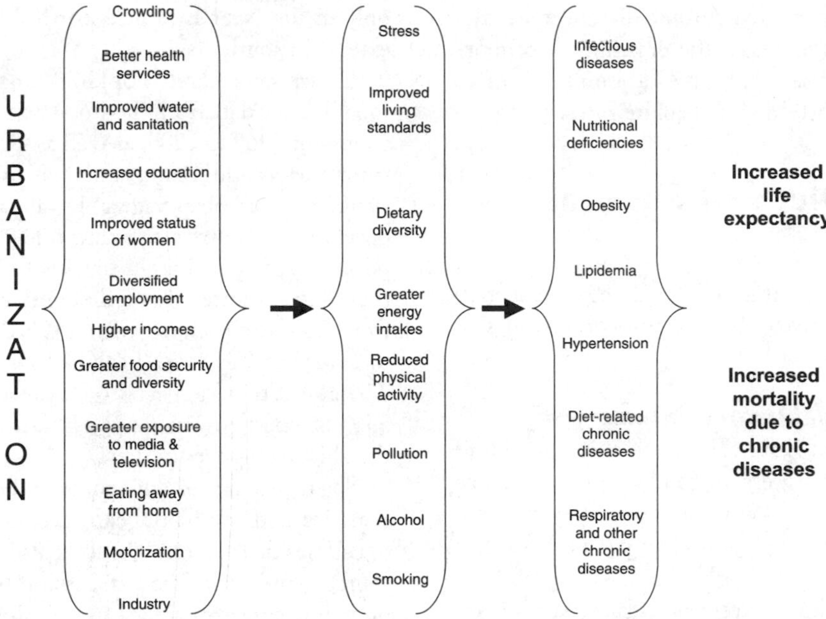

Figure 3. The links between urbanization and increased mortality due to chronic diseases.

needed for sustained economic growth.[42] The growth sectors of the economy, manufacturing and services, are usually found in cities where they "benefit from agglomeration economies and ample markets for inputs, outputs, and labor, and where ideas and knowledge are rapidly diffused."[42] In developed countries, economic growth and structural transformation accompanied urbanization. The modernization of agriculture in these countries reduced the number of agricultural jobs and forced people to look for jobs in non-agricultural industries that were generally in cities. In all regions of the world except sub-Saharan Africa, urbanization has been associated with rising per capita income.[42] A reason given by the World Bank for the pattern of "urbanization without growth" in Africa is the "distorted incentive that encouraged migrants to move to cities to exploit subsidies rather than in response to opportunities for more productive employment."[42]

Between 1950 and 2020, virtually all of the increases in population in the world will be in developing countries and in urban areas.[42] The areas where the largest increases in urban population are expected to occur by 2020 are those that are least urbanized today: sub-Saharan Africa, east asia, and Pacific and south Asia. Europe and Central Asia, Latin America and the Caribbean; the Middle East and North African regions, which are further along the "urban transition," will grow less rapidly.

Urbanization and the emergence of diet-related chronic diseases are intimately related. As Gopalan[50] noted, "[t]he escalation of nutrition-related diseases is, to a considerable extent, an urban phenomenon." Figure 3 describes the pathways that link the conditions of urban living to the emergence of diet-related chronic diseases as public health problems. Cities generally offer better services than rural areas, including health services, water, sanitation, education, electricity, transportation, and other amenities.[42,45] For example, 83% of the urban population in developing countries was supplied with water in 1994, compared with 70% in rural areas.[8] Similarly, sanitation coverage for 1994 was 63% in urban areas, compared with just 21% in rural areas.[8] The "agglomeration" of cities makes it more cost effective to deliver services; in addition, urban dwellers are politically more powerful and hence more effective in demanding assistance from governments. Cities offer more employment opportunities, enjoy higher incomes, and have greater availability and variety of foods. Women's status improves in urban settings.[51]

These factors lead to improved living standards and to reduced rates of nutritional deficiencies. However, the nature of the diet changes. Foods become more energy dense, and more calories are consumed. Eating away from home and exposure to advertisements also affect patterns of intake. The fast food industry, both local and international, is expanding rapidly and contributing to dietary change. Physical activity is reduced in urban areas because most jobs are not as energy demanding as are agricultural jobs in rural areas.[52] Transportation replaces walking, and sedentary actvities, such as television watching, increase. Also, city dwellers experience more stress than rural residents, and alcohol and smoking use are increased in cities.

Cities have more air pollution than rural areas because of industry and motor vehicle use, which results in higher rates of respiratory and other related chronic diseases.[53] The incidence of infectious diseases appears not to differ markedly between urban and rural areas.[51] While better living standards and health and sanitation services may exert downward pressure on disease rates, crowding may do the opposite.

As a result of these influences, life expectancy in urban areas is increased relative to rural areas, but at the same time, age-specific, diet-related chronic disease morbidity is also increased. This increases the prominence of mortality due to chronic diseases, both as a proportion of all causes of death and in terms of absolute rates.

Changes in Diet and Physical Activity

We now turn to the nature of the changes in dietary intake and physical activity that are the cornerstones of the nutrition transition.

Food Security and Dietary Intake

Food Balance Sheet Data. The Food and Agriculture Organization tracks progress in food security. Balance sheet data from its sixth World Food Survey indicate that the dietary energy supply, on a per person basis, has increased in most of the world from 1969–1971 to 1990–1992.[54] The striking exception is sub-Saharan Africa, where the average availability of calories declined by 100 kcal/person, from a baseline value of 2140 kcal/person. It is now the region of the world with the lowest dietary energy supply, as Asian countries have moved ahead. As a result of political and economic instability, dietary energy supply values in the transition economies of eastern Europe and the former Soviet Union declined from 3400 kcal/person in 1978–1981 to 3230 in 1990–1992; however, these are still very high levels of availability.

The percentage of the dietary energy supply from fat is increasing in all regions of developing countries except in sub-Saharan Africa. No developing region has yet reached the high levels observed in industrialized countries and transition economies, 36.4% and 27.3%, respectively. The highest values in developing countries were observed in Latin America and the Caribbean (25.6%) and in the Near East and north Africa (21.3%). Levels stagnated in sub-Saharan Africa at 18.1%, but remained greater that those of Asia in 1990 to 1992. Asia may have already overtaken sub-Saharan Africa by now, since levels have been rising fast since the 1980s, particularly in east and southeast Asia. The percentage of energy from fat was 17.1% in east and southeast Asia and 16.1% in south Asia in 1990 to 1992.

Comparison of Food and Agriculture Organization data for 1969–1971 and 1990–1992 reveals important changes in the proportional composition of fat. The proportion of fat calories derived from vegetable oils and fats increased in all developing country regions; increases also occurred in industrialized countries and economies in transition. The largest change occurred in Latin America; in 1969–1971, vegetable oils and fats contributed 29.8% of fat calories, increasing to 44.0% in 1990–1992. In most regions the proportion of fat calories from other non-vegetable sources and from animal sources declined. The proportion of fat calories from animal sources increased only in the Near East and north Africa and, to a lesser extent, in south Asia.

Drewnowski and Popkin[55] analyzed country-level food balance data from the Food and Agriculture Organization for 1962 to 1990, as well as GNP per capita figures from the World Bank, and concluded that the global availability of cheap vegetable oils and fats has allowed developing countries to achieve levels of fat intake only possible before at higher levels of income; for example, their data indicated that a diet deriving 20% of its energy from fat was associated with a GNP per capita of $1900 in 1962, but only $900 (both in 1993 US dollars) in 1990. The global trend appears to be toward a value of 30% to 35% of energy from fat.[55] Urbanization is accelerating the shift to higher-fat diets.

Sugar is an important source of dietary energy in Latin America and the Caribbean, accounting for about 16% of calories in 1990 to 1992. It is also an important energy source in industrialized nations and transition economies, providing approximately 13% of calories. Values for 1990 to 1992 for the Near East, north Africa, and south Asia were approximately 9% of calories and were lowest in sub-Saharan Africa (4.1% of calories) and east and southeast Asia (3.8% of calories). Compared with 1969 to 1971 values, the per capita supply of sugar in 1990 to 1992 decreased somewhat in industrialized nations (13.9% vs. 13.1%), remained stable in south Asia (9.6% vs. 9.5%), and increased in the rest of the world.

Drewnowski and Popkin[55] characterized the above changes as a "global paradox" in the making and write:

> Wealthy industrialized nations in North America and the European Union spend significant sums of money to convince their citizens to replace dietary fats with a simpler diet based on grains, vegetables, and fruit. Paradoxically, developing countries use their growing incomes to replace their traditional diets, rich in fibers and grains, with diets that include a greater proportion of fats and caloric sweeteners.

Dietary Surveys. Food balance sheet data provide information at the aggregate level and measure potential rather than actual average consumption. For the latter and for information about variability in consumption, we must turn to dietary survey results. These data are difficult to obtain but are available for several countries, including China and Brazil. Guo et al.[56] have documented remarkable changes in dietary intake using panel data for the years 1989, 1991, and 1993 for 5600 Chinese adults aged 20 to 45 years in 1989. In each survey, household food inventory and 24-hour dietary recall information were obtained for 3 consecutive days on the same individuals. In just 2 to 4 years, considerable change occurred. The proportion of adults with high-fat diets, measured as >30% fat, >10% saturated fat, or ≥300 mg of cholesterol per day, increased sharply from 1989 to 1993 among all income groups. This was due to large increases in fat intake, particularly vegetable oils and fats, and in animal foods. Associated with these changes were decreases in the consumption of course grains, potatoes, and carotene-poor vegetables. Diets became more diverse as more adults incorporated meat, eggs, edible oils, and carotene-rich vegetables into the diet.

Patterns of intake have also changed dramatically in Brazil.[57] In general, the consumption of staple cereals and starchy roots, beans, pork meat, and animal fat (lard and butter) has declined, whereas consumption of chicken, eggs, milk and dairy products, and vegetable oils and fats has increased. The consumption of polyunsaturated fatty oils has increased, and that of dietary cholesterol has decreased. Total carbohydrate intake has declined, and the importance of fat as a source of calories has increased. A greater share of total protein is provided by animal sources. The consumption of green and other vegetables and of fruits has increased. Other changes include increased consumption of food away from home and increased supermarket shopping, which favors increased food variety and use of processed foods.

Dietary diversity has increased in both China and Brazil, suggesting that not all of the changes that are occurring should be viewed negatively. Vitamin and mineral intake have undoubtedly improved in both countries. While the consumption of vegetable oils and fats has increased in both countries, animal fat consumption decreased in Brazil but not in China. Thus, saturated fat and cholesterol intake increased in China and not in Brazil. However, total fat consumption increased in both countries. Analyses of food balance sheet data from China and Brazil corroborate these conclusions.

Food Security Projections. Projections of food production and consumption for the year 2020 provide good and bad news according to the International Food Policy Research Institute.[58] Worldwide, per capita availability of food will increase by about 7% between 1993 and 2020, from approximately 2700 calories per person per day to about 2900 calories. China and east Asia are projected to have the largest increases. Nevertheless, the projected increase in sub-Saharan Africa will increase values to only 2300 calories per person per day in 2020, "just barely above the minimum required for a healthy and productive life."[58] Despite significant advances in south Asia, that region and sub-Saharan Africa will be the "locus of hunger in the developing world."[58]

The demand for cereals to feed livestock will increase dramatically, especially in economically vigorous developing countries such as China, in response to strong demand for livestock products.[58] Between 1993 and 2020, the demand for cereals in developing countries will double in the case of animal feed and will increase by 50% for direct human consumption. The International Food Policy Research Institute projects that cereal production in developing countries will be insufficient to meet the demand and that, as a result, net import of cereals will more than double in developing countries by 2020. The area of concern is again sub-Saharan Africa, where the gap between population and food production will continue to increase into 2020. The shortfall will need to be covered by food aid, but rising cereal prices and increased demand from developing countries with the ability to pay will likely decrease availability and interest among donor nations.

The projected growth in the demand for food is in great measure driven by the rising economies and populations of developing countries. The growth in production needs to occur by means of increases in crop yields of cereals, and not through expansion of the area under cultivation.[58] This is feasible but exceedingly difficult because of declining soil fertility, growing water scarcity, weather fluctuations, and climate change. New technologies, in particular biotechnology, are expected to boost food production levels, but realizing this potential requires careful study of risks and benefits and consumer acceptance of this analysis. Also, for biotechnology to help poor farmers in developing countries, there needs to be public sector investment in research relevant to their needs currently, and most research is funded by private corporations and largely concentrated on the agricultural sector of industrial nations.[59]

Physical Activity

There are at present limited data about worldwide trends in physical activity. From other evidence, however, we presume that levels of physical activity around the world are declining and that they will continue to do so. The situation in industrialized countries, a possible reflection of the direction in which developing countries are headed, is alarming. Most occupations today in industrialized nations demand little physical activity and the extent of leisure-time physical activity is low. For example, using a strict criterion of being sedentary (i.e., no exercise, recreation, or physical activity other than work during the previous month), the Centers for Disease Control and Prevention report that 40% of adults in the United States were sedentary in 2004.[60] Also, 33% of US high school students did not meet recommended levels of moderate or strenuous physical activity (males, 26.9%; females, 40.1%).[60] Few data are available from developing countries; among Chilean university students 18 to 25 years of age, 61% were classified as having sedentary lifestyles.[61]

The occupational distribution in most developing countries has changed dramatically because of the transition and urbanization caused by economic development. Over time, the proportion of workers employed in energy intensive activities of the agricultural sector has declined as many have shifted to jobs in industry and services.[52,62] The China Health and Nutrition Survey has provided an opportunity for assessing short-term trends in occupational physical activity among adults 20 to 45 years of age.[63] These data show that occupational activity is more strenuous in rural than in urban areas. In 1991, 55% of urban residents had sedentary occupations compared with 12% of rural residents. On the other hand, only 11% of urban residents participated in strenuous activities compared with 77% of rural residents. In just the span of 2 years, from 1989 to 1991, the percentage of urban residents in sedentary occupations rose from 39% to 55%. On the other hand, rural residents reported a higher proportion of sedentary occupations in 1989 compared with 1991, 17% versus 12%, respectively. Unfortunately, information about leisure-time physical activity was not collected.

Discussion

We have documented the nutrition and epidemiologic transitions in developing countries and identified factors driving these transitions. There are few data about overt chronic disease morbidity. Instead, we rely on mortality statistics. A surprising finding is that the age-specific probability of death from noncommunicable diseases among adults is greater in developing than in industrialized countries. Death rates by specific cause are less reliable. In general, rates for ischemic heart disease and stroke are lower in developing regions than in industrialized countries. However, rates are expected to rise in all developing country regions except sub-Saharan Africa. By 2015, CVD will be the leading cause of death in developing countries, accounting for 35% of deaths. Incidence rates for some cancers are already greater in developing countries, and the rates of others, such as breast, colon, rectal, prostate, and lung cancer, are rising. By 2020 cancer will account for 14% of all deaths in developing countries.

The paucity and poor quality of the information available from developing countries are limiting factors. The registration of cause of death is notoriously deficient. Data concerning risk factors such as hypertension and hypercholesterolemia generally come from studies in nonrepresentative populations. Although national nutrition surveys have provided data on obesity, these are mainly for women and young children and are not generally available for the more prosperous countries of the developing world. Information about patterns of physical activity is rare. Data on the national food supply of countries provide estimates of average availability; data about actual consumption patterns by socioeconomic group are rarer. Assessments of current status in terms of mortality, morbidity, or risk factors must therefore be interpreted with caution; that of trends, even more so.

Nonetheless, there remains no doubt that the nutrition and epidemiologic transitions are at an advanced stage in all regions of the developing world except south Asia and sub-Saharan Africa. Sub-Saharan Africa is experiencing a resurgence of child malnutrition and mortality. Food security is threatened by declines in per capita food production, and AIDS has become a modern plague. Other emerging infectious diseases remain a concern. Political instability and ethnic conflict have unleashed famines and displaced millions of people. Economic prospects remain bleak. In India, on the other hand, the economy and public health are improving, albeit slowly. India boasts a large middle, urban class—a group that is experiencing a surge in chronic diseases such as type 2 DM. China is experiencing explosive economic growth, rapid urbanization, and pronounced epidemiologic change. Many other Asian countries, such as Indonesia, Thailand, and Malaysia, are also developing rapidly. Latin America and the Caribbean, as well as the Middle East and north Africa, are already far into the nutrition transition and will likely continue to evolve in that direction.

Economic development, particularly urbanization, is driving the demographic, epidemiologic, and nutrition transitions. The population of developing countries is aging rapidly, as early childhood mortality from undernutrition and infection has declined in importance and more people are surviving to old age. The dietary energy supply has increased in developing countries, and more of the calories are in the form of fat. Greater availability of vegetable oils, rather than increases in animal fat, accounts for this change. Processed foods have become more important in the diets, and eating away from home is becoming more common. More sugar and less fiber are consumed. On the other hand, diets have become more diverse, particularly in urban areas, with a greater variety of fruits and vegetables. Thus, the increased incomes and greater food diversity of urban areas present opportunities for counseling and nutrition education. Few data are available, but we may assume that physical activity has declined, as jobs become less energy demanding, use of cars and buses replaces walking, and more time is spent watching television. Not surprisingly, obesity among women, and likely in men and school-age children, is now common in developing countries except in sub-Saharan Africa and south Asia. In more advanced developing countries, obesity is as common among poorly educated women and in villages as it is among women with better education in cities. In these countries, obesity is no longer just a problem in urban areas and of the rich, but of society in general. While information on blood pressure and lipid levels is mostly from nonrepresentative samples, the populations studied, such as those of INCLEN,[30] included rural and urban areas and were drawn from a wide range of socioeconomic status. Values for these populations from developing countries, while lower than values for selected European countries, are not unlike those found in the United States. Type 2 DM is already very common in many developing countries and is increasing at alarming rates.

Reflecting on the body of evidence reviewed, we draw four general recommendations for developing countries:

- Increase awareness among decision makers that diet-related chronic diseases are important public health problems.
- Develop multisectoral programs and policies aimed at the prevention of noncommunicable diseases.
- Invest in training professionals to address the new

epidemiology and invest in operations research aimed at developing effective interventions.
- Maintain efforts to eradicate nutritional deficiencies.

To increase national awareness of the importance of noncommunicable diseases, national data are desperately needed. It is recommended that national health surveys collect data about risk factors for chronic diseases and related morbidities, and not be limited to infectious diseases and nutritional deficiencies; such surveys should also sample school-age children, men, and the elderly. It would be ideal to use similar methods across countries because consistency of methods would facilitate comparisons across countries and regions. National-level data are essential for constructing regional and social maps of noncommunicable diseases that serve to identify groups at higher risk. To the extent that these emerging problems are widespread in all sectors of the population, it will then be easy to argue for policies and programs to address them. Decision makers, the public health sector, research and academic institutions, and the public at large must be exposed to the findings and made aware of their implications.

Developing countries need to take decisive action to bring under control the epidemic of noncommunicable diseases. A broad range of policies and programs across multiple sectors is required. Examples might include agricultural policies that influence the food basket and the prices of its items, urban development policies that influence the availability of parks and recreational facilities, educational policies about content to be taught to children with an emphasis on the promotion of physical education, and educational campaigns about healthy living aimed at the public at large.

Developing countries lack the manpower and experience to tackle the new problems effectively. In general, public health workers are not trained to deal with the new epidemiology. There is also a lack of adequately trained professionals at academic, research, and training institutions. Developing effective interventions has been a difficult and laborious undertaking in industrialized countries and has resulted only in limited success. Strategies effective in developed countries need to be tested for relevance in other settings. Developing countries need to invest in research, particularly operations research aimed at improving program effectiveness.

The eradication of nutritional deficiencies, particularly those that affect women and young children, and of infectious and parasitic diseases associated with poverty, must remain a high priority for at least two reasons: 1) because of their impact on mortality and human capital;[64,65] and 2) if the developmental origins hypothesis[10] proves to be correct, the elimination of fetal and infant undernutrition will contribute, over the long run, to the future amelioration of noncommunicable diseases. The relative priorities given to old and emerging problems will have to be based on country-specific data. In countries such as Chile, where undernutrition in children is now very low, remaining programmatic efforts should be focused on "pockets of undernutrition," specific populations with high rates of undernutrition.

New developments in industrialized countries offer a glimpse of a better future. In the United States and other countries, there is increasing interest in healthy living, particularly among individuals with higher incomes and educational levels. Many have changed their diets to consume less fat and sugar and to include more fiber and nutrient-rich grains, fruits, and vegetables. Exercise is popular among those of higher socioeconomic status, and obesity has become a marker of social class because it is now more prevalent among the poor and in minorities.[22] The clinical management of chronic disease has improved, and a range of effective options, from pharmaceuticals such as cholesterol-lowering drugs to heart bypasses and other surgeries, is now readily available. With these developments comes the promise of longer lifespans with declining age-specific disability— in other words, the possibility of healthy aging. Indeed, improvements in diet and lifestyle, including reductions in tobacco use, have already produced positive results in many industrialized countries. There have been dramatic reductions in mortality from CVD in the past few decades in Australia, Canada, Finland, New Zealand, and the United States.[8] We hope that this future awaits developing countries as well.

References

1. Last JM, ed. *A Dictionary of Epidemiology*. 3rd ed. New York: Oxford University Press; 1995; 208 pp.
2. Murray CJL, Lopez AD, eds. *The Global Burden of Disease*. Boston: Harvard University Press; 1996; 1022 pp.
3. World Health Organization: International Statistical Classification of Diseases and Related Health Problems, 10th Revision. Available at: http://www3.who.int/icd/vol1htm2003/fr-icd.htm. Accessed March 30, 2006.
4. World Health Organization/Food and Agriculture Organization. *Diet, Nutrition and the Prevention of Chronic Diseases. Report of a Joint WHO/FAO Consultation*. WHO Technical Report Series 916. Geneva: World Health Organization; 2003.
5. Steyn NP, Mann J, Bennett PH, et al. Diet, nutrition and the prevention of type 2 diabetes. Public Health Nutr. 2004;7:147–165.
6. Zimmet PZ, McCarty DJ, de Courten MP. The global epidemiology of non-insulin dependent diabetes mellitus and the metabolic syndrome. J Diabetes Complications. 1997;11:60–68.
7. King H, Aubert RE, Herman WH. Global burden of diabetes, 1995–2025. Prevalence, numerical estimates, and projections. Diabetes Care. 1998;21: 1414–1431.

8. World Health Organization. *The World Health Report 1998—Life in the 21st Century: A Vision for All.* Geneva: World Health Organization; 1998.
9. Neel JV. Diabetes mellitus: a "thrifty" genotype rendered detrimental by "progress"? Am J Hum Genet. 1962;14:353–363.
10. Barker DJP. *Mothers, Babies and Disease in Later Life.* London: BMJ Publishing Group; 1994; 180 pp.
11. Gluckman P, Hanson M. *The Fetal Matrix: Evolution, Development and Disease.* Cambridge, UK: Cambridge University Press; 2004; 272 pp.
12. Willet WC, Lenart ER. Dietary factors. In: Mason J, Ridker PM, Gaziano JM, Hennekens CH, eds. *Prevention of Myocardial Infarction.* New York: Oxford University Press; 1996; 351–383.
13. Reddy KS, Katan MB. Diet, nutrition and prevention of hypertension and cardiovascular disease. Public Health Nutr. 2004;7:167–181.
14. Murray CJL, Lopez AD, eds. *Global Health Statistics.* Boston: Harvard University Press; 1996; 1010 pp.
15. World Cancer Research Fund. *Food, Nutrition and the Prevention of Cancer: A Global Perspective.* Washington, DC: American Institute for Cancer Research, 1997.
16. Zheng W, Gustafson DR, Sinha R, et al. Well-done meat intake and the risk of breast cancer. J Natl Cancer Inst. 1998;90:1724–1729.
17. Shriver SP, Bourdeau HA, Gubish CT, et al. Sex-specific expression of gastrin-releasing peptide receptor: relationship to smoking history and risk of lung cancer. J Natl Cancer Inst. 2000;92:24–33.
18. Plaisted CS, Istfan NW. Metabolic abnormalities of obesity. In: Blackburn GL, Kanders BS, eds. *Obesity: Pathophysiology, Psychology and Treatment.* New York: Chapman & Hall; 1994; 80–97.
19. Kanders BS, Peterson FJ, Lavin PT, Norton DE, Istfan NW, Blackburn GL. Long-term health effects associated with significant weight loss: a study of the dose-response effect. In: Blackburn GL, Kanders BS, eds. *Obesity: Pathophysiology, Psychology and Treatment.* New York: Chapman & Hall; 1994; 167–184.
20. Institute of Medicine Committee on Prevention of Obesity in Children and Youth. *Preventing Childhood Obesity: Health in the Balance.* Washington, DC: National Academies Press; 2005.
21. World Health Organization. *Obesity: Preventing and Managing the Global Epidemic.* Report of a WHO Consultation on Obesity. Geneva: World Health Organization; 1998.
22. Martorell R, Kettel KL, Hughes ML, Grummer-Strawn LM. Obesity in women from developing countries. Eur J Clin Nutr. 2000:54:247–252.
23. Martorell R, Kettel KL, Hughes ML, Grummer-Strawn LM. Overweight and obesity in preschool children from developing countries. Int J Obes Relat Metab Disord. 2000:24:959–967.
24. Hamill PCC, Drizch TA, Johnson CL, Reed RB, Roche AF, Moore WM. Physical growth: National Center for Health Statistics percentiles. Am J Clin Nutr. 1979;32:607–629.
25. National Heart, Lung, and Blood Institute: The Seventh Report of the Joint National Committee on Prevention, Detection, Evaluation, and Treatment of High Blood Pressure (JNC VII). Available at: http://www.nhlbi.nih.gov/guidelines/hypertension/jncintro.htm. Accessed March 30, 2006.
26. van den Hoogen PC, Feskens EJM, Nagelkerke NJD, Menotti A, Nissinen A, Kromhout D, for the Seven Countries Study Research Group. The relation between blood pressure and mortality due to coronary heart disease among men in different parts of the world. N Engl J Med. 2000;342:1–8.
27. National Heart, Lung, and Blood Institute: Primary Prevention of Hypertension: Clinical and Public Health Advisory from the National High Blood Pressure Education Program. Available at: http://www.nhlbi.nih.gov/health/prof/heart/hbp/pphbp.htm. Accessed March 30, 2006.
28. Cutler JA, Follmann D, Allender PS. Randomized trials of sodium reduction: an overview. Am J Clin Nutr. 1997;65(2 Suppl):643S–651S.
29. Harsha DW, Lin PH, Obarzanek E, Karanja NM, Moore TJ, Caballero B, for the DASH Collaborative Research Group. Dietary approaches to stop hypertension: a summary of study results. J Am Diet Assoc. 1999;99(8 Suppl):S35–S39.
30. INCLEN Multicentre Collaborative Group. Risk factors for cardiovascular disease in the developing world: a multicentre collaborative study in the International Clinical Epidemiology Network (INCLEN). J Clin Epidemiol. 1992;45:841–847.
31. Berrios X, Koponen T, Huiguang T, Khaltaev N, Puska P, Nissinen A. Distribution and prevalence of major risk factors of noncommunicable disease in selected countries: the WHO Inter-Health Programme. Bull World Health Organ. 1997;75:99–108.
32. National Heart, Lung, and Blood Institute: Third Report of the Expert Panel on Detection, Evaluation, and Treatment of High Blood Cholesterol in Adults (Adult Treatment Panel III). Available at: http://www.nhlbi.nih.gov/guidelines/cholesterol/atp_iii.htm. Accessed March 30, 2006.
33. Castelli WP, Anderson K, Wilson PW, Levy D. Lipids and risk of coronary heart disease. The Framingham Study. Ann Epidemiol. 1992;2:23–28.
34. Katan MB, Zock PL, Mensink RP. Dietary oils, serum lipoproteins, and coronary heart disease. Am J Clin Nutr. 1995;61(6 Suppl):1368S–1373S.
35. Zock PL, Katan MB. Trans fatty acids, lipoproteins, and coronary risk. Can J Physiol Pharmacol. 1997;75:211–216.
36. Friedwald WT, Levy RI, Fredrickson DS. Estimation of the concentration of low-density lipoprotein

cholesterol in plasma, without use of the preparative ultracentrifuge. Clin Chem. 1972;18:499–502.

37. Ford ES, Mokdad AH, Giles WH, Mensah GA. Serum total cholesterol and awareness, treatment and control of hypercholesterolemia among US adults: findings from the National Health and Examination Survey, 1999 to 2000. Circulation. 2003;107: 2185–2189.
38. Gelbard A, Haub C, Kent MM. World population beyond six billion. Popul Bull. 1999;54:1–44.
39. Omran AR. The epidemiologic transition. A theory of the epidemiology of population change. Milbank Mem Fund Q. 1971;49:509–538.
40. Olshansky SJ, Carnes B, Rogers RG, Smith L. Infectious diseases—New and ancient threats to world health. Popul Bull. 1997;52:1–52.
41. Olshansky SJ, Ault AB. The fourth stage of the epidemiologic transition: the age of delayed degenerative diseases. Milbank Q. 1986;64:355–391.
42. The World Bank. *Entering the 21st Century*. World Development Report 1999/2000. New York: Oxford University Press; 2000.
43. Pan American Health Organization. *Health in the Americas, 1998 Edition*. Volume I; Scientific Publication No. 569. Washington, DC: Pan American Health Organization; 1998.
44. Popkin BM. The nutrition transition in low-income countries: an emerging crisis. Nutr Rev. 1994;52: 285–298.
45. World Health Organization/Nutrition for Health and Development. *Progress and Prospects on the Eve of the 21st Century*. Geneva: World Health Organization; 1999.
46. United Nations Children's Fund. *The State of the World's Children 1998*. New York: Oxford University Press; 1998.
47. United Nations Development Programme. *Human Development Report 1999*. New York: Oxford University Press; 1999.
48. Fritschel H, Mohan U. *Pushing Back Poverty in India. News and Views*. Washington, DC: International Food Policy Research Institute; 1999.
49. Fan S, Hazell P, Thorat S. *Linkages Between Government Spending, Growth, and Poverty in Rural India*. Research Report 110. Washington, DC: International Food Policy Research Institute; 1999.
50. Gopalan C. Nutrition and development transition: lessons from the Asian experience. Bull Nutr Found India. 1999;20:1–5.
51. Ruel MT. Urbanization in Latin America: constraints and opportunities for child feeding and care. Food Nutr Bull. 2000;21:12–24.
52. Popkin BM. Urbanization, lifestyle changes and the nutrition transition. World Dev. 1999;27: 1905–1916.
53. DeSouza RM. *Household Transportation Use and Urban Air. Pollution: A Comparative Analysis of Thailand, Mexico and the United States*. Washington, DC: Population Reference Bureau; 1999.
54. Food and Agriculture Organization of the United Nations. *The Sixth World Food Survey 1996*. Rome, Italy: Food Agriculture Organization; 1996.
55. Drewnowski A, Popkin BM. The nutrition transition: new trends in the global diet. Nutr Rev. 1997; 55:31–43.
56. Guo Z, Popkin BM, Zhai F. Patterns of change in food consumption and dietary fat intake in Chinese adults, 1989–1993. Food Nutr Bull. 1999;20: 344–353.
57. de Oliveira SP. Changes in food consumption in Brazil. Arch Latinoam Nutr. 1997;47(2 Suppl 1):22–24.
58. Pinstrup-Anderson P, Pandya-Lorch R, Rosegrant MW. *The World Food Situation: Recent Developments, Emerging Issues, and Long-term Prospects*. Food Policy Report. Washington, DC: The International Food Policy Research Institute; 1997.
59. Pinstrup-Anderson P. Modern biotechnology and small farmers in developing countries. IFPRI Res Persp. 1999;21:3.
60. Centers for Disease Control and Prevention: Health, United States, 2004. Available at: http://www.cdc.gov/nchs/data/hus/hus04.pdf. Accessed October 20, 2005.
61. Chiang-Salgado MT, Casanueva-Escobar V, Cid-Cea X, et al. [Cardiovascular risk factors in Chilean university students]. Salud Publica Mex. 1999;41: 444–451.
62. Popkin BM. Population, development and nutrition: overview. In: Sadler M, Strain JJ, Caballero B, eds. *The Encyclopedia of Human Nutrition*. London: Academic Press. 1998;1562–1572.
63. Paeratakul S, Popkin BM, Ge K, Adair LS, Stevens J. Changes in diet and physical activity affect the body mass index of Chinese adults. Int J Obes Relat Metab Disord. 1998;22:424–431.
64. Martorell R. Results and implications of the INCAP Follow-up Study. J Nutr. 1995;125:1127S–1138S.
65. Fogel RW, Helmchen LA. Economic and technological development and their relationships to body size and productivity. In: Caballero B, Popkin BM, eds. *The Nutrition Transition: Diet and Disease in the Developing World*. San Diego: Academic Press; 2002; 9–24.

66 Food Insecurity, Hunger, and Undernutrition

David L. Pelletier, Christine M. Olson, and Edward A. Frongillo

Recent decades have witnessed some fundamental changes in the way that food insecurity, hunger, and undernutrition are understood within scientific and policy communities. In previous eras, these three problems were typically viewed as a causal or chronological continuum, with food insecurity representing a situation of inadequate access to food due to social and economical circumstances, hunger representing the immediate physiological manifestation of inadequate intake, and undernutrition representing the physical consequences of chronically or acutely inadequate intake. Such a view has various distorting effects on how each is measured and on notions of their prevalence, causes, consequences, and appropriate policy responses. This chapter describes the current understanding of the nature of each of these problems, their relationships with each other, what is known about prevalence, causes, and consequences, and policy implications. For convenience, the food security situation in developed and developing countries is described in separate sections. An important conclusion of the chapter, however, is that the current understandings of these problems are global in the sense that they apply to all settings, and they suggest that the range of potentially effective program and policy options is broader, and more complicated, than previously recognized.

Food Insecurity and Hunger in Food-Rich Countries: The United States as a Case Example

Nature of the Problem

Although food insecurity and hunger have long been nutrition concerns among poorer countries, these problems have reemerged as nutrition concerns for food-rich countries such as the United States. The term "hunger" is familiar and understood by most nutrition professionals, but the term "food insecurity" is relatively new and not well understood, particularly as it relates to the circumstances in food-rich countries. This section of the chapter will briefly describe food insecurity and its measurement and prevalence in the United States, and then review its consequences in food-rich countries.

In 1989, an expert panel convened by the American Institute of Nutrition for the Life Sciences Research Organization identified food insecurity and hunger as core indicators of an individual's nutritional state.[1] This group put forth what have become consensus definitions of food insecurity and hunger. Food insecurity is the "limited or uncertain availability of nutritionally adequate and safe foods or limited or uncertain ability to acquire acceptable foods in socially acceptable ways." Thus, food insecurity is a broad concept that encompasses availability and access to food, as well as the certainty of food availability and access; it includes the sufficiency, nutritional quality, and safety of food; and, finally, it is also concerned with cultural and social acceptability of available and accessible food and the means by which this food is acquired. Hunger, a narrower and more severe form of deprivation, is "the painful or uneasy sensation caused by a lack of food." It is a potential, although not necessary, consequence of food insecurity.[1]

Food insecurity is experienced primarily at two different levels of social organization: the household or family eating unit and the individual level. Hunger is generally used to describe an experience of food deprivation at the level of the individual. Interest is growing in the concept of community food security. The Community Food Security Coalition[2] has defined community food security as "the state in which all persons obtain a nutritionally adequate, culturally acceptable diet at all times through local non-emergency sources."

Radimer et al[3] have described food insecurity and hunger at the household and individual levels as managed processes in which inadequate means to obtain food results in anxiety about household food supply. This situation leads to the use of coping tactics, such as getting additional food in unusual ways, stretching food or food money, and restricting the food intake, all of which have emotional manifestations for the household and its individual members. The household food manager, generally a woman in US society, has some control over the sequence in which the various components of food insecurity are experienced and who experiences them. Thus, adults and children in the same household will experience different components of food insecurity at different times and to different degrees. Nonetheless, there is a general sequence to the phenomenon: household-level food insecurity, with the depletion of household food supplies and anxiety, is generally experienced first; the quantity and quality of women's food intake, as well as the quality of the household food supply, are affected next; and, finally, the quantity and quality of children's food intake are affected. This basic understanding of the sequenced nature of the phenomenon has been incorporated into instruments for measuring the problem.

Measurement

The comprehensive plan for the National Nutritional Monitoring and Related Research Program set in motion a series of collaborative efforts across government agencies, academia, and the private sector to create a measure of food insecurity and hunger that could be used annually to assess the prevalence of food insecurity and hunger in the US population.[4,5] The process of developing this measure is well described in the nutrition literature[6] and has been of interest to groups in other food-rich countries wishing to undertake the development of measures for national, state, or local level nutrition monitoring. The development and testing of questionnaire items by two groups, the Community Childhood Hunger Identification Project, sponsored by the Food Research and Action Center,[7] and the Division of Nutritional Sciences at Cornell University,[8] was critical to this effort.[6] In April 1995, the US Census Bureau administered the 18-item food-security scale to 45,000 households in its regular Current Population Survey. With data from this survey and methods from item-response theory (Rasch modeling), the scale was further refined, cut-points in the scale for differentiating levels of severity of the phenomena were defined, and categories of responses representing food security, food insecurity without hunger, food insecurity with moderate hunger, and food insecurity with severe hunger were created.[6]

The US Household Food Security Survey Module is

- **"We worried whether our food would run out before we got money to buy more." Was that often, sometimes, or never true for you in the last 12 months?**
- **"The food that we bought just didn't last and we didn't have money to get more." Was that often, sometimes, or never true for you in the last 12 months?**
- **"In the last 12 months did you or other adults in the household ever cut the size of your meals because there wasn't enough money for food?**
- **"In the last 12 months were you ever hungry, but didn't eat, because you couldn't afford enough food?**
- **(For households with children) In the last 12 months did any of the children ever not eat for a whole day because there wasn't enough money for food?**

Figure 1. Examples of questions from the 18-item core food security survey module. (From Bickel G, Nord M, Price C, et al. *Guide to Measuring Household Food Security.* Alexandria, VA: US Department of Agriculture, Food and Nutrition Service; March 2000.)

an 18-item scale with a 12-month time reference.[9] Figure 1 contains examples of items from the Food Security Survey Module. The scale has been shown to have good reliability, with a reliability coefficient of 0.81 for households with children and 0.74 for all households (extreme values that would inflate the reliability coefficient were omitted).[10] In addition, responses to the Current Population Survey items follow a pattern similar to those found in administration of the same items to samples from diverse populations, including racial and ethnic minorities.[11] Scale scores are significantly related to the poverty income ratio (income relative to the poverty line), weekly food expenditures, and the food sufficiency question in the expected ways, thus indicating validity.[10] The Food Security Survey Module has now been administered to participants in the Current Population Survey conducted by the US Census Bureau for the US Department of Labor, Bureau of Labor Statistics, for 10 years (1995–2004)[12] and has been incorporated in many other surveys.

In 2004, a National Research Council expert panel was asked to conduct an independent, two-phase review of the conceptualization and method of measuring food insecurity and hunger in the US population. A report for phase 1 of the project has been issued.[13] This report confirmed the importance of continuing to measure food insecurity in the US population. It urged additional research on the concept and definition of hunger and its relation to food insecurity. The report also noted that prevalence surveys may not be a good mechanism for evaluating food assistance programs. Although the panel suggested that the US Department of Agriculture explore alternate household surveys, it recommended that "USDA should continue to measure food insecurity as currently conducted using the Food Security Supplement to the CPS."[13]

Prevalence

In 2004, 11.9% of US households were food insecure: 8.0% were food insecure without hunger, and 3.9% were food insecure with hunger.[12] About 36 million persons lived in these food insecure households. Food insecurity differs by household characteristics in expected ways. Households with incomes below the official poverty line have a prevalence that is more than three times the national average. Central city and rural households have higher prevalence than do suburban households. Black and Hispanic households have a prevalence of 23.7% and 21.7%, respectively, and 33.0% of households headed by a single woman with children are food insecure.

From 1995 through 1999, there was a downward trend in the prevalence of household-level food insecurity in the United States. From 1999 to 2004, there has been a steady increase of over one full percentage point (10.1%–11.9%) in the prevalence of food insecurity.

Consequences

The early ethnographic research of Radimer et al.[3] suggest that individual household members experience food insecurity differently, with adults experiencing negative consequences before children. The available research tends to support this hypothesis. For example, Rose and Oliveira,[14] using data from the Continuing Survey of Food Intake by Individuals for 1989–1991, found food insufficiency (a more severe phenomenon than food insecurity) significantly associated with low intakes of eight nutrients, including energy, magnesium, and vitamins A, E, C, and B_6 in adult women but not in preschoolers (ages 0–5 years). These results remain when the analyses are controlled for other confounding variables. A group of researchers in Canada led by McIntyre[15] specifically examined this hypothesis in a study of 141 low-income single mothers with at least two children living in the Atlantic provinces of Canada. These investigators found widespread food insecurity, with 78% of households experiencing the condition. They also found consistently lower dietary intakes in mothers compared with their children. Across the month, as the money to purchase food became less available, this gap widened, supporting the findings of Radimer et al.[3] that mothers compromise their own nutritional status to feed their children.

Lower dietary intakes of essential nutrients and important food groups among food-insecure adults have been confirmed in local[16] and national surveys,[17] including the work of Rose and Oliveira,[14] as cited earlier. Dixon et al.[17] have provided the first biochemical evidence from a national survey showing that both young and older adults from food-insufficient households have lower blood levels of vitamin A and other carotenoids. Although the health effects of low dietary intakes and biochemical indicators of nutritional status may not be immediately apparent, over the long-term they could result in increased risk of ill health. Numerous investigators have demonstrated a significant association in adults between food insecurity and poorer self-rated health and poorer functional health status.[18,19] Similar associations have been found in the elderly[20,21] and among person with diabetes.[22]

In 2004, 19% of children in the United States lived in food-insecure households.[12] The bulk of research done to date indicates that food insecurity is associated with poorer nutritional status in children, as well as poorer health, mental and psychological functioning, and cognitive and academic achievement. Casey et al.[23] found no differences in the nutrient intakes of low-income food-sufficient and low-income food-insufficient children participating in the Continuing Survey of Food Intakes by Individuals from 1994 to 1996, but low-income food-insufficient children had lower energy and carbohydrate intakes and higher cholesterol intakes than high-income food-sufficient children. Kaiser et al.[24] studied 211 Mexican-American preschoolers ages 3 to 6 and found significantly lower Food Guide Pyramid scores ($P < 0.006$) in children from households with severe hunger compared with children from households without severe hunger. The proportion of children meeting the recommended servings for milk ($P < 0.003$) and meat ($P < 0.06$) was lower. Also, among Hispanic fifth graders in California, Matheson et al.[25] found significantly lower mean body mass index (BMI) among those from food-insecure households compared with those from food-secure households ($P < 0.04$).

Several studies have examined the association between measures of physical health and food insecurity. Cook et al.[26] interviewed the parents of children ages 36 months and younger who visited emergency rooms and clinics in urban medical centers in five states and Washington, DC. They found that food-insecure children had an adjusted odds-ratio for being in fair or poor health that was nearly twice as large as that of children from food-secure households. The risk of being hospitalized since birth was almost one-third larger among the children from food-insecure households.

Using the National Health and Nutrition Examination Survey (NHANES III), Alaimo et al.[27] found that food-insufficient preschool and elementary school-age children are more likely to be in fair or poor health. After controlling for confounding factors, including poverty status, food-insufficient children were significantly more likely to have poorer health status. Food-insufficient middle-income children (family income between 130% and 350% of the federal poverty line) were just as likely to be in poor health as food-insufficient low-income children (family income less than or equal to 130% of the federal poverty line). Both food-insufficient groups were more likely to be in poor health than food-sufficient children in either income group. These results indicate that food insufficiency is associated with poor health that goes beyond poverty.

One study specifically examined hunger and its correlates on homeless and low-income housed preschool and school-age children in Worcester, Massachusetts.[28]

Among both preschool and school-age children, severe hunger was associated with higher levels of chronic illness and internalizing behavior problems. Severe hunger was also associated with higher levels of anxiety and depression among school-age children.

Two papers by Kleinman et al.[29] and Murphy et al.[30] demonstrate a relationship between hunger and risk of hunger, as measured by the Community Childhood Hunger Identification Project scale and psychosocial problems in children, as measured by the Pediatric Symptom Checklist. The positive relationship of increasing psychosocial problems with the increasing severity of food insecurity and hunger remains even when controlling for available measures of the socioeconomic status of the household.[31] Using the NHANES III data, Alaimo et al.[32] found that household-level food insufficiency was associated with having seen a psychologist and having difficulty getting along with other children in 6- to 11-year-olds, controlling for confounding variables. Food-insufficient teenagers were more likely to have seen a psychologist, have been suspended from school, and have had difficulty getting along with other teenagers. Food insufficiency was also associated with increased risk of suicide in teenagers.[33] Moving to children's cognitive and academic performance, we find some disturbing effects of food insufficiency. After adjusting for poor health and poverty status, 6- to 11-year-old food-insufficient children in NHANES III had significantly lower arithmetic scores and were more likely to have repeated a grade level.[32] Using data on 3500 children ages 0 to 12 years from the 1997 Child Development Supplement to the Panel Study of Income Dynamics, Reid[34] found a relationship between the number of years a child had lived in a food-insecure family and letter word, passage comprehension, and calculation scores.

A recent paper that examined a range of nutritional outcomes associated with food insecurity, including dietary intake expressed as the Healthy Eating Index, blood levels of selected nutrients, and BMI in children, adolescents, and adults contradicts some of the findings of other authors. Using NHANES III data, Bhattacharya et al.[35] found that food insecurity did not add any predictive power for poor nutritional outcomes beyond poverty in children ages 2 to 5. In school-age children, neither poverty nor food insecurity was associated with poor nutritional outcomes, whereas both were predictive of poor outcomes in adults and the elderly. These investigators, however, used a grouping of items to measure food insecurity that has questionable validity and reliability. Previous research has shown that the items used by these investigators as measures of food insecurity in NHANES III are not understood by respondents, calling into question the researchers' conclusions.[36]

One of the most controversial and confusing associations between a measure of health status and food insecurity is that found between obesity and food insecurity. Olson et al.[31,37] were among the first to show that BMI was significantly higher ($P < 0.05$) for women in food-insecure households compared with women in food-secure households (28.2 vs. 25.6). Also, 37% of the women in the households with the least severe level of food insecurity had BMIs greater than 29 compared with 26% of women in food-secure households. Controlling for the woman's height, income level, educational level, single parent status, and employment status in the statistical analysis, food insecurity was still positively related to BMI ($P < 0.06$). Women in food-insecure households were approximately two BMI units heavier than women in food-secure households. Women in households where hunger was present did not differ on BMI or obesity from women in food-secure households. This association between obesity and food insecurity in women has been replicated by Townsend et al.[38] using Continuing Survey of Food Intake by Individuals data and by Basiotis[39] using NHANES III data. Investigators using several state-level data sets have also found the association,[40,41] whereas one group using New York State and Louisiana Behavioral Risk Factor Surveillance System data for 1 year has not found an association.[42] Recently, a smaller survey of Mexican-American mothers in California also demonstrated the association.[43] The association in men is equivocal, with one study finding no association[38] and another finding the association in women.[41]

A potential relationship of hunger and food insecurity to obesity in childhood was first highlighted by Dietz.[44] He described an obese 7-year-old African-American girl whose family fed her high-fat foods at the end of the month when the money for food was running out. This original case study has been followed by several studies using large national data sets[23,45] and one smaller study.[24] With the possible exception of non-Hispanic older girls, in whom there was an indication that food insecurity was positively associated with overweight ($P < 0.10$),[45] food insecurity and hunger were not related to increased overweight and obesity in US children in the research that has been done to date to address the issue.

All of the studies described previously are cross-sectional with data for the two major constructs collected at the same point in time. Thus, all are constrained in specifying the direction of causality between the two constructs. Longitudinal data and analyses are needed to make inferences about the direction of the causality.

In recognition of the health correlates of food insecurity, the nutrition objective for Healthy People 2010 include increasing the prevalence of food security among US households to 94% of all households.[46] Also, the US Action Plan on Food Security lays out a number of priority actions and strategies to achieve this public health goal.[47]

Food Insecurity and Hunger in Developing Countries

Nature of the Problem

The concept of food security first gained international prominence with the World Food Conference of 1974.

It has been a powerful and useful concept, as evidenced by the 200 definitions of food security that have emerged since then.[48] The most commonly cited definition is "access by all people at all times to enough food for an active, healthy life."[49] This definition emphasizes that food security is relevant for individuals, implies each individual's entitlement and right to food, requires sufficient and sustainable access to food, and has consequences. Despite its merits, this definition or any single definition understates the complexity of food security issues in the developing world.[50] This complexity is reflected in the three significant shifts in thinking about food security that have occurred in the past 25 years: 1) from the global and national level to the household and individual level, 2) from a food-first to a livelihood perspective, and 3) from objective to subjective understandings.[48]

Food security can be considered at various levels, including global, regional, national, provincial, community, household, and individual. A simplified conceptual framework for food security from the global and the national level to the household and the individual level is presented in Figure 2. This framework illustrates what is meant by food security that differs at each level; a different lens is needed to understand food security at each level. At the global level, food security concerns the overall availability of food. At the national level, food security also concerns availability, which results from the balance of importing and producing food. At the household level, food security concerns the availability and access to food by the household, which results from household production and availability from the market or others in the community. At the individual level, food security concerns the use or consumption of food, which results from its availability to and access by the household and also the distribution within the household.[51] "An individual person is food secure when his or her consumption of food is sufficient, secure (not vulnerable to consumption shortfalls), and sustainable."[52]

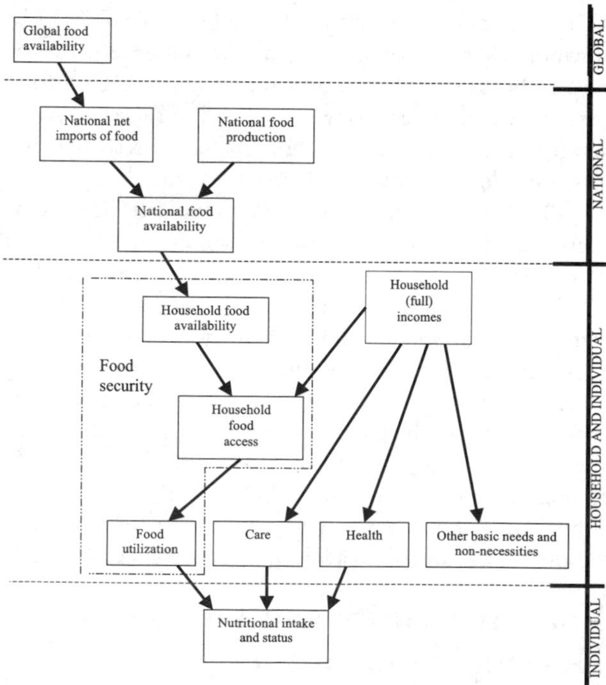

Figure 2. Simplified conceptual framework for food security from the global and the national to the household and the individual. (From Smith 1998[52]; used with permission from Elsevier.)

Food is a fundamental need in that each individual must have access to necessary nutrients to survive and to participate actively in society. Previously, it was assumed that food was a primary need, meaning that the need for food would take precedence over other needs. In recent years, however, it has been recognized that food is only one of the needs that people must attempt to meet. The term "livelihood security" has emerged to capture the understanding that households often make trade-offs to ensure their long-term viability as productive and reproductive units.[48] Livelihood security refers to the stocks and flows of assets and cash to meet basic needs, offset risk, ease shocks, and meet contingencies.[50,53] People may go hungry in the present to preserve assets and future ability to make their living. They may forgo eating now to preserve seed for future planting or to save an animal for future use. These are examples of people going hungry in the present to avoid or lessen going hungry in the future.[54] Livelihood security implies other trade-offs as well. For example, people may forgo some food to be able to buy medication to treat illness.

Food insecurity is a form of deprivation. Just as with poverty, when thinking about food insecurity, one can refer to both the conditions of deprivation and the feelings of deprivation.[54] Whereas previously, the tendency was to consider food security solely as referring to the adequacy of food or nutrients in objective terms, increasingly, the understanding now is that the subjective experience of individuals is central. From this understanding comes the view that the relevant food security is that which is actually perceived by a household or individual rather than that which is decided on by researchers or policy makers, given that households will behave according to their perception and not according to indicators defined by outsiders.[54] Important categories of behaviors potentially influenced by one's perceptions of food insecurity are investment (e.g., in productive assets, education, and children), risk avoidance (e.g., regarding adoption of new agricultural technologies or management practices), and survival strategies (e.g., rural-urban migration, diversification of livelihood strategies).

Taken together, these three shifts in thinking about food security shape our current understanding of the nature of the problem in developing countries. Food security is not just about national food supply and prices. Food security instead must be considered differently at each level of social organization. At the household and individual levels, food security is "concerned with the complexities of livelihood strategies in difficult and uncertain environments, and with understanding how people themselves respond to perceived risks and uncertainties."[54] Food security is thus a multilevel and multidimensional phenomenon. This complexity has important implications for how food security is assessed and for efforts to improve food security.

Measurement

At the global and national levels, food security has primarily been measured by estimating "the number of people whose food intake does not provide enough calories to meet their basic energy requirements."[55] The Food and Agriculture Organization of the United Nations (FAO) refers to these people as the undernourished. The FAO uses undernourishment to represent those with chronic food insecurity. Estimates are made from information on food production, trade, and stocks; figures for total population and distribution by age and gender; and distribution of consumption.[55] The method involves calculating the amount of energy available in a country and an average minimum energy requirement for the total population, adjusting for inequality in access to food, and then constructing the distribution of the food supply within the country. These calculations are intended to "produce an estimate of the number of people in each country whose average caloric intake falls below the minimum required to keep the body going and perform light activity."[55]

A critique of the FAO method found that it largely reflects national food availability and does not adequately reflect people's ability to access food.[52] Therefore, this method yields a direct measure of food security at the national level if it is defined in terms of national food availability (Figure 2). But the FAO method does not yield an accurate measure of food security at the household or individual level because it does not adequately reflect access to and use of food. The critique showed that this limitation results in misclassification of food security with respect to differentiating geographical locations or detecting changes over time.[52]

As an outcome of the 1996 World Food Summit, a program has been established called the Food Insecurity and Vulnerability Information and Mapping System to provide better information about global and national food security. It is coordinated by an interagency working group with the FAO serving as secretariat. The program draws on many existing information systems, such as crop forecasting and early warning systems, household food security and nutritional information systems, and vulnerability assessment and mapping systems.[55,56]

How best to measure household and individual food security is the subject of much debate, partly because of the difficulty of defining it. At the household and individual levels, food security has been most often measured indirectly. Food security affects dietary intake and, ultimately, nutritional status and physical well-being, as well as other outcomes. While measures of dietary intake of individuals can assess some aspects of food security such as energy insufficiency and nutrient inadequacy, they do not assess the cognitive and affective components of uncertainty (expressed as anxiety), unacceptability, or unsustainability. For example, current intake may be adequate, but food insecurity still may be experienced because of concern over future intake. Alternatively, intake may be inadequate, but only temporarily so as to protect supplies and prevent future food insecurity. Growth status is also used as an indicator, but again does not assess most of the components of food security. Furthermore, growth status is an indirect outcome because it also depends on factors such as health and child care.

Food security is also related to available economical and social resources. Precursors such as income or total expenditure are correlated with energy sufficiency, but they only capture this component of food insecurity and are quite indirect.[57] Food-related management or "coping" strategies have also been used to assess food insecurity.[48,58] Management strategies result from and affect the experience of food insecurity and may be useful as early indications of future food insecurity. The presence or absence of particular management strategies, however, often is not indicative of food security, and measures of management strategies do not include all components of the experience of food insecurity.

Several other approaches have been used to develop measures of household and individual food security. Chung et al.[59] used ethnography in India to understand local perceptions, early signs, coping strategies, and intrahousehold decision-making related to food security, and then to develop locally defined measures. Ethnography was also used in rural Nepal to help develop culturally appropriate and valid quantitative instruments for assessing and making operational household food security and for constructing scales of past food supply, current food stores, and adequacy of future food supply.[60] Several simple tools and techniques for assessing problems and situations at the community level have been developed as part of the Rapid Rural Appraisal and the similar but more action-oriented Participatory Rural Appraisal. These often involve focus groups and in-depth interviews to understand the food security situation and to help develop quantitative measures.[61-64] The Food Economy Approach monitors household food security and early warning of food crises by quantifying household access to food in normal years and the effects of external shocks on this access.[65] Results include an estimate of the shortfall in food income that people are likely to face, the costs of coping in terms of depletion of assets and dislocation of families, and the likely effects of different levels and forms of assistance. Phillips and Taylor[41] developed a method for assessing household food security that combines a household questionnaire with a quasi-expert analysis system. Davies[53] developed an approach to food security monitoring that uses field agents, in-depth interviews, Rapid Rural Appraisal techniques, and more conventional surveys to understand the local livelihood systems and develop indicators for tracking livelihood vulnerability. These indicators are monitored annually and used to predict needs and develop appropriate interventions.

Because the closer or more direct a measure is to the phenomenon of interest, the better that measure will be, it is important to measure the experience of food insecurity itself, including whatever its key components are in a given location.[11] This experience could be objectively and definitively measured by observing in detail a household over time.[11,66] Because such an approach is not feasible for a large number of households, this experience can instead be measured subjectively by assessing not only aspects of the availability of, access to, and use of food, but also how a person feels about it (e.g., anxiety, worry) and what a person thinks about it (e.g., perceptions, social acceptability). Because these manifestations are overt, we can tap into them to directly measure the experience of food insecurity in a comprehensive manner.

One way to develop direct measures that include these components and can complement existing measures is to base them on an in-depth understanding of the experience of food insecurity at the household level, as was used successfully to develop the US Food Security Survey Module. Although the US measure itself may not be applicable to many developing countries, the approach is applicable, with the potential for developing improved measures of household food security on the basis of an in-depth understanding of food insecurity at the household level.[67,68] Recently, this approach has been used in Indonesia[69] and Bangladesh[70] to develop experience-based measures of food insecurity. Furthermore, the Food and Nutrition Technical Assistance Project has sponsored studies in Burkina Faso, Bangladesh, and several other countries to examine the development and validation of such measures, what aspects of food insecurity are common across locations and cultures, and when measures should be developed locally from in-depth understanding versus adapting existing measures. The results from this project demonstrate that experience-based measures are valid for differentiating households both at a given time and with changes over time, that developing such measures is feasible in programmatic settings, and that many, but not all, aspects of the experience of food insecurity are common across locations and cultures.[71-73]

Prevalence

Information about the prevalence of food insecurity at the global, regional, and national levels is primarily available from FAO estimates of undernourishment. According to these estimates, nearly 815 million people or 17% of people in developing countries are undernourished (Table 1). Because of its large population, Asia has by far the largest number of undernourished people. Sub-Saharan Africa has by far the largest prevalence of undernourishment at 33%. As explained earlier, these estimates are likely to be an accurate reflection of food availability

Table 1. Prevalence of Undernourishment in Developing Countries

Region	Undernourished in Total Population (2000–2002)	
	Number	**Prevalence**
	(millions)	(%)
Asia and Pacific	519.0	16
Latin America and Caribbean	52.9	10
Near East and North Africa	39.2	10
Sub-Saharan Africa	203.5	33
All developing countries	814.6	17

Used with permission from Food and Agriculture Organization of the United Nations. *The State of Food Insecurity in the World.* Rome: FAO; 2005.

at the global, regional, and national levels, but not of food security at the household or individual levels.

Consequences

Food insecurity adversely affects well-being in many ways. Mechanisms that bring about such effects may be biological, acting through decreased nutrient intake, or social and behavioral, acting through, for example, compromised time and energy for and attention to care of self and dependents. Some adverse effects of food insecurity include infants with low birth weight and high risk of mortality, mothers who cannot adequately provide human milk for their infants, children with impaired cognitive and neurological development that leads to reduced learning capacity and school performance, and adults with low work productivity and capacity to be food secure. The cycle is completed as these adults have children.[75] Another set of consequences is a range of behavioral responses to uncertainty (including investment, risk avoidance, and survival strategies) and the experience of stress, alienation, deprivation, and adverse family and social interactions.[76]

Undernutrition

Nature of the Problem

Undernutrition, as manifested by deviations from normal growth in early childhood, is a problem primarily in developing countries, and these will be emphasized in this section. Scientific understandings of the nature and causes of undernutrition, and its potential solutions, have evolved significantly in the last 50 years and have had enormous (often negative) effects on the design of programs, policies, and research. Briefly summarizing this evolution of thought is important, not out of mere historical curiosity, but because, to this day, we continue to experience paradigm shifts.

From mid-century through the 1960s, the major focus was on protein deficiency. Based on the earlier description of kwashiorkor by Williams[77] and the prevailing nutrient deficiency paradigm during that time in nutritional sciences, attention was directed toward estimating human requirements for protein and individual amino acids under varying physiological states and conditions of health and disease prevalent in developing countries. Simultaneously, various other disciplines (e.g., animal and agricultural sciences, food science), development agencies, and governments sought to develop and implement technological and food-based means for increasing animal protein or essential amino acids in the food supplies and diets in developing countries. This protein era came to an unusually rapid end in the 1970s, at least in the expert communities, with the downward revision of estimated protein requirements,[78] but the protein focus continues to influence thinking and food and nutrition policy in many countries even today. This episode has also negatively affected nutrition's image within scientific and development communities, an impact that reverberates to this day, resulting from the perception that nutritionists directed attention to protein deficiency and then changed their minds after many other scientists and institutions had redirected their work to help close the protein gap.

For a field of scientific and applied work that has experienced the dramatic and damaging effects of such a paradigm shift, the nutrition community has since revealed a surprising propensity to again shift and re-shift its focus of research and intervention strategies. This shifting focus includes the era of the energy gap in the 1960s and 1970s,[79,80] multisectoral nutrition planning, applied nutrition programs, nutrition surveillance in the 1970s and 1980s,[81,82] and micronutrient deficiencies in the 1990s.[81] By the 1990s (and continuing to the present) the discourse in international nutrition included a wide array of problems and causes (e.g., growth faltering, low birth weight, maternal undernutrition, iodine, vitamin A, iron and zinc deficiencies, diarrhea, HIV and other infectious diseases, inadequate infant and child feeding practices, female time constraints, limited household income and agricultural production, food insecurity, environmental degradation, and urbanization) and a wide array of partial solutions (e.g., growth monitoring, supplementary feeding, breast-feeding and complementary feeding, nutrition education, oral rehydration, child spacing, fortification, vitamin A, iron and multiple-nutrient supplementation, income generation, food aid, home gardening, and agricultural intensification). Such a situation would be a cause for concern for any development issue, but it is particularly challenging for nutrition because its problems are multisectoral and addressing them requires understanding, trust, and cooperation with diverse line ministries such as health, agriculture, education, and finance. Rather than generating a coherent and understandable approach to the problem, nutrition's history has contributed to the perception among many policy makers and planners that the nutrition problem is too complicated, that it has created a fragmentation of effort across international and government agencies, and that it has failed to generate a consensus within the nutrition community itself about priority problems, actions, and strategies.

In an effort to respond to this situation in the early 1990s, the nutrition section of the United Nations Children's Fund (UNICEF) developed and promoted an inclusive conceptual framework for organizing scientific knowledge and experience, fostering a common understanding and developing coherent strategies for addressing them (Figure 3). Some of the key features of this framework and the nutrition strategy of which it was a part[83] follow:

- Malnutrition is a biological manifestation of inadequate dietary intake and disease, but these are deeply rooted in a set of underlying and basic causes related to social and economical development. As such, malnutrition should not be viewed as distinct from other developmental problems, but rather as a reflection of them. This reframing of the problem permits a more constructive dialog about nutrition within various sectors.
- This framework makes explicit the assumptions underlying various approaches to malnutrition so that they can be questioned and debated. This is in contrast to the tendency among specialized scientists, professionals, or institutions that implicitly assumes that malnutrition is due to lack of food, health care, education, breast-feeding, agricultural production, or some other factor of particular interest to those actors or institutions.
- The framework explicitly recognizes that the relative importance of the three underlying causes of malnutrition (food, health, and care) can vary widely across households, communities, and countries. This context specificity implies that universal causes and solutions do not exist and that the binding constraints must be assessed and acted upon in each setting. From this perspective, the list of specific causes and proposed solutions noted earlier can be viewed as an asset rather than a problem if they are viewed as a menu of possibilities whose relevance needs to be assessed in each setting. This requires a highly decentralized approach to assessment, analysis, and action, as opposed to national or global solutions, as in the past. The potential impact of such an approach has been documented by the Iringa Nutrition Program in Tanzania, which gave rise to the UNICEF strategy and was repeated in Thailand, Indonesia, and Vietnam.[84-86]

This unified framework has contributed enormously to fostering a shared understanding and a basis for communication across disciplines and sectors concerning the nature of malnutrition and ways to address it. Much work

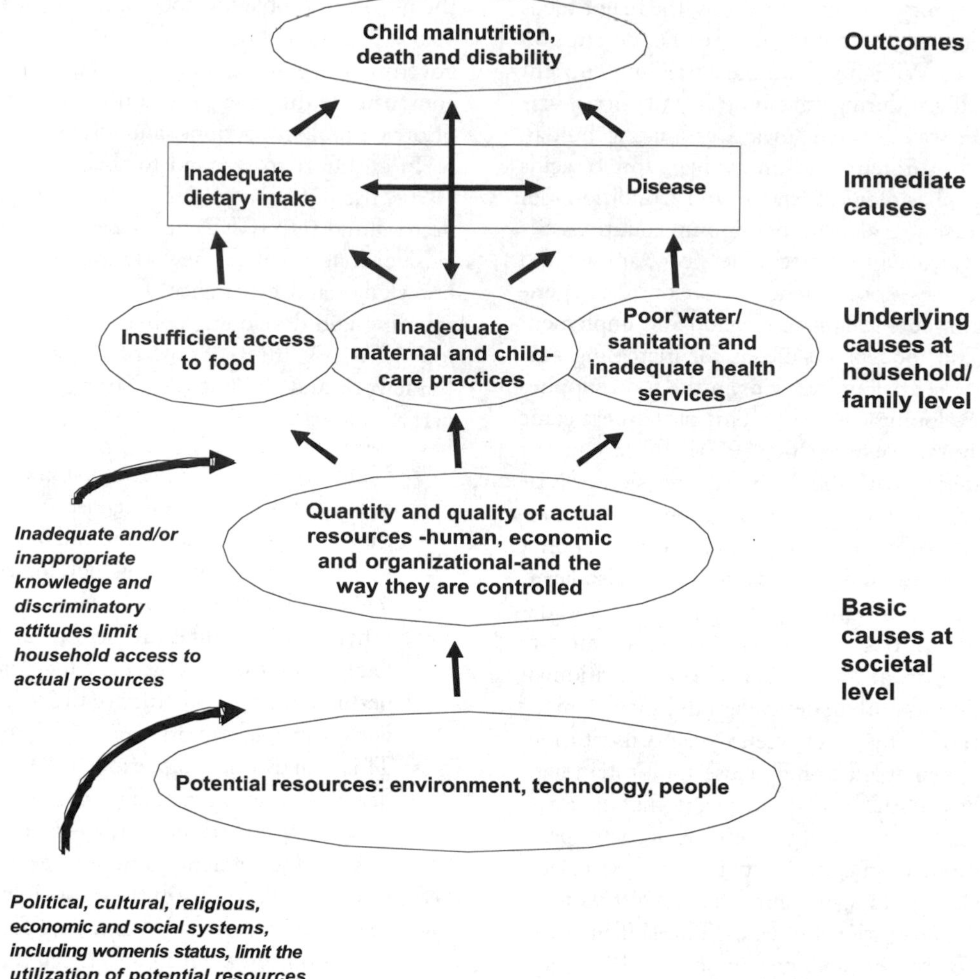

Figure 3. UNICEF conceptual framework for the causes of malnutrition. (Used with permission from UNICEF. *The State of the World's Children 1998.* New York: UNICEF; 1997; p. 24.)

is still required, however, to counter or accommodate the continued tendency for specialized scientists, professionals, and institutions to single out and promote (in the context of research, policy development, and programs) that part of the framework that suits their particular interests and agendas even when the context suggests that other actions may be more appropriate.[86]

Measurement

In light of the current understanding of the nature of the problem, it is apparent that the traditional approach to nutritional assessment is limited to measuring the physical manifestations of the problem (clinical, anthropometric, and biochemical indicators) and some of the immediate causes related to dietary intake. These physical indicators may be adequate for estimating the magnitude of the problem, but the principle of context specificity requires additional methods and approaches for assessing the broader nutrition situation that includes consideration of food, health, and care, and such basic causes as the level and control of resources at household, community, and national levels. An important area for future research is the development of practical methods and approaches for doing so, with recognition of the distinctive requirements and possibilities at national, district, and community levels.[87]

For the purposes of this chapter, attention will be restricted to anthropometric indicators that reveal the prevalence and trends in undernutrition at the national level among preschool children.[88] These include height-for-age that indicates the cumulative effects of malnutrition in the life of the child; weight-for-height that indicates recent nutritional experiences (typically weeks or months); and weight-for-age that reflects the combined effects of recent and longer-term conditions. These indicators are considered to be sensitive to the immediate and underlying causes of malnutrition, as depicted in Figure 3, although they are not specific to any particular cause. In other words, they do not reveal the relative importance of dietary intake (e.g., energy, protein, iron, zinc, vitamin

A, or overall diversity), infectious disease, food insecurity, inadequate health environment and health services, low birth weight, child-care practices, income constraints, or disparities in resource control. These factors are part of the assessment of the larger nutrition situation, as distinct from the anthropometric indicators that merely reflect the severity and extent of the problem, distribution across geographical and social groups, and trends over time.

Prevalence

Tables 2 and 3, respectively, list the prevalence (percentage) of preschool children with low weight-for-age and height-for-age by region or subregion and over time. For the developing world as a whole, 22.7% of preschoolers were estimated to be underweight in 2005, and 26.5% were estimated to be stunted (low height-for-age). The estimates for 1990 were 30.1% and 37.9%, respectively, figures that indicate considerable improvement in some regions over the two decades.

In 1990, south Asia and southeast Asia were noted for having the highest prevalences of underweight and stunting, with sub-Saharan Africa having intermediate levels and Latin America having the lowest levels of these three major regions. The data reveal, however, that the direction and rate of change varies across regions (Tables 2 and 3). For example, the prevalence of underweight among preschool children declined substantially in east Asia, southeast Asia, and south-central Asia from 1990 to 2005, and it remained relatively low in Latin America/Caribbean and north Africa during this period. The prevalence in regions of sub-Saharan Africa, however, remained more or less constant or increased. In general, the trends in stunting parallel those for underweight, although in eastern and west Africa they did not rise to the same extent that underweight did. The more limited estimates of wasting (low weight-for-height) in 2005 revealed high prevalence in Asia and west and middle Africa, intermediate levels in the remainder of Africa, and very low levels in western Asia, Latin America, and the Caribbean. The net result of these changes is that the prevalence of undernutrition in eastern and west Africa, as measured by underweight and stunting, now exceeds that in east and southeast Asia and is similar to or approaching that in south Asia. In terms of numbers of children affected, however, the Asian regions remain by far the most affected.

Data and experience from the United States can be used to illustrate the near absence of undernutrition, as manifested in child anthropometrics, while at the same time illustrating the universal applicability of the UNICEF conceptual framework for understanding its causes. Data from NHANES III (1988–1991) reveal that the prevalence of low height-for-age (below the fifth percentile) is 4% to 5% throughout the period for those ages 2 months to 11 years.[89] These values have remained essentially unchanged since NHANES I (1971–1974), and the lack of a secular trend in height-for-age is confirmed with data from the Pediatric Nutrition Surveillance System over the same period.[89] The NHANES III data reveal that populations with a high prevalence of poverty, such as Mexican Americans, are found to have prevalence in the same range as the general population. Although these data suggest that undernutrition is not elevated at the

Table 2. Prevalence of Underweight* Among Preschool Children† by Region, 1990–2005

United Nations Regions	1990	1995	2000	2005‡
All of Africa	23.6%	23.9%	24.2%	24.5%
North Africa	12.3%	10.9%	9.7%	8.6%
East Africa	26.7%	27.9%	29.2%	30.6%
West Africa	27.8%	27.5%	27.1%	26.8%
Middle Africa	27.8%	26.9%	26.1%	25.3%
Southern Africa	14.0%	13.9%	13.7%	13.6%
All of Asia	35.1%	31.5%	27.9%	24.8%
East Asia	18.5%	13.2%	9.3%	6.5%
South-central Asia	49.6%	45.2%	40.8%	36.5%
Southeast Asia	35.2%	31.2%	27.4%	23.9%
Western Asia	12.9%	12.1%	11.3%	10.6%
Latin America and Caribbean	8.7%	7.3%	6.1%	5.0%
All	30.1%	27.3%	24.8%	22.7%

* Underweight is defined as a weight-for-age ≤2 standard deviations of the median value of the National Center for Health Statistics and World Health Organization international growth reference.
†Ages 0–5 years.
‡Projected.

Table 3. Prevalence of Stunting* Among Preschool Children by Region, 1990–2005, and of Wasting† in 2005

United Nations Regions	1990	1995	2000	2005†	Wasting in 2005‡
All of Africa	36.9%	36.1%	35.2%	34.5%	9.5%
North Africa	27.4%	24.4%	21.7%	19.1%	8.0%
East Africa	44.4%	44.4%	44.4%	44.4%	8.7%
West Africa	34.7%	33.8%	32.9%	32.0%	10.2%
Middle Africa	42.2%	40.0%	37.8%	35.8%	11.9%
Southern Africa	25.4%	25.0%	24.6%	24.3%	6.6%
All of Asia	41.1%	35.4%	30.1%	25.7%	8.9%
East Asia	30.0%	21.5%	14.8%	10.0%	8.9%
South-central Asia	50.8%	45.2%	39.7%	34.5%	13.3%
Southeast Asia	41.8%	36.8%	32.1%	27.7%	8.7%
Western Asia	25.0%	21.7%	18.7%	16.1%	3.9%
Latin America and Caribbean	18.3%	15.9%	13.7%	11.8%	1.5%
All	37.9%	33.5%	29.6%	26.5%	8.3%

* Stunting is defined as a height-for-age ≤2 standard deviations of the median value of the National Center for Health Statistics and World Health Organization international growth reference.
† Projected.
‡ Wasting is based on the same criterion as applied to the weight-for-height reference.

population level, there is a recognized syndrome of "inorganic failure-to-thrive" observed in clinical practice. Most of these cases are associated with inattentive or inappropriate parenting, neglect, or abuse. In other words, they are attributable to problems associated with care in the UNICEF framework (Figure 3).

Consequences

The consequences of undernutrition in developing countries have been the subject of study for several decades, and the cumulative evidence suggests that undernutrition has pervasive effects on human performance, health, and survival.[90] This includes effects on morbidity,[91] mortality,[92,93] intrauterine growth,[94] cognitive and social development,[95,96] physical work capacity,[97] productivity,[98] and economical growth.[99] In several cases, the magnitude of these effects has been unexpected. For instance, a meta-analysis of eight prospective studies revealed that the relative risk of child mortality is 8.4 for the severely underweight (<60% of reference weight) but is also substantial for less severe forms: 4.6 for the moderately underweight (60%–69% of reference) and 2.5 for the mildly underweight (70%–79% of reference).[93] Given the high prevalence of the mild and moderate forms, these results suggest that 56% of child deaths are due to malnutrition (via the potentiation of infectious disease), of which 83% is due to mild-to-moderate forms. These estimates are much higher than the 2% to 5% previously assumed[100] and have stimulated renewed interest in the role of nutrition in child survival policies and programs. More recent studies have confirmed the importance of underweight as an underlying cause of child mortality[101] and demonstrated that underweight increases cause-specific mortality due to neonatal disorders, diarrhea, pneumonia, and malaria.[102,103] As another example of the expanding knowledge about the consequences of undernutrition, on the basis of an extensive empirical analysis of historical trends, Fogel[99] concluded that improvements in nutritional status and health accounted for most of the economical growth in Europe during the 18th and 19th centuries, a finding with important implications for contemporary populations in developed and developing countries. This body of work led to a Nobel Prize in economics for Fogel and North in 1993.

In part because of the broader recognition of the consequences and importance of hunger, food insecurity, and undernutrition, these three problems play a prominent role in the Millennium Development Goals, a set of eight development goals advanced by the United Nations in 2000 and since ratified by over 190 United Nation member states[104] with the aim of achieving numerical targets by 2015. The first of these goals is to eradicate extreme poverty and hunger, with the target of reducing by half the proportion of people whose income is less than one dollar a day and the proportion who suffer from hunger. The hunger target is to be measured by two indicators: the prevalence of underweight children and the proportion of the population below minimum dietary energy consumption. In addition to these explicit goals and targets related to nutrition, goal number 3 (reduce child mortality by two-thirds) and goal number 5 (improve maternal health) have important linkages to nutrition.

Although the Millennium Development Goals are a significant recognition at the international level of the importance of reducing hunger, food insecurity, and malnutrition, achieving them requires a firm understanding of the nature of these problems, and, as described in earlier sections, this has not always been the case in the past. The implications of this are examined in the next section.

Policy Implications

Food insecurity and undernutrition are the behavioral or biological manifestations of problems rooted in the social world, from the individual and household levels to the community, organizational, national, and international levels. A wide range of scientific disciplines may be drawn upon to maximize the possibility of finding effective and sustainable solutions. Even a solution seemingly as simple as vitamin A supplementation requires an understanding of the behavior of households, communities, clinic workers, program managers, and policy makers.[105] Thus, a scientific approach for addressing these problems must include, but go well beyond, the biological sciences that have formed the core of the discipline of nutrition. This section on policy implications is based on this broad perspective.

The evolution of thought concerning food security and undernutrition in developed and developing countries has some commonalities with significant policy implications. The main commonality is the recognition that the causes of these problems, though strongly related to poverty in a global sense, are actually highly contextual, multilevel, and easily misunderstood. This is evident in the fact that in the United States not all of the food insecure are living in poverty, and not all of the poor are food insecure. Similarly, in developing countries, child malnutrition is common even among households with ample food resources as a result of suboptimal health conditions or caring practices.

Thus, we now recognize that food security and undernutrition are imbedded in, and arise out of, various social, economical, and ecological conditions that vary over time and place. These conditions range from the individual and household levels to the community, national, and international levels, and the coping strategies and behaviors of individual and households are highly responsive to various microcontextual factors. Moreover, these coping strategies and behaviors (including responses to external interventions or policy changes) are strongly influenced by the ways in which reality is experienced by the food insecure and undernourished. A good example is the risk avoidance and risk management strategies of poor households, which discourage them from adopting new crop varieties or making other changes in their livelihood strategies, despite the fact that such changes may appear desirable and rational from a technical (outsider's) perspective. In such a case, the effectiveness of a crop promotion policy may be significantly enhanced by simultaneously taking actions to minimize the real and perceived risks, such as providing insurance against crop losses in the first few seasons.

Although some of these principles have been known for some time, a major reason that policies and programs are ineffective or create unintended consequences is that their design and implementation does not adequately assess, anticipate, and embrace the coping strategies and likely responses of the population. In the "triple A" terms used in the UNICEF nutrition strategy (assessment, analysis, and action), food insecurity and undernutrition may persist because of faulty assessment and analysis (i.e., failing to properly understand the contextual, multilevel, and subtle causes, coping strategies, and responses in a particular setting) or because the actions are not consistent with what we have learned through assessment and analysis. Examples of actions that do not reflect sound assessment and analysis are abundant and include: 1) supplementary food distribution programs in settings where food shortages are not the problem[106]; 2) nutrition education approaches that ignore the constraints (and assets) of poor households[107]; 3) promotion of food production (or transition out of welfare programs) by poor households regardless of labor constraints and market realities[108]; and 4) attempts to develop national health, nutrition, or other programs in the face of marked and well-known variations in ecological, cultural, and economical conditions.[87] Addressing the relationship between assessment, analysis, and action is especially important at this time because of the changes in macrocontextual factors described later.

Hunger, food insecurity, and undernutrition remain widespread problems in the world, especially in developing countries but even in food-rich countries such as the United States. Of equal importance is that these problems and our efforts to address them are being affected by profound changes in some macrocontextual factors such as the decline of the welfare state, the weakened role of the nation state, political and administrative decentralization in many countries, globalization and trade liberalization, rapid urbanization, the spread of HIV/AIDS, the nutrition transition, agricultural and human biotechnology, environmental degradation, and civil conflict. Some of the changes may create opportunities for progress, but many of them can only be viewed as enormous and unprecedented challenges. The nature and intensity of these changes in the macro context demand that policy analysis and policy formation related to food security and nutrition take explicit account of those changes. This is true for policy analysis at national levels and, under decentralization, is also true at local levels, which does not imply a naive expectation that macro policies will be shaped solely in the name of improved nutrition (though food and nutrition can and should be one of the justifications for advocating more equitable policies). Rather, in the meantime, efforts and strategies to improve nutrition should take into account the macro realities that do exist. For example, a major challenge is to rethink the most appropriate roles and relationships among markets, civil society, and governments and to critically examine whether and how communities have or might develop the capacity to address concerns arising from several simultaneous processes: retreat of the welfare state, administrative decentralization within countries, and global economical integration that challenges the autonomy and sovereignty of nation states and localities.

These trends suggest the need for significant changes in the training, research, and practice designed to assess and address food and nutrition disparities within and among countries and communities.[109] An important reason for faulty assessment, analysis, and action in the past, especially in food security and nutrition, is disciplinary, professional, and bureaucratic specialization that influences what is assessed or analyzed, how this is done, and the nature of preferred solutions. This tendency has its origins in the discipline-based nature of university training programs, the specialized nature of research, partial approaches to policy analysis, and some powerful institutional forces in practice settings at the community, national, and international agency levels. At this stage it is not clear whether, or to what extent, this is even recognized to be a problem by academic, governmental, and nongovernmental institutions.[110]

Another weakness within the food and nutrition practice communities in the world is the object of our assessment, analysis, and action. By and large, the main object has been estimating the prevalence of problems, cause-and-effect relationships (e.g., the influence of income, food, and health care on food consumption or nutritional status), and intervention-effect relationships. Our research and training have given relatively little attention, however, to assessment, analysis, and strategy development related to the social, political, and institutional processes that mediate, obstruct, or underlie all causes, potential interventions, and effects. The scientific literature on these topics is well developed,[111-113] and a small but growing body of work in nutrition has taken this direction in recent years, which is a positive sign for the maturation or expansion of the field.[114-122] Continued expansion in this direction will be important for the continued evolution of our field from a science of nutrition to a science and practice of public nutrition.[123]

References

1. Anderson S. Core indicators of nutritional status for difficult-to-sample populations. J Nutr Educ. 1990;120:1559–1600.
2. Gottlieb R, Fisher A. Community food security and environmental justice: searching for a common discourse. Agric Human Values. 1996;3(3):23–32.
3. Radimer KL, Olson CM, Greene JC. Understanding hunger and developing indicators to assess it in women and children. J Nutr Educ. 1992;24(Suppl): 36S–45S.
4. Food and Consumer Service and National Center for Health Statistics. Papers and proceedings. In: *Conference on Food Security Measurement and Research.* Alexandria, VA: USDA; 1995.
5. U.S. Department of Health and Human Services and Department of Agriculture. Ten year comprehensive plan for the National Nutrition Monitoring and Related Research Program. Fed Regist. 1993; 58(111):322772.
6. Carlson SJ, Andrews MS, Bickel GW. Measuring food insecurity and hunger in the United States: development of a national benchmark measure and prevalence estimates. J Nutr Educ. 1999; 129(Suppl):510S–516S.
7. Wehler CA, Scott RI, Anderson JJ. The Community Childhood Hunger Identification Project: a model of domestic hunger demonstration project in Seattle, Washington. J Nutr Educ. 1992;24(Suppl): 29S–35S.
8. Kendall A, Olson CM, Frongillo E Jr. Validation of the Radimer/Cornell measures of hunger and food insecurity. J Nutr Educ. 1995;125:2793–2801.
9. Bickel G, Nord M, Price C, et al. *Guide to Measuring Household Food Security.* Alexandria, VA: U.S. Department of Agriculture, Food and Nutrition Service; March 2000.
10. Hamilton WL, Cook JT, Thompson WW. *Household Food Insecurity in the United States in 1995: Summary Report of the Food Security Measurement Project.* Alexandria, VA: Food and Consumer Service, USDA; 1997.
11. Frongillo E. Validation of measures of food insecurity and hunger. J Nutr Educ. 1999;129(Suppl): 506S–509S.
12. Nord M, Andrews M, Carlson S. *Household Food Security in the United States 2004.* Economic Research Report No 8. Washington, DC: USDA; 2005.
13. National Research Council. *Measuring Food Insecurity and Hunger, Phase 2 Report.* Panel to Review US Department of Agriculture's Measurement of Food Insecurity and Hunger. Committee on National Statistics, Division of Behavioral and Social Sciences and Education, Washington, D.C.: The National Academics Press, 2005.
14. Rose D, Oliveira V. Nutrient intakes of individuals from food-insufficient households in the United States. Am J Public Health. 1997;87:1956–1961.
15. McIntyre L, Glanville NT, Raine KD, et al. Do low-income lone mothers compromise their nutrition to feed their children? CMAJ. 2003;168(6): 686–691.
16. Kendall A, Olson CM, Frongillo E Jr. Relationship

of hunger and food insecurity to food availability and consumption. J Am Diet Assoc. 1996;96:96.

17. Dixon LB, Winkleby MA, Radimer K. Dietary intakes and serum nutrients differ between adults from food-insufficient and food-sufficient families: Third National Health and Nutrition Examination Survey, 1988–1994. J Nutr. 2001;131:1232–1246.
18. Pheley AM, Holben DH, Graham AS, et al. Food security and perceptions of health status: a preliminary study in rural Appalachia. J Rural Health. 2002;18:447–454.
19. Stuff J, Casey PH, Szeto KL, et al. Household food insecurity is associated with adult health status. J Nutr. 2004;134:2330–2335.
20. Sahyoun N, Basiotis PP. Food insufficiency and the nutritional status of the elderly population. In: *Nutrition Insights.* Washington, DC: USDA, Center for Nutrition Policy and Promotion; 2000.
21. Lee JS, Frongillo EA Jr. Nutritional and health consequences are associated with food insecurity among US elderly persons. J Nutr. 2001;131:1503–1509.
22. Nelson K, Cunningham W, Andersen R, et al. Is food insufficiency associated with health status and health care utilization among adults with diabetes? J Gen Intern Med. 2001;16(6):404–411.
23. Casey PH, Szeto K, Lensing S, et al. Children in food-insufficient, low-income families. Prevalence, health and nutrition status. Arch Pediatr Adolesc Med. 2001;155:508–514.
24. Kaiser LL, Melgar-Quinonez HR, Lamp CL, et al. Food insecurity and nutritional outcomes in preschool-age Mexican-American children. J Am Diet Assoc. 2002;102:924–929.
25. Matheson DM, Varady J, Varady A, et al. Household food security and nutritional status of Hispanic children in fifth grade. Am J Clin Nutr. 2002;76: 210–217.
26. Cook JT, Frank DA, Berkowitz C, et al. Food insecurity is associated with adverse health outcomes among human infants and toddlers. J Nutr. 2004; 134:1432–1438.
27. Alaimo K, Olson CM, Frongillo EA Jr. Food insufficiency, family income, and health in US preschool and school-aged children. Am J Public Health. 2001;91:781–786.
28. Weinreb L, Wehler C, Perloff J, et al. Hunger: its impact on children's health and mental health. Pediatrics. 2002;110(4):1–9.
29. Kleinman RE, Murphy JM, Little M. Hunger in children in the United States: potential behavioral and emotional correlates. Pediatrics. 1998;101:1–6.
30. Murphy JM, Wehler CA, Pagano ME. Relationship between hunger and psychosocial functioning in low-income American children. J Am Acad Child Adolesc Psychiatry. 1998;37:163–170.
31. Olson CM. Nutrition and health outcomes associated with food insecurity and hunger. J Nutr Educ. 1999;129(Suppl):521S–542S.
32. Alaimo K, Olson CM, Frongillo EA Jr. Food insufficiency and American school-aged children's cognitive, academic and psychosocial development. Pediatrics. 2001;108:44–53.
33. Alaimo K, Olson CM, Frongillo EA. Family food insufficiency, but not low family income, is associated with dysthymia and suicide symptoms in adolescents. J Nutr. 2002;132:719–725.
34. Reid LL. *The Consequences of Food Insecurity for Child Well-Being: An Analysis of Children's School Achievement, Psychological Well-Being, and Health.* Vol. Working Paper 137. Chicago, IL: Joint Center for Poverty Research; 2000.
35. Bhattacharya J, Currie J, Haider S. Poverty, food insecurity and nutritional outcomes in children and adults. J Health Econ. 2004;23:839–862.
36. Alaimo K, Olson CM, Frongillo EA Jr. Importance of cognitive testing for survey items: an example from food security questionnaires. J Nutr Educ. 1999;31:269–275.
37. Frongillo E, Olson CM, Rauschenbach BS, et al. *Nutritional Consequences of Food Insecurity in a Rural New York State County.* Vol. Discussion Paper no. 1120–97. Madison, WI: Institute for Research on Poverty, University of Wisconsin-Madison; 1997.
38. Townsend MS, Peerson J, Love B, et al. Food insecurity is positively related to overweight in women. J Nutr. 2001;131:1738–1745.
39. Basiotis PP, Lino M. Food insufficiency and prevalence of overweight among adult women. Fam Econ Nutr Rev. 2003;15:55–57.
40. Adams EJ, Grummer-Strawn L, Chavez G. Food insecurity is associated with increased risk of obesity in California women. J Nutr. 2003;133:1070–1074.
41. VanEenwyk J. Self-reported concern about food security associated with obesity-Washington 1995–1999. Morb Mortal Wkly Rep. 2003;52(35): 840–842.
42. Larai BA, Siega-Riz AM, Evenson KR. Self-reported overweight and obesity are not associated with concern about enough food among adults in New York and Louisiana. Prev Med. 2003;38: 175–181.
43. Crawford PB, Townsend MS, Metz DL, et al. How can Californians be overweight and hungry? Calif Agric. 2004;58(1):12–17.
44. Dietz WH. Does hunger cause obesity? Pediatrics. 1995;95:766–767.
45. Alaimo K, Olson CM, Frongillo EA Jr. Low family income and food insufficiency in relation to overweight in US children. Arch Pediatr Adolesc Med. 2001;155:1161–1167.
46. Office of Disease Prevention and Health Promotion, US Department of Health and Human Ser-

vices. *Healthy People 2010*. Available at www.health.gov/healthypeople.
47. Interagency Working Group on Food Security and Food Security Advisory Committee. *U.S. Action Plan on Food Security. Solutions to Hunger*. Washington, DC: USDA; 1999.
48. Maxwell D. Measuring food insecurity: the frequency and severity of "coping strategies." Food Policy. 1996;21(3):291–303.
49. World Bank. *Poverty and Hunger: Issues and Options for Food Security in Developing Countries*. Washington, DC: World Bank; 1986.
50. Maxwell S, Frankenberger T. *Household Food Security: Concepts, Indicators, Measurements*. A technical review. New York and Rome: United Nations Children's Fund and International Fund for Agricultural Development; 1992.
51. Riely F, Mock N, Cogill B. *Food Security Indicators and Framework for Use in the Monitoring and Evaluation of Food Aid Programs*. Arlington, VA: Food Security and Nutrition Monitoring (IMPACT) Project, for the U.S. Agency for International Development; 1997.
52. Smith L. Can FAO's measure of chronic undernourishment be strengthened? Food Policy. 1998; 23(5):425–445.
53. Davies S. *Adaptable Livelihoods: Coping with Food Insecurity in the Malian Sahel*. London: Macmillan Press; 1996.
54. Maxwell S. Food security: a post-modern perspective. Food Policy. 1996;21(2):155–170.
55. Food and Agriculture Organization (FAO). *State of Food Insecurity in the World*. Rome: Food and Agriculture Organization; 1999.
56. Anonymous. *Food Insecurity and Vulnerability Mapping System*, 2000. Accessed December 29, 2000, at http://www.fivims.net.
57. Haas J, Sypher B, Sypher H. Do shared goals really make a difference? Manage Commun Q. 1992;2: 166–179.
58. Maxwell D, Ahiadeke C, Levin C. Alternative food-security indicators: revisiting the frequency and severity of "coping strategies." Food Policy. 1999;24:411–429.
59. Chung K, Haddad L, Ramakrishna J, et al. *Identifying the Food Insecure: the Application of Mixed-method Approaches in India*. Washington, DC: International Food Policy Research Institute; 1997.
60. Gittelsohn J, Mookherji S, Pelto G. Operationalizing household food security in rural Nepal. Food Nutr Bull. 1998;19(3):210–222.
61. Freudenberger Schoonmaker K. *Rapid Rural Appraisal (RRA) and Participatory Rural Appraisal (PRA): A Manual for CRS Field Workers and Partners*. Washington, DC: Catholic Relief Services; 1999.
62. Nyborg I, Haug R. *Food Security Indicators for Development Activities by Norwegian NGOs in Mali, Ethiopia and Eritrea*. Aas, Norway: Centre for International Environment and Development Studies (NORAGRIC), Agricultural University of Norway; 1994.
63. Nyborg I, Haug R. Measuring household food security: a participatory process approach. Forum Dev Stud. 1995;1:29–59.
64. Gervais S, Bryson J, Freudenberger K. *Africare Field Manual on the Design, Implementation, Monitoring and Evaluation of Food Security Activities*. Washington, DC: Africare; 1999.
65. Boudreau T. The food economy approach: a framework for understanding rural livelihoods. In: *Relief and Rehabilitation Network Paper*. London: Overseas Development Institute; 1998.
66. Hamelin AM, Habicht JP, Beaudry M. Food insecurity: consequences for the household and broader social implications. J Nutr Educ. 1999;129(Suppl): 525S–528S.
67. Eilerts G. *Food Security Measurement in the United States: New Ideas for Third-world Assessments?* Rome: Food Insecurity and Vulnerability Information and Mapping Systems, Food and Agriculture Organization, United Nations; 1999.
68. Wolfe WS, Frongillo E Jr. *Building Household Food Security Measurement Tools from the Ground Up*. Food and Nutrition Technical Assistance (FANta) Project. Washington, DC: Academy for Educational Development; 2000.
69. Studdert LJ, Frongillo EA Jr, Valois P. Measuring household food insecurity in Java during Indonesia's economic crisis. J Nutr. 2001;131:2685–2691.
70. Frongillo EA, Chowdhury N, Ekström EC, et al. Understanding the experience of household food insecurity in rural Bangladesh leads to a measure different from that used in other countries. J Nutr. 2003;133:4158–4162.
71. Frongillo E, Nanama S. *Development and Validation of an Experience-based Tool to Directly Measure Household Food Insecurity Within and Across Seasons in Northern Burkina Faso*. Food and Nutrition Technical Assistance Project. Washington, DC: Academy for Educational Development; 2004.
72. Coates J, Wee P, Houser R. *Measuring Food Insecurity: Going Beyond Indicators of Income and Anthropometry*. Food and Nutrition Technical Assistance Project. Washington, DC: Academy for Educational Development; 2003.
73. Food and Nutrition Technical Assistance Project. *Measuring Household Food Insecurity Workshop Report: April 15–16, 2004*. Washington, DC: Food and Nutrition Technical Assistance Project, Academy for Educational Development; 2004.
74. Food and Agriculture Organization of the United Nations. The State of Food Insecurity in the world.

Rome: Food and Agriculture Organization of The United Nations, 2005.

75. Tweeten L, Gleckler J. *Food Security Discussion Paper. Prepared for U.S. Agency for International Development.* Washington, DC: International Science and Technology Institute; 1992.
76. Hamelin AM, Beaudry M, Habicht JP. Characterization of household food insecurity in Quebec: food and feelings. Soc Sci Med. 2002;54:119–132.
77. Williams C. A nutritional disease of childhood associated with a Maize diet. Arch Dis Child. 1933; 8:423–433.
78. World Health Organization. *Energy and Protein Requirements.* Report of a joint FAO/WHO ad hoc expert committee, WHO technical report series. Vol. 522. Geneva, Switzerland: FAO/WHO; 1973.
79. Food and Agriculture Organization. *Manual on Food and Nutrition Policy.* Rome: FAO; 1969.
80. Reutlinger S, Selowsky M. *Malnutrition and Poverty: Magnitude and Policy Options.* World Bank staff occasional papers. Baltimore: Johns Hopkins University Press; 1976.
81. Levinson J. Multisectoral nutrition planning: a synthesis of experience. In: Pinstrup-Andersen P, Pelletier DL, Alderman H, eds. *Enhancing Child Nutrition: An Agenda for Action.* Ithaca, NY: Cornell University Press; 1995; 262–282.
82. World Bank. *Enriching Lives: Overcoming Vitamin and Mineral Malnutrition in Developing Countries.* Washington, DC: World Bank; 1994.
83. UNICEF. *Strategy for Improved Nutrition of Children and Women in Developing Countries.* UNICEF policy review. New York: UNICEF; 1991.
84. United Nations Administrative Coordinating Committee and S.o.N. (ACC/SCN). *How Nutrition Improves.* Geneva, Switzerland: WHO; 1996.
85. Sternin M, Sternin J, Marsh D. *Scaling Up a Poverty Alleviation and Nutrition Program in Vietnam.* In: Marchione TJ, ed. *Scaling Up, Scaling Down: Overcoming Malnutrition in Developing Countries.* Singapore: Gordon and Breach Publishers; 1999.
86. Pelletier D. *Toward a Common Understanding of Malnutrition: Assessing the Contributions of the UNICEF Conceptual Framework.* In: *World Bank/UNICEF Assessment of Contributions to Nutrition Policy.* Washington, DC: 2000.
87. Pelletier D. The role of information in enhancing child growth and nutrition: a synthesis. In: Pinstrup-Andersen P, Pelletier DL, Alderman H, eds. *Beyond Child Survival: Enhancing Growth and Nutrition in Developing Countries.* Ithaca, NY: Cornell University Press; 1995; 304–334.
88. WHO. *The Use and Interpretation of Anthropometry.* In: *WHO Technical Report Series.* Geneva, Switzerland: WHO; 1995.
89. LSRO. *Third Report on Nutrition Monitoring in the United States.* Washington, DC: LSRO; 1995.
90. United Nations and Standing Committee on Nutrition. *Nutrition: A Foundation for Development.* Geneva, Switzerland: 2002.
91. Lanata CF, Black RE. Diarrheal and respiratory diseases. In: Semba R, Bloem M, eds. *Nutrition and Health in Developing Countries.* Totawa, NJ: Humana Press; 2001.
92. Pelletier DL, Frongillo EA Jr, Habicht JP. Epidemiologic evidence for a potentiating effect of malnutrition on mortality. Am J Public Health. 1993; 83:1130–1133.
93. Pelletier DL, Frongillo EA Jr, Schroeder DG, et al. The effects of malnutrition on child mortality in developing countries. Bull World Health Organ. 1995;73(4):443–448.
94. Kramer A. Determinants of low birth weight: methodological assessment and meta-analysis. Bull World Health Organ. 1987;65(5):663–737.
95. Pollitt E, Gorman KS, Engle PL. Early supplementary feeding and cognition. Monogr Soc Res Child Dev. 1993;Serial 235,58(7):1–122.
96. Grantham-McGregor S. A review of the studies of the effect of severe malnutrition on mental development. J Nutr Educ. 1995;125(85):2233S–2238S.
97. Haas JD, Murdoch S, Rivera J, et al. Early nutrition and later physical work capacity. Nutr Rev. 1996; 54(2 Pt 2):S41–S48.
98. Haddad L, Bouis H. The impact of nutritional status on agricultural productivity: wage evidence from the Philippines. Oxf Bull Econ Stat. 1990;53(1): 45–68.
99. Fogel R. Economic growth, population theory, and physiology: the bearing of long-term processes on the making of economic policy. Am Econ Rev. 1994;84(3):369–395.
100. World Bank. *Investing in Health.* Washington, DC: World Bank; 1993.
101. Pelletier DL, Frongillo EA Jr. *Changes in child survival are strongly associated with changes in malnutrition in developing countries.* J Nutr. 2003;133: 107–119.
102. Caulfield L, de Onis M, Blossner M, et al. Undernutrition as an underlying cause of child deaths associated with diarrhea, pneumonia, malaria, and measles. Am J Clin Nutr. 2004;80(1):193–198.
103. Black R, Morris S, Bryce J. Where and why are 10 million children dying each year? Lancet. 2003;361: 2–10.
104. United Nations Development Programme (UN DP). *Human Development Report, 2003. Millennium Development Goals: A Compact Among Nations to End Human Poverty.* New York: Oxford University Press; 2003.
105. Garza C, Pelletier D (eds). *Beyond Nutritional Recommendations: Implementing Science for Healthier Populations.* In: 14th annual Bristol-Myers Squibb/ Mead Johnson Nutrition Research Symposium.

in the Rift Valley lowlands of SNNPR to 29.90% among pastoralists in Ayssaita, Afar Region.[6] Temporal changes in malnutrition also occur. For example, in the besieged city of Melange in Angola, the prevalence of acute malnutrition decreased from 32% to 8% within a 4-month period.[5] It may also remain high in long-term camp situations, such as in Kakuma refugee camp in Kenya, where the prevalence of acute malnutrition was reported to be 17.2% in April 2001, at least 20 years after the camp was opened.[7] However, not all emergencies are characterized by increases in acute malnutrition. For example, among refugees and returnees in Kosovo and neighboring countries, the level of acute malnutrition remained well below 5% throughout the crisis. In some situations, micronutrient deficiency diseases may be a greater public health priority than acute malnutrition. Between 2000 and 2003, outbreaks of scurvy were reported in Afghanistan, while levels of acute malnutrition remained relatively low, between 3% and 12%.[3] However, in almost all situations of complex emergencies, there will be an increase in nutritional risk as a result of either a deterioration in the general public health or food security situation or social disturbances affecting caregiving behaviors. This increase is largely due to the fact that malnutrition itself is influenced by a range of conditions, including the widely recognized underlying causes of malnutrition—food insecurity, poor health environment, inadequate access to health services, and poor social and care environment. This is best described by the well-recognized conceptual model of causes of malnutrition (Fig. 1). The combined effect of a failure in all three groups of underlying causes of malnutrition, which commonly occurs in acute emergencies, is far greater than the sum of their individual effects of each—that is, there is a multiplicative effect rather than an additive effect.[8,9] Therefore, analysis and understanding of each of these causes are critical in all complex emergencies.

Malnutrition, Nutritional Risk, Food Insecurity, and Famine

Increased nutritional risk and elevated malnutrition and mortality rates are undoubtedly a frequent characteristic of complex emergencies, but diagnosing a situation as a famine is more ambiguous.[10] This is because famines do not generally appear uniformly and with common characteristics. Famine is defined as the advanced stages of food insecurity linked with the exhaustion of household coping strategies and threat of destitution, which is accompanied by localized health crises, increased prevalence of malnutrition, and, consequently, elevated morbidity and mortality. Famines are precipitated by a wide range of natural and man-made shocks within any given country or region. Food insecurity may cause the affected population to become destitute, which may in turn precipitate distress migration and, consequently, a localized public health crisis where the displaced population settles. At this stage, not only does acute malnutrition increase because of food insecurity, but also because of increased exposure to disease, thus multiplying the combined impact of malnutrition and morbidity on mortality.[8,9] In practice, diagnosis of famine remains problematic. For example, the crisis that occurred throughout the southern Africa region during 2001–2002 was initially reported as "a regional food crisis." Two years of drought and widespread harvest failure caused serious food insecurity, but there was generally no widespread malnutrition and mortality. However, extremely high levels of acute malnutrition and mortality were reported for confined geographic areas, and the situation was later described as famine.[11] Therefore, it is practically more useful to assess both the outcomes of famine (malnutrition, morbidity, mortality, loss of livelihood) and the underlying causes of malnutrition that contribute to increased nutritional risk and risk of dying. It is this type of analysis that is required for

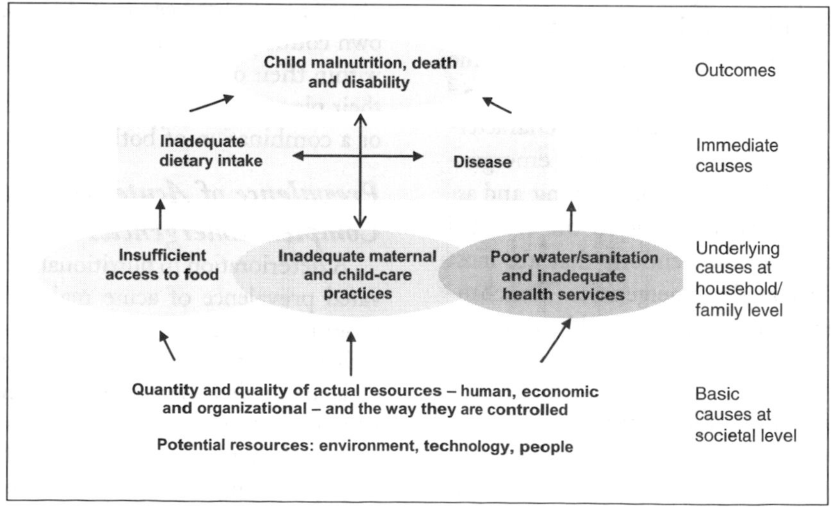

Figure 1. Conceptual framework of causes of malnutrition. (Adapted with permission from UNICEF. *The State of the World's Children 1998*. New York: UNICEF; 1998.)

planning and implementing strategic humanitarian responses.

Historical Perspective of Food and Nutrition Responses

The origins of current food relief and nutritional assistance programs can be traced to famine relief programs in Biafra and Bangladesh in the 1960s and early 1970s.[3] Emergency nutrition interventions during this early period were largely based on the provision of large quantities of supply-driven food commodities and medical interventions designed to treat malnutrition. The latter were based on the premise that malnutrition was a result of protein deficiency, and were therefore focused on the provision of high-protein foods, often in the form of dried milk. Since these early programs, scientific knowledge and understanding of the physiology of malnutrition have led to profound improvements in treatment protocols. Furthermore, there is better understanding of the broader political and social context of vulnerability in crisis situations and its implications on the nutritional situation. This improved conceptual understanding has allowed policies and practices in assessment and response to evolve from a narrow focus on protein-energy malnutrition and its treatment to a more problem-solving approach, which has been termed public nutrition.[2] The range of assessment tools and response options are described in the next sections.

Assessment and Analysis Tools for Measuring the Extent and Severity of the Nutritional Situation

Assessing Nutritional Status: Individual and Population Levels

In emergencies, the two-stage random 30-cluster nutrition survey is a well-established and standardized tool for estimating the prevalence of acute malnutrition among children younger than 5 years of age. Acute malnutrition is measured using the National Center for Health Statistics/World Health Organization/Centers for Disease Control and Prevention weight-for-height reference, with the standard cut-offs of less than -3 standard deviation scores for severe acute malnutrition and less than -2 standard deviation scores for global acute malnutrition (Table 1). Children with nutritional edema, as indicated by bilateral swelling, are classified as severely malnourished. In general, the *Z*- score index is used for survey purposes and percentage of the median is used for targeting. Nutrition surveys usually include estimates of mortality rates, referred to as crude mortality rate (number of deaths per 10,000 per day), and mortality rates for children younger than 5 years of age. In addition, the prevalence of acute malnutrition should be interpreted on the basis of a review of the underlying causes as either part of the survey tool or through qualitative investigations, such as rapid rural appraisal. These findings may be used to determine and design relief programs, to prioritize affected groups or geographic areas (target scarce resources), to plan nutritional interventions, and for monitoring and evaluation.

Table 1. Classification of Acute Malnutrition Using *Z*- Score and Percentage of the Median

	Global Acute Malnutrition	Severe Acute Malnutrition
Z- score	< -2 *Z* score or edema	< -3 *Z*- score or edema
Percentage of the median	<80% of the median or edema	<70% or edema

The anthropometric measurement of mid-upper arm circumference (MUAC) for children ages 1 to 5 years is a useful tool for nutritional screening, specifically for referral to selective feeding programs, but is not recommended for the estimating prevalence of acute malnutrition unless the MUAC measurements are correlated to reference values for height (or length)[12] or age.[13] The use of unadjusted MUAC continues because it is a simple measurement requiring no adjustments, and because some studies have reported that it is a better index than weight-for-height in predicting mortality. There is also evidence to suggest that MUAC may better reflect acute changes in muscle mass than the weight-for-height index, and it preferentially selects younger children.[14] The International Committee of the Red Cross routinely uses an index called the QUAC stick for assessments of nutritional status; this is a height stick that classifies nutritional status by relating the child's arm circumference measurement to his or her height.[15]

During the past decade, experience has shown that undernutrition among adults and adolescents is often a public health priority in emergencies. Increasingly, agencies have included these population groups in nutrition surveys, but there considerable debate continues on the appropriate indices and cutoff criteria. For adults the body mass index (BMI or weight/height^2) remains the recommended index.[16] However, large individual variations in body shape, particularly the relative leg length for different ethnic groups, can alter individual BMI by as much as 4 kg/m^2.[17] These differences can be corrected by using the Cormic Index,[16] although this is not routine practice.[18] Arm span and knee height can be used as proxies for height among the elderly, although their relationships with height for different ethnic groups have not been established.[18] WHO recommends the use of sex-specific MUAC cutoffs of 22 cm for women and 23 cm for men for chronic energy deficiency. Although MUAC, in conjunction with clinical criteria (ability to stand, edema, and dehydration), is often proposed as a tool for rapid assessment for adults and older people, the outcomes of these

Table 2. Guidelines to Assist in Decision to Implement Nutrition Programs

Prevalence of Malnutrition (<−2 *Z*-score or edema)	General Ration	Interpretation and Selective Feeding Intervention
Malnutrition rate ≥20% or 10%–19% with aggravating factors*	Advocate for general ration of 2100 kcal	Serious: Blanket and targeted supplementary feeding, therapeutic feeding
Malnutrition rate >10%–19% or 5%–9% with aggravating factors		Alert: Targeted supplementary feeding and therapeutic feeding
Malnutrition rate <10% with no aggravating factors		Acceptable: No need for population-level intervention (individual attention for malnourished)

* Aggravating factors to consider are crude mortality rate >1; inadequate general food ration; epidemic of measles, shigella, or other important communicable disease; severe and inadequate shelter.

different MUAC cutoffs in relation to mortality and morbidity are not known. More research is needed to validate these MUAC criteria so that useful tools are available both for nutrition surveys and for individual targeting of adults and adolescents in emergencies. For adolescents, the variable age for the onset of puberty complicates measures of nutritional status. The limited evidence available also suggests that extended weight-for-height charts are poor predictors of mortality, and the available BMI charts for adolescents have not yet been validated.[19]

Interpretation: Benchmarks and Decision-Making Frameworks

To determine the severity of any given situation, the estimated prevalence of acute malnutrition is compared with benchmarks that have been developed based on studies conducted among emergency-affected populations. These objective comparisons are useful for reviewing trends for surveillance, for making international comparisons, and for advocacy purposes. Decision-making frameworks that combine benchmarks of nutritional status with aggravating factors (e.g., mortality, morbidity, access to food) have been proposed and used to inform practitioners on the most appropriate interventions (Table 2).

However, this utility of this framework may be limited in some contexts. For example, the prevalence of acute malnutrition may remain consistently higher than the benchmark of, for example, 10% to 19% proposed for implementing emergency supplementary feeding programs (SFPs).[20] Alternatively, the prevalence of acute malnutrition may remain within the normal range (i.e., less than 5% to 10%) but the associated mortality rate may be elevated (i.e., crude mortality rate of more than 1 per 10,000 per day). Despite the widespread assumption that the relationship between the prevalence of acute malnutrition and the mortality rate is linear,[21] there are many examples of emergencies where this is not applicable. For example, Figure 2 shows the rates of malnutrition and crude mortality from 15 different surveys conducted in Ethiopia in 2002. Almost half (6/15) of the surveys reported a prevalence of malnutrition that exceeded the benchmark for acute malnutrition (15%), but reported associated mortality rates that fell well below the mortality benchmark for emergencies (crude mortality rate of 1 per 10,000 per day). A further limitation of this decision-making framework is that it is too prescriptive and does not describe possible non-food interventions that may improve the population's nutritional status or encourage more innovative interventions tailored to the context. Although practitioners and decision-makers tend to focus on the single outcome of the prevalence of acute malnutrition, a review of the entire distribution is required to better understand how the entire sample has been affected.[8,9,22]

Assessing Nutritional Risk: Nutritional Surveillance and Food Security Assessments

Nutritional surveillance monitors changes in nutritional status over time for the purposes of problem identification and advocacy, timely warning and intervention,

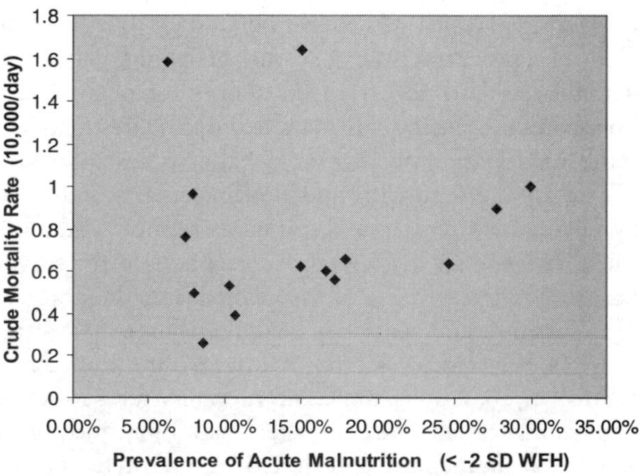

Figure 2. Malnutrition and mortality rates from nutrition surveys in Ethiopia (August to December 2002). (Data from Hedlund 2003.[6])

resource allocation and targeting, and program monitoring. Nutritional surveillance can also contribute to policy development. In emergencies, usually one or more of the following three methodologic approaches are used: representative nutrition surveys conducted every 2 to 12 months, clinic-based surveillance data (based on existing growth monitoring data), and a purposively selected sentinel-site food security and nutritional surveillance system. These approaches all have advantages and drawbacks. Regularly conducted nutrition surveys are relatively resource intensive but do provide valid and reliable data. Clinic-based surveillance potentially strengthens the capacity of existing clinics, although the data may not be representative or timely. Sentinel-site surveillance provides timely and relevant data but cannot be extrapolated to the wider population.

Nutritional status is limited as an early warning indicator because it is generally considered to be a late indicator of deterioration in the nutritional situation. Nonetheless, an analysis of trends can reveal deviations from normal patterns. In recent years there have been moves toward exploring other indicators of nutritional risk, such as dietary diversity.

It is important for assessments and analyses to consider all types of vulnerability that affect nutritional risk. Nutritional vulnerability is most appropriately assessed using nutritional surveys as described above. Vulnerability to food insecurity and the disruption or loss of livelihoods is preferentially assessed using food security and livelihood assessment methods. Some examples of these include the household economy approach, livelihood assessments, and the World Food Programme's (WFP) Vulnerability Assessment and Mapping.[23-25] These methods are less standardized than nutrition surveys, but many of the available methods share the same conceptual understanding of food security and use similar data-collection tools. In general, they identify and disaggregate information using different livelihood or food economy groups and use qualitative methods of investigation (rapid appraisal procedures) to investigate the food security situation. Components of food security that are considered include access to food, food availability, and, in some situations, food utilization. An analysis of the changes in food security and livelihood brought about as a result of the acute crisis is a critical factor for designing the appropriate response.

Addressing the General Nutritional Needs of Populations

There is no single intervention to address the complex problems found in communities exposed to the wide range of nutritional risks relating to food insecurity, inadequate maternal and child care, and poor public health that occur in complex emergencies. A range of intervention strategies are required that are based on a process of assessment, analysis, and prioritization (as described above) and are, in most cases, unique to a given situation.

Food Security Interventions and Protection of Livelihoods

The overriding goals of the response are reflected in the Sphere Minimum Standards of Disaster Response on Food Security, Nutrition and Food Aid. The first Nutrition Standard states, "The nutritional needs of the population shall be met," while the first Food Security Standard states, "People have access to adequate and appropriate food and non-food items in a manner that ensures their survival, prevents erosion of assets and upholds their dignity."[26] These standards reflect both the right to adequate food and freedom from hunger. The food security standard proposes how this should be achieved and emphasizes the importance of upholding dignity and protecting livelihoods and the importance of interventions building on local efforts and using participatory approaches.

Addressing food insecurity and protecting livelihoods has become a recognized component of a nutritional response in complex emergencies because these are critical for protecting and supporting nutrition, albeit through indirect pathways.[27] Increasingly, a range of food security interventions are applied that help people meet their food needs, earn income, and protect their assets.[28,29] Examples of these food security or livelihood support measures are shown in Table 3.

Different contexts determine which types of strategies are required. For example, for non-displaced populations whose livelihoods are relatively intact, the interventions described in Table 3 may be appropriate. In contrast, for populations displaced to camps, both refugees and internally displaced persons, the opportunities for such innovative interventions may be limited due to lack of land or employment opportunities. The process of prioritizing different interventions is a careful balance between relatively top-down, short-term responses intended to save lives and reduce mortality (e.g., provision of general food assistance) and longer-term solutions that protect and support people's livelihoods, which indirectly save lives and aim to preserve people's dignity. This concept is illustrated through the recent Darfur case study (below), which combines both direct food assistance and food security and livelihood interventions.

Case Study: Darfur, Sudan, 2004

The Darfur region in Sudan has an estimated population of just over 6 million. In 2003, region-wide conflict erupted, which involved armed militias systematically attacking rural villages, killing, looting, and raping civilians. As a result, more than 1 million people fled their homes and became internally displaced, while an estimated 170,000 fled across the border to Chad. Outside the main towns, insecurity and threats of violence restricted peo-

Table 3. Examples of Food Security Projects in Emergency Contexts

Definition: Food security exists when all people at all times have physical and economic access to sufficient, safe and nutritious food for a healthy and active life (World Food Summit Plan of Action, paragraph 1, 1996).

Agricultural Production

- Distribution of seeds, tools, and fertilizer (Longley et al., 2002[30])
- Seed vouchers and fairs: brings together sellers and buyers (Remington et al., 2002[31])
- Training and education in relevant skills
- Livestock interventions: animal health services; emergency de-stocking; restocking of livestock; distribution of livestock fodder and nutritional supplementation; and provision of alternative water sources (Aklilu and Wekesa, 2002[32])
- Distribution of fishing nets and gear, or hunting implements
- Promotion of food processing, milling, and fortification
- Local agricultural extension and veterinary services (Jones et al., 1998[33])

Income and Employment

- Cash or Food-for-Work (CFW) provides food-insecure households with opportunities for paid work that at the same time produce outputs of benefit to themselves and the community (Peppiatt et al., 2001[34]).
- Income-generating schemes allow people to diversify their sources of income in small-scale, self-employment business schemes.

Market Interventions

- Support of market infrastructure (e.g., transportation to allow producers to take advantage of distant markets)
- De-stocking: livestock purchase usually from pastoralists in times of drought (Aklilu and Wekesa, 2002[32])
- Fair price shops: sale of goods at controlled or subsidized prices

Food or cash vouchers: for exchange in shops for food and other goods (Harvey, 2005[35])

Microfinance Projects

- Credit and saving schemes; grants, loans, cattle or other livestock banks, cooperative savings accounts (Jacobsen, 2004[36])

ple's access to markets, agricultural land, and employment opportunities and therefore seriously undermined their livelihoods and food security. In this context, the priority interventions were the provision of basic services of those displaced to camps, including the provision of a nutritionally adequate rations, shelter, water and sanitation, immunization, and other public health interventions. However, food assistance programs must also endeavor to reach the rural food-insecure population of Darfur as well as the internally displaced persons in the main towns. Therefore, the priority is also to ensure that sufficient quantities of food are available on local markets and that there is safe access to these markets for both buyers and sellers. Support to food security, both for internally displaced persons and those remaining in rural areas, is also important. One example is the provision of fodder for donkeys, which are a household necessity in Darfur for water collection and general transport. Other priorities include support for access to cooking fuel by providing protection for women to allow them to safely collect firewood, as well as the promotion of fuel-efficient cooking techniques. Prioritization of humanitarian response in this context clearly illustrates the careful balance that must be struck between alleviating the immediate suffering of internally displaced persons and thereby saving lives, and preventing further suffering and excess deaths among the rural population by supporting livelihoods. The needs of both groups are entirely different in type, scale, and severity, but nevertheless represent humanitarian needs that must be addressed as part of an impartial humanitarian response.[37]

General Food Assistance

General food distribution, or the provision of dry food rations known as a food basket, is the most common strategy for ensuring that the nutritional needs of the affected population are met. A well-established body of best practice exists for the planning, distribution, and targeting of nutritionally adequate food rations.[38,39] A nutritionally adequate ration is calculated on an average per-capita energy requirement basis. An initial planning figure of 2100 kcal (8.8 MJ) per person per day is used, which is adjusted to suit the specific conditions of the crisis.[39] These adjustments are determined by the ambient temperature, demographic profile, activity levels, and the health status of the population. The recommended amount of total fat and protein in the ration is calculated based on the percentage of energy each provides; 10% to 12% of energy should be obtained from protein and 17% of energy from fat. Nutritionally adequate rations must also provide a source of micronutrients, and it is the policy of several international organizations, including WFP, to provide fortified food commodities, such as iodized salt, oil fortified with vitamin A, and fortified blended food, which contains a range of micronutrients. In addition, general food rations should be culturally acceptable and safe for human consumption, should include a variety of foods, should be digestible by children, should be fuel efficient, and should be easy to store and prepare. Although a variety of foods are recommended, including a cereal grain or flour, pulses, vegetable oil, blended food, and salt, shortfalls in donor pledges and logistical difficulties in practice frequently lead to breaks in the food aid pipeline and shortages of particular commodities for distribution.

In the design of food assistance programs, consideration is also given to supporting food preparation and cooking processes at the household level. Whole-grain cereal has limited digestibility for young children and older persons, and therefore this staple food needs to be provided as flour. It is the policy of WFP and the United Nations High Commission for Refugees to provide either milled flour or milling equipment during the initial response to a crisis to facilitate food preparation and cooking. However, milled flour tends to have a shorter shelf-life, is more difficult to transport and store, and is more expensive than whole grain. The availability of fuel for cooking is often a problem. Frequently, rations may be sold or exchanged to obtain cooking fuel, pay for milling costs, or access a range of food items not provided in the ration.

Targeting strategies and distribution mechanisms are planned to ensure that the food ration reaches the affected communities in the most efficient and effective way. Targeting is closely linked with the assessment process, which determines both the worst-affected geographic areas and the worst-affected population groups within these areas. Defining and then accessing these specific population groups are challenging. The distribution system for food aid is complex and divided into a number of stages, from donor country to port, to a centralized main warehouse, then to extended-distribution warehouses, and finally to local distribution points, where it reaches the affected community. Usually, rations are distributed directly to household heads through local leaders (if necessary, newly appointed leaders), or through community groups. The WFP policy is to distribute food directly to women-in the household rather than to the male head of household.

Public Health Interventions

Malnutrition may be caused or exacerbated by disease; therefore, a range of public health strategies are required to promote and protect health. In the emergency phase the priorities include initial assessment, public health surveillance, control of communicable diseases and epidemics (diarrheal diseases, measles, acute respiratory infections, and malaria), water and sanitation, and shelter and site planning.[4,17,40,41] Other specific issues of direct relevance to nutrition include curative health care, child health care, HIV/AIDS, and psychosocial and mental health care. The prevailing HIV/AIDS epidemic in southern Africa is undermining the ability of communities to recover from famine, as it directly affects able-bodied adults who are the most productive in terms of food security.[42] Delivery of essential health services, including immunization campaigns, water, and sanitation, has greatly improved in camp settings, but emergencies that affect wide geographic areas or are conflict related pose greater logistical and security challenges.[43]

Targeting the Physiologically Vulnerable

Specific population groups are recognized as physiologically more vulnerable in most situations. Children younger than 5 years of age are generally always considered the most physiologically vulnerable. Other nutritionally vulnerable subgroups include infants, pregnant and lactating women, older persons, and those living with a chronic illness. However, in complex emergencies, a flexible appreciation of vulnerability is necessary, as nutritional risk is influenced by other important determinants that require a broad, context-specific analysis of vulnerability beyond physiologic risk.

Infants. It is well recognized that exclusive breast-feeding for a duration of 6 months reduces morbidity and mortality from a range of infectious diseases.[44] In complex emergencies, due to additional risks such as compromised hygiene and care practices, poor sanitation and overcrowding, a lack of access to clean water and cooking fuel for safe preparation and a lack of regular supply replacement feeding carries even greater risks.[45] Adherence to World Health Assembly legislation is frequently compromised, and unsolicited donations of breast milk substitutes are frequently reported.[46] A number of interagency and agency-specific policies and guidelines that address the protection of, promotion of, and support for exclusive breast-feeding in complex emergencies have been developed and endorsed,[47] but the application of these policies in practice is often poor, constrained by a lack of institutional memory and available expertise, as well as a failure in agency leadership and coordination.[38] Where the prevalence of breast-feeding practices is already poor and national policies are inadequate to protect exclusive breast-feeding, such as in Iraq, implementing an appropriate response to meet the nutritional needs of infants in crisis situations may be challenging (see the case study below).

Case Study: Challenges for the Protection and Promotion of Breast-feeding in Iraq

Studies conducted in Iraq prior to 2003 indicated a low prevalence of breast-feeding practices and a high acceptability of the use of infant formula among Iraqi women. For example, a study conducted in Baghdad in 1977 found that 58.7% of the women exclusively breast-fed their children during the first 6 months. A later survey conducted in 2002 by UNICEF revealed that only 7% of infants less than 6 months of age were breast-fed. In addition, reports from health clinics suggested that severe malnutrition was associated with bottle feeding in northern Iraq.[40]

A major factor contributing to the low prevalence of breast-feeding was the systematic inclusion of free infant formula in the food ration under the Oil-For-Food Program since the early 1990s. In 1994, the Iraqi legislature drafted a national code for the protection and promotion of breast-feeding that included discontinuing the free distribution of infant formula in the general ration. The code was approved by the cabinet and submitted to the president's office for endorsement, and as a consequence infant formula was removed from the food ration. A significant increase in the market price of commercially available formula followed shortly. Public demonstrations took place to protest the removal of infant formula from the food basket, and the president's office withdrew the decision to implement the national code despite strong support by the Ministry of Health and the United Nations for its endorsement.

Following the 2003 war and subsequent change in regime in Iraq, aid agencies were confronted with numerous challenges as they strived to adhere to international guidelines on infant feeding. The first challenge was the effective promotion of breast-feeding in a context where breast-feeding was not common practice. This was complicated by the influx of unsolicited donations of infant formula and the absence of any policies or regulations for their control. Secondly, it was well recognized that many women who had previously not breast-fed may have been eligible to receive ongoing supplies of breast milk substitutes; however, this needed to be carried out with appropriate mechanisms in place to support counseling, safe use of breast milk substitutes, and follow-up, especially given the additional risks associated with artificial feeding. These included lack of access to clean water and an associated increase in the incidence of diarrhea, and to the fact that instructions on donated products were often in English or Arabic and rarely in the local Kurdish language. Thirdly, agencies were challenged with setting up a system to manage the donations of breast milk substitutes because unsolicited donations included some brand-name products, which provided free advertising and an opportunity to build a new market for some manufacturers. In recognition of some of these challenges, a Policy on the Use of Infant Formula in Iraq was drawn up in May 2003,[49] stating that "no UN agency, NGO or bilateral donor should distribute [breast milk substitutes] directly to families" in Iraq. (A. Borrel and R. Ndunge, unpublished case study)

The increase in prevalence of HIV/AIDs has brought new challenges, specifically in relation to policies and interventions to provide adequate nutritional support to infants of HIV-positive women. The United Nations recommends exclusive breast-feeding for the first 6 months for all women who are HIV-negative or whose status is unknown. Only if replacement feeding is acceptable, feasible, affordable, sustainable, and safe is avoidance of breast-feeding recommended for HIV-positive women.[42] If the above conditions are not met, exclusive breast-feeding is recommended during the first months of life and should then be discontinued as soon as it is feasible. In many emergency situations, HIV testing is limited, HIV status is rarely known, and there are inadequate resources to provide replacement feeding with adequate support and monitoring,[51] and therefore responses for infants under these conditions are frequently inadequate.

Pregnant and Lactating Women. The nutritional requirements for women during pregnancy and lactation are higher than the population average.[52] Consequently, macronutrient (food) and micronutrient (iron and folic acid) supplements are usually provided to all pregnant and lactating women during pregnancy and for the first 6 months of breast-feeding through emergency SFPs or maternal-child health care clinics. If food resources are scarce, only some pregnant and lactating women are targeted: those with a MUAC of less than 21 to 23 cm.[53] Evidence of the impact of providing macronutrient and micronutrient supplements to women for this short period is limited. Poor impact may be a result of intrahousehold distribution patterns, ambiguity of the outcomes to be measured, a lack of opportunity to improve prepregnancy nutritional status, and limited possibilities for integrating nutrition interventions with other public-health programs.

Older People. The nutritional risks that older people normally face are likely to be exacerbated in complex emergencies because of the loss of support systems as a result of family separations or the disruption of informal and formal social networks. Increased nutritional risk for older people may be a result of lack of access to health care, exposure to the cold, psychological stress, constraints on food preparation,[54] a lack of mobility, limited employment opportunities, lack of access to land, food, and basic services, and psychosocial trauma.[55] Nutritional interventions to support older persons essentially comprise only a food supplement. There is a lack of universally accepted targeting criteria and a poor awareness of the specific nutritional needs of older persons.

Chronic Illness, Including HIV/AIDS. Food supplements are frequently targeted to individuals with disabilities, those with chronic illnesses, those receiving treatment for tuberculosis, and, increasingly, persons with HIV/AIDS. The purpose of the ration is to address household food security, to meet additional nutritional requirements, and to improve compliance with treatment regimens.

More recently, regional and national food insecurity have frequently been associated with epidemics of HIV/AIDS, especially in the context of localized drought or conflict. At the household level, high mortality among the most productive members limits recovery from food insecurity.[42] At the individual level, malnutrition and HIV/AIDS are inextricably linked. Malnutrition, reduced food intakes, and micronutrient deficiencies are associated with more rapid disease progression of HIV/AIDS. People with HIV/AIDS are at increased risk of malnutrition because of increased nutritional requirements, reduction in dietary intake, nutrient malabsorption, and metabolic changes.[56] Nutrition interventions potentially have a wide range of benefits on HIV-related outcomes, but their impact depends on the type of intervention, the length of time that it is given, and the underlying vulnerability of the infected person. In general, HIV-affected persons should consume 10% to 15% more energy and 50% to 100% more protein a day. Furthermore, micronutrient supplements, specifically vitamins A, B, C, and E, have been shown to have beneficial effects on morbidity and other outcomes in HIV-affected persons.[57] However, nutritional supplements alone are insufficient and must be combined with other intervention such as counseling, care, and food security. In the absence of testing and treatment of HIV/AIDS, the targeting of these combined interventions remains problematic. Documentation and institutional experience of effective strategies are limited.

Challenges for Understanding Vulnerability and Accessing Other High-Risk Groups

There are three main challenges associated with identifying and accessing high-risk groups in complex emergencies that relate to the assessment and design of interventions.

First, despite the recognition that a variety of social groups are physically and socially vulnerable, disproportional assistance is often provided to children and other physiologically vulnerable groups. This is partly because many survey instruments and standardized intervention strategies have been adopted from development aid, where the risks are relatively stable.[58] In emergencies, the relative risk between different age and social groups is dynamic, changing both with locality and over time. In emergencies, understanding vulnerability and identifying the highest-priority groups require the use of sophisticated epidemiologic studies, and these also need to be combined with wider political and social analyses.

Second, unless the underlying causes of the vulnerability are addressed, the effectiveness of any emergency nutrition intervention will be undermined. Therefore, the design of nutritional interventions to support older people, HIV-affected persons, and unaccompanied children needs to be combined with a strong community-based component that strengthens and rebuilds social support systems within crisis-affected communities, as well as medical referral mechanisms. This is challenging, particularly in situations where normal social support networks are severely disrupted.

Third, the necessary mechanisms for effectively accessing these at-risk groups are often problematic, and setting up multiple parallel systems of support may not be the most cost-effective strategy. Some agencies, such as the International Committee of the Red Cross, therefore, increase the general food rations to ensure that food meets the additional requirements of at-risk groups. In some situations, where there is either inadequate analysis or delivery mechanisms to reach the priority groups, food assistance is channeled for pragmatic reasons through institutions such as schools, hospitals, and orphanages, despite the well-recognized limitations of reaching the most vulnerable though these mechanisms.

Addressing and Treating Malnutrition

Preventing and Addressing Micronutrient Deficiency Diseases

The major risk factors for micronutrient deficiency diseases in complex emergencies include the provision of a general food ration that consists of a limited number of commodities (cereals, oil, and pulses) and in some circumstances even a single commodity ration (cereal), and a lack of access to markets or production systems that allow populations to access a diverse range of foods. The provision of fortified food commodities is therefore not feasible, and a high incidence of diarrhea exists due to a poor public health environment. Consequently, a range of micronutrient deficiency diseases, including vitamin A, iron, and iodine deficiency disorders, are common, and other micronutrient deficiency diseases specific to emergencies, such as pellagra, scurvy, and beriberi, are frequent public health priorities in complex emergencies.[3] A range of strategies are required to address micronutrient deficiency diseases, including food fortification, food-based approaches, and supplementation, but in most circumstances prioritization of one or more of these is necessary, depending on the context and type of deficiencies.

Food Fortification. Food fortification in emergencies is most commonly applied through the provision of fortified food commodities or through fortification at the level of camp or community mills. According to WFP policy, food aid commodities that must be fortified include vegetable oil with vitamin A, salt with iodine, and blended food with multiple micronutrients.[59] Blended food is a precooked blend of cereals and pulses fortified with a range of micronutrients based on Codex Alimentarius guidelines.[60] The acceptability of this blended food is good, and because its resale value is far less than that for other food aid commodities, it is generally consumed by beneficiaries and not sold.

Increasingly, efforts are being made to fortify cereals through local milling initiatives. For example, in Malawi maize flour was fortified with niacin to combat niacin deficiency among Mozambican refugees.[61] While these local-level initiatives have huge potential, many operational constraints exist, such as poor quality control, maintaining the supply of fortificant, and poor acceptability.[59] Two potential mechanisms for household-level fortification include the use of "sprinkles" (a powdered micronutrient supplement that is added to food after preparation)[62] and the use of iron pots for cooking[63] as novel strategies for reducing anemia. However, there is an insufficient evidence base yet to justify implementing these strategies on a large scale.

Improving Access to Foods Rich in Micronutrients. The provision of a fresh food commodity that is rich in the relevant micronutrients, such as pulses, groundnuts, red palm oil, fruits, and vegetables, can be a strategy to address one or more deficiencies. For example, the distribution and consumption of groundnuts protected Mozambican refugees in Malawi against pellagra.[61] However, this strategy is often costly and logistically difficult, and foods need to be culturally acceptable. The use of animal-source foods to improve micronutrient status is well documented,[64] and livestock, veterinary, and market interventions, increase access to animal-source foods, potentially play a key role in the response to nutritional crises. However, the feasibility of these interventions is often limited by a lack of access to land, insecurity, and lack of employment opportunities. The impact of these interventions for improving nutritional status has rarely been documented. Although studies have demonstrated that iron-fortified commodities such as candies,[66] fish sauce,[66] and fat-based spreads[67] are effective in reducing anemia among some population groups, there is limited evidence to suggest that these interventions are feasible and effective as large-scale public health interventions in emergencies.

Supplementation. The distribution of micronutrient supplements may be effective in controlling micronutrient deficiency diseases in the short term, when routine health services are not functional or food-based approaches are not feasible or are still being investigated (see the scurvy case study below).[68] Vitamin A supplementation is routinely provided every 4 to 6 months for all children 6 to 59 months of age to prevent vitamin A deficiency and to reduce the risk of mortality and other sequelae of measles.[69] Vitamin A supplementation is often conducted in conjunction with measles or other vaccination campaigns. Two other supplements likely to be increasingly important in emergencies in the future are multiple micronutrient supplements for women[70,71] and zinc.[72,73]

Case Study: Vitamin C Supplementation to Address Scurvy in Afghanistan

In March 2002, reports of symptoms and increased mortality of a hemorrhagic fever outbreak in western Afghanistan were confirmed to be due to a large-scale epidemic of scurvy. Aid workers and health professionals had not reported the disease as scurvy initially because they were unfamiliar with the nonspecific clinical symptoms and because the disease was most commonly associated with populations living in refugee camps, who were entirely reliant on food rations. A survey estimated that the prevalence (based on clinical symptoms) was 6.3% and determined that the attack rates peaked each year at the end of winter (i.e., February to March). The risk factors for scurvy for populations living in the rural mountainous areas include the consumption of a limited range of foods, lengthy winters, continuing drought, and a general depletion of household assets. A number of potential interventions were considered, including supplementation, food-based fortification, and food security interventions to address and prevent future outbreaks of scurvy. A large-scale vitamin C supplementation was prioritized largely because of its timeliness and rapid impact compared with other intervention strategies. A 3-month supply of vitamin C tablets was distributed to family members in 827 villages in high-risk areas. Based on a follow-up monitoring visit, it was concluded that acceptability and compliance of supplements were good and there were no reports of further cases of scurvy during the winter of 2002–2003. The follow-up assessment also highlighted the need to explore long-term measures such as the use of locally appropriate interventions for increasing access to high-vitamin C foods. This case study confirms that non-refugee populations in crisis situations are also at risk of scurvy, and that as a short-term response, vitamin C supplementation for a 3-month period can be an effective preventive measure for scurvy on a large scale.[74]

Addressing Moderate Acute Malnutrition

SFPs aim to contribute to reducing mortality among populations where there is an elevated level of moderate acute malnutrition. A food supplement and basic health care are given to moderately malnourished children and other nutritionally vulnerable groups. If the prevalence of acute malnutrition is extremely high or if general rations are not yet established, "blanket" SFPs are established as a preventive strategy to all members of a population group, usually all children younger than 5 years of age and all pregnant and lactating women. A daily supplement consisting of a fortified, blended food mixed with oil and providing 500 to 1200 kcal is given in the form of an on-site meal or a dry take-home premix. The indicators for assessing the effectiveness of emergency SFPs include reporting the average weight gain (in grams per kilogram body weight per day), the length of stay (in days), and the number of children who have recovered, died, been transferred to a hospital or other program, or defaulted (defined as those leaving the program prior to recovery). Although there is no definite consensus on a methodology, program coverage is another important indicator.[75,76] Greater coverage, higher recovery rates, and lower default rates are associated with dry take-home SFPs.[78]

The impact of SFPs in addressing elevated levels of moderate malnutrition in non-emergency situations,[78] and in complex emergencies,[79] has been challenged. The coverage of SFPs is frequently low because of poor access and acceptability among the populations they aim to reach. Poor security conditions and long distances limit access, and cultural factors such as ethnicity, trust, stigma, cultural taboos, and traditional child care practices reduce acceptability.[68] Changes in the prevalence of acute malnutrition are rarely attributable to SFPs alone and are just as likely to be a result of changes in the broader underlying causes. Despite these well-recognized problems, SFPs continue to be perceived by many agencies as the most pragmatic response to addressing elevated levels of acute malnutrition.

Management and Treatment of Severe Acute Malnutrition

The management and treatment of severe malnutrition is conducted in therapeutic feeding programs according to universally recognized guidelines and protocols.[80-82] Traditionally, treatment is undertaken in inpatient health facilities and temporary structures during large-scale emergencies, but more recent approaches to treatment combine inpatient with outpatient or home-based treatment.

Treatment protocols for inpatient facilities are implemented in four distinct phases, generally referred to as stabilization, transition, recovery, and follow-up. During the first three phases, low-protein F75 and F100 therapeutic milks, which are fortified with minerals and vitamins, are given in small, frequent meals according to body weight for about 4 weeks. Solid foods, using local ingredients if possible, are introduced gradually as the child recovers. Hypothermia, hypoglycemia, electrolyte imbalances, and underlying complications are systematically managed and treated from admission, and the child's weight and progress are monitored daily.[83]

There is increasing evidence to show that severely malnourished infants younger than 6 months and adults also respond well to treatment. Severe malnutrition among infants younger than 6 months of age can be successfully addressed using the supplementer suckling technique, which carefully combines supplementing breast-feeding with diluted F100, thereby still protecting and promoting breast-feeding but also providing an additional supplement for catch-up growth.[83] Good recovery rates have been reported for severely malnourished adults in therapeutic feeding programs in Sudan, Somalia, and Angola despite the associated challenges, such as relatively poorer compliance, increased risk of population displacement, and higher rates of underlying chronic illnesses among adults.[84]

During the past decade, improved practices and reduced mortality rates have been achieved in Tops even under the most difficult circumstances. This is largely a result of the timely revision of protocols and guidelines based on new scientific research, the wide dissemination of WHO guidelines, and standardized indicators for measuring performance and outcomes. However, the progress that has been achieved is mostly relevant to centralized, inpatient settings such as hospitals or refugee camps. In many complex emergencies, agencies and governments face a number of operational challenges that render a centralized inpatient approach inappropriate.[85] Some of these challenges are: coverage of the programs is frequently reported to be as low as 10% to 20%[32]; compliance is low because women are not in a position to remain in the inpatient facilities for the required 4- to 6- week period, leaving other siblings without a caregiver; the high risk of cross-infection; and the high costs associated with medical and dietary regimens and high staff-to-patient ratios. Building on previous experience of developing protocols for decentralized community-based settings,[86] home-based treatment regimens using ready-to-use therapeutic foods are under development.[87] Community therapeutic care, which stipulates inpatient care during the first phase of treatment only for children with complications and a home-based treatment regimen for all others, is becoming increasingly well accepted as a more effective approach where access to health facilities is limited.[88,89] The community therapeutic care approach aims to achieve greater coverage through more decentralized outpatient treatment centers and relies heavily on a community outreach and follow-up component; it has been implemented and the outcomes have been documented in a number of countries, including Ethiopia, Malawi, and Sudan[90] (see the case study below). Some design issues remain unresolved; therefore, guidelines for community therapeutic care have not yet been universally endorsed.

Case Study: Community-Based Therapeutic Care in Ethiopia

The vast majority of the population in South Wollo, Ethiopia, is chronically food insecure and lives in relatively densely populated, inaccessible mountainous terrain. After a deterioration in the food security situation as a result of the drought in 2002–2003, a nutrition survey conducted by an international aid agency, Concern Worldwide, in collaboration with the Amhara Region Disasters, Preparedness, and Prevention Bureau, in December 2002 reported a global acute malnutrition rate of 17.2% and a severe acute malnutrition rate of 3.1% (weight-for-height, Z-scores). A simultaneous multiagency crop assessment reported that the harvest was only 25% of normal and estimated that 50% of the population was in need of food aid.

In response to the high prevalence of acute malnutrition, Concern Worldwide implemented a large-scale SFP providing a biweekly ration of FAMIX (a local blended food) distributed through 19 decentralized sites and targeted 13,000 children and 3500 pregnant or lactating mothers. The community therapeutic care program targeting an estimated 2500 severely malnourished children was integrated into the SFP. The program consisted of an outpatient therapeutic program, a facility for inpatient care (local hospital), and an outreach program. The outpatient treatment consisted of a weekly health check, provision of ready-to-use therapeutic food supplies according to weight, standard medical treatment, and basic nutrition education for caregivers. The approach aimed to achieve a timely response, high coverage, and integration into existing health structures and services.

The outcome indicators for the program compare favorably with the Sphere Project's universally accepted standards for therapeutic care. For example, the proportion of children who recovered was 74.5%, the proportion who defaulted was 9.7%, and 7.5% died (Sphere targets for these same indicators are more than 75%, less than 15%, and less than 10%). Relatively low average weight gain (4.4 g/kg/d compared to a target of more than 8 g/kg/d) and long length of stay (81 days compared with a target of less than 30 days) represent some of the outstanding challenges for community therapeutic care. After 3 months of implementation, coverage was estimated as 77.5%.

This case study highlights the fact that good outcome indicators can be achieved through the community therapeutic care approach. The effectiveness of the program can be partly attributed to partnership with local health structures such as the hospital and placing a greater emphasis and resources on outreach workers. The major challenges that remain for the program include more innovative, sustainable, and local solutions for improving logistical access food and medical supplies; greater integration into the existing food security, water, and sanitation interventions; and sustaining community and Ministry of Health support for the program.[91,92]

Policy Development, Application of Best Practices, and Capacity

During the past several decades, learning in the emergency nutrition sector has been fostered by two main processes: recognition of a much broader definition of nutrition and the strengthening of interagency collaboration and sharing of knowledge and skills. Up until the 1980s, the sector primarily focused on malnutrition as an outcome, and advances had been predominantly technical. Then an important paradigm shift occurred in the policy domain, analogous perhaps to the expansion of the pure medical perspective into a public health perspective. Theories of famine and causal models of mass undernutrition that arose in the early 1980s[10,93,94] began to influence the field of emergency nutrition. This represented an important shift in focus from the outcome of malnutrition at the individual level to a broader, population-based discipline that took into account perspectives and expertise from economists, agriculturists, epidemiologists, and anthropologists. Some agencies have since adopted these broader frameworks into their policies, providing the tools and rationale to intervene during earlier stages of crises. By the end of the 1980s, there had been a critical confluence of two bodies of knowledge, one in the technical domain and the other in policy. Furthermore, learning in the sector was facilitated and strengthened through frequent interagency conferences, workshops, and the development of an interagency field magazine. The preconditions for the development of a public nutrition sector in complex emergencies was then present.[95]

Policy development and application have continued to play a key role in influencing food and nutrition responses in complex emergencies. Different United Nations agencies have made public their commitments to addressing specific aspects of emergency nutrition in emergencies. For example, UNICEF's Core Corporate Commitments refer to their commitment to provide essential nutrition services, including therapeutic feeding and vitamin A supplements,[96] and WFP's recent policy specifically emphasizes a greater role for nutrition within their food aid assistance responses, including the role of fortification for addressing micronutrient deficiencies.[60] The lead technical United Nations agencies are responsible for developing state-of-the-art technical guidelines.[53,83] Interagency initiatives have also played a critical role in policy development, such as the Ad Hoc Group on Infant Feeding in Emergencies, which has focused on policies and guidelines for the protection and support of breastfeeding in emergencies.[97] A wide range of practical and operational guidelines also exist, and memoranda of understanding developed between the United Nations agencies define the different operational roles and responsibilities of the different agencies.[98,99] Despite the wide array of policies that exist, there are inconsistencies in the application and adherence to these policies for a number of reasons. This includes some ambiguity and discrepancies between the different agency-specific guidelines, a general lack of awareness of policies because of rapid agency staff turnover, lack of systematic mechanisms that ensure adherence to policies and standards, and a relatively rapid revision of policies based on new evidence. These challenges are to some extent being overcome through a number of ongoing processes, including the preliminary institutionalization of policies and guidelines within national structures and governments; a commitment to adhere to a set of minimum standards by nongovernmental organizations, specifically through the Sphere Project[100] (see below); and recognition of the need to further professionalize the sector of emergency nutrition, particularly in crisis-affected countries. Evaluations of humanitarian responses have shown that few organizations have adequately qualified nutritionists working in emergencies—that is, professional nutritionists in key management positions with specific skills and knowledge to design and implement appropriate food and nutrition interventions in emergencies. Professional training initiatives can no longer be left to ad hoc training initiatives within the operational agencies themselves, but need to be systematically incorporated into academic curricula, particularly within the national training and academic institutions located in crisis-affected countries themselves.

Sphere Project: Minimum Standards in Food Security, Food Aid, and Nutrition

An important interagency initiative that has contributed to improved practice in humanitarian response over the past decade is the Sphere Project. Through a global consultative process, the Sphere Project has developed a set of minimum standards and related key indicators for different sectors, including food security, nutrition, and food aid. The cornerstone of the Sphere Project is the Humanitarian Charter, which is based on the principles and provisions of international humanitarian law, international human rights law, and refugee law. The Humanitarian Charter reasserts the rights of emergency-affected populations to life with dignity. The minimum standards and their related indicators are considered by some to be a practical interpretation of what these rights mean in the context of humanitarian response (i.e., it aims to link human rights with standards for operation). The most recent revision of the Sphere Project (2004) attempts to incorporate relevant human rights principles and values into the Sphere Standards as reflected in the Humanitarian Charter, including the right to life with dignity, nondiscrimination, impartiality, and participation. Although the minimum standards potentially establish a mechanism for transparency and accountability, ensuring their implementation will require more reflection on the precise modes and mechanisms of accountability.[101]

Conclusions

Nutrition in emergencies has evolved from a narrowly defined technical sector focusing on the treatment of malnutrition to a multidisciplinary approach to reducing nutritional risk and thereby supporting nutrition and preventing malnutrition. This has required broadening the concept of nutrition to encompass a much greater breadth and understanding of the wider political, economic, and social influences on nutrition in emergencies and has now been termed public nutrition.

Significant technical progress has been accomplished within the sector. There is greater consensus, awareness, and application of analytical tools and frameworks for assessing food security and nutritional risks. The quality and standardization of nutritional surveys have improved, especially in countries that have endorsed their own national guidelines based on universally accepted best practice. Significant progress has been achieved in learning the etiology and treatment of severe malnutrition and its application in emergency health services.

Although acute malnutrition among children is widely recognized as the most common characteristic of complex emergencies in the past, nutritional risk among other age groups and other outcomes such as micronutrient deficiencies are increasingly recognized as equally important. Consequently, analytical frameworks need to broaden their concept of nutritional vulnerability and risk to incorporate all three groups of underlying causes; this will require both qualitative studies and epidemiologic data. Furthermore, as a result of the multicausal nature of malnutrition, direct nutrition interventions as described in this chapter should rarely be implemented in isolation of integrated health and food security programs. Health care and food security programs may be necessary to ensure adequate nutrition, but each on its own is insufficient to protect the nutrition of populations.

The design and delivery of food and nutrition interventions in complex emergencies are frequently constrained by the characteristic breakdown of local infrastructure, including government, civil society, and community networks. Humanitarian agencies also face difficulties in identifying and accessing the most vulnerable groups, particularly in contexts where vulnerability is influenced by a complex number of determinants, not just physiologic. Poor security and lack of access to the affected populations, rapidly changing situations, and a lack of timely and representative information for appropriate decision making are all critical challenges for designing appropriate nutrition responses.

The promotion and support of national capacity and of developing professional leadership in the countries directly affected by crises, within both the technical and policy domains, will be critical toward achieving more effective responses in future nutritional crises.

References

1. *Nutrition Information in Crisis Situations* (formerly RNIS). Geneva: United Nations Standing Committee on Nutrition, 1993–2005.
2. Young H. Public nutrition in emergencies: an overview of debates, dilemmas and decision-making. Disasters. 1999;23:277–292.
3. Young H, Borrel A, Holland D, et al. Public nutrition in complex emergencies. Lancet. 2004;364: 1899–1909.
4. Salama P, Spiegel P, Talley L, et al. Lessons learned from complex emergencies over past decade. Lancet. 2004;364:1801–1813.
5. Borrel A, Salama P. Public nutrition from an approach to a discipline: Conern's nutrition case-studies in complex emergencies. Disasters. 1999;24: 326–342.
6. Hedlund K. *Ethiopia: Mortality Rates Baseline 2000–2003*. Addis Ababa, VAM: World Food Programme, 2003.
7. International Rescue Committee. *Anthropometric Survey: Somali Bantu (New Arrivals): Kakuma Refugee Camp*. Nairobi: International Rescue Committee, 2003.
8. Young H, Jaspars S. *Nutrition Matters: People, Food and Famine*. London: IT Publications, 1995.
9. Young H, Jaspars S. Nutritional assessments, food security and famine. Disasters. 1995;19:26–36.
10. de Waal A. *Famine that Kills: Darfur, Sudan, 1984–85*. Clarendon Paperbacks, 1989.
11. Devereux S. The Malawi Famine of 2002. IDS Bulletin. 2002;33:70–78.
12. Mei Z, Yip R, Grummer-Strawn LM, et al. Development of a research child growth reference and its comparison with the current international growth reference. Bull WHO. 1998;152:471–480.
13. de Onis M, Habicht JP. Anthropometric reference data for international use: recommendations from a World Health Organization Expert Committee. Am J Clin Nutr. 1996;64:650–658.
14. Briend A, Garenne M, Maire B, et al. Nutritional status, age and survival: the muscle mass hypothesis. Eur J Clin Nutr. 1989;43:715–726.

15. Sommer A, Loewenstein MS. Nutritional status and mortality: a prospective validation of the QUAC stick. Am J Clin Nutr. 1975;28:287–292.
16. Collins S, Duffield A, Myatt M. *Adults: Assessment of Nutritional Status in Emergency-Affected Populations*. Administrative Committee on Coordination/ Sub-Committee on Nutrition, 2000.
17. Salama P, Collins S. An ongoing omission; adolescent and adult malnutrition in famine situations. ENN Field Exchange. 2000;18(5).
18. Busolo D. *Assessment of Adults and Older People in Emergencies: Approaches, Issues and Priorities*. Washington DC, 2002.
19. Woodruff B A, Duffield A. *Adolescents. Assessment of Nutritional Status in Emergency-Affected Populations*. Geneva: Administrative Committee on Coordination/Sub-Committee on Coordination, 2000.
20. Médecins sans Frontières. *Nutrition Guidelines*. Paris: Médecins sans Frontières, 1995.
21. Nieburg P, Person-Karell B, Toole MJ, et al. Malnutrition-mortality relationships among refugees. J Refugee Studies. 1992;5:247–256.
22. Yip R, Scanlon K. The burden of malnutrition: population perspective. *J Nutr.* 1994;124: 2043S–2046S.
23. Seaman J, Clark P, Boudreau T, et al. *The Household Economy Approach: A Resource Manual for Practitioners*. London: Save the Children, 2000.
24. Young H, Jaspars S, Brown R, et al. *Food Security Assessments in Emergencies: A Livelihoods Approach*. London, Overseas Development Institute, 2001.
25. VAM/WFP. *Comprehensive Food Security and Vulnerability Assessment Thematic Guidelines, 2005*.
26. Project TS. Chapter 3 in *Food Security, Nutrition and Food Aid.* Oxford: Oxfam UK, 2004.
27. Longley C, Maxwell D. *Livelihoods, Chronic Conflict and Humanitarian Response: A Synthesis of Current Practice*. Working Paper 182. London: Overseas Development Institute, 2003.
28. Harvey P. *Cash Vouchers in Emergencies*. London: Overseas Development Institute, 2005.
29. Lautze E. *More Than Seeds and Tools; An Overview of OFDA Livelihood Interventions 1964–2002*. Boston, MA: Feinstein International Famine Center, 2003.
30. Longley C, Dominguez C, Saide MA, et al. Do farmers need relief seed? A methodology for assessing seed systems. Disasters. 2002;26:343–355.
31. Remington TJ, Maroko J, Walsh S, et al. Getting off the seeds-and-tools treadmill with CRS seed vouchers and fairs. Disasters. 2002;26:316–328.
32. Aklilu A, Wekesa M. Drought, *Livestock and Livelihoods: Lessons from the 1999–2001 emergency response in the pastoral sector in Kenya. Humanitarian Practice Network Discussion Paper 40.* London: Overseas Development Institute; 2002.
33. Jones B, Deemer B, Leyland TJ, et al. *Community-Based Animal Health Services in Southern Sudan: The Experience So Far.* Nairobi: Community-based Animal Health and Participatory Epidemiology Unite (CAPE), Organization for African Union;1998.
34. Peppiatt D, Mitchell J, Holzman P. Cash Transfers in Emergencies: Evaluating Benefits and Assessing Risks. London: Humanitarian Practice Network, Overseas Development Institute; 2001.
35. Harvey P. *Cash Voucher in Emergencies. HPG Discussion Paper.* London: Humanitarian Policy Group, Overseas Development Institute; 2005.
36. Jacobsen K *Supporting Displaced Livelihoods with Microcredit and Other Income Generating Programs: Findings from the Alchemy Project, 2001–2004.* Medford, MA; Feinstein International Famine Center, Tufts University; 2004.
37. Young H, Osman MA, Aklilu Y, et al. *Livelihoods Under Seige.* Medford, MA: Feinstein International Famine Center, Tufts University, 2005.
38. Jaspars S. *Solidarity and Soup Kitchens: A Review of Principles and Practice for Food Distribution in Conflict.* Humanitarian Policy Group, Overseas Development Institute & Nutrition Works, Public Nutrition Resource Group, 2000.
39. *Food and Nutrition Needs in Emergencies.* Geneva, United Nations High Commissioner for Refugees, United Nations Children's Fund, World Food Programme, World Health Organization, 2002.
40. Salama P, Assefa F, Talley L, et al. Malnutrition, measles, mortality, and the humanitarian response during a famine in Ethiopia. JAMA. 2001;286: 563–571.
41. Médicins sans Frontières. *Refugee Health. An Approach to Emergency Situations.* London: Macmillan, 1997.
42. de Waal A, Whiteside A. New variant famine: AIDS and food crisis in southern Africa. Lancet. 2003;362:1234–1237.
43. Connoly MGM, Ryan MJ, Salama P, et al. Communicable diseases in complex emergencies; impact and challenges. Lancet. 2004;364:1974–1983.
44. WHO. *Infant and Young Child Nutrition: Global Strategy on Infant and Young Child Feeding.* Geneva: WHO, 2002.
45. Kelly M. Infant feeding in emergencies. Disasters. 1993;17:110–121.
46. Borrel A, Taylor A, McGrath M, et al. From policy to practice: challenges in infant feeding in emergencies during the Balkan crisis. Disasters. 2001;25: 149–163.
47. Seal A, Taylor A, Gostelow L, et al. Review of policies and guidelines on infant feeding in emergencies: common ground and gaps. Disasters. 2001; 25.
48. Scherbaum SH. *Infant Nutrition in North Iraq.* Ernahrungs Umschau, 2003.
49. Tolvanen M, Kumar S. *Policy on the Use of Infant*

Formula in Iraq. Nutrition Co-ordination Sector for Iraq Emergency, 2003.

50. UNAIDS, FAO, et al. *HIV and Infant Feeding. Framework for Priority Action, 2003.*
51. Leyenaar J. Human immunodeficiency virus and infant feeding in complex humanitarian emergencies: priorities and policy considerations. Disasters. 2004; 28:1–15.
52. WHO. *The Management of Nutrition in Major Emergencies*. Geneva, World Health Organization, United Nations High Commissioner for Refugees, International Federation of Red Cross and Red Crescent Societies, World Food Programme, 2000.
53. WHO. *Field Guide on Rapid Nutritional Assessment in Emergencies*. World Health Organization Regional Office for the Eastern Mediterranean, 1995.
54. Vespa J, Watson F. Who is nutritionally vulnerable in Bosnia-Hercegovina? Br Med J. 1995;311: 652–654.
55. Pieterse S, Ismail S. Nutritional risk factors for older people. Disasters. 2003;27:16–36.
56. Piwoz EG. *Nutrition and HIV/AIDS: Evidence, Gaps and Priority Action*. Washington DC: USAID/ SERA, 2004.
57. Piwoz EG, Preble EA. *HIV/AIDS and Nutrition. A Review of the Literature and Recommendations for Nutritional Care and Support in Sub-Saharan Africa*. Washington DC: USAID, 2000.
58. Davies A. *Targeting the Vulnerable in Emergency Situations—Adults Last*. 1995.
59. WFP. *Micronutrient Fortification: WFP Experiences and Ways Forward. Policy Issues*. Rome: WFP, 2004.
60. Codex Alimentarius. *Guidelines on Formulated Supplementary Foods for Older Infants and Young Children CAC/GL08-1991*. Rome, Joint FAO/WHO Food Standards Programme Codex Alimentarius Commission, 1991.
61. Malfait P, Moren A, Dillon JC, et al. An outbreak of pellagra related to changes in dietary niacin among Mozambican refugees in Malawi. Int J Epidemiol. 1993;22:504–511.
62. Nyamsuren M, Emary C, Bat G, et al. *Integrated Programming Including Home-Based Fortification Using "Sprinkles" Is an Effective Strategy for Addressing Anemia in Mongolian Children.* Peru: International Nutritional Anemia Consultative Group (INACG), 2004.
63. Adish A. Effect of consumption of food in iron cooking pots on iron status and growth of young children: a randomized trial. Lancet. 1999;353: 712–716.
64. Allen LH. Interventions for micronutrient deficiency control in developing countries; past, present and future. J Nutr. 2003;133:3875S–3878S.
65. Sari M, Bloem M, de Pee S, et al. Effect of iron-fortified candies on the iron status of children aged 4–6 years in East Jakarta, Indonesia. Am J Clin Nutr. 2001;73:1034–1039.
66. Van Thuy P, Berger J, Nakanishi Y, et al. Regular consumption of NaFeEDTA-fortified fish sauce improves iron status and reduces the prevalence of anemia in anemic Vietnamese women. Am J Clin Nutr. 2003;78:284–290.
67. Lopriore C, Guidoum Y, Briend A, et al. Spread fortified with vitamins and minerals induces catch-up growth and eradicates severe anemia in stunted refugee children aged 3–6 years. Am J Clin Nutr. 2004;80:973–981.
68. Cheung E, Mutahar R, Assefa F, et al. An epidemic of scurvy in Afghanistan: assessment and response. Food Nutr. Bull. 2003;24:247–255.
69. Nieburg P, Waldman RJ, Leavell R, et al. Vitamin A supplementation for refugees and famine victims. Bull WHO. 1988;66:689–697.
70. UNICEF. *Micronutrients to Enhance Foetal and Infant Survival, Growth and Development; Workshop to Review Effectiveness Trials*. Bangkok: UNICEF, 2004.
71. Friis H, Gomo E, Nyazema N, et al. Effect of multimicronutrient supplementation on gestational length and birth size; a randomized, placebo-controlled, double-blind effectiveness trial in Zimbabwe. Am J Clin Nutr. 2004;80:178–184.
72. Bhutta ZA, Nizami SQ, Isani Z. Zinc supplementation in malnourished children with persistent diarrhea in Pakistan. Pediatrics. 1999;103:42–51.
73. Black RE. Zinc deficiency, infectious disease and mortality in the developing world. J Nutr. 2003;133: 1485S–1489S.
74. Cheung ER, Mutahar R, Assefa F, et al. An epidemic of scurvy in Afghanistan; assessment and response. Food Nutr Bull. 2003;42:247–255.
75. Shoal J. *Good Practice Review 2*. Emergency Supplementary Feeding Programmes, Relief and Rehabilitation Network, Overseas Development Institute, 1995.
76. *UNHCR/WFP Guidelines for Selective Feeding in Emergency Situations.* United Nations High Commissioner for Refugees, World Food Programme, 1999.
77. Vautier F, Hildebrand K, Dedeurwaeder M, et al. Dry supplementary feeding programmes: an effective short-term strategy in food crisis situations. Trop Med Int Health. 1999;4:875–879.
78. Beaten GH, Glassman H. Supplementary feeding programs for young children in developing countries. Am J Clin Nutr. 1982;35:864–916.
79. Dick B. Supplementary feeding for refugees and other displaced communities: questioning current orthodoxy. Disasters. 1986;10:53–64.
80. Ashworth A, Schofield C. Latest developments in the treatment of severe malnutrition in children. Nutrition. 1998;14:24445.

81. Golden MHN. *Severe Malnutrition*. Oxford University Press, 1996.
82. *Management of Severe Malnutrition: A Manual for Physicians and Other Senior Health Workers*. World Health Organization, 1999.
83. Golden BE, Corbett M, McBurney R, et al. Malnutrition: trials and triumphs. Trans R Soc Trop Med Hyg. 2000;94:12–13.
84. Collins S, Myatt M, Golden B. The dietary treatment of severe malnutrition in adults. Am J Clin Nutr. 1998;68:193–199.
85. Collins S. Changing the way we address severe malnutrition during famine. Lancet. 2001;358: 498–501.
86. Khanum S, Ashworth A, Huttly SR. Controlled trial of three approaches to the treatment of severe malnutrition. Lancet. 1994;344:1728–1732.
87. Diop el H, Dossou N, Ndour MM, et al. Comparison of the efficacy of a solid ready-to-use food and a liquid, milk-based diet for the rehabilitation of severely malnourished children: a randomized trial. Am J Clin Nutr. 2003;78:302–307.
88. Collins S, Sadler K. Outpatient care for severely malnourished children in emergency relief programmes: a retrospective cohort study. Lancet. 2002;360:1824.
89. Khara T, Collins S. *Community-Based Therapeutic Care (CTC)*. Dublin, Ireland, Emergency Nutrition Network, Valid International, Concern Worldwide, 2004.
90. Collins S. *Community-Based Therapeutic Care: A New Paradigm for Selective Feeding in Nutritional Crises*. London: Overseas Development Institute, 2004.
91. Khara T, Collins S. *Community-Based Therapeutic Care*. Dublin: The Field Exchange, Emergency Nutrition Network; 2004.
92. Collins S. *Community-Based Therapeutic Care: A New Paradigm for Selective Feeding in Nutritional Crises. HPN Network Paper 48*. London: Humanitarian Practice Network, Overseas Development Institute; 2004.
93. Sen A. *Poverty and Famines: An Essay on Entitlement and Deprivation*. Oxford: Clarendon Press, 1981.
94. Swift J. Why are rural people vulnerable to famine? *IDS Bulletin*. 1989;20:8–15.
95. Borrel A. *A Mapping of Learning Processes within the Emergency Nutrition Sector*. London: ALNAP, ODI, 1999.
96. *UNICEF Core Corporate Commitments in Emergencies*. New York: UNICEF, 2000.
97. Ad Hoc Group on Infant Feeding in Emergencies. *Infant Feeding in Emergencies. Policy, Strategy and Practice*. Dublin: Emergency Nutrition Network, 1999.
98. *Memorandum of Understanding between United Nations High Commissioner for Refugees (UNHCR) and United Nations Children's Fund (UNICEF)*, 1996.
99. *Memorandum of Understanding between the Office of the United Nations High Commissioner for Refugees (UNHCR) and the World Food Programme (WFP)*, 2002.
100. Sphere Project. Food security, nutrition and food aid. Chapter 3 in *Humanitarian Charter and Minimum Standards of Disaster Response*. Oxford: Oxfam, 2004.
101. Young H, Taylor A, Way SA, et al. Linking rights and standards: the process of developing "rights-based" minimum standards on food security, nutrition and food aid. Disasters. 2004;28:142–159.

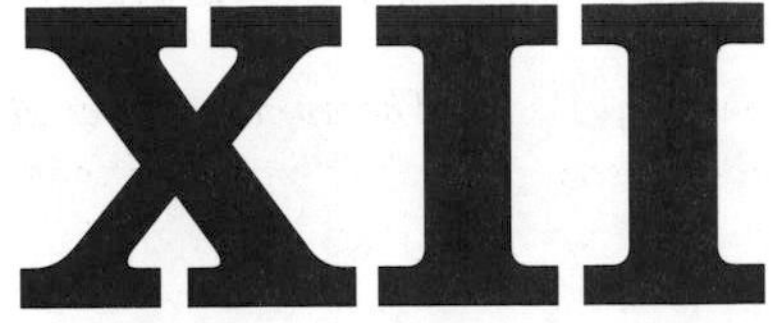

XII Emerging Issues

68 Foodborne Infections and Food Safety

Robert V. Tauxe and Marguerite A. Neill

The concept that food can cause human illness dates back to antiquity. The germ theory of disease and, since the late 1800s, the microbiologic identification of predominantly bacterial agents laid the groundwork for the concept that food could be made safer by interventions limiting pathogen growth and survival. Improved water sanitation, better animal husbandry practices, pasteurization of milk, and the widespread use of refrigeration have contributed to the steep decline in foodborne illnesses during the 20th century in the United States and other industrialized nations.[1,2]

Following on the heels of these achievements, however, has come a different set of issues in food safety during the last two decades of the 20th century. A far broader array of agents have come to be recognized as significant contributors to foodborne disease, including newly emergent bacterial pathogens and previously undescribed viruses and parasites. Several nondiarrheal human illnesses have been shown to have an infectious etiology that is foodborne in origin. In the natural evolution of analyses of food safety, their conceptual framework has become more dynamic, and at present the aim of such assessments is to define acceptable levels of risk.

This chapter will focus on newer developments in foodborne illness, including the expanded spectrum of human disease, recently described causative agents, changes in the epidemiology of foodborne disease, and current progress in prevention. It is beyond the scope of this chapter to include a comprehensive description of clinical manifestations, diagnosis, and treatment, and the reader is referred elsewhere.[3,4]

Causative Agents

Diverse etiologic agents are capable of causing diarrhea or other forms of foodborne disease in humans (Table 1). Infectious agents include bacteria, viruses, and parasites, each with their own ecologic niche in nature. These agents may be normal inhabitants of animal gastrointestinal tracts, soil, or water ecosystems. For some, the primary host is human, and for many others, the reservoir is in other animals. Their pathogenic properties for humans may be the result of evolutionary changes conferring selective survival advantages.

Prions (proteinaceous infectious particles) are novel transmissible agents that do not contain any nucleic acids. Prions cause a group of diseases known as the transmissible spongiform encephalopathies (TSE); in animals, TSE can be transmitted following oral inoculation with a species-specific prion protein. An epidemic in Great Britain of bovine spongiform encephalopathy (BSE or "mad cow disease") has been followed by an increase in humans of a fatal degenerative neurologic disease, new variant Creutzfeldt-Jakob disease, which is probably related to the consumption of BSE-contaminated foods.

In addition to infectious microorganisms, other enti-

Table 1. Classification of Etiologic Agents of Foodborne Disease

Infectious
Bacteria
Viruses
Parasites
? Prions
Noninfectious
Nonbacterial toxins
Chemicals
Poisonous mushrooms
Heavy metals

ties are capable of causing foodborne disease. Nonbacterial toxins produced by dinoflagellates can cause paralytic shellfish poisoning and ciguatera. Chemical causes of foodborne illness include histamine, the causative agent of scombroid fish poisoning. Extremely serious clinical illness results from the consumption of poisonous mushrooms, and clinical manifestations range from delirium to gastroenteritis with hepatorenal failure. Species of mushrooms that produce amatoxins and phallotoxins are causes of the latter form of illness. Heavy metals, including copper, zinc, tin, and cadmium, have caused acute nausea, vomiting, and abdominal cramps within 1 hour of consuming contaminated food.

Unfortunately, there is no 1:1 correspondence of an etiologic agent to a specific clinical scenario, and there can be considerable overlap among the categories in considering the etiologies of a patient's illness. The usefulness of this classification is to remind clinicians of all causes of a clinical illness with a possible foodborne etiology to ensure that appropriate questions are asked of the patient to ascertain whether significant exposures have occurred.

Types of Illness

Diarrhea and vomiting are most often considered the main manifestations of foodborne disease, but it is now recognized that a much wider range of human illness can be seen. Foodborne disease can present as an acute illness with a main manifestation of vomiting, diarrhea, sepsis, jaundice, or paralysis, or as a chronic illness with persistent diarrhea, neurologic findings, or chronic anemia (Table 2). Common among these different forms of illness is an initial step in pathogenesis that takes place at the mucosal surface of the gastrointestinal tract. This may range from adherence and colonization by a bacterial pathogen to viral replication within an enterocyte to absorption of a nonbacterial toxin.

The features of acute enteric illness following ingestion of contaminated food may be quite varied. Clues to the diagnosis are to discern the type of symptoms, their relative predominance in the context of the illness, and their intensity. Patients who experience nausea and vomiting with onset within 1 to 6 hours of a meal have likely ingested foods contaminated with a preformed toxin from either *Staphylococcus aureus* or *Bacillus cereus*. The vomiting is abrupt in onset and is intense, lasting for a few hours and resolving within a day with no specific therapy. Diarrhea is a less common component. Staphylococcal food poisoning was a major form of foodborne disease recognized during the middle of the 20th century.

An illness consisting of vomiting and diarrhea without abdominal cramping is usually due to norovirus or rotavirus. Rotavirus occurs commonly in young children but may affect adults as well. Community-wide outbreaks of norovirus infections have been a particular challenge in wintertime.

Watery diarrhea accompanied by abdominal cramp-

Table 2. Clinical Spectrum of Illness in Foodborne Disease and Examples of Common Causative Agents

Type of Illness	Examples of Causative Agents
Acute enteric illness	
Nausea and vomiting within 6 hours	*Staphylococcus aureus*, *Bacillus cereus*
Vomiting and diarrhea	Rotavirus, norovirus
Diarrhea and abdominal cramping	ETEC, EPEC, *Clostridium perfringens*
Diarrhea and fever	Non-typhoidal Salmonellae, Vibrio
Bloody diarrhea	*Escherichia coli* O157:H7, *Campylobacter jejuni*, *Shigella* ssp *Vibrio parahemolyticus*
Enteric fever	*Salmonella* Typhi, *Brucella*
Acute sepsis	*V. vulnificus*
Acute hepatitis	Hepatitis A virus
Acute pseudoappendicitis	*Yersinia enterocolitica*, *Y. pyseudotuberculosis*
Acute neurological illness	
Paralysis	Botulism, Paralytic shellfish poisoning, Guillain-Barré syndrome
Paresthesias	Scombroid, ciguatera
Meningitis	*Listeria monocytogenes*
Chronic enteric illness	
Diarrhea >3 weeks	*Giardia*, *Crypstosporidium*, *Cyclospora*, Brainerd diarrheal syndrome
Chronic neurologic illness	
Seizures (neurocysticercosis)	*Taenia solium*
Congenital abnormalities	*Toxoplasma gondii*
Encephalitis (AIDS patients)	*T. gondii*
Chronic anemia	Hookworm
Vitamin B_{12} deficiency	*Diphyllobothrium latum*

ing, typically but not invariably without fever, may be due to specific types of diarrheagenic *Escherichia coli* (enterotoxigenic *E. coli* [ETEC], enteropathogenic *E. coli* [EPEC])[5] or *Clostridium perfringens*. ETEC are a major cause of diarrhea worldwide and are the most frequently implicated pathogen in travelers' diarrhea. EPEC was originally described as a causative agent of nursery outbreaks in the 1940s and is relatively uncommon in the developed world today. In the developing world, EPEC are a significant cause of diarrhea in infants, particularly at the time of weaning.

Fever accompanying abdominal cramps and diarrhea suggests an inflammatory or invasive diarrhea. When the diarrhea is not bloody, this is most commonly associated with non-typhoidal salmonellae in the developed world.[6] Bloody diarrhea accompanied by moderately severe cramping and/or abdominal pain indicates a serious infection and should be treated as a medical emergency. In the developed world, causative agents include *Campylobacter jejuni*[7,8] and *E. coli* O157:H7.[9] *Vibrio parahaemolyticus* infection is common in Japan and along coasts of the United States.[10] In the developing world, other infectious causes of bloody diarrhea include *Shigella flexneri*, *Shigella dysenteriae*, and *Entamoeba histolytica*.

Enteric fever is the designation for an illness characterized by fever for several days with headache, malaise, anemia, and splenomegaly. When the causative agent is *Salmonella* Typhi, the illness is referred to as typhoid fever. *Brucella* can cause a similar syndrome. Typhoid fever is extremely uncommon in the United States today but remains common in the developing world, and most currently reported cases are acquired through overseas travel. It is now recognized that a few non-typhoidal *Salmonella* species can cause a similar illness in immunocompromised persons.[6]

Sepsis (fever, chills, hypotension) is a very infrequent form of foodborne disease. A specific association exists with sepsis from *Vibrio vulnificus* infection in persons with underlying liver disease, particularly alcoholic cirrhosis.

Jaundice with nausea and anorexia can be the manifestation of acute infectious hepatitis. As a foodborne illness, this may be due to hepatitis A virus infection. The overall incidence of hepatitis A in the developed world is considerably lower than that in the developing world or in countries whose economies are in transition, and it is decreasing rapidly where immunization is routine.[11] Infection early in childhood is often asymptomatic or unaccompanied by jaundice and confers lifelong immunity. Infection in adulthood is more frequently clinically symptomatic and is usually more serious. Hepatitis A is the most common travel-related illness that is preventable by vaccine.

Focal abdominal pain and fever, mimicking appendicitis, is often how infections with *Yersinia enterocolitica* or *pseudotuberculosis* present; these infections are rare in the United States, and have been more commonly described in Europe.[12,13]

A variety of acute neurologic illnesses may be manifestations of a foodborne infection. Muscle weakness leading to frank paralysis may be due to botulism or paralytic shellfish poisoning;[14] Guillain-Barré syndrome has a similar presentation. This latter entity is now recognized in many cases as being a postinfectious complication of antecedent *C. jejuni* infection.[8] Paresthesias (a tingling sensation in the skin) can occur in scombroid poisoning (histamine fish poisoning). Paresthesias occurring several hours after fish consumption, accompanied by reversal of hot and cold sensations in the mouth, abdominal cramps, vomiting, and diarrhea are suggestive of ciguatera.[14] A distinctive feature of this illness is the propensity for pain in the extremities to persist for months to years after the acute illness.

Acute meningitis (fever, headache, photophobia) can be a manifestation of foodborne disease when the causative illness is *Listeria monocytogenes*.[15] In contrast to many of the microorganisms already mentioned, *L. monocytogenes* is an opportunistic pathogen that mainly affects those with a compromised immune system. Such immune compromise can be physiologic (associated with pregnancy), age related (infancy, the elderly), due to an underlying malignancy (either diagnosed and being treated or not yet diagnosed), or due to HIV infection. Recently, a febrile diarrheal illness in normal individuals has been noted in several listeriosis outbreaks; however, the overall frequency of *Listeria* as a cause of diarrhea is not yet known.

Chronic forms of enteric illness, such as diarrhea for more than 3 weeks, can be a form of foodborne disease from particular pathogens. In addition to *Giardia*, two recently described parasites, *Cryptosporidium* and *Cyclospora*, cause chronic diarrhea.[16,17] The prolonged diarrheal illness known as Brainerd diarrhea, which is associated with drinking raw milk, remains of unknown etiology but which is causes a distinctive debilitating illness.[18]

Chronic neurologic illness can result from foodborne infection, often following months to years after the initial infection. Seizures can result from the cyst forms of the pork tapeworm, *Taenia solium*, in the central nervous system. Neurocysticercosis is the most common cause of seizures worldwide.[19] A variety of congenital abnormalities (e.g., blindness, microcephaly, mental retardation) are associated with congenital toxoplasmosis. A form of encephalitis has been seen in AIDS patients as a consequence of reactivation of the latent cyst forms of *Toxoplasma gondii*.

Pathogenic Mechanisms

The mechanisms by which foodborne illness develops are best characterized for bacterial causes. Presently, there are four main mechanisms by which bacterial enteric pathogens cause disease, and recent progress has suggested a fifth mechanism (Table 3). Some organisms produce illness after a period of growth in food during which a toxin is elaborated. Ingestion of this preformed toxin can produce excessive vomiting shortly after consumption, such as from *S. aureus* or *B. cereus* contamination, or frank paralysis,

Table 3. Pathogenic Mechanisms in Bacterial Foodborne Disease

Mechanism	Organism
Preformed toxin	*Staphylococcus aureus*
	Bacillus cereus
	Clostridium botulinum
Toxin secretion within the GI tract	*Escherichia coli* 0157:H7 and other Shiga-toxin producing *E. coli*
	Enterotoxigenic *Escherichia coli*
	Vibrio cholerae O1, O139
Cell penetration	*Campylobacter jejuni*
	Salmonella
Cell invasion	*Shigella*
	Yersinia enterocolitica
Adherence and signal transduction	Enteropathogenic *E. coli*

as in botulism. Other ingested pathogens may secrete a toxin following attachment to and colonization of a particular section of the gastrointestinal tract. ETEC produce a toxin closely related to cholera toxin from *Vibrio cholerae*; both toxins cause a net secretion of water and electrolytes, resulting in watery diarrhea. By contrast, *E. coli* O157:H7 produces Shiga toxin (closely related to that from *Shigella dysenteriae* type 1), which causes cell death and results in bloody diarrhea.

Apart from toxin production, two other mechanisms of disease induction are well recognized. Both *Salmonella* and *C. jejuni* can penetrate the mucosal layer of the gastrointestinal tract without causing cell death. Pathogens that invade the mucosal layer and cause cell death include *Shigella* and *Y. enterocolitica*. Bloody diarrhea is more common among pathogens with this latter mechanism of action.

Recent work to elucidate the pathogenic basis for EPEC-associated diarrhea has suggested a mechanism distinct from those already described. EPEC have been shown to produce certain attachment factors, including several secreted proteins. The interaction of these proteins with the cell surface receptor appears to initiate a series of events involving signal transduction. This leads to changes in cellular ion fluxes, with subsequent secretion of water and electrolytes into the lumen of the gastrointestinal tract.

Some bacterial pathogens have overlapping mechanisms of pathogenicity, and not all members of a genus may have the same mechanism of causing diarrhea. Grouping organisms by their mechanism of action nonetheless serves a number of purposes: 1) to function as an existing framework for classifying new pathogens, 2) to discern genetic relationships among diverse bacterial species, and 3) to use as a basis to predict the therapeutic usefulness of new therapies.

Epidemiology

The epidemiology of foodborne disease is a complex interplay of the expression of a pathogen's virulence traits, host susceptibility, physical characteristics of the contaminated food, geographic location, and season of the year. Some pathogens have a predilection for particular foods, usually resulting from an overlap between their ecologic niche and the harvest and/or processing environment for the food (Table 4).

Substantial changes occurred in the epidemiology of foodborne disease in the United States in the last half of the 20th century. In the early 1900s, milk-borne tuberculosis, staphylococcal food poisoning, and typhoid fever were the main forms of foodborne disease.[2] Today, the spectrum of causative organisms, risk factors for enteric infection, and types of food involved are vastly different.[20] Use of antimicrobials in food animals has selected for increasingly resistant strains of *Campylobacter* and *Salmonella*.[21] Changes in diet in the United States have occurred because of recognition of the relationship between diets rich in saturated fat and subsequent cardiovascular disease. This has led many Americans away from the traditional meat and potatoes diet of the 1950s to a diet that emphasizes fresh fruits and vegetables, grains, and fish and poultry. Changes in food distribution systems have led to an "end of seasonality" for many fresh fruits and vegetables. Commodities formerly considered "exotic" are now routinely available in most grocery stores in the United States, and they are likely to have arrived within several days of harvest or production elsewhere in the world. Consumption of prepared, preprocessed, or ready-to-eat foods from commercial establishments has increased, providing a context in which transmission from food handlers has been seen with moderate frequency, particularly with cold food items requiring hand contact. Substantial demographic changes also have occurred, with increases in populations with an increased susceptibility to particular pathogens.

Surveillance

The purpose of surveillance for foodborne disease is to monitor disease trends over time, to implement and monitor the effectiveness of interventions for control, and to detect outbreaks. Disease reporting is usually laboratory based, with the isolation or detection of a pathogen in the clinical microbiology laboratory. In general, only a small fraction of actual illnesses are reported, but this can vary considerably among pathogens according to the severity of illness and the ease of and access to laboratory testing.[20] For *Salmonella*, this has been estimated directly from surveys of populations and laboratories; an estimated 38 illnesses occur for every one that is diagnosed and re-

Table 4. Etiology of Foodborne Disease Outbreaks by Food, Season, and Geographic Predilection

Etiology	Foods	Season	Geographic Predilection
Bacterial			
Salmonella	Beef, poultry, eggs, dairy products, produce	Summer, fall	None
Staphylococcus aureus	Ham, poultry, egg salads, pastries	Summer	None
Campylobacter jejuni	Poultry, raw milk	Spring, summer	Higher in California and Hawaii
Clostridium botulinum	Vegetables, fruits, fish, honey (infants)	Summer, fall	None
Clostridium perfringens	Beef, poultry, gravy, Mexican food	Fall, winter, spring	None
Shigella	Egg salads, lettuce	Summer	None
Vibrio parahaemolyticus	Shellfish	Spring, summer, fall	Coastal states
Bacillus cereus	Fried rice, meats, vegetables	Year-round	None
Yersinia enterocolitica	Milk, tofu, pork chitterlings	Winter	Unknown
Vibrio cholerae O1	Shellfish	Variable	Tropical, Gulf Coast, Latin America
V. cholerae non-O1	Shellfish	Unknown	Tropical, Gulf Coast
Shiga toxin-producing *Escherichia coli*	Beef, raw milk, fresh produce	Summer, fall	Northern states
Viral			
Norwalk-like agents	Shellfish, salads	Year-round	None
Chemical			
Ciguatera	Barracuda, snapper, amberjack, grouper	Spring, summer (in Florida)	Tropical reefs
Histamine fish poisoning (scombroid)	Tuna, mackerel, bonito, skipjack, mahi-mahi	Year-round	Coastal
Mushroom poisoning	Mushrooms	Spring, fall	Temperate
Heavy metals	Acidic beverages	Year-round	None
Monosodium-L-glutamate	Chinese food	Year-round	None
Paralytic shellfish poisoning	Shellfish	Summer, fall	Temperate coastal zones
Neurotoxic shellfish poisoning	Shellfish	Spring, fall	Subtropical

Adapted from Fry et al., 2005[3]; copyright 2005, with permission from Elsevier.

ported.[22] Some pathogens are transmitted exclusively through food (e.g., *Trichinella spiralis*), whereas others may be transmitted most often through water (e.g., *Giardia*) or by person-to-person spread (e.g., *Shigella*), and only occasionally through food. A recent analysis took many of these aspects into consideration in developing new estimates of the burden of foodborne disease on health in the United States.[23] Approximately 76 million illnesses were estimated to have occurred annually, with 325,000 hospitalizations and 5000 deaths. *Salmonella*, *Listeria*, and *Toxoplasma* were responsible for 83% of deaths from known pathogens. A provocative estimate from this analysis, however, was that unknown pathogens accounted for 75% of all illnesses and 60% of deaths. These disease estimates were based on data from several sources not used in previous estimates. They contain a number of assumptions, including estimates of the total number of illnesses for each pathogen, the proportion of pathogen transmission that is foodborne, and the incidence of acute gastroenteritis with unknown agents. Continued refinements in surveillance will test the validity of these assumptions.

A new surveillance program of the Centers for Disease Control and Prevention, FoodNet,[24] develops population-based estimates and tracks the trends of known foodborne pathogens. The FoodNet sites now have nearly 14% of the US population within the surveillance network, and important trends are emerging in the 9 years since FoodNet's inception.[25] *Campylobacter*, initially the highest-incidence pathogen, has shown substantial geographic variation among the participating sites. The most recent data for 2004 show a marked decline in incidence of *Campylobacter* infection since 1996, to below that for *Salmonella*.[25] The incidence of *Listeria, Y. enterocolitica,* and *E. coli* O157:H7 infections also has declined during the surveillance period and may indicate the success of current disease prevention efforts aimed at multiple points along the "farm to fork" continuum. Limitations to the FoodNet data include whether the population within the 10 surveillance sites is truly representative of the US population in terms of demographics and risk factors and the fact that the system can capture information only on persons for whom diagnostic specimens were submitted. However, FoodNet represents a significant advance over traditional public health surveillance and provides more substantial estimates of the disease burden from particular foodborne pathogens.

PulseNet, developed under the auspices of the Centers for Disease Control and Prevention, is a relatively new system of laboratory-based electronic surveillance of foodborne bacterial infections.[26] After *E. coli* O157:H7, *Listeria*, or *Salmonella* are isolated from an ill patient, the bacterial strain is sent to state public health laboratories, where a pulsed-field gel electrophoresis analysis is done. The pulsed-field gel electrophoresis "fingerprint" of that bacterial strain is stored, analyzed, and compared electronically with a national database of such "fingerprints." In this manner, PulseNet has been instrumental in identifying and investigating many geographically dispersed outbreaks. Because the typical interval between specimen collection and pulsed-field gel electrophoresis analysis is 7 to 14 days, PulseNet does not yet function as an early warning system; however, this system has proven extraordinarily useful in detecting outbreaks that would otherwise have been missed until they were much bigger and in facilitating epidemiologic investigations of them. Food testing laboratories in the US Food and Drug Administration and Department of Agriculture have joined the network, making it possible to link patterns isolated from ill people with those of isolates from foods. Adoption of the same laboratory protocols in Canada, Europe, Japan, and other regions is making it easier to identify and investigate international outbreaks.[27]

Another, albeit sobering, aspect of surveillance is that it needs to be viewed as the first line of defense in a bioterrorist event. Food processing today has increasingly centralized production and wide geographic distribution, which may have economic advantages but which makes the food supply more vulnerable. Discussions of bioterrorism preparedness have often focused on airborne agents (e.g., anthrax), but more recently, consideration has been given to scenarios involving the food supply. An unheralded attack may well resemble an unintentional outbreak, and is very likely to be identified and investigated with standard public health procedures. Agricultural biosecurity will also need to be a component of the bioterrorism preparedness portfolio. A strong public health infrastructure with surveillance systems capable of functioning internationally is likely to be the most effective defense against both naturally occurring epidemic disease and bioterrorism-related events. The importance of robust public health surveillance in supporting both the public health and national security interests cannot be overemphasized.

Table 5. Populations at Increased Risk of Infection and Clinical Illness from Foodborne Pathogens

Infants
Pregnant women
Persons over age 60 years
Persons with HIV infection
Alcoholics
Transplant recipients (bone marrow, solid organ)
Persons receiving cancer chemotherapy
Persons receiving immunosuppressive drugs, including steroids

The Challenges of Special Populations

As epidemiologic investigations of outbreaks have delineated new and/or emerging pathogens as causative agents of foodborne disease, so too have new risk factors been defined for the acquisition of infection. The identification of groups with an increased risk for clinical illness following exposure is one of the most notable trends in foodborne disease epidemiology (Table 5). The magnitude of increased risk and the spectrum of pathogens differ among these groups. Young infants are particularly at risk for enteric infections, although they do not eat the foods that adults eat. *Y. enterocolitica* infections may offer a model for how indirect exposure can happen; bottle-fed infants get this infection when their caregiver is also cleaning pork intestines and likely transfers the organism to the infants' bottle via their unwashed hands.[28] Persons over 60 years of age may have an increased susceptibility to infection irrespective of other risk factors such as malignancy. The aging of the US population, along with that in western Europe and several other countries, has clear-cut public health implications in underscoring the need for ensuring a safe food supply. Advances in clinical medicine have created populations that never previously existed, for example, transplant recipients and those receiving immunosuppressive drugs. The epidemic of HIV infection has irrevocably changed modern society in numerous ways. With respect to foodborne pathogen exposures, HIV-infected patients are more likely to become ill, have a more severe illness, and have extra-intestinal or unusual clinical manifestations.

These at-risk populations were previously estimated to constitute 10% to 20% of the population,[29] but today the percentage is thought to be even higher. Many persons within these categories have no or only limited perception of their increased risk for foodborne disease. Although educational efforts seem a logical approach to disease prevention, this is often easier said than done. Some educational efforts, even when specifically targeted and culturally appropriate, have had disappointing results.[30] Because educational efforts alone may be insufficient to reduce risk and because even one organism may represent an infective dose for some populations, additional measures of protection need to be built into the food supply. Making food safe from farm to table is a joint responsibility of the food industry, the regulators, and the consumers. Technologic interventions such as pasteurization of milk and retort canning of vegetables have long played a critical role in making food safer. Irradiation is an example of a new supplemental intervention to enhance food safety.[31,32]

New Infectious Agents

Several infectious agents were added to the list of foodborne pathogens during the closing decades of the 20th century. Common to their "discoveries" was the magic combination of astute recognition of clinical illness and dogged epidemiologic investigation backed up by intensive laboratory investigation. The yield from this combined approach ranged from new information for an "old" pathogen (the foodborne nature of *Listeria* transmission) to the discovery of a truly new pathogen (*E. coli* O157:H7).

E. coli O157:H7 was first discovered as a human pathogen in 1982. It is now recognized as the most common cause of bloody diarrhea in North America and western Europe and has caused outbreaks on an unprecedented scale that have strained clinical and public health resources.[9] Hemolytic uremic syndrome may develop as a complication of this infection, and this is the most common cause of acute renal failure in childhood. Diverse food vehicles, including undercooked ground beef, alfalfa sprouts, unpasteurized juice, unpasteurized milk, and lettuce, have transmitted this infection.[33]

Salmonella has appeared in a variety of forms and foods. In the 1980s, a worldwide pandemic of *Salmonella* serotype Enteritidis infections began that continues today. This pandemic is related particularly to eggs, as this type of *Salmonella* colonizes the ovaries of hens so that the internal contents of the eggs they lay are contaminated with *Salmonella*.[34] In the late 1990s, two highly resistant strains of *Salmonella*, serotype Typhimurium defined type 104 and serotype Newport with the multi-drug-resistant AmpC gene appeared in the United States in cattle and in people. While they have been transmitted through various foods, they are most strongly associated with dairy-cattle and foods derived from them, such as lean ground beef and unpasteurized milk.[35,36] These two strains now represent 11% of human salmonellosis in the United States and are not controlled by current measures.

Two newly described parasitic causes of foodborne disease include *Cryptosporidium* and *Cyclospora*. Originally considered a veterinary pathogen, *Cryptosporidium* had only on rare occasions been described as a human pathogen prior to 1980. This changed considerably with the advent of the HIV epidemic, in which HIV-infected patients, mainly those with extremely low CD4 lymphocyte counts, developed severe and unremitting watery diarrhea from *Cryptosporidium*. Contaminated water accounts for a larger proportion of transmission of this pathogen than contaminated foods.[37] A waterborne outbreak in Milwaukee in 1993 affected more than 400,000 persons and illustrated the vulnerability of some municipal water supplies.[38]

Contaminated raspberries from Guatemala were the source for numerous outbreaks of diarrhea in 1996 in both the United States and Canada. Recognition of outbreaks was facilitated by extremely high attack rates (often greater than 80%) and a notably severe diarrheal illness. Yet these aspects were at odds with the largely negative coprodiagnostic testing. More intensive laboratory investigation ultimately identified *Cyclospora* as the causative agent.[17]

Novel foodborne diseases have been described for which there is incomplete understanding of the pathogenic agent. Brainerd diarrhea is the designation for a chronic diarrhea syndrome that originally occurred in Brainerd, Minnesota. Illness was associated with raw milk consumption and was both severe and long lasting, with diarrhea for more than 1 year in many patients.[18]

New variant Creutzfeldt-Jakob disease is a dementing, ultimately fatal illness that occurred in otherwise healthy young and middle-aged adults, mainly in the United Kingdom in the late 1990s.[39] Pathologic changes in the brains of these patients and characterization of the prions in them indicated that this disease is a form of a TSE.[40] The human cases were recognized after an epidemic of BSE in the United Kingdom that had occurred approximately 6 years earlier. It is likely that changes in rendering practices allowed meat and bonemeal to remain infectious with the BSE prion agent, and that subsequent foodborne transmission to cattle ensued when these were used in feeds. The link is thought to be that the BSE agent, crossed the species barrier and the human new variant Creutzfeldt-Jacob disease cases resulted from acquisition of infection through consumption of BSE-contaminated beef or beef-derived products.[41]

Different Risks in Food Production

There are marked differences in food production practices today compared with those earlier in the 20th century. Agricultural products and food animals used to be raised in smaller groupings, and food products used to be usually only seasonally available to a population in the immediate vicinity of the harvest. Food technologies that are now commonplace (e.g., aquaculture, extended shelf-life products) did not even exist. Today, the scale of production within the food industry has markedly increased; for example, hamburger may be ground in lots of several thousand pounds. Finished products are distributed over a much broader geographic region, and even raw materials may be transported in bulk over considerable distances. A large-scale outbreak of salmonellosis was the result of a tanker truck being used to transport pasteurized ice cream premix immediately after it had transported raw eggs contaminated with *Salmonella*. The subsequently contaminated ice cream product was distributed over the entire continental United States.[42]

Foodborne outbreaks due to fresh produce have increased markedly in the last three decades as the consumption of fresh produce increased and as produce imported from around the world became available.[43] This means that the health of the consumer in the United States is now linked directly to the sanitary conditions of field workers and the food safety systems of many countries.

Low-level contamination of a foodstuff may cause outbreaks that are difficult to detect because a relatively small number of cases may be dispersed over a broad geographic area. Newer food processing technologies may affect the survival and growth of microorganisms within the processing environment. Stresses (temperature, acidity, salt, sanitizers) may select for traits conferring survival advantages to the foodborne pathogen or may alter competing microflora in a manner that facilitates pathogen survival. Efforts to enhance food safety must have built-in mechanisms to continually evolve, because challenges from new pathogens, new vehicles of transmission, and new risk factors will undoubtedly continue to arise.

Vaccine Prospects

Of the microbial agents commonly recognized as being transmitted by food, only three have an effective licensed human vaccine for prevention: hepatitis A, *Salmonella* Typhi, and *V. cholerae* O1. Typhoid and cholera occur at such exceedingly low rates in the United States that vaccination is not warranted; however, travelers to high-risk countries are advised to get typhoid immunization. Hepatitis A vaccination increasingly is being used to control local outbreaks or more broadly in states with high case rates. Some institutions and commercial establishments have chosen to provide hepatitis A vaccine for food handlers and others involved in food preparation. Rotavirus vaccine had been approved for use in infants in the United States, but within 1 year it was noted to be associated with intestinal intussusception and was withdrawn from the market. A new rotavirus vaccine has recently been approved.

An experimental human vaccine for *E. coli* O157:H7 has been developed that induces antibody to the O157 lipopolysaccharide. Vaccine constructs have been developed for *Shigella* and *Salmonella* that have been tested in animal models. Considerable work remains to be done to demonstrate their safety and efficacy.

Many foodborne pathogens are colonizers of animal digestive tracts. These include *E. coli* O157:H7 and ETEC in cattle and *Salmonella* and *Campylobacter* in poultry. Another avenue of pursuit in vaccine development has been the development of animal vaccines. Whether for humans or animals, the ultimate success of a vaccine will rest with defining the target group to be immunized, accessing that group consistently, and ensuring high vaccination rates.

Prevention

Surveillance for foodborne disease has become the ultimate cornerstone for preventive efforts. In recent years, the major focus of outbreak investigations triggered by surveillance has been to ascertain a root cause for how a food became contaminated—whether as a raw product, during processing, or afterward. The findings are then used to devise control strategies to reduce or eliminate the problem of pathogen contamination. In the eyes of most public health authorities, surveillance has been transformed from a slow, paper-pushing effort to one that is dynamic, interactive, and increasingly Web based.

Similarly, the field of prevention has seen rapid progress in recent years, as the food industry has embraced the need for reducing the contamination of foods before they reach the final consumer. Food processing equipment manufacturers now routinely consider microbiologic outcomes in their designs, and the processes themselves are being overhauled to produce products that are microbiologically safer, as well as tasty, nutritious, and economically sound.

Much of the prevention of foodborne diseases occurs before the food is prepared and served. Minimizing contamination starts on the farm, field, or fishery, where good practices may reduce the likelihood of contamination even before harvest. After harvest, our industrialized food supply offers many points at which contamination can be prevented or eliminated. A safety engineering approach that identifies those points and sets controls in place to guarantee that they are effectively used is becoming the new standard throughout the food industry. This Hazard Analysis Critical Control Point (HACCP) approach is geared to prevent contamination before it occurs, rather than to inspect for contamination that has already occurred.[44] The HACCP program depends on continuous monitoring of steps in food processing that are critical in preventing the introduction, survival, or outgrowth of pathogens (such as temperature or pH), as well as those that reduce the pathogens burden (such as retort canning, pasteurization, high-pressure treatment, or irradiation). It is essential that documentation of the measurements of the parameter considered critical for control be recorded. Deviation from the accepted parameters for process control requires corrective action, which must also be documented. HACCP is well established for processed foods exposed to an adequate kill step. HACCP is being implemented in meat and poultry processing plants, and seafood and food service operations have modified HACCP programs. A HACCP approach for other commodities such as fresh produce is currently being debated.

Future Directions

Unpredictably but reliably, new foodborne diseases will continue to emerge. The constantly changing food supply will continue to offer opportunities for pathogens to infect us through new and unsuspected routes. Enhanced public health vigilance, investigation of unexplained outbreaks, and microbiologic and food science research will continue to be critical components of food safety. The globalization of the food supply will need to be matched by the expanded collaborative surveillance networks around the world and by a commitment in many countries to address the identified hazards. Surveillance will increasingly include monitoring the circulation of human pathogens among animals and plants and those present in foods to provide an integrated view of the ecologies that drive them. The inappropriate uses of antibiotics in agriculture to promote growth and prevent disease will diminish, and with it the threat of antimicrobial-resistant strains of food-associated bacteria and viruses such as avian influenza should decrease. The growing science of probiotics, at both the animal and human level, offers the hope of broad-scale prevention of infection by bolstering the resistance of gut flora to colonization by external pathogens.

The future of food safety lies in the joint efforts of consumers, food producers, public health authorities, and government. One major step in this direction is the recognition of a "farm to fork" continuum. Ensuring a safe food supply depends on efforts all along that continuum. Improved consumer education is needed that targets specific populations and/or food practices and that results in consistent and long-lasting behavioral change, but education by itself is insufficient. Safer processing is critical at animal slaughter and food fabrication plants, and more critical pathogen control technologies, such as pasteurization, irradiation, and pressure treatment, will be needed for foods likely to be contaminated with deadly pathogens. Introducing safer practices in animal husbandry, fresh vegetable production, and shellfish harvesting will have long-term benefits for public health. Introducing safety specifications into purchase contracts can rapidly make the concerns of consumers and retailers heard all the way back at the primary producers. The food industry and governmental authorities need to adapt to both the global marketplace and to pathogens, for which national boundaries are irrelevant. Because much of the burden of foodborne disease is preventable, it is a reasonable expectation that scientifically based efforts can significantly reduce that burden and improve human health.

References

1. Centers for Disease Control and Prevention (CDC). Safer and healthier foods. MMWR Morb Mortal Wkly Rep. 1999;48:905–913.
2. Tauxe RV, Esteban EJ. Advances in food safety and the prevention of foodborne diseases in the United States. In: Ward J, Warren C, eds. *A Safer Healthier America: The Advancement of Public Health in the 20th Century*. New York: Oxford University Press; 2006; in press.
3. Fry AM, Braden CR, Griffin PM, Hughes JM. Foodborne disease. In: Mandell GL, Bennett JE, Dolin R, eds. *Principles and Practice of Infectious Diseases*. 6th ed. Philadelphia: Elsevier Churchill-Livingstone; 2005; 1286–1300.
4. Butterton JR, Calderwood SB. Acute infectious diarrheal diseases and bacterial food poisoning. In: Kasper DL, Braunwald E, Fauci AS, Hauser S, Longo D, Jameson JL, eds. *Harrison's Principles of Internal Medicine*. 15th Ed. New York: McGraw-Hill; 2001;834–839.
5. Nataro JP, Kaper JB. Diarrheagenic *Escherichia coli*. Clin Microbiol Rev. 1998;11:142–201.
6. Goldberg MB, Rubin RH. The spectrum of *Salmonella* infections. Infect Dis Clin North Am. 1988;2: 571–598.
7. Allos BM, Blaser MJ. *Campylobacter jejuni* and the expanding spectrum of related infections. Clin Infect Dis. 1995;20:1092–1101.
8. Mishu B, Ilyas AA, Kosli CL, et al. Serologic evidence of previous *Campylobacter jejuni* infections in patients with the Guillain Barré syndrome. Ann Intern Med. 1993;118:947–953.
9. Tarr PI. *E. coli* O157:H7: clinical, diagnostic and epidemiological aspects of human infection. Clin Infect Dis. 1995;20:1–10.
10. Daniels NA, MacKinnon L, Bishop R, et al. *Vibrio parahaemolyticus* in the United States, 1973–1998. J Infect Dis. 2000;181:1661–1666.
11. Centers for Disease Control and Prevention: National Center for HIV, STD, & TB Prevention: Viral Hepatitis. Available at: http://www.cdc.gov/hepatitis. Accessed August 1, 2005.
12. Ostroff SM, Kapperud G, Lassen J, et al. Clinical features of *Yersinia enterocolitica* infections in Norway. J Infect Dis. 1992;166:812–817.
13. Nuorti JP, Niskanen T, Hallanvuo S, et al. A widespread outbreak of *Yersinia pseudotuberculosis* O:3 infection from iceberg lettuce. J Infect Dis. 2004;189: 766–774.
14. Underman AE, Leedom JM. Fish and shellfish poisoning. Curr Clin Top Infect Dis. 1993;13:203–225.
15. Lorber B. Listeriosis. Clin Infect Dis. 1997;24:1–11.
16. Guerrant RL, Bobak DA. Bacterial and protozoal gastroenteritis. N Engl J Med. 1991;325:327–340.
17. Herwaldt BL, Ackers ML, for the *Cyclospora* Working Group. An outbreak in 1996 of cyclosporiasis

associated with imported raspberries. N Engl J Med. 1997;336:1548–1556.
18. Mintz ED. Brainerd diarrhea turns 20: a riddle wrapped in a mystery inside an enigma. Lancet. 2003: 362:2037–2038.
19. White AC. Neurocysticercosis: a major cause of neurological disease worldwide. Clin Infect Dis. 1997; 24:101–115.
20. Hedberg CW, MacDonald KL, Osterhom MT. Changing epidemiology of foodborne disease: a Minnesota perspective. Clin Infect Dis. 1994;18: 671–682.
21. Anderson AD, Nelson JM, Rossiter S, Angulo FJ. Public health consequences of use of antimicrobial agents in food animals in the United States. Microbial Drug Resist. 2003;9:373–379.
22. Voetsch AC, Van Gilder J, Angulo FJ, et al. FoodNet estimate of the burden of illness caused by nontyphoidal *Salmonella* infections in the United States. Clin Infect Dis. 2004;38(suppl 3):S127–S134.
23. Mead PS, Slutsker L, Dietz V, et al. Food related illness and death in the United States. Emerg Infect Dis. 1999;5:607–625.
24. Centers for Disease Control and Prevention: FoodNet—Foodborne Diseases Active Surveillance Network. Available at: http://www.cdc.gov/foodnet. Accessed August 1, 2005
25. Centers for Disease Control and Prevention (CDC). Preliminary FoodNet data on the incidence of infection with pathogens transmitted commonly through food—10 sites, United States, 2004. MMWR Morb Mortal Wkly Rep. 2005;54:352–356.
26. Centers for Disease Control and Prevention: PulseNet. Available at: http://www.cdc.gov/pulsenet. Accessed August 1, 2005.
27. Centers for Disease Control and Prevention (CDC). *Escherichia coli* O157:H7 infections associated with ground beef from a U.S. military installation, Okinawa, Japan, February 2004. MMWR Morb Mort Wkly Rep. 2005;54:40–42.
28. Lee LA, Gerber AR, Longsway DR, et al. *Yersinia enterocolitica* O:3 infections in infants and children, associated with the household preparation of chitterlings. New Engl J Med. 1990;322:984–987.
29. Council for Agricultural Science and Technology. *Foodborne Pathogens: Risks and Consequences: Task Force Report*. Ames, Ia: Council for Agriculture Science and Technology; 1994.
30. Mouzin E, Mascola L, Tormey MP, Dassey DE. Prevention of *Vibrio vulnificus* infections: assessment of regulatory educational strategies. JAMA. 1997; 278:576–578.
31. Osterholm MT, Potter ME. Irradiation pasteurization of solid foods: taking food safety to the next level. Emerg Infect Dis. 1997;3:575–577.
32. Tauxe RV. Food safety and irradiation: protecting the public from foodborne infections. Emerg Infect Dis. 2001;7(suppl 7):516–521.
33. Rangel JM, Sparling PH, Crowe C, et al. Epidemiology of *Escherichia coli* O157:H7 outbreaks in the United States, 1982–2002. Emerg Infect Dis. 2005; 11:603–609.
34. Patrick ME, Adcock PM, Gomez TM, et al. *Salmonella* enteritidis infections in the United States, 1985–1999. Emerg Infect Dis. 2004;10:1–7.
35. Glynn M, Bopp C, Dewitt W, et al. The emergence of multidrug resistant *Salmonella enterica* serotype typhimurium DT104 infections in the United States. New Engl J Med. 1998;328:1333–1338.
36. Gupta A, Fontana J, Crowe C, et al. The emergence of multidrug-resistant *Salmonella enterica* serotype Newport resistant to expanded-spectrum cephalosporins in the United States. J Infect Dis. 2003;188: 1707–1716.
37. Roy SL, Delong SM, Stenzel SA. Risk factors for sporadic cryptosporidiosis among immunocompetent persons in the United States from 1999 to 2001. Clin Infect Dis. 2004;42:2944–2951.
38. MacKenzie WR, Hoxie NJ, Proctor ME, et al. A massive outbreak in Milwaukee of *Cryptosporidium* infection transmitted through the public water supply. N Engl J Med. 1994;331:161–167.
39. Will RG, Zeidler M, Stewart GE, et al. Diagnosis of new variant Creutzfeldt-Jakob disease. Ann Neurol. 2000;47:575–582.
40. Bruce ME, Will RG, Ironside JW, et al. Transmissions to mice indicate that "new variant" CJD is caused by the BSE agent. Nature. 1997;389: 498–501.
41. Brown P, Will RG, Bradley R, et al. Bovine spongiform encephalopathy and variant Creutzfeldt-Jakob disease: background, evolution, and current concerns. Emerg Infect Dis. 2001;7:6–16.
42. Hennessy TW, Hedberg CW, Slutsker L, et al. A national outbreak of *Salmonella enteritidis* infections from ice cream. N Engl J Med. 1996;334: 1281–1286.
43. Sivapalasingam S, Friedman CR, Cohen L, Tauxe RV. Fresh produce: a growing cause of outbreaks of foodborne illness in the United States. J Food Protect. 2004;67:2342–2353.
44. Doores S. *Food Safety: Current Status and Future Needs*. Washington, DC: American Society for Microbiology Press; 1999; 1–28.

69
Food Biotechnology

Charles R. Santerre

Over the past decade (1996–2006), more than 1 billion acres (400 million hectares) have been planted with crops that were developed using modern biotechnology. These crops have been grown in 21 countries by 8.5 million farmers.[1] Although more than 50 biotech crops have been developed, corn (45% of the crop is transgenic), cotton (76%), and soybean (85%) have seen the fastest rate of adoption in the United States. Support for modern biotechnology has come from thousands of scientists, including 25 Nobel Prize winners and numerous professional organizations, including the Institute of Food Technologists,[2] Society of Toxicology,[3] American Medical Association,[4] American Dietetic Association,[5] International Food Information Council,[6] Council for Agricultural Science and Technology,[7] and Food and Agriculture Organization of the United Nations,[8] among others.

To meet the challenge of a growing world population over the past century, agriculture has increased crop density and yields through conventional breeding, chemical fertilizers, pesticides, and mechanization, and has reduced postharvest spoilage through improved processing, storage, and distribution. The agriculture industry has done an outstanding job of feeding the world's inhabitants. Between 1960 and 2000, the global population doubled to 6 billion people; at the same time, agricultural output more than doubled. The "Green Revolution" was a term coined by William Gaud, director of the US Agency for International Development, in 1968 to highlight the improvements in agriculture that started around 1945. The improvements have helped agriculture to meet the needs of an expanding world population. The person often credited with being the "Father of the Green Revolution" is Norman Borlaug, who won the Nobel Peace Prize in 1970 for his efforts to develop wheat varieties that have fed over 1 billion people.[9]

To meet the dietary needs of a population that is predicted to reach 8 to 9 billion by mid-century, agriculture must continue to bring innovations forward. In addition, an increase in productivity is expected to occur on less acreage because many farm fields are being displaced by urban growth. In 1900, about 40% of the US population lived on the farm; today it is about 2%. Therefore, technological advances will need to offset the increasing population, the decreasing farm acres, and, desire of consumers to have "designer" foods that allow for improved health during an ever-increasing lifespan.

Along with increased production, improvements in food processing and distribution have provided an increasing array of food choices for consumers. Consumers in 1960 could select from about 6000 food items in grocery stores, but today's consumers have more than 30,000 choices. Along with the increasing variety of food products, the availability of perishable foods has also increased. Many fresh fruits and vegetables that were once available only seasonally can now be purchased throughout the year.

Around the world, people are consuming more animal products as their standard of living improves. Because it takes 10 calories of wheat to produce 1 calorie of meat, as populations move away from a vegetarian diet, crop productivity must also increase. Many scientists agree that in light of growing demand for meat, poultry, and fish products, increasing agricultural output exclusively through conventional breeding will not be possible. Modern biotechnology needs to be used in conjunction with conventional breeding to meet projected dietary needs around the world.

Modern Biotechnology

Modern biotechnology is a process for enhancing the traits of a crop by the direct transfer of one or more genes that typically are obtained from another species. After gene splicing, a transformed plant will produce one or more additional proteins and express one or more beneficial traits. Modern biotechnology differs from conventional breeding in the way that the genetic makeup is enhanced. Conventional breeding is limited to like species in which half of the genes are provided by each parent. Modern biotechnology is more precise and predictable than conventional breeding because it does not require that 50% of the genes be provided by each parent. In both modern biotechnology and conventional breeding, the overall objective is to improve a crop's traits.

For the purposes of this chapter, we will limit our discussion regarding modern biotechnology to the process of inserting DNA (or genes) into a plant cell that can then be grown into an entire plant. After this process is successfully completed, the transformed plant will express one or more proteins that are either new to the species or are expressed at a higher concentration than previously found in the species.

Genetic Engineering

Using techniques that employ restriction enzymes (enzymes to cut DNA at precise locations) and DNA ligases (enzymes that join DNA segments), a recombinant DNA (rDNA) molecule can be created.[10] In this chapter we will discuss rDNA biotechnology-derived foods (or more simply "biotech crops"). Through the use of cutting and joining techniques, we can splice DNA into a bacterial plasmid through a process called transformation. Next, we produce many copies of the DNA fragments so that we can improve our chances of adding this DNA into the target plant's genome. The DNA that we will add to our plant cells will have the gene or genes that we want to transfer, plus a gene that will allow us to separate the transformed cells from those that did not acquire the DNA. The new protein that is used to select the transformed cells is called a selectable marker. One commonly used selectable marker will make our transformed cells resistant to a specific antibiotic. Thus, antibiotic can be added to our cell culture, and only those cells that have been transformed will grow and multiply.

Two methods are commonly used for moving our DNA fragments into the target plant cells.[11] For monocots, such as corn, rice, and other cereal grains, a microprojectile bombardment technique is used to transform cells. First, the DNA that we want to incorporate is coated onto microscopic pellets made of gold or tungsten. Next, these pellets are blasted into the target plant cells. Then, the surviving cells are grown in a culture medium that contains antibiotic (if the selectable marker conferred antibiotic resistance). Finally, the transformed cells are regenerated into plantlets and evaluated. (This explanation is simplified, and it has taken many years to refine each step in this process.)

The method commonly used to transform dicots, such as tomato, potato, and soybean, employs a common soil bacterium called *Agrobacterium tumefaciens*. In nature, this bacterium is known to cause crown gall in plants. This bacterium can infect plant cells by attaching and forming a bridge that allows it to pass some of its DNA to the infected plant cell. Scientists have hijacked the bacteria's machinery and use it to transfer genes into the target plant cells. As described previously, the transformed cells are separated from the nontransformed cells using a selectable marker, and then the transformed cells are regenerated and plants produced.

Crops Approved in the United States

The beginning of this revolution in agriculture has resulted from numerous technical advances, but a ruling by the US Supreme Court (*Diamond v. Chakrabarty*, 447 US 303) in 1980 was critical to allowing this technological advance to bring us biotech crops. The Supreme Court upheld a patent claim by Chakrabarty, who had developed a number of bioengineered organisms that were capable of breaking down crude oil. His intent was to use these transformed organisms for environmental remediation after an oil spill. The court's ruling, which allowed the patenting of transformed organisms, opened the door for biotech companies to realize a profit from their development of biotech organisms, including crops. The agriculture industry is not the only one to benefit from this ruling: more than 25% of the 20 most popular pharmaceuticals are produced using bioengineered organisms.[12]

The first food to be produced using biotech organisms was cheese made from a bioengineered protein called chymosin. Historically, cheese was made using a protein mixture (rennin) that was taken from the forth stomach of milk-fed calves. Rennin, which contains chymosin, coagulates the casein at the start of cheese making. Since approval by the US Food and Drug Administration (FDA) in 1990, much of the cheese consumed in the United States has been produced using bioengineered chymosin that is made by fermentation. Cheese made using the biotech chymosin is acceptable for consumers who follow Kosher or Halal dietary practices.

As of 2005, many transgenic crops have been approved in the United States, including cotton, corn, sugar beet, wheat, canola, rice, cantaloupe, soybean, tomato, flax, potato, radicchio, squash, and papaya.[13] Traits that have been added to these crops include tolerance to herbicides; resistance to insects and/or viruses; delayed ripening/softening; addition of male sterility; increased lysine, oleic acid (C18:1 n-9), or lauric acid (C12:0); and addition of phytase. Most of these first-generation biotech crops have been targeted to producers, but next-generation crops will increasingly provide benefits more apparent to consumers.

Examples of Enhanced Crops

Generally, when a gene is added to a crop, an additional protein is produced; by understanding the function of the new protein, we can understand the enhanced trait that has been gained. The first crop to make it through the regulatory process was the FlavrSavr™ tomato (developed by Calgene Inc.).[14] The scientists at this company wanted to slow the softening process that occurs as tomatoes ripen. They thought that this would allow tomatoes to develop a deep red color with improved flavor development before harvest. To accomplish this, the gene that codes for the enzyme polygalacturonase was inserted backwards. Transformed tomatoes produce less polygalacturonase during ripening as a result of this transformation. Polygalacturonase causes pectin to break down; this is one of the factors that cause tomatoes to soften. In addition, tomatoes that produce less polygalacturonase have a longer shelf life, so spoilage is reduced.[15] Because a high percentage of fresh produce is lost to spoilage, attempts to slow or delay ripening can benefit producers, retailers, and ultimately consumers. The FlavrSavr™ tomato was approved by the FDA in 1994, but because this variety was not agronomically superior for a number of traits, it is no longer produced.

Bt corn was first grown in 1996, and this variety was enhanced by the addition of a gene from the common soil bacterium *Bacillus thuringiensis*. Bt corn produces a protein that is toxic to certain insects.[16] When insect pests such as the European corn borer eat this plant, the protein (called a cry protein to represent its crystalline nature) binds in their gut and forms crystals or spear-like structures that punch holes in their gut lining, which leads to massive infection and death. Because most other insects, animals, and humans have digestive systems that function in a different manner, this protein is digested without causing harm. The European corn borer can reduce crop yields by 20% in some parts of the country; nationally, it has been estimated to reduce yields by 5%. Another popular crop that uses the Bt trait is Bt cotton, also introduced in 1996.

One other crop first grown in 1996 is the Roundup-Ready™ soybean.[17] This crop was given a gene that allows it to resist the herbicide glyphosate (Roundup™). Glyphosate kills weeds by inhibiting the enzyme 5-enolpyruvylshikimate-3-phosphate synthase (EPSPS), which is necessary for the production of aromatic amino acids (tyrosine, phenylalanine, and tryptophan). Without these amino acids, the plant cannot survive because it cannot produce vital proteins. Roundup-Ready soybeans will produce additional amounts of this enzyme and as a result will have a greater tolerance for glyphosate after spraying. Weeds are undesirable because they compete for water, sunlight, and nutrients. In addition, some weeds produce seeds that can contaminate the harvested product, so there is good reason for minimizing their presence in the field. Application of glyphosate in the field has increased due to the popularity of Roundup-Ready crops, and glyphosate is less toxic and not as environmentally persistent as the herbicides it displaced.

Regulatory Oversight

The FDA regulates transgenic crops under the Food, Drug and Cosmetic Act and the Public Health Service Act (Figure 1). Review of these crops is currently voluntary, but all biotech crops in the marketplace have completed this review. Some contend that biotech crops should be regulated using the precautionary principle, which is intended to guarantee their safety. However, in the United States, biotech crops are regulated based on the standard of substantial equivalence.[2] This standard uses existing crops as the basis for determining whether a new crop will be "as safe" or "substantially equivalent" to those crops that have a history of safety and are currently in the marketplace. For a crop to be considered substantially equivalent it must contain levels of those nutrients typically found in that crop, and it should not contain significantly greater amounts of naturally occurring contaminants, such as solanine (potatoes) or psoralens (celery).[18] In addition, it should not contain a new protein likely to cause foodborne allergies. For proteins that are introduced from a non-food source, it is nearly impossible to ensure that the new protein will not cause an allergy in at least one individual. However, a series of predictive tests are used to determine whether the protein is likely to have the same characteristics as a food allergen.[19] The tests measure whether the protein is resistant to breakdown during digestion or processing and whether it has structural similarities to known allergens, and predict allergenic potential using in vitro and in vivo tests. When testing has been completed, if the new crop contains a protein that is allergenic and not commonly associated with that plant species, then the food derived from this must be labeled. Currently, all biotech crops in stores are substantially equivalent and do not require labeling unless sold in a country that has mandatory labeling (e.g., European Union, Japan, South Korea, Australia, New Zealand).[2] In the decade since the first biotech crops were planted, not a single adverse event can be attributed to a food derived from a biotech crop. This is an impressive track record given that an estimated two-thirds of all processed foods contain an ingredient from a biotech crop, and millions of consumers have been eating these foods for more than 10 years.

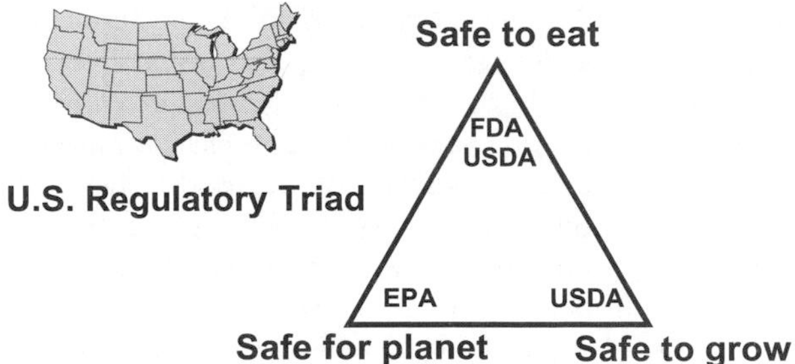

Figure 1. US regulatory triad. FDA: US Food and Drug Administration; USDA, US Department of Agriculture; EPA, US Environmental Protection Agency.

Those who promote the precautionary principle would like many years of testing to ensure the safety of biotech crops. Use of the precautionary principle to regulate foods would likely cause more harm then good. This principle assumes that foods developed using conventional breeding techniques are free from risk; that delays in adoption of these crops will not have negative impacts on human health; and that current testing techniques can guarantee absolute safety of a new crop. Each of these assumptions is incorrect. For example, most of the crops consumed today contain chemicals that can cause injury at high levels. Potatoes that are allowed to turn green when exposed to sunlight often have higher levels of a toxic glycoalkaloid called solanine. Celery will produce psoralens that can sensitize the skin and produce a rash following exposure to sunlight. Peanuts produce proteins that can cause anaphylaxis in a few sensitized individuals. Although conventional breeding has reduced solanine levels in modern potatoes, some conventionally bred celery, which had higher levels of psoralens, had to be removed from the marketplace because workers were found to have a higher incidence of skin rashes after harvesting this crop. It is safe to say that there is nothing that we eat that is free of risk. An excessive delay in the adoption of a biotech crop may pose greater risk to human health than releasing a crop after reasonable review. For instance, Golden Rice is a variety of rice that has higher β-carotene and iron concentrations. Current estimates suggest that up to 2 million deaths occur each year from vitamin A deficiency. Therefore, a protracted review process may cost more lives. In the future, crop failures similar to the one that led to the Irish potato famine in the 1840s may be avoided if the systems for evaluating new crops are refined. The fungus *Phytophthora infestans* caused the blight that led to the Irish potato famine.[12] Scientists are exploring genetic modifications that can prevent a similar disaster.

Another example in which modern biotechnology may be used to prevent a crop failure can be seen in the papaya industry. The papaya industry in Hawaii was being devastated by ringspot virus, which was threatening to destroy the entire industry. Scientists at Cornell University developed two varieties resistant to this virus. Due to genetic modification, 60% of the papayas currently grown in Hawaii are resistant to this virus, and this industry is now producing fruit at 1992 production levels.

In addition to review by FDA, all transgenic crops must be reviewed by the Animal and Plant Health Inspection Service of the US Department of Agriculture before planting in the greenhouse or field.[20] If the crop will produce a pesticide (e.g., Bt corn), it must also be approved by the Environmental Protection Agency. With the advent of transgenic livestock and poultry, the US Department of Agriculture will play a greater role in the review process.

It is impossible to guarantee the safety of any crop, whether it is derived from conventional techniques or modern biotechnology. When trying to assess the safety of a biotech crop, difficulties arise when testing a whole food that are not seen when testing a food ingredient.[21] When food ingredients are tested for safety, test animals can be exposed to higher concentrations, and then the results can be extrapolated to human exposure levels. However, whole foods cannot be tested for safety in the same manner because increasing the amount of a whole food will likely cause a nutritional deficiency. Therefore, increasing the intake of a single dietary component can cause deleterious effects due to nutrient imbalance rather then due to toxicity of the food. This is one reason that using the substantial equivalents principle is more appropriate for the regulation of biotech crops than the precautionary principle.

Foodborne Allergens

Because biotech crops produce one or more additional proteins, it is important to avoid introducing a food allergen into the new biotech crop.[22] A review of this topic can be found in another chapter of this book (Chapter 47).

One of the first incidents to demonstrate the importance of evaluating new biotech crops for allergenicity occurred after the development of a new soybean variety. Scientists at Pioneer Seed Co. were attempting to improve the protein quality of soybeans by adding a gene from the Brazil nut that would increase the levels of methionine in the soybean. Because their soybean received multiple copies of the gene from the Brazil nut, the new protein represented approximately 10% of the total protein. Scientists at the University of Nebraska found that individuals who were allergic to the Brazil nut were also allergic to this new soybean.[23] As a result, Pioneer Seed Co. discontinued development and never attempted to market the new soybean.

This incident helped to improve the methods used to screen biotech crops. To date, there has not been a single incident of a new food allergy that can be attributed to a genetic transformation.

Most scientists and food regulators would agree that foods created using modern biotechnology are not inherently risky due to the process by which they were created; however, each crop should be evaluated on its own merits. Just like for the soybean that was given a gene from a Brazil nut, it was not the process of moving the gene that made the soybean allergenic to certain individuals; rather, it was the specific gene that was moved.

Mycotoxins in Corn

Mycotoxins, which are produced by some molds, are problematic in corn. If corn is stressed by drought, hail, wind, or insect pests, it becomes more susceptible to molds that can produce mycotoxins. So, logically, if the stress factors are reduced during growth in the field, then mold growth would be reduced as well as mycotoxin content. Munkvold et al.[24] reported that Bt corn grown in Iowa had consistently less *Fusarium* ear rot than a conventional variety. In addition, the transgenic corn had lower levels of fumonisin (a toxic mycotoxin). This suggests that because Bt corn experiences less damage from insect pests, it may be safer than conventional corn in terms of mycotoxin content.

Environmental Impact

A study of the environmental impact after 9 years (1996–2004) of biotech crop plantings found that these crops have reduced the footprint of agriculture by 14% due to reduced pesticide applications.[25] Primarily due to Bt crops, pesticide application has decreased by 6% since 1996, which is equivalent to the elimination of 1514 rail cars of pesticide active ingredient. In addition, less fuel consumption (because the need to apply pesticides has decreased) and less tillage (due to better management of weeds) have both reduced greenhouse gas emissions by 1.8 billion liters. In 2004, this was the equivalent of removing 5 million cars from the road for 1 year.

In 1999, Cornell University researchers[26] conducted a laboratory experiment and reported that 44% of monarch butterfly larvae died after consuming milkweed leaves that were dusted with pollen from a certain type of Bt corn. This report caused a fury of activity as researchers at a number of institutions attempted to determine whether these results were also seen in the field. The Environmental Protection Agency[27] summarized these findings and reported that: 1) pollen does not drift more than 1 m from cornfields at levels that would be toxic to larvae; 2) corn pollen shed and monarch breeding generally do not overlap in most habitats; 3) larvae typically feed on the underside of milkweed leaves, where pollen concentrations are even lower than on the top surface of leaves; 4) corn pollen does not remain on milkweed leaves for very long as it is quickly blown or washed away; 5) reduced use of broad-spectrum insecticides (which results when Bt corn is grown) is beneficial to insects such as the monarch butterfly that do not feed on corn; 6) and monarch butterfly populations were increasing as Bt crops were being planted at increasing rates. In summary, monarch butterflies are more likely to be benefited by Bt corn.

Future Crops

Golden Rice, a transgenic rice developed by Ingo Potrykus and Peter Beyer, has increased levels of β-carotene (a vitamin A precursor) and iron. It was created by adding genes from a daffodil and a bacterium (*Erwinia uredovra*). Vitamin A deficiency has been blamed for up to 2 million deaths per year, and iron deficiency affects 1.9 billion people worldwide. Critics maintain that β-carotene levels are too low to effectively reduce vitamin A deficiency, which affects an estimated 180 to 250 million children annually. The Recommended Daily Allowance for vitamin A for children 1 to 3 years of age is 0.3 mg/d; each gram (dry weight) of Golden Rice contains 1.6 to 2.0 mg of β-carotene. If one assumes that the Retinol Activity Equivalence is between 4 and 12 and the bioavailability of β-carotene in Golden Rice is 50% to 100%, then a child must consume 1.3 to 10 lb/d (dry weight) to meet the Recommended Daily Allowance. However, it would take only 0.4 to 3 lb/d to prevent deficiency, and it may be possible to increase β-carotene levels by three- to five-fold, according to the developers.[28]

Although critics may be correct that Golden Rice may not be immediately ready to benefit malnourished individuals, it does represent a "proof of concept" and carries the promise of the future as this technology advances. Since we have recently celebrated the 100-year anniversary of the beginning of human flight, it is not difficult to recall the naysayers from a century ago saying, "If man were meant to fly..."

As seen with Golden Rice, we are already getting a preview of the second generation of biotech crops[29]—for example, Golden Mustard with higher levels of β-carotene; soybeans and corn with higher levels of α-tocopherol; strawberries with higher vitamin C content; rice that has been modified to have higher concentrations of iron plus added cysteine and phytase to improve bioavailability; soy and/or canola with stearidonic acid (C18:4 n-3), which can more efficiently be converted to EPA (C20:5 n-3) compared with α-linoleic acid (C18:3 n-3); crops with EPA (C20:5 n-3), DHA (C22:6 n-3), and conjugated linoleic acid, which can be used in animal feeds; canola with lower saturated fat; cottonseed and palm oils with higher oleic acid (C18:1 n-9) and lower palmitic acid (C16:0) content; rice with higher lysine content; rice and soybeans with higher methionine content; sweet potatoes with increased levels of essential amino acids; soybeans that contain human milk proteins for producing infant formulas; soybeans with lower raffinose levels to reduce gastric distress; tomatoes with higher lycopene content; and enhanced levels of healthy phytochemicals in soybeans, tomatoes, and oilseeds. With all of these "designer" crops in the pipeline, there are an equal number of new crops that will have improved quality, improved functional properties, and reduced or eliminated allergens.

As a result of modern biotechnology, there will also be many new challenges.[30] The regulatory oversight of transgenic animals is already facing government agencies. The first transgenic salmon is undergoing review. This salmon, produced by Aqua Bounty Inc., has added a gene from ocean pout that increase the salmon's feeding rate, thereby causing it to grow twice as fast. This could be an important development if the feed conversion for this popular fish was enhanced. Another challenge will involve the physical separation of crops that are grown for food from those that are grown to produce pharmaceuticals[31] or non-food compounds such as polymers or industrial chemicals.

Consumer Acceptance and Labeling

American consumers have been mostly accepting of biotech crops, unlike European consumers. An attitudinal survey of US consumers found that 62% felt that biotechnology would provide benefits to them or their families within the next 5 years.[32] Sixty-nine percent of respondents were likely to purchase biotech tomatoes or potatoes that have been "protected from insect damage and required fewer pesticide applications." Unfortunately, only 36% were aware that biotech crops were available in supermarkets.[32,33]

Ninety percent of consumers who received approximately 50 minutes of training on biotechnology would eat or serve biotech crops to their family, and 90% believed that they or their family would benefit from these crops within the next 5 years.[34] Prior to training, 31% felt that these crops were properly regulated; following training, 83% felt this way. It is apparent from this research that when consumers receive sound, science-based information, they are more accepting of biotechnology.

As mentioned, the FDA does not require special labeling for foods derived from biotech crops if the crop is substantially equivalent to its existing counterpart. However, some contend that labeling should be mandated; they believe that consumers have a "right to know." A survey of consumers provides conflicting results. On the one hand, a number of surveys have shown that when asked whether biotech foods should be labeled, a high percentage of consumers indicated that these foods should be labeled. On the other hand, when asked an open-ended question that forced respondents to indicate what additional information should be provided on labels, only 2% indicated that food labels should indicate when a food product contains a biotech ingredient.[26] It would be safe to say that when prompted, consumers would like biotech crops to be labeled; however, it is not an issue that rises very high on their radar screens.

It has been estimated that 70% to 75% of processed foods contain a biotech ingredient; therefore, it is questionable whether mandatory labeling would provide useful information for consumers.[35] Manufacturers are concerned that a mandatory label will scare away their customers. One reason that irradiated products have not been widely produced is that manufacturers do not want to add the mandated logo (radura) and the label statement that are required by the 1958 Food Additive Amendments of the Food, Drug and Cosmetic Act.

With the increased production and sale of biotech crops, it is unlikely that consumers can totally avoid these foods/ingredients, but they can select "organic" foods that restrict the use of biotech crops. In 1990, Congress passed the Organic Foods Production Act, which limits the use of certain practices in the production of "organic" crops. Prohibited items include chemical fertilizers, sewage sludge, animal hormones, and synthetic pesticides. Three "natural" pesticides are still allowed (rotenone, pyrethrin, Bt). Although some consumers believe that "organic" foods are superior to conventionally grown crops, Secretary of Agriculture Dan Glickman stated that "organic" foods are not safer or more nutritious then their conventionally produced counterparts. It will be interesting to see whether "organically produced" crops will eventually become less safe and less nutritious as second- and third-generation biotech crops start to appear in the marketplace.

Table 1. Potential Benefits of Crop Biotechnology

- Increased total yields due to:
  - Reduced pest damage
  - Reduced weed competition
  - Increased resistance to viral infestations
  - Increased tolerance of environmental stress
  - Increased yield
- Improved nutrient content
- Reduced allergens, pesticides, mycotoxins, and natural toxins
- Extended shelf life
- Improved flavor and quality
- Extended growing seasons
- Reduced cost
- Reduced environmental impact from agriculture

The European Union, Zambia, and the World Trade Organization

The European Union, which currently comprises 25 member countries, imposed a moratorium on the planting of new biotech varieties between 1998 and 2004. After 2004, there was significant resistance by a number of European countries, which imposed their own bans. The countries that instituted bans included Germany, France, Austria, Italy, Greece, and Luxembourg. In 2003, three countries (the United States, Canada, and Argentina) brought a case to the World Trade Organization contending that these bans violated fair trade policies. In early 2006, the World Trade Organization issued a preliminary finding that there was no scientific justification for the European Union's refusal of biotech crops. The decision was hailed by C.S. Prakash of the AgBioWorld Foundation, who said, "This favorable ruling gives European farmers the option to use safe, approved and proven tools to grow food crops, and gives consumers the right to choose those foods in grocery stores."[36] However, it is not likely that European consumers will be rushing to the market to purchase biotech crops, because they still have concerns about the safety of these crops. Some have suggested that their resistance may be due to past controversies that formed an association between food safety and new technologies (i.e., the Chernobyl meltdown and "mad cow disease").

A troubling episode occurred in 2002 in Zambia, where President Levy Mwanawasa's government ordered the United Nations World Food Programme to remove 35 ktons of biotech corn that was provided as relief for 3 million starving Zambians[37] who were suffering through a severe drought. Although some contend that Zambian officials were concerned about the loss of European markets for their crops from possible contamination, others have indicated that Zambia's main exports are cotton and tobacco not corn. In addition, Zambia does have the option of grinding the seed to render it infertile. Antibiotech groups praised Zambia's "bold decision" to assert its sovereignty. In 2005, President Mwanawasa declared a national food disaster due to continued drought and "appeal[ed] for donor assistance."

Future Directions

We are experiencing and will continue to experience many benefits from food biotechnology. However, with these advances, we will also be faced with challenges as we gain a better understanding of the technology that is before us. The potential benefits (Table 1) are numerous and include increased total yields (from reduced insect pests, viral damage, and weed competition, to increased productivity); improved nutrient content (including phytochemicals and reduced anti-nutrients); reduced toxins and toxicants (from reduced pesticides, allergens, mycotoxins, and naturally occurring toxins); extended shelf life; improved flavor and quality; increased tolerance to extreme growing conditions; reduced cost; and reduced environmental impact from production and processing.

Modern biotechnology does not make newly developed crops inherently more risky than crops developed using conventional breeding, so each new crop should be evaluated based upon its own merits. Regulatory review should permit adequate evaluation of new biotech crops without adding unnecessary hurdles. A review that requires excessive premarket testing may discourage the development of minor crops that will not bring the same financial returns as major crops.

References

1. International Service for the Acquisition of Agri-Biotech Applications (ISAAA). *Global Status of Commercialized Biotech/GM Crops*. 2005. Available at: http://www.isaaa.org.
2. Institute of Food Technologists. IFT Expert Report on Biotechnology. Food Technology. 2000;54:8–10.
3. Society of Toxicology. *The Safety of Genetically Modified Foods Produced Through Biotechnology*. 2002. Available at: http://www.toxicology.org/ai/gm/GM_Food.asp.
4. American Medical Association. *Council on Scientific Affairs Report: Genetically Modified Crops and Foods*. 2000. Available at: http://www.ama-assn.org/ama/pub/category/13595.html.
5. American Dietetic Association. Position of the American Dietetic Association: agricultural and food biotechnology. J Am Diet Assoc. 2006;106:285–293.
6. International Food Information Council. *Food Biotechnology*. 2004. Available at: http://www.ific.org/food/biotechnology/index.cfm.
7. Chassy BM, Parrott WA, Roush R. *Crop Biotechnology and the Future of Food: A Scientific Assessment*. CAST Commentary (QTA 2005-2). Available at: http://www.cast-science.org/cast/src/cast_top.htm.
8. Food and Agriculture Organization. *Electronic Forum on Biotechnology in Food and Agriculture: Summary Conference 5*. 2001. Available at: http://www.fao.org/documents/show_cdr.asp?url_file=/docrep/004/y2729e/y2729e00.htm.
9. *Norman Borlaug Biography*. 2006. Available at: http://nobelprize.org/peace/laureates/1970/borlaug-bio.html.
10. McHughen A. *A Consumer's Guide to GM Food From Green Genes to Red Herrings*. New York: Oxford University Press, 2000.
11. Mackey MA, Santerre CR. Biotechnology and our food supply. Nutrition Today. 2000;35:120–128.
12. DeGregori TR. *Genetically Modified Nonsense*. 2000. Available at: http://www.iea.org.uk/env/gmo.htm.
13. FDA-CFSAN. *List of Completed Consultations on Bioengineered Foods*. 2005. Available at: http://www.cfsan.fda.gov/~lrd/biocon.html.
14. Redenbaugh K, Hiatt W, Martineau B, et al. Regulatory assessment of the FlavrSavr tomato. Trends Food Sci Tech. 1994;5:105–110.
15. Kramer M, Sanders R, Bolkan H, et al. Postharvest evaluation of transgenic tomatoes with reduced levels of polygalacturonase: processing, firmness and disease resistance. Posthar Biol Tech. 1992;1:241–255.
16. Gianessi LP, Carpenter JE. *Agricultural Biotechnology: Insect Control Benefits*. 1999. National Center for Food and Agricultural Policy. Available at: http://www.ncfap.org/reports/biotech/insectcontrolbenefits.pdf.
17. Gianessi LP, Carpenter JE. *Agricultural Biotechnology: Benefits of Transgenic Soybeans*. 2000. National Center for Food and Agricultural Policy. Available at: http://www.ncfap.org/reports/biotech/rrsoybeanbenefits.pdf.
18. National Research Council and Institute of Medicine. *Safety of Genetically Engineered Foods*. Washington DC: National Academy of Sciences, 2004.
19. Taylor SL. Protein allergenicity assessment for products derived through plant biotechnology. Annu Rev Pharmacol Toxicol. 2002;42:99–112.
20. National Research Council. *Environmental Effects of Transgenic Plants*. Washington DC: National Academy of Sciences, 2002.
21. Chassy BM. Food safety assessment of current and future biotechnology products. In: Thomas JA, Fuchs RL, eds. *Biotechnology and Safety Assessment*. San Diego, CA: Academic Press, 2002:87–117.

22. Taylor SL, Hefle SL. Food allergy assessment for products derived through plant biotechnology. In: Thomas JA, Fuchs RL, eds. *Biotechnology and Safety Assessment.* San Diego, CA: Academic Press, 2002: 326–347.
23. Nordlee JA, Taylor SL, Townsen JA, et al. Identification of Brazil nut allergen in transgenic soybeans. N Engl J Med. 1996;334:688–692.
24. Munkvold GP, Hellmich RL, Rice LG. Comparison of fumonisin concentrations in kernels of transgenic Bt maize hybrids and nontransgenic hybrids. Plant Disease. 1999;83:130–138.
25. Brookes G, Barfoot P. *GM Crops: The Global Socioeconomic and Environmental Impact—The First Nine Years 1996–2004.* 2005. Available at: http://www.pgeconomics.co.uk/pdf/globalimpactstudyfinal.pdf.
26. Losey JE, Raynor LS, Carter ME. Transgenic pollen harms Monarch larvae. Nature. 1999;399:214.
27. Environmental Protection Agency. *Bt Biopesticides Registration Action Document.* 2000. Available at: http://www.epa.gov/scipoly/sap/2000/index.htm.
28. Potrykus I, Beyer P. *AgBioWorld.* Available at: http://www.agbioworld.org/biotech-info/topics/goldenrice/how_much.html.
29. Mackey MA, Fuchs RL. Plant biotechnology products with direct consumer benefits. In: Thomas JA, Fuchs RL, eds. *Biotechnology and Safety Assessment.* San Diego, CA: Academic Press, 2002:118–142.
30. Pew Initiative on Food and Biotechnology. *Future Fish: Issues in Science and Regulation of Transgenic Fish.* 2002. Available at: http://pewagbiotech.org/research/fish/fish.pdf.
31. Rogers KK. *The Potential of Plant-Made Pharmaceuticals.* 2003. Available at: http://www.mpt.monsanto.com/potential/potential.pdf.
32. International Food Information Council. *April 2003 IFIC Survey: Americans' Acceptance of Food Biotechnology Matches Growers' Increased Adoption of Biotech Crops.* Available at: http://www.ific.org/research/upload/IFIC-Survey-Americans-Acceptance-of-Food-Biotechnology-Matches-Growers-Increased-Adoption-of-Biotech-Crops.pdf.
33. Hallman WK, Hebden WC, Cuite CL, et al. *Americans and GM Food: Knowledge, Opinion, and Interest in 2004.* Food Policy Institute, Cook College Rutgers–The State University of New Jersey (Publication No. RR-1104–007), 2004.
34. Santerre CR, Machtmes KL. The impact of consumer food biotechnology training on knowledge and attitude. J Am Col Nutr. 2002;21:174S–177S.
35. Bren L. *Genetic Engineering: The Future of Foods.* FDA Consumer Publication No. FDA04–1332C, 2003:1–8.
36. Clapp S. WTO rules against Europe in biotech case. Food Chemical News. 2006;48:1–3.
37. Rao, CK. *Junk Science and Inept Politics Compound Nature's Wrath in Zambia.* Foundation for Biotechnology Awareness and Education, 2005. Available at: http://www.fbae.org/Channels/Biotech_basics/junk_science_and_inept_politics.htm.

70

Bioactive Components in Foods and Supplements for Health Promotion[a]

Paul M. Coates and John A. Milner

Introduction

Belief in the medicinal powers of food and its components is not a new concept but has been handed down from generation to generation. Almost 2500 years ago, Hippocrates suggested, "Let food be thy medicine and medicine be thy food." Today, consumers are bombarded by claims about the ability of foods and their constituents to modify health and/or the risk of chronic disease. Undeniably, strategies that use foods and dietary supplements to optimize nutrition for achieving one's "genetic potential," for improving physical and cognitive performance, and for reducing the risk of chronic diseases are highly commendable and appropriate, particularly in this era of mounting health care costs. Although defining the most effective use of foods or their isolated components will not be simple, there is mounting scientific evidence to believe that such a personalized approach is feasible.

Why Foods and Dietary Supplements?

The putative health-promoting effects of bioactive components are often first identified by observational or ecologic studies in populations with certain food preferences. Examples of this include the observations that populations consuming large quantities of oily fish have lower population burdens of cardiovascular disease, or that populations consuming large quantities of soy have lower rates of certain cancers. These observations usually have led to investigation and characterization of the bioactive principles responsible for these effects in vitro or in animal models—in the examples above, long-chain polyunsaturated fatty acids and isoflavones, respectively.[1,2] Frequently, these components have been isolated and characterized and then studied in various preclinical models in an attempt to better understand their mechanisms of action outside of the food matrix. Many of these isolated components are marketed as dietary supplements. In the United States, for example, the use of dietary supplements is very high, with more than 50% of Americans consuming dietary supplements on a regular basis. By far the largest component of the US dietary supplement market comprises vitamins, minerals, and other nutrient supplements, although botanical dietary supplements (e.g., echinacea, ginseng, ginkgo) are also commonly consumed.

In some instances, the health effects of individual components as part of foods have been borne out when single ingredients have been used as dietary supplements; however, in other cases, such as with tomatoes, it is the presence of the multiple components of the food matrix that is important in bringing about the desired response.[3] It is possible—but not automatically true—that the health benefit of a food component will be realized by consuming it as a supplement with one or more active components. Generally speaking, when consumers opt for a food-based and/or supplement-based choice for promoting health or for reducing the risk of chronic disease, they expect several features to be in place: 1) the products are known to be safe, because they have been in use in the

[a]The opinions expressed are those of the authors and do not constitute official policy of the National Institutes of Health.

human diet for long periods; 2) there are proven benefits; and 3) there is reasonable consistency in the products from batch to batch and over time. Research on all of these issues is needed, particularly as it relates to dietary supplements.

An Evidence-Based Approach to the Literature

Several questions arise about how to document the health benefits and risks of nutrients. Are ecologic studies, in which particular patterns of food intake are associated with health benefits and low apparent risk for harm, sufficient to make informed decisions for proposing dietary change to populations or individuals? Are randomized, controlled, double-blind clinical trials most appropriate? Because genomics is increasingly recognized to modify the response to food components, would haplotype-specific trials rather than randomized trials be a better way to evaluate health effects? Do we have reliable biomarkers of disease progression or surrogate end points for chronic diseases? Can an evidence-based approach sift through the relevant, available literature in a systematic fashion (Figure 1) and, based on the totality of the evidence, assist researchers, policymakers, clinicians, and ultimately consumers in making decisions about the role of bioactive food components in health promotion?

Dietary Modifiers and Biologic Responses

Numerous reviews extolling the merits and possible risks associated with bioactive food components have surfaced in recent years.[1,4,5] Collectively, more than 500 dietary compounds have been identified as potential modifiers of human health. Both essential and nonessential allelochemicals arising from plants, along with zoochemicals occurring in animal products, fungochemicals from

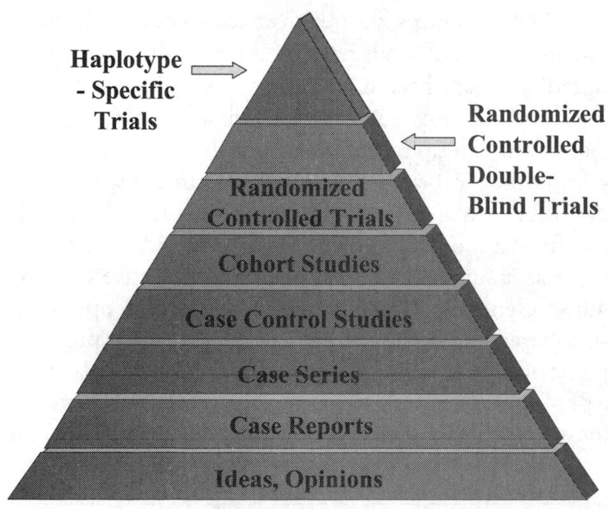

Figure 1. Pyramid of evidence.

mushrooms, and bacterochemicals from bacteria, may be physiologically relevant modifiers of health. Compounds encompassing such diverse categories as minerals, amino acids, carbohydrates, fatty acids, carotenoids, dithiolthiones, flavonoids, glucosinolates, isothiocyanates, and allyl sulfurs may influence multiple pathways associated with growth, development, and disease resistance. For example, garlic (*Allium sativum*) has been valued for its medicinal properties for centuries. It has been suggested that garlic can reduce the risk of heart disease and cancer,[6,7] serve as a source of antioxidants and thereby reduce tissue damage,[8] and influence immunocompetence[9] and possibly mental function.[10] Such data suggest that the health implications of bioactive food components may be extremely widespread and are likely not explained by a single cellular mechanism.

Population and Personalized Experimental Designs

The study of nutritional genomics has the potential to identify definitively which components in foods bring about either positive or negative consequences, and to clarify their relevant mechanisms of action and, most importantly, when they can be manipulated to optimize growth and development and reduce disease risk.[11] Knowledge about how diet-induced phenotypic responses depend on an individual's genetic background (nutrigenetics), the expression of genes (epigenomics and transcriptomics), changes in the amounts and activities of proteins (proteomics), and shifts in small-molecular-weight compounds (metabolomics)—collectively referred to as "-omics"—will be key to separating responders from nonresponders.

Polymorphisms

It is now recognized that close to 30,000 genes are found in the human genome. Single nucleotide polymorphisms (SNPs) occurring in a gene coding sequence are of particular interest because they may cause an amino acid substitution and therefore alter the biologic function of a protein. For example, an SNP in the human gene encoding the low-density lipoprotein receptor results in a A370T codon substitution that leads to asparagine being replaced by serine; this change is associated with higher plasma cholesterol levels and an increased risk of developing cardiovascular disease. Genomic data for humans and mice (including SNPs, expressed sequence tags, gene expression patterns, and cluster assemblies) and cytogenetic information are increasingly available through a number of databases; these provide opportunities to evaluate genomics as a factor in explaining the variations in response to food components in terms of human growth, development, performance, and health. Examples of these databases can be found at http://www.ncgr.org; www.jgi.doe.gov; http://www.gmod.org;

http://www.genome.gov; http://www.ebi.ac.uk; and http://www.nugo.org.

Increasingly, genetic polymorphisms are thought to have a role in determining the response to foods and their components. Unfortunately, although this area is receiving increased attention, it remains unclear whether these polymorphisms are directly linked to outcome. Nevertheless, it is certainly plausible that polymorphic differences have contributed to the inconsistencies among studies of the health effects of dietary components. In a random sample of participants in the Alpha-Tocopherol, Beta-Carotene Cancer Prevention (ATBC) study, for example, the low prevalence of polymorphisms in genes coding for the activation (phase I) enzymes CYP1A1 (0.07) and CYP2E1 (0.02) and the high prevalence in genes coding for detoxification (phase II) enzymes GSTM1 (0.40) and NQO1 (0.20)[12] may have influenced the outcomes and conclusions of the study. Further, in a nested case-control study within the ATBC study, glutathione peroxidase 1 (hGPX1), a selenium-dependent enzyme involved in the detoxification of hydrogen peroxide, was found to have a polymorphism exhibiting a proline to leucine replacement at codon 198. This polymorphism conferred a relative risk for lung cancer of 1.8 for heterozygotes and 2.3 for homozygous variants compared with homozygote wild types.[13]

Several common genetic polymorphisms may also modulate cancer and cardiovascular disease risk through their influence on folate metabolism, including polymorphisms of the methylenetetrahydrofolate reductase (*MTHFR*) gene. Substituting C for T at nucleotide 677 in the MTHFR gene (C677T) results in reduced conversion of 5,10-methylene tetrahydrofolate to 5-methlene-tetrahydrofolate, the form of folate that circulates in plasma. Individuals with the TT genotype have been reported to be at a decreased risk of colorectal adenomas when they had high (more than 5.5 ng/mL) plasma folate and at increased risk when they had low (5.5 ng/mL or less) plasma folate concentrations.[14] Another common polymorphism is an A-to-C transition at nucleotide 1298 (A1298C), which leads to the replacement of glutamine by alanine and results in mild hyperhomocysteinemia. The MTHFR SNP A1298C is more prevalent than the MTHFR SNP C677T among south Indian Tamils and has recently been associated with an increased risk of myocardial infarction, although results have been mixed.[15] Part of the inconsistency in results may relate not just to the intake of folate, but also to the intake of other vitamins, methyl donors, or other factors that influence DNA stability.

Polymorphisms in the vitamin D receptor (VDR) gene have been linked to bone health and to the risk of some types of cancer. Common polymorphisms include BsmI, TaqI in intron 8 and exon 9, and a poly-A site in the 3′ end of the gene. The femoral and vertebral bone mineral density was greater in children with the homozygous recessive (bb) version of the VDR polymorphism BsmI compared with those with the dominant genotype (BB). Likewise, BsmI B and short poly-A polymorphisms in the 3′ end of the VDR gene have been associated with increased breast cancer risk, with a trend for increasing risk with increasing number of BsmI B alleles or short (S) poly-A alleles.[16]

Literally millions of SNPs occur within the human genome, making it unlikely that a single base change will be found that is sufficient to account for a number of chronic diseases. However, because genetic variants are often inherited together in segments of DNA called haplotypes that are shared by a majority of the human population, they may be useful in deciphering the genetic differences that make some people more susceptible to disease than others, and likewise how diet will affect their susceptibility. The International HapMap Project (http://www.hapmap.org/) may be particularly useful in teasing out genetic differences that determine the response to specific foods and their components.

Epigenomics and Dietary Exposure

Evidence already exists that the transcriptional silencing of genes by DNA methylation plays a crucial role in a number of disease states.[17] Genes involving cell-cycle regulation, DNA repair, angiogenesis, and apoptosis are all inactivated by the hypermethylation of their respective 5′ CpG islands. Key regulatory genes—including E-cadherin, pi-class glutathione S-transferase, the tumor suppressors cyclin-dependent kinases (CDKN2) and phosphatase gene (PTEN), and insulin-like growth factor (IGF-II) targeted histone acetylation and deacetylation—are influenced by DNA hypermethylation. Although folate intake is recognized to influence DNA methylation patterns, other nutrients such as selenium can also have an impact.[18] Restoring proper methylation may represent a fundamental process by which selected nutrients can influence gene expression. Recently, Fang et al.[19] have provided evidence indicating that feeding genistein and related soy isoflavones can reactivate methylation-silenced genes, partially through a direct inhibition of DNA methyltransferase.

Bioactive Components and Transcriptomics

A fundamental action of several bioactive food components is that they serve as regulators of gene expression and/or modulate gene products. Typically, increasing intensity and duration of the exposure increases the number of gene expressions that are influenced.[20,21] Thus, dose and duration of exposure become fundamental considerations in interpreting findings from microarray studies. Although most studies are simple snapshots of genomic expression changes that can help to identify important possible targets, they must be interpreted cautiously because of inherent biological variability.[22]

Molecular Targets

The era of molecular nutrition holds promise for not only increasing our understanding of the specific site(s) of action of food components, but also the development of a "nutritional preemption" strategy that will incorporate bioactive food components at points of initiation and progression of pathways that lead to unhealthy or lethal conditions. Success with this strategy will depend on early predictors of the response to food components rather than gross phenotypic changes (Figure 2). Similar to the US Department of Agriculture's pyramid for dietary guidance, it is likely that the early predictive biomarkers will not be at the apex because of the lateness of the observation, but instead will be focused at the base, where they will be more specific and timelier for preemptive strategies. Molecular biomarkers (the "-omics" approach) will likely offer the sensitivity and reliability to evaluate dietary exposures and to provide invaluable insights into behaviors of specific molecular targets and predictors of individual responsiveness to dietary change.[5] These biomarkers must be readily accessible, easily and reliably assayed, differentially expressed in normal and diseased conditions, directly associated with disease progression, modifiable, and—most importantly—predictive (see Figure 2). The future of biomarkers of nutritional exposures, effect, and susceptibility likely resides in the enhanced use of molecular technologies to help distinguish responders from nonresponders.

Complementary and overlapping mechanisms appear to account for the response to bioactive food components in foods or dietary supplements (Figure 3). These biologic responses encompass such diverse functions as promoting the activity of detoxification enzymes, serving as an antioxidant, shifting hormonal homeostasis, influencing cellular energetics, regulating cell division, and participating in cellular differentiation. Since the responses may occur simultaneously, it is difficult to determine which is most important in dictating the change in health. Figure 3 demonstrates some of the plausible processes by which dietary components may influence health outcomes. The

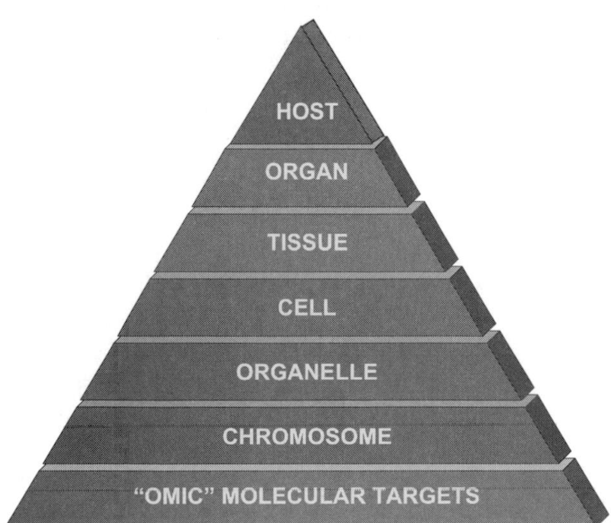

Figure 2. Predictive biomarkers of response to bioactive components.

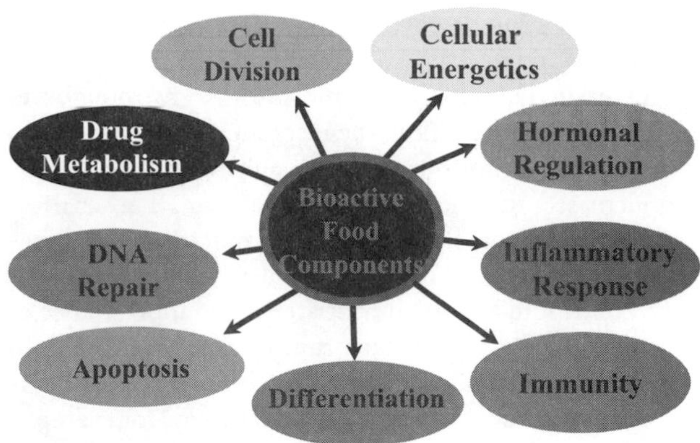

Figure 3. Diagram depicting how diet may influence several health-related processes.

ability of several nutrients to influence the same or multiple biologic processes raises issues about possible synergy—as well as antagonistic interactions—that may occur within and among foods.[23,24]

DNA Instability

A host of factors can contribute to DNA instability and ultimately to cellular proliferation. Endogenous agents, including methylating and reactive oxygen species arising during normal cellular respiration, can lead to DNA damage. Some nutrients, such as unsaturated fatty acids and iron, may influence this process by promoting the formation of the damaging agents, whereas other components (e.g., some flavonoids and folate) may function to enhance endogenous repair mechanisms.[25] Support for this comes from the observation that an aqueous fraction of Fushimi sweet pepper increases repair against UV-induced cyclobutane pyrimidine dimers in human fibroblasts.[26] Other data point to the need for folate in maintaining normal DNA synthesis and repair.[27,28] Some dietary components may also retard repair, as has been suggested following alcohol exposure.[29] Unquestionably, DNA replication is central to cell growth, development, and generation of tissues and organs. Recent advances in understanding replication machinery have revealed striking conservation of the components involved in the DNA replication processes from yeast to humans, thus raising the possibility of using various models to test the site of action of nutrients.[30]

Cellular Proliferation and Death

Cell homeostasis is regulated by a delicate balance among proliferation, growth arrest, differentiation, and apoptosis (programmed cell death). Although vitamin A has been repeatedly linked to differentiation, other nutrients such as vitamin D can also be involved.[31] Dysregulation of apoptosis frequently accompanies a wide array of conditions, including cancer, neurodegeneration, autoimmunity, and heart disease. Diverse nutrients, including plant sterols, selenium, and even butyrate arising from fermentable fibers, may promote apoptosis.[32,33]

Inflammation and Immunonutrition

The immune system represents a primary defense against invading pathogens, non-self components, and cancer cells. Inflammation is a basic process by which the body reacts to infection, irritations, or other injuries and is recognized as a type of nonspecific immune response. The inflammatory processes, including the release of pro-inflammatory cytokines and the formation of reactive oxygen and nitrogen species, are critical factors driving this process and can be influenced by several dietary components. Although pro-inflammatory actions are usually followed almost immediately by anti-inflammatory responses, excessive production of pro-inflammatory cytokines may lead to chronic inflammation. The ability of bioactive food components, including zinc, epigallocatechin gallate, and omega-3 fatty acids, appears to be mediated through unique molecular targets.[34-37]

The immune system protects against infection by producing specific antibodies in response to antigens. Vaccine-specific serum antibody production, delayed-type hypersensitivity response, vaccine-specific or total secretory IgA in saliva, and the response to attenuated pathogens are classic markers that can be influenced by dietary habits. Markers, including natural killer cell cytotoxicity, oxidative burst of phagocytes, lymphocyte proliferation, and the cytokine pattern produced, have also surfaced as potential predictors of immunocompetence. Because no single marker permits firm conclusions to be made about the ability of diet to modulate the entire immune system, combining markers appears to be a suitable strategy. It is also clear that excesses of some nutrients can enhance the immune system, whereas other food components can have detrimental effects.[38]

In addition to influencing immunocompetence, the availability of nutrients can influence angiogenesis. In adipose tissue, vascular endothelial cells provide oxygen and nutrients to the growing mass of adipocytes. In fact, the formation of new blood vessels from existing ones often precedes adipogenesis. Insights into how food components alter angiogenesis may be particularly useful in combating the growing global incidence of obesity. Likewise, the importance of angiogenesis in tumor growth and metastasis serves as additional justification for examining the impact of diet on this process. It is known that vascular endothelial cell proliferation, migration, and capillary formation can be stimulated by several angiogenic growth factors, as well as by eicosanoids synthesized from omega-6 fatty acids.[39] Lipoxygenase and cyclooxygenase products of omega-6 fatty acid metabolism are angiogenic in in vitro assays. The activity of both of these enzymes can be suppressed by the consumption of resveratrol, found in grapes, or omega-3 fatty acids, occurring in fish.[39,40] Likewise, genistein, found in soybean products, and selenium, found in fish and grains, have been reported to influence angiogenesis.[41]

Summary of Molecular Targets

Collectively, overwhelming evidence demonstrates that a variety of nutrients can influence a number of key intracellular targets. Determining which one of these targets is most important in altering tumor growth will not be a simple task. Likewise, unraveling the multitude of interactions among nutrients with these key events makes the challenge even more daunting. Finally, interindividual differences, probably reflecting genetic polymorphisms, can mask the response to a nutrient and thereby complicate this undertaking to an even greater extent. Nevertheless, deciphering the role of diet is fundamental to optimizing health. Access to this information should help resolve the inconsistencies within the literature and provide clues to strategies that may be developed to assist individuals in improving their health.

Biomarkers and Long-Term Intervention

Scientifically sound intervention studies must be viewed as the cornerstone for establishing nutrition guidance. Unfortunately, the number of long-term intervention studies that would be needed to adequately define the needs for bioactive food components is likely impractical in terms of speed of discovery and cost. Alternative procedures that use validated and sensitive biologic markers will need to be developed to assist in determining who might benefit most and who might be placed at risk, and the minimum quality of the food and/or component needed to bring about the intended response. To assess whether a food or its constituent has a physiologic effect, stringent experimental design characteristics must be followed, including appropriateness of controls, randomization of subjects, blinding, statistical power of study, presence of bias, attrition rates, recognition and control of confounding factors (e.g., weight change or nutrition status), and appropriateness of statistical tests and comparisons. Each of these factors must become the mainstay for all clinical investigations. These same factors must also be considered in the conduct of preclinical investigations.

The question arises whether typical intakes of these dietary components are sufficient to bring about these effects and how frequently these food components must be consumed. Combs and Gray[42] emphasized that the responses in antioxidant status, drug metabolism, and cell proliferation to a bioactive food component (in this case, selenium) were highly dependent on total intakes/exposures. Therefore, the development of "intended use" models represents a logical approach for determining the quantity of a food component needed for health promotion within specific segments of society, while building on the belief that not every individual will benefit from the same type of nutritional preemption strategies. There is also evidence that individuals do acclimate and accommodate to inadequacies in the food supply, and therefore the biologic response cannot be considered constant.[43] It is known that drug resistance frequently involves an induction mechanism, thereby reducing or eliminating the response.[44] Since bioactive food components have molecular targets, as at least some of which are identical to those of specific drugs, it is logical to assume that there is adjustment to their biologic consequences as well.

Increasing the consumption of a wide variety of fruits, vegetables, and whole grains daily continues to be advocated as a practical strategy for consumers to optimize health and to reduce the risk of chronic diseases. The superiority of food blends is evident from the enhanced antioxidant potential achieved by combining multiple fruits rather than simply providing individual portions.[45] Exposure to food blends may also result in synergistic response by modifying multiple biologic processes. For example, because quercetin and genistein block different phases of the cell cycle, their combined use is more effective in inhibiting the growth of human ovarian carcinoma cells than either provided alone.[46] This has significance for dietary supplements, in which the effects of individual constituents, as well as combinations of them, outside the food matrix will need to be carefully studied.

Omega-3 Fatty Acids as an Example

For more than 25 years, clinical studies have provided data on the potential health benefits of consuming polyunsaturated fatty acids (PUFAs) and particularly omega-3 fatty acids. Dietary omega-3 fatty acids may come from fish and fish oils (chiefly eicosapentaenoic acid [EPA] and docosahexaenoic acid [DHA]); plant sources such as canola oil, walnuts, soybeans, and flaxseed, primarily as alpha-linolenic acid (ALA); and, most recently, some novel genetically modified plants with exaggerated amounts of EPA and DHA.[47]

Results of several studies have suggested that long-chain omega-3 fatty acid intake is associated with reduced risk of numerous diseases, including cardiovascular disease, stroke, certain cancers, immune disorders, asthma, and neurologic disorders; rarely, however, has causality been established. Recently, a series of evidence-based reports about the health effects of omega-3 fatty acids were developed by scientists in the Evidence-Based Practice Centers at Tufts-New England Medical Center, RAND-Southern California, and the University of Ottawa (summarized at http://ods.od.nih.gov/FactSheets/Omega3FattyAcidsandHealth.asp#ref). The primary goal of these reports was to assess the nature and quality of the evidence relating omega-3 consumption from foods and supplements to health outcomes such as cardiovascular disease prevention and treatment. The reports systematically reviewed the evidence from numerous lines of inquiry. Systematic review of the randomized, controlled trials of the effects of omega-3 fatty acids on cardiovascular disease risk factors[48-50] showed that there is considerable heterogeneity in treatment effects. It is apparent from these and other reports that the speciation of the bioactive components must be considered, along with the multiple interactions with other dietary/environmental factors that may influence the overall response. For example, it is recognized that omega-3 fatty acids are not all equivalent in bringing about a biologic response and that confounders such as the total omega-6 fatty acid intake may influence the magnitude of the response.[51-53]

Which Risk Factor Is Most Important?

There was a strong, consistent, dose-dependent beneficial effect on plasma triglyceride levels (10% to 30% lowering) that was generally significant across studies.[48] In addition, there was a small but significant beneficial effect on systolic and diastolic blood pressure (about 2 mmHg decrease). There were possible beneficial effects on coronary artery restenosis after angioplasty, exercise capacity in patients with coronary atherosclerosis, and heart rate variability, especially in patients with recent myocardial infarction. There were nonsignificant increases in low-density lipoprotein and high-density lipoprotein cholesterol, and no consistent effects on carotid intimal-medial thickness; on blood levels of apolipoproteins, lipoprotein (a), hemoglobin A1c, glucose, insulin, C-reactive protein; or on any measures of hemostasis. A conclusion from these analyses is that if cardiovascular disease benefits of omega-3 fatty acids exist, they are not well explained by their effects on the cardiovascular disease risk factors examined, unless the overall benefit is due to the accumulation of small effects on several of them (e.g., triglycerides, blood pressure). Furthermore, it is obvious that whatever criteria are used, all individuals do not respond identically to the same intervention strategy.

Generalizability of Information for Prevention and Treatment

A fundamental question remains: do pathologic evaluations reflect what occurs normally?[54] In addition, questions remain about the generalizability of information across various populations. Is it appropriate to extrapolate information about omega-3 fatty acids in the prevention of cardiovascular disease in unselected populations (primary prevention) from data obtained on prevention in patients with previous cardiovascular disease events (secondary prevention)? To date, there is strong evidence that omega-3 fatty acid consumption in patients who have suffered myocardial infarction can reduce the risk of subsequent cardiovascular events and all-cause mortality, although the data regarding primary prevention in otherwise unselected subjects are less secure.

Likewise, information about the potential role of omega-3 fatty acids in one condition may not be sufficient for judging their importance in another condition. For example, in type 2 diabetes mellitus, omega-3 fatty acids reduce serum triglycerides but have no effect on total cholesterol, high-density lipoprotein cholesterol, or low-density lipoprotein cholesterol; there is insufficient evidence to draw conclusions regarding their role in altering insulin resistance. In rheumatoid arthritis, one measure (tender joint count) appears to be improved, but there is no obvious effect on other clinical outcomes. For most of the other indications in which omega-3 fatty acids have been suggested to have benefits (e.g., inflammatory bowel disease, renal disease, bone density or fractures, need for anti-inflammatory or immunosuppressive drugs), there are insufficient data to draw firm conclusions.[55]

Health Consequences of Omega-3 Fatty Acids as a Model

The example of omega-3 fatty acids illustrates the challenges in documenting the health effects of bioactive food components. Overall, there is considerable potential for the role of omega-3 fatty acids in fish or in dietary supplements to reduce the risk of cardiovascular events in previously affected patients, but the data are less certain in the context of primary prevention. Even though for some treatment effects the results were positive, there was considerable heterogeneity in the data. This undoubtedly reflects differences in experimental design (e.g., background diets, form and dose of intervention, duration of exposure, inclusion/exclusion criteria for subjects), but it also reflects genetic differences among subjects, a topic dealt with earlier in this chapter. In any event, the evidence-based approach will allow us to more clearly delineate research directions and strategies for the future. In the case of omega-3 fatty acids, for example, more research is needed in well-designed primary prevention settings to determine the form (i.e., food vs. supplements), dose, duration, and subject selection where health effects can be assessed. The effects of omega-3 fatty acids in other settings need much more investigation. This does not mean that omega-3 fatty acids are without effect in these settings, but it does mean that the data are insufficient to make firm recommendations.

Future Directions

In the setting of the health effects of bioactive components of foods and dietary supplements, it is important to remember that the effect sizes are very likely to be small and perhaps realized only over a long time. This could explain why it has been difficult in intervention trials to document the putative benefits of food-based ingredients (e.g., omega-3 fatty acids) found in epidemiologic studies. Most reports included a small number of subjects who were studied for only short periods. There was considerable heterogeneity in the interventions used and the outcomes measured. There was little indication, however, of serious adverse events, although these studies may not have been sufficiently powered to detect rare events. Systematic review of the literature using appropriate analytic tools can be valuable in judging the state of science, in detecting modest effects (both positive and negative), and in leading to the development of recommendations. Recommendations may include what further research is necessary and what research designs are the most appropriate to pursue; they may also include messages for the public about health-promoting dietary habits or supplementation.

Research in nutrition and health must give greater attention to understanding the basic molecular mechanisms by which bioactive components influence cellular processes. Well-coordinated, multidisciplinary efforts among scientists—including nutrition scientists, molecular biologists, geneticists, statisticians, and clinical cancer researchers—will be needed to advance this molecular approach to nutrition and health. Many research questions and issues will need to be addressed for this approach to become a reality. For example, can the impact of a nutrient be evaluated by the use of a single molecular target, or do multiple targets need to be evaluated simultaneously to predict a response? What interactions are critical in modifying the response to bioactive food components? Additional attention on the importance of the time and duration of exposures on the overall response is needed. Key to moving this science forward will be the identification and validation of biomarkers that can be used to assess intake, effect, and susceptibility.

The development and implementation of a successful multidisciplinary effort that emphasizes a molecular approach to nutrition and health will take motivation, dedication, and specialized training. While the challenges to this research are enormous, the potential rewards in terms of improving health are also enormous.

References

1. Schmidt EB, Arnesen H, de Caterina R, et al. Marine n-3 polyunsaturated fatty acids and coronary heart disease. Part I. Background, epidemiology, animal data, effects on risk factors and safety. Thromb Res. 2005;115:163–170.
2. Sarkar FH, Li Y. Soy isoflavones and cancer prevention. Cancer Invest. 2003;21:744–757.
3. Kim Y, DiSilvestro R, Clinton S. Effects of lycopene-beadlet or tomato-powder feeding on carbon tetrachloride-induced hepatotoxicty in rats. Phytomedicine. 2004;11:152–156.
4. Kanadaswami C, Lee LT, Lee PP, et al. The antitumor activities of flavonoids. In Vivo. 2005;19: 895–909.
5. Milner JA. Molecular targets for bioactive food components. J Nutr. 2004;134:2492S–2498S.
6. Khanum F, Anilakumar KR, Viswanathan KR. Anticarcinogenic properties of garlic: a review. Crit Rev Food Sci Nutr. 2004;44:479–488.
7. Blomhoff R. Dietary antioxidants and cardiovascular disease. Curr Opin Lipidol. 2005;16:47–54.

8. Banerjee SK, Mukherjee PK, Maulik SK. Garlic as an antioxidant: the good, the bad and the ugly. Phytother Res. 2003;17:97–106.
9. Kyo E, Uda N, Kasuga S, Itakura, Y. Immunomodulatory effect of aged garlic extract. J Nutr. 2001;131: 1075S–1079S.
10. Yamada N, Hattori A, Hayashi T, et al. Improvement of scopolamine-induced memory impairment by Z-ajoene in the water maze in mice. Pharmacol Biochem Behav. 2004;78:787–791.
11. Davis CD, Milner J. Frontiers in nutrigenomics, proteomics, metabolomics and cancer prevention. Mutat Res. 2004;551:51–64.
12. Woodson K, Ratnasinghe D, Bhat NK, et al. Prevalence of disease-related DNA polymorphisms among participants in a large cancer prevention trial. Eur J Cancer Prev. 1999;8:441–447.
13. Ratnasinghe D, Tangrea JA, Andersen MR, et al. Glutathione peroxidase codon 198 polymorphism variant increases lung cancer risk. Cancer Res. 2000; 60:6381–6383.
14. Jiang Q, Chen K, Ma X, et al. Diets, polymorphisms of methylenetetrahydrofolate reductase, and the susceptibility of colon cancer and rectal cancer. Cancer Detect Prev. 2005;29:146–154.
15. Angeline T, Jeyaraj N, Granito S, et al. Prevalence of MTHFR gene polymorphisms (C677T and A1298C) among Tamilians. Exp Mol Pathol. 2004; 77:85–88.
16. Ingles SA, Garcia DG, Wang W, et al. Vitamin D receptor genotype and breast cancer in Latinas (United States). Cancer Causes Control. 2000;11: 25–30.
17. Ross SA. Diet and DNA methylation interactions in cancer prevention. Ann NY Acad Sci. 2003;983: 197–207.
18. Davis CD, Uthus EO. Dietary folate and selenium affect dimethylhydrazine-induced aberrant crypt formation, global DNA methylation and one-carbon metabolism in rats. J Nutr. 2003;133:2907–2914.
19. Fang MZ, Chen D, Sun Y, et al. Reversal of hypermethylation and reactivation of p16INK4a, RARbeta, and MGMT genes by genistein and other isoflavones from soy. Clin Cancer Res. 2005;11: 7033–7041.
20. El-Bayoumy K, Sinha R. Molecular chemoprevention by selenium: a genomic approach. Mutat Res. 2005;591:224–236.
21. Prima V, Tennant M, Gorbatyuk OS, et al. Differential modulation of energy balance by leptin, ciliary neurotrophic factor, and leukemia inhibitory factor gene delivery: microarray deoxyribonucleic acid-chip analysis of gene expression. Endocrinology. 2004; 145:2035–2045.
22. Zakharkin SO, Kim K, Mehta T, et al. Sources of variation in Affymetrix microarray experiments. BMC Bioinformatics. Aug. 29, 2005;6:214.
23. Kensler TW, Curphey TJ, Maxiutenko Y, et al. Chemoprotection by organosulfur inducers of phase 2 enzymes: dithiolethiones and dithiins. Drug Metabol Drug Interact. 2000;17:3–22.
24. Ikeda N, Uemura H, Ishiguro H, et al. Combination treatment with 1-alpha, 25-dihydroxyvitamin D3 and 9-cis-retinoic acid directly inhibits human telomerase reverse transcriptase transcription in prostate cancer cells. Mol Cancer Ther. 2003;2:739–746.
25. Fenech M. The Genome Health Clinic and Genome Health Nutrigenomics concepts: diagnosis and nutritional treatment of genome and epigenome damage on an individual basis. Mutagenesis. 2005;20:255–269.
26. Nakamura Y, Tomokane I, Mori T, et al. DNA repair effect of traditional sweet pepper Fushimitogarashi: seen in suppression of UV-induced cyclobutane pyrimidine dimer in human fibroblast. Biosci Biotechnol Biochem. 2000;64:2575–2580.
27. Beetstra S, Thomas P, Salisbury C, et al. Folic acid deficiency increases chromosomal instability, chromosome 21 aneuploidy and sensitivity to radiation-induced micronuclei. Mutat Res. 2005;578:317–326.
28. Friso S, Choi SW. Gene–nutrient interactions in one-carbon metabolism. Curr Drug Metab. 2005;6: 37–46.
29. Hong YC, Lee KH, Kim WC, et al. Polymorphisms of XRCC1 gene, alcohol consumption and colorectal cancer. Int J Cancer. 2005;116:428–432.
30. Mathers JC. The biological revolution: towards a mechanistic understanding of the impact of diet on cancer risk. Mutat Res. 2004;551:43–49.
31. Dong X, Lutz W, Schroeder TM, et al. Regulation of relB in dendritic cells by means of modulated association of vitamin D receptor and histone deacetylase 3 with the promoter. Proc Natl Acad Sci USA. 2005; 102:16007–16012.
32. Awad AB, Fink CS. Phytosterols as anticancer dietary components: evidence and mechanism of action. J Nutr. 2000;130:2127–2130.
33. McEligot AJ, Yang S, Meyskens FL Jr. Redox regulation by intrinsic species and extrinsic nutrients in normal and cancer cells. Annu Rev Nutr. 2005;25: 261–295.
34. Philpott M, Ferguson LR. Immunonutrition and cancer. Mutat Res. 2004;551:29–42.
35. Cunningham-Rundles S, McNeeley DF, Moon A. Mechanisms of nutrient modulation of the immune response. J Allergy Clin Immunol. 2005;115:1119–1128.
36. Li R, Huang YG, Fang D, et al. (−)-Epigallocatechin gallate inhibits lipopolysaccharide-induced microglial activation and protects against inflammation-mediated dopaminergic neuronal injury. J Neurosci Res. 2004;78:723–731.
37. Calder PC. Polyunsaturated fatty acids and inflammation. Biochem Soc Trans. 2005;33:423–427.

38. Calder PC, Kew S. The immune system: a target for functional foods? Br J Nutr. 2002;88(Suppl 2): S165–S177.
39. Rose DP, Connolly JM. Regulation of tumor angiogenesis by dietary fatty acids and eicosanoids. Nutr Cancer. 2000;37:119–127.
40. Kaga S, Zhan L, Matsumoto M, et al. Resveratrol enhances neovascularization in the infarcted rat myocardium through the induction of thioredoxin-1, heme oxygenase-1 and vascular endothelial growth factor. J Mol Cell Cardiol. 2005;39:813–822.
41. Su SJ, Yeh TM, Chuang WJ, et al. The novel targets for anti-angiogenesis of genistein on human cancer cells. Biochem Pharmacol. 2005;69:307–318.
42. Combs GF Jr, Gray WP. Chemopreventive agents: selenium. Pharmacol Ther. 1998;79:179–192.
43. Young VR, Gucalp C, Rand WM, et al. Leucine kinetics during three weeks at submaintenance-to-maintenance intakes of leucine in men: adaptation and accommodation. Hum Nutr Clin Nutr. 1987; 41:1–18.
44. Kohno K, Uchiumi T, Niina I, et al. Transcription factors and drug resistance. Eur J Cancer. 2005;41: 2577–2586.
45. Liu RH. Potential synergy of phytochemicals in cancer prevention: mechanism of action. J Nutr. 2004; 134(12 Suppl):3479S–3485S.
46. Shen F, Weber G. Synergistic action of quercetin and genistein in human ovarian carcinoma cells. Oncol Res. 1997;9:597–602.
47. Nichols PD, Mansour P, Robert S, et al. Alternate sources of long-chain omega-3 oils. Asia Pac J Clin Nutr. 2005;14(Suppl):S112.
48. Balk E, Chung M, Lichtenstein A, et al. *Effects of Omega-3 Fatty Acids on Cardiovascular Risk Factors and Intermediate Markers of Cardiovascular Disease.* Evidence Report/Technology Assessment No. 93 (Prepared by Tufts-New England Medical Center Evidence-based Practice Center under Contract No. 290-02-0022). AHRQ Publication No. 04-E010-2. Rockville, MD: Agency for Healthcare Research and Quality, March 2004.
49. Wang C, Chung M, Lichtenstein A, et al. *Effects of Omega-3 Fatty Acids on Cardiovascular Disease.* Evidence Report/Technology Assessment No. 94 (Prepared by Tufts-New England Medical Center Evidence-based Practice Center, under Contract No. 290-02-0022). AHRQ Publication No. 04-E009-2. Rockville, MD: Agency for Healthcare Research and Quality, March 2004.
50. Jordan, H, Matthan N, Chung M, et al. *Effects of Omega-3 Fatty Acids on Arrhythmogenic Mechanisms in Animal and Isolated Organ/Cell Culture Studies.* Evidence Report/Technology Assessment No. 92 (Prepared by Tufts-New England Medical Center Evidence-based Practice Center under Contract No. 290-02-0022). AHRQ Publication No 04-E011-2. Rockville, MD: Agency for Healthcare Research and Quality, March 2004.
51. Leitzmann MF, Stampfer MJ, Michaud DS, et al. Dietary intake of n-3 and n-6 fatty acids and the risk of prostate cancer. Am J Clin Nutr. 2004;80: 204–216.
52. Gago-Dominguez M, Yuan JM, Sun CL, et al. Opposing effects of dietary n-3 and n-6 fatty acids on mammary carcinogenesis: the Singapore Chinese Health Study. Br J Cancer. 2003;89:1686–1692.
53. Luan J, Browne PO, Harding AH, et al. Evidence for gene–nutrient interaction at the PPARgamma locus. Diabetes. 2001;50:686–689.
54. Prentice RL, Willett WC, Greenwald P, et al. Nutrition and physical activity and chronic disease prevention: research strategies and recommendations. J Natl Cancer Inst. 2004;96:1276–1287.
55. MacLean CH, Mojica WA, Morton SC, et al. *Effects of Omega-3 Fatty Acids on Lipids and Glycemic Control in Type II Diabetes and the Metabolic Syndrome and on Inflammatory Bowel Disease, Rheumatoid Arthritis, Renal Disease, Systemic Lupus Erythematosus, and Osteoporosis.* Evidence Report/Technology Assessment No. 89 (Prepared by Southern California/RAND Evidence-based Practice Center under Contract No. 290-02-0003). AHRQ Publication No. 04-E012-2. Rockville, MD: Agency for Healthcare Research and Quality, March 2004.

PRESENT KNOWLEDGE IN
NUTRITION

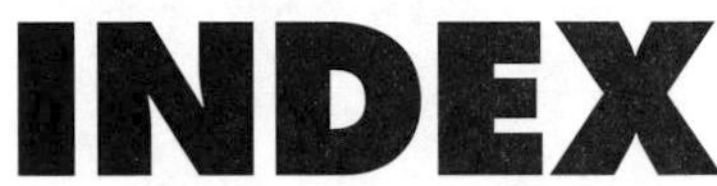

INDEX

Page numbers followed by a t indicate a table, those followed by f indicate a figure.

A

B

C

D

E

F

G

H

O

P

Q

R

S

T

U

V

W

X

Z